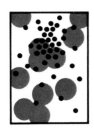
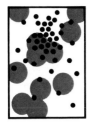
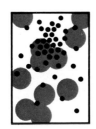

ATLAS OF DIAGNOSTIC CYTOPATHOLOGY

Barbara F. Atkinson, M.D.
Professor and Chairman
Department of Pathology and Laboratory Medicine
The Medical College of Pennsylvania
Philadelphia, Pennsylvania

• *With over 1500 full-color illustrations* •

W. B. SAUNDERS COMPANY
Harcourt Brace Jovanovich, Inc.

Philadelphia London Toronto Montreal Sydney Tokyo

W. B. SAUNDERS COMPANY
Harcourt Brace Jovanovich, Inc.

The Curtis Center
Independence Square West
Philadelphia, Pennsylvania 19106

Library of Congress Cataloging-in-Publication Data

Atlas of diagnostic cytopathology/[edited by] Barbara F. Atkinson.
   p.   cm.

Includes index.

ISBN 0–7216–3528–8

1. Cytodiagnosis—Atlases.   I. Atkinson, Barbara F.

[DNLM: 1. Cells—pathology—atlases.   2. Cytodiagnosis—atlases.   QY 17 A8805]

RB43.A84   1992

616.07′582—dc20

DNLM/DLC   92–11624

Editor: Jennifer Mitchell
Developmental Editor: Leslie E. Hoeltzel
Designer: Joan Wendt
Cover Designer: Megan Costello Connell
Production Manager: Peter Faber
Manuscript Editors: Karen Neff and David Prout
Illustration Coordinator: Walt Verbitski
Page Layout Artist: W. B. Saunders Staff
Indexer: Linda Van Pelt

Atlas of Diagnostic Cytopathology   ISBN 0–7216–3528–8

Last digit is the print number: 9   8   7   6   5   4   3   2   1

To Bill, Nancy and George, Mom and Dad—
With love and thanks.

CONTRIBUTORS

BARBARA F. ATKINSON, M.D.
Professor and Chairman
Department of Pathology and Laboratory
  Medicine
Medical College of Pennsylvania
Philadelphia, Pennsylvania
  Respiratory Cytology

NIRMALA BATHEJA, M.D. (MIAC)
Instructor, Pathology
Mt. Sinai School of Medicine
New York, New York
Attending Pathologist
Mt. Sinai Hospital Medical Center
New York, New York
  General Cytologic Principles

SANDRA H. BIGNER, M.D.
Professor of Pathology
Duke University Medical Center
Durham, North Carolina
  *Stereotactic Biopsy of the Central Nervous
  System*

SALLY-BETH BUCKNER, B.A.
Department of Cellular Pathology
Armed Forces Institute of Pathology
Washington, D.C.
  General Cytologic Principles

PETER C. BURGER, M.D.
Professor of Pathology
Duke University Medical Center
Durham, North Carolina
  *Stereotactic Biopsy of the Central Nervous
  System*

EDMUND S. CIBAS, M.D.
Assistant Professor of Pathology
Harvard Medical School
Boston, Massachusetts

Director, Cytology Laboratory
Brigham and Women's Hospital
Boston, Massachusetts
  *Effusions (Pleural, Pericardial, and
  Peritoneal) and Peritoneal Washings;
  Cerebrospinal Fluid Cytology*

JEAN M. COLANDREA, M.D.
Director of Cytopathology
St. Agnes Hospital
Baltimore, Maryland
  Urinary Cytology

BARBARA S. DUCATMAN, M.D.
Assistant Professor of Pathology
Harvard Medical School
Boston, Massachusetts
Director, Cytopathology Laboratory
Beth Israel Hospital
Boston, Massachusetts
  *Fine Needle Aspiration of the Liver and
  Pancreas; Fine Needle Aspiration of the
  Kidneys, Adrenals, and Retroperitoneum;
  Fine Needle Aspiration of the Breast*

HORMOZ EHYA, M.D.
Professor of Pathology
Hahnemann University School of Medicine
Philadelphia, Pennsylvania
Director of Cytopathology
Hahnemann University Hospital
Consultant Pathologist
Wills Eye Hospital
Philadelphia, Pennsylvania
  Ocular Cytology

LORI J. ELWOOD, M.D.
Deputy Chief of Cytopathology Section
NCI/NIH
Bethesda, Maryland
  Urinary Cytology

JAMES M. ENGLAND, M.D., PH.D.
Associate Professor of Pathology
The Medical College of Pennsylvania
Philadelphia, Pennsylvania
General Cytologic Principles

ALLAN H. FRIEDMAN, M.D.
Professor of Pediatrics
Duke University Medical Center
Durham, North Carolina
Stereotactic Biopsy of the Central Nervous System

MICHAEL D. GLANT, M.D.
Clinical Associate Professor of Pathology
Indiana University School of Medicine
Indianapolis, Indiana
Medical Director
Diagnostic Cytology Laboratory, Inc., and
  Aspiration Biopsy Clinic
Indianapolis, Indiana
Staff Pathologist
Humana Women's Hospital
Indianapolis, Indiana
Aspiration Biopsy of Lymph Nodes: Reactive and Primary Neoplasia; Salivary Glands, Head and Neck, and Skin Aspiration Cytology

LINDA GREEN, M.D.
Assistant Professor
Baylor College of Medicine
Houston, Texas
Staff Pathologist, Physician-in-Charge of Fine
  Needle Aspiration Cytology and Flow
  Cytometry
Veterans Affairs Medical Center
Houston, Texas
Gastrointestinal Cytology

CAROLYN ERNST GROTKOWSKI, M.D.
Associate Professor of Pathology
Medical College of Pennsylvania
Philadelphia, Pennsylvania
Vice Chairman and Director of Anatomic
  Pathology
Medical College Hospitals
Philadelphia, Pennsylvania
Thyroid Aspiration Cytology

L. PATRICK JAMES, M.D.
Director, Anatomic Pathology
St. Joseph Hospital
Denver, Colorado
Fine Needle Aspiration of Soft Tissue and Bone

CHRISTINE KING, CT(ASCP)
Laboratory of Pathology
National Cancer Institute
National Institutes of Health
Bethesda, Maryland
Urinary Cytology

DOUGLAS C. KING, M.S. CT(ASCP), MIAC
General Supervisor
Diagnostic Cytology Laboratory, Inc.
Indianapolis, Indiana
Aspiration Biopsy of Lymph Nodes: Reactive and Primary Neoplasia; Salivary Glands, Head and Neck, and Skin Aspiration Cytology

IBRAHIM RAMZY, M.D.
Professor of Pathology
Professor of Obstetrics-Gynecology
Baylor College of Medicine
Houston, Texas
Senior Attending and Chief of Anatomic
  Pathology
The Methodist Hospital
Houston, Texas
Ovarian Aspiration Cytology

MARY R. SCHWARTZ, M.D.
Associate Professor
Department of Pathology
Baylor College of Medicine
Houston, Texas
Associate Attending
The Methodist Hospital
Houston, Texas
Ovarian Aspiration Cytology

JAN F. SILVERMAN, M.D
Professor
East Carolina University School of Medicine
Greenville, North Carolina
Director of Cytology
Pitt County Memorial Hospital
Greenville, North Carolina
Respiratory Cytology

PHILIP T. VALENTE, M.D.
Assistant Professor of Pathology and Obstetrics
  and Gynecology
University of Texas Health Science Center at
  San Antonio
San Antonio, Texas
Director of Cytology
Medical Center Hospital and Audie L. Murphy
  Memorial Veterans Hospital
San Antonio, Texas
Gynecologic Cytology

SCOTT WANG, M.D.
Assistant Professor of Pathology
Medical College of Pennsylvania—
    Allegheny Campus
Philadelphia, Pennsylvania
Chairman of Pathology
Newport Hospital
Newport, Rhode Island
    Fine Needle Aspiration of the Orbit

G. FRED WORSHAM, M.D.
Clinical Assistant Professor of Pathology
Medical University of South Carolina
Charleston, South Carolina
Chairman of Pathology and Director of
    Laboratories
Roper Hospital
Charleston, South Carolina
    Thin Needle Biopsy of the Prostate

PREFACE

Atlas of Diagnostic Cytopathology was planned and written with two goals in mind: to help those learning cytopathology for the first time, including cytotechnology students and pathology residents, and to provide a resource for those who have experience in cytopathology but are faced with a difficult diagnostic dilemma.

For students, we have organized each chapter to begin with an overview of the topic, including the types of preparations and the most important diagnostic features of that specimen type. Each contributor was requested to share his or her favorite diagnostic rules and "tips." Because this is an atlas, we have not presented extensive diagnostic information on each topic; rather, we refer the student to a textbook of cytopathology for detailed didactic information. To that end, and for further reading on individual topics, a bibliography has been provided at the end of each chapter.

For the difficult diagnostic challenges, most chapters present panels of pictures of comparative lesions. In this way, many of the unusual entities are pictured and their diagnostic criteria discussed. In each chapter we have included all the basic lesions plus many of the more unusual lesions occurring at that site.

The figure legends are detailed, and the figures and legends have been designed so that they can stand by themselves or can be used in addition to the text of a chapter. Thus there is some duplication of information in the text and the figure legends, which reinforces the material, but the pictures themselves are instructive because of their clear presentation of findings. Diagnoses are grouped under pertinent headings for easy referral, and differential diagnoses are usually grouped at the end of chapters. For purposes of thoroughness of discussion, at times the interpretation of a figure may go beyond what can actually be seen on that particular figure. For example, a diagnosis may not be apparent from one field alone. If overall cellularity needs to be assessed in order to arrive at the diagnosis, this additional information is given in the figure legend. We have also tried to indicate the most difficult differential diagnosis and to assess how the distinctions can be made.

We believe that *Atlas of Diagnostic Cytopathology* fills the need for a comprehensive atlas in this rapidly growing field. I thank all who have contributed to this book for their careful work and their excellent pictures, and I hope that both students and practitioners find it useful.

BARBARA F. ATKINSON, M.D.

ACKNOWLEDGMENTS

Many very busy and excellent diagnostic cytopathologists and cytotechnologists have worked hard and contributed their best Kodachromes and most helpful diagnostic guidelines to make the *Atlas of Diagnostic Cytopathology* possible. I cannot begin to express appropriate thanks to each of them for their high level of expertise and their devotion to this project. A project like this is too big for one person, and all the authors have been patient, considerate, and supportive as the work progressed. All have been dedicated to producing the finest possible atlas, and their efforts show in the final product.

Many people at the Medical College of Pennsylvania (MCP) were instrumental in making the *Atlas* possible and thus deserve special thanks. Carolyn E. Grotkowski, M.D., and James M. England, M.D., Ph.D., are my key support system, make my life easier, and keep the department going (the Department of Pathology and Laboratory Medicine). Terry Neeson, C.T.(A.S.C.P.), Cytopathology Supervisor, has always been supportive, gives above and beyond necessity, and keeps our diagnostic service going smoothly. Sheila Gillespie, my administrative assistant, helps me finish everything, even when it looks impossible. Many others at MCP deserve my thanks as well and are in my thoughts.

I would also like to recognize with thanks the many people at W. B. Saunders who have supported the book. Richard Zorab, who first interested me in this project, Jennifer Mitchell, Pathology Editor, and especially Leslie Hoeltzel, Development Editor, who has been essential throughout the writing and production phases of this book. Many others have devoted considerable time and energy to various aspects of the project; I think they all have done an excellent job.

I would also like to heartily thank all of the many fellows, residents, cytotechnologists, and cytotechnology students with whom I have worked. They are the ones who really taught me cytopathology. To paraphrase a cliche, you learn only by being forced to explain "why." You may think you know, but teaching is the final test. Teaching smart, probing students, residents, and fellows is the final test as well as the biggest thrill. I hope that *Atlas of Diagnostic Cytopathology* succeeds in explaining some of those "whys."

BARBARA F. ATKINSON, M.D.

CONTENTS

C • H • A • P • T • E • R

4

EFFUSIONS (PLEURAL, PERICARDIAL, AND PERITONEAL) AND PERITONEAL WASHINGS 195

Edmund S. Cibas

C • H • A • P • T • E • R

5

CEREBROSPINAL FLUID CYTOLOGY .. 239

Edmund S. Cibas

C • H • A • P • T • E • R

6

STEREOTACTIC BIOPSY OF THE CENTRAL NERVOUS SYSTEM 265

Sandra H. Bigner, Allan H. Friedman, and Peter C. Burger

C • H • A • P • T • E • R

7

GASTROINTESTINAL CYTOLOGY 283

Linda Green

C • H • A • P • T • E • R
19

Hormoz Ehya

C·H·A·P·T·E·R

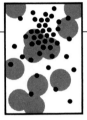

1

GENERAL CYTOLOGIC PRINCIPLES

Sally-Beth Buckner

James M. England

Nirmala Batheja

The cytologic appearance of benign, atypical, premalignant, and malignant processes must be thoroughly understood by all those engaged in rendering cytologic diagnoses. In addition, cellular changes associated with degeneration, infectious agents, and reparative or reactive atypia may be superimposed on benign or malignant processes and must be taken into account when making a diagnostic decision. Although diagnostic subtleties exist for each site and specimen type, there are common cytologic criteria that aid in arriving at an accurate diagnosis of benignity or malignancy. This chapter focuses on diagnostic criteria based on the morphology of cellular components, cells, cellular growth patterns, and the background milieu. It must be kept in mind that accurate cytologic diagnoses depend not only on knowledge of diagnostic criteria but also on a clear, internal frame of reference, which is established with practical experience.

NUCLEUS

The morphology of the nucleus is of the utmost importance in cytologic evaluation, since it not only reflects the overall biosynthetic activity of the cell but also evinces genetic alterations that appear to be the common denominator of neoplastic transformation. Thus, changes in nuclear morphology reflect alterations in genome function as well as genome structure. In the case of malignancy, genetic alterations may be important in oncogenesis, e.g., chemical or physical mutagenesis, oncogene activation, and growth-suppressor gene inactivation, or may be a reflection of the genetic instability of transformed cells, which is thought to be an underpinning of tumor progression.

Nuclear characteristics are manifested in the chromatin and in the nuclear envelope. Chromatin is composed of DNA and DNA-associated proteins. It is these DNA-associated proteins that stain with hematoxylin, yielding the characteristic purple or purple-black nuclei observed on slides stained by the modified Papanicolaou method. Chromatin has both transcriptionally active and inactive components—euchromatin and heterochromatin, respectively. The heterochromatin stains darkly with hematoxylin; the euchromatin stains faintly. Heterochromatin is located predominantly near the inner membrane of the nuclear envelope (the chromatinic rim) and in the chromatinic network throughout the nucleus. Euchromatin is located primarily in the so-called cleared, or lightly stained, portion of the nucleus.

In general, heterochromatin and euchromatin are uniformly distributed in benign cells. Chromatin granules in the chromatinic network are small and evenly distributed throughout the nucleus. This pattern is often referred to as smooth or bland. Chromocenters, i.e., clumps of heterochromatin that appear disassociated from the nuclear background, are set against the uniform chromatin pattern. As benign cells become more transcriptionally active, the heterochromatin generally becomes more granular but still maintains an even distribution. Patterns that comprise moderately sized or large granules that are evenly distributed are referred to as moderately granular or coarsely granular, evenly distributed chromatin. This even distribution of chromatin, cytologically observed as a uniform arrangement of heterochromatin and euchromatin, is a key feature in distinguishing benign from malignant cells.

In cells from the uterine cervix, moderately granular, evenly distributed chromatin is seen in atypical repair and squamous intraepithelial lesions (cervical intraepithelial neoplasia [CIN] or dysplasia). Classically, the degree of granularity increases as the severity of the squamous intraepithelial lesion (SIL) increases. Theoretically, high-grade SIL (CIN III or carcinoma in situ) contains coarsely granular, evenly distributed heterochromatin or so-called salt and pepper chromatin, although in practice this is not always observed.

Chromatin patterns in malignancy are variable and, depending on cell type, range from a bland or uniform distribution to a coarsely granular, uneven distribution. In the latter, classic pattern, large, clear areas of hypochromatic euchromatin are adjacent to dense areas of heterochromatin. The chromatin granules and the interfaces between euchromatin and heterochromatin are irregular, angular, and crisp, whereas they are round and smooth in benign cells or blurred and hazy in degenerating cells.

The nuclear envelope complex consists of an inner and outer membrane and a nuclear lamina, which is adherent to the inner surface of the inner membrane. Chromosomes are bound to the nuclear lamina, and the heterochromatin attached to the nuclear lamina is known as the chromatinic rim. In benign cells, the chromatinic rim is of uniform thickness along the entire circumference of the nucleus. The chromatin and its cytoplasmic-nuclear interfaces are sharp and crisp. In degeneration and malignancy, there is an uneven distribution of chromatin along the chromatinic rim. In degeneration, the chromatin and its interfaces are blurred and hazy, whereas in malignancy they are classically sharp, crisp, angular, and irregular. The latter pattern is attributed to the increased amount of chromatin material and an aberrant pattern of chromatin activation and inactivation in the malignant nucleus.

The contour of the nuclear envelope also reflects the biologic activity of the cell. In benign quiescent cells, the outer membrane is smooth and round to oval in shape. In synthetically active or reactive cells, the outer membrane is wavy or undulating, reflecting the increased nuclear membrane surface area that accommodates the increased flux of macromolecules to and from the nucleus. In reversible cellular injury, cytologic changes are largely dependent on the disruption of ionic and fluid homeostasis, and consequently, an influx of water occurs that results in cellular and nuclear swelling. Because of this, the nuclear membrane develops a round shape and a smooth center. In addition, clumping of heterochromatin occurs; this is apparently a result of a reduction in intracellular pH. In irreversible cell injury, striking changes in nuclear morphology occur ranging from shrinkage (pyknosis) to nuclear dissolution (karyolysis, karyorrhexis). In malignant cells, the contour of the nuclear membrane is variable, ranging from round and smooth in some cell types to the classic malignant pattern, which is angular, with acute angles and points. The angularities are irregular and sharp, and are not caused by compression from vacuoles or other nuclei.

NUCLEOLI

Nucleoli are the sites where ribosomal RNAs and proteins are assembled into immature ribosomes and as such reflect the level of cellular protein synthetic activity. This means that cells that are actively synthesizing protein have large, prominent nucleoli, e.g., reactive and reparative, and tumor cells. It must be remembered that prominent nucleoli indicate active protein synthesis, i.e., they are not pathognomonic of malignancy. Nucleoli form in association with the nucleolar organizer regions on the satellites of the five pairs of acrocentric chromosomes. Although the potential for 10 nucleoli exists in benign cells, six nucleoli is the maximum practically observed.

Nucleoli have acidophilic (red) staining properties, are generally round to oval in shape in benign cells, and can be irregularly shaped in atypical reparative and malignant cells. Disparities in terms of nucleolar size and shape within a single nucleus generally do not occur in benign cells but can be features of malignancy. For example, a malignant cell containing six nucleoli can have two small, round nucleoli and four large, irregular nucleoli. Disparities in nucleolar number among cells within the same tissue fragment are other criteria of malignancy. A low nucleolar to nuclear size ratio generally favors benignity. This ratio often increases in malignancy and is sometimes a key criterion in diagnosing malignancy, especially in fluids. As a rule of thumb, when prominent nucleoli are present in specimens from the female genital tract, there are only two diagnostic choices—repair reaction or invasive malignancy. Squamous intraepithelial lesions generally do not possess nucleoli.

NUCLEAR TO CYTOPLASMIC RATIO

The ratio of nuclear area to total cellular area (N/C ratio) conveys information concerning the maturity and biologic activity of a cell. In general, the degree of cellular maturity and the N/C ratio are inversely proportional, i.e., the more mature the cell, the lower the N/C ratio; conversely, the more immature the cell, the higher the N/C ratio. For example, superficial and intermediate squamous cells of the uterine cervix are mature epithelial cells; they have very small nuclei and large amounts of cytoplasm and thus low N/C ratios. On the other hand, parabasal cells are more immature squamous epithelial cells with higher N/C ratios than superficial or intermediate cells because of smaller amounts of cytoplasm and larger nuclei. In the urinary bladder and ureter, umbrella or surface cells are mature transitional cells that have low N/C ratios. Despite the fact that they can have multiple large nuclei, the low N/C ratios of these cells derive from their copious cytoplasmic volume. However, immature transitional cells obtained by sampling the underlying urothelium during instrumentation have much higher N/C ratios than surface urothelial cells. Therefore, cytologists must learn the degree of variation that exists in normal and reactive cell populations to correctly assess abnormally high N/C ratios and the possibility of malignancy. One must be familiar with the appearance of benign and reactive cells for each cell type to be able to judge the normal N/C ratio for that cell. Again, an internal frame of reference for each cell type must be learned.

Nuclear to cytoplasmic ratios generally increase in atypical processes and malignancy as a result of nuclear enlargement and a decrease in cellular maturation. Slight increases are observed in inflammatory atypia. Higher than normal N/C ratios are characteristic of squamous intraepithelial lesions, repair, and malignancy.

CYTOPLASMIC DIFFERENTIATION

The cytoplasm not only contains components that carry out general metabolic functions common to all cells but also contains components that enable cells to carry out specialized structural and functional activities. It is these specific components that confer the distinctive phenotype that is characteristic for a given cell type. In cytologic preparations, benign cells generally retain the same shape and cytoplasmic characteristics that they possess in histologic sections, especially if they are mechanically exfoliated. For example, mature stratified squamous epithelial cells and transitional cells are polygonal in shape and possess abundant transparent cytoplasm. In contrast, immature stratified squamous epithelial cells and transitional cells are rounder in shape and possess a smaller amount of dense cytoplasm. Hepatic cells retain their polygonal shape and possess a moderate amount of granular cytoplasm. Glandular cells retain their columnar shape or appear in a "honeycomb" configuration when viewed en face. Mucin-producing glandular cells are often distended and can possess light, frothy cytoplasm. Cells that spontaneously exfoliate into a fluid environment tend to lose their characteristic shape and become round.

Cytoplasmic staining properties reflect the biologic activity of cells and suggest the presence of specialized cellular constituents. Cells engaged in active protein synthesis generally stain basophilically (blue-green) with the modified

Papanicolaou stain, presumably because of the higher concentration of ribosomes in the cytoplasm. Relatively inactive cells generally stain eosinophilically (pink) and keratinized cells stain orangeophilically (bright orange, although there is a gradation from slightly orange to pumpkin orange to dense yellow). As examples, parabasal, columnar, squamous metaplastic, and mesothelial cells (metabolically active cells) generally have basophilic cytoplasm; superficial cells (metabolically inactive cells) can have eosinophilic cytoplasm; dyskeratocytes, parakeratotic cells, and keratinized squamous carcinoma cells have orangeophilic cytoplasm. These staining properties are subject to variation and may be altered by cellular thickness, degenerative and drying artifacts, improper dye penetration, or poor staining technique. The direct detection of specific cytoplasmic constituents is made possible by the use of histochemical and immunohistochemical techniques. The latter is extensively employed to detect specific antigens, e.g., intermediate filaments, hormones, and lineage-specific antigens, and facilitates the classification of cells in cytologic preparations. Patterns of shape and cytoplasmic contents often enable the cytologist to determine the origin of normal cells and the histogenic type of tumor cells.

DEGREE OF TUMOR CELL DIFFERENTIATION

In cytologic preparations, cells from a well-differentiated tumor tend to retain the shape and cytoplasmic characteristics of their benign counterparts, enabling identification of the histogenic type of tumor. Cells from well-differentiated squamous cell carcinoma usually have an extremely hard (dense) cytoplasm, polygonal cell shape, and orangeophilic staining. Cells from well-differentiated adenocarcinoma generally possess a columnar shape and can contain cytoplasmic vacuoles indicative of mucin production. The cells are usually arranged in an altered honeycomb configuration or in glandular configurations, such as three-dimensional papillary tissue fragments or acinar morulae with peripherally located nuclei. Cells from well-differentiated hepatic carcinoma generally retain the cytoplasmic characteristics of normal hepatocytes but lose the normal architectural relationship to portal triads. Cells from low-grade transitional cell carcinoma retain a normal or near normal cellular morphology but exhibit aberrant growth patterns, e.g., papillary groupings. Well-differentiated tumors often contain abundant specialized cytoplasmic constituents, e.g., mucin in adenocarcinoma, keratin in squamous cell carcinoma, myoglobin in skeletal muscle tumors, and melanin in melanoma.

In contrast, cells from a poorly differentiated tumor generally possess few specific markers that allow classification as to histogenic type. In such cases, diagnosis relies more heavily on cell size, the amount of cytoplasm, N/C ratios, nuclear shape, chromatin patterns, chromasia, the degree of nuclear crowding and overlap, and the site of specimen and clinical history. In some cases, immunohistochemistry and ultrastructural analysis may be informative.

Poorly differentiated squamous cell carcinoma sheds pseudosyncytial groupings of cells that exhibit marked nuclear crowding and overlap. The nuclei are irregular in shape, and the chromatin is often dense, granular, and hyperchromatic. Cells from poorly differentiated adenocarcinoma generally have round to oval nuclei with a more finely granular chromatin. The cells possess variable amounts of granular or diffusely vacuolated cytoplasm; large mucin vacuoles can be present. Both poorly differentiated squamous cell carcinoma and adenocarcinoma can possess prominent nucleoli, but prominent nucleoli are generally more numerous in adenocarcinoma.

Small-cell carcinoma of the lung is composed of small cells with large nuclei and very high N/C ratios. It is sometimes difficult to observe the tiny rim of cytoplasm. The nuclei are round to irregular in shape, possess hyperchromatic granular chromatin that is evenly distributed, and generally have no or very small nucleoli. The cells are arranged in aggregates in sputum specimens or in pseudosyncytia in bronchial brushings, washings, and aspirates. Nuclear molding and crowding are characteristic findings.

CELL NUMBER

The number of cells present in a cytologic preparation increases in proportion to the vigor of mechanical exfoliation and the degree of dysplasia or anaplasia in a neoplastic lesion. The latter correlates with the loss of cellular cohesion associated with high-grade SIL and poorly differentiated tumors. For example, low-grade SIL of the uterine cervix (CIN I, or mild dysplasia) can exfoliate only a few cells, whereas thousands of abnormal cells can exfoliate from high-grade SIL (CIN III, CIS). Because cellular cohesion is of central importance in epithelial cell function, i.e., covering biologic surfaces, a loss of cohesion in neoplasia can be interpreted as a diminution of a specialized cellular function.

CELLULAR CONFIGURATION

Cellular configuration is largely dependent on the method of sampling. Physiologic or spontaneous exfoliation usually results in single cells or small aggregates (clusters) of cells. Benign cells that are mechanically exfoliated can be single, in aggregates, or in tissue fragments. Benign tissue fragments usually consist of sheets of cells that have well-defined cellular borders. In epithelial groups, one nucleus can affect the shape of a neighboring nucleus. This phenomenon is termed nuclear molding and indicates that the cells were present in vivo within the same epithelial tissue fragment, in contrast to adventitiously aggregating after exfoliation.

Malignant cells, regardless of sampling method, can be present singly, in cellular aggregates, or in tissue fragments. Malignant tissue fragments generally appear as pseudosyncytial groups rather than as sheets of cells (in cytologic preparations, pseudosyncytial groups appear to lack well-defined cellular borders and, therefore, appear to be syncytial). The nuclei of malignant cells in pseudosyncytial groupings exhibit disorientation, crowding, and loss of polarity (polarity is recognized as an orderly orientation of nuclei in the same tissue fragment).

Three-dimensional tissue fragments are sometimes difficult to differentiate from loose, adventitious aggregates of cells. A true tissue fragment, i.e., a group of cells that maintain the relationship that they had in vivo, generally possesses a well-defined outer border, which is composed of the cytoplasm of contiguous cells. In contrast, an aggregate of cells generally possesses an outer border that has a random appearance as a result of the random agglutination of individual cells. In addition, true tissue fragments are composed solidly of cells, whereas cellular aggregates can possess gaps, or "windows," between individual cells.

Nuclear molding is present in true tissue fragments but not in cellular aggregates.

The following are examples of cellular configurations commonly observed in various body sites. In the female genital tract, benign superficial, intermediate, and parabasal cells are generally observed singly; however, sheets can also be present, exhibiting rather abundant cytoplasm and well-defined cell borders. Parabasal cells from post-menopausal women are often exfoliated in sheets, as are endocervical and squamous metaplastic cells from reproductive-age females. Parabasal cells from post-menopausal women can also be observed in pseudo-syncytial groupings. Endometrial cells are observed either in loose aggregates or in tissue fragments with a three-dimensional appearance; these cells spontaneously exfoliate from the uterine cavity during menses, "tumble" down the endocervical canal, and finally end in the vaginal pool. Cellular configurations aid in the differential diagnosis of endocervical versus endometrial adenocarcinoma. Endocervical adenocarcinoma is generally observed in sheets or pseudo-syncytial groupings, whereas endometrial adenocarcinoma is often observed as small, round, single cells and three-dimensional tissue fragments.

Benign sputum specimens contain singly exfoliated columnar cells. The presence of tissue fragments of glandular morphology in sputum specimens (that are *not* post-bronchoscopy specimens) generally is abnormal and indicates either hyperplasia or carcinoma. On the other hand, benign bronchial brushings and washings typically contain single cells, aggregates of cells, and tissue fragments composed predominantly of columnar cells. Malignant cells from a squamous cell carcinoma in sputum specimens are exfoliated singly, in aggregates, or in small pseudosyncytia. Squamous carcinoma cells in bronchial brushings or washings appear singly, in aggregates, and in larger syncytial groupings as a result of mechanical exfoliation. Adenocarcinoma cells in sputum specimens can appear singly, in aggregates, and in "classic" adenocarcinoma configurations, i.e., papillary tissue fragments or acinar formations. These glandular configurations can appear in bronchial brushings and washings, but pseudosyncytial groupings are more prevalent.

Single transitional cells are the rule of thumb in benign voided urine specimens. Tissue fragments are abnormal in voided urine and indicate a need for further patient follow-up. Urothelial fragments can be observed, however, when prior instrumentation has occurred or if inflammation or calculi are present. Conversely, tissue fragments are normally present in specimens from the urinary tract that are obtained by instrumentation. Therefore, it is of the utmost importance that the observer knows the correct specimen type and has an accurate clinical history.

Body cavity fluids normally contain mesothelial cells that spontaneously exfoliate singly, in aggregates, and, rarely, in small tissue fragments. The presence of numerous large tissue fragments in a body cavity fluid is abnormal and indicates the possibility of atypical mesothelial proliferation, mesothelioma, or metastatic carcinoma. It must be noted, however, that peritoneal washings normally contain tissue fragments as a result of mechanical exfoliation. Because the washing technique lifts whole layers of mesothelial cells from the peritoneal surface, the presence of tissue configurations is not necessarily an abnormal finding.

In cytologic samples obtained by fine needle aspiration, the number of cells (cellularity), cellular configurations, cellular cohesiveness, and prominent nucleoli are useful diagnostic criteria. In general, fine needle aspirations of benign lesions contain only a few cells that represent the normal constituents of the aspirated site. These cells are observed singly, in clusters, or in sheets with well-defined cell borders. The cells present in aspirations of malignant lesions generally exhibit high cellularity; exfoliate as numerous single, isolated cells (indicating loss of cohesion) or in pseudosyncytial groupings (indicating abnormal growth patterns); or possess prominent nucleoli (indicating increased protein synthetic activity). A criterion for malignancy that can carry over from exfoliative cytologic examination is pleomorphism among cells, especially within a group. Well-differentiated malignancies in fine needle aspirations are difficult to diagnose because cellular pleomorphism is often minimal. Tumor cellularity, however, is an extremely helpful diagnostic feature, coupled with small variations in nuclear size, a small degree of nuclear crowding, and nuclear overlap.

SLIDE BACKGROUND

The slide background can alert the cytologist to the possibility of an inflammatory or malignant process. Especially in the female genital tract, a clean background usually indicates a benign smear; however, the possibility of an intraepithelial lesion, an exophytic keratinizing carcinoma, or a metastatic carcinoma cannot be excluded. Inflammation generally indicates a host response to an etiologic agent, a foreign entity or substance, or an abnormal physiologic process. It alerts the cytologist to conduct a careful search for the cause of the inflammation, which may or may not be detectable in the cytologic specimen. Acute inflammation that is associated with a granular-appearing precipitate of cell debris, perinuclear halos, and an increase in the maturation of squamous cells should alert the cytologist to conduct a careful search for the presence of trichomonads. Trichomonads, however, may be present without eliciting any host response. Tumor diathesis, i.e., necrotic cellular debris and hemolyzed blood, is associated with invasive carcinoma, although invasive carcinoma can be present without evidence of necrotic debris or hemolyzed blood. Structures that are foreign to a particular body site can yield useful information. The presence of psammoma bodies in peritoneal fluid from a woman is highly suggestive of ovarian carcinoma. Reactive mesothelial proliferations rarely spontaneously shed psammoma bodies. Conversely, the presence of psammoma bodies in peritoneal washings cannot be considered highly suggestive of that tumor, since psammoma bodies can be part of a reactive mesothelial process mechanically abraded by the washing technique.

CLINICAL HISTORY

Finally, an accurate and thorough clinical history is essential for the proper evaluation of a cytologic specimen. If a clinical history is not available, the cytologic specimen should not be evaluated until a history is obtained. Very often, the clinical history provides the bit of information that enables the cytologist to render the correct diagnosis in a difficult case. Although it is the responsibility of the clinician to provide a history, it is the responsibility of the cytologist to insist on it and seek it when it is not given.

The cytologic characteristics discussed above are the parameters that are most commonly observed in daily laboratory practice. Unfortunately, classic criteria are not present in all cases. The cytologist must thoroughly observe the changes that are present, weigh them against expected findings, and make the most accurate diagnosis possible. It is important to remember that a gynecologic smear is a screening test. Although it may not always be possible to make a definitive diagnosis, it is essential to identify women who need to have additional studies or careful follow-up. The worst mistake in Papanicolaou smear evaluation is to miss a significant lesion. In contrast, the role of cytologic evaluation is different for specimens obtained for definitive diagnosis, e.g., needle aspirations and pulmonary and gastrointestinal tract specimens. In these cases, a diagnosis of malignancy often leads to definitive treatment; therefore, the cytologist must be conservative until convinced that malignancy exists. If there are too few abnormal cells present, or if cells that are present are abnormal but the cytologist is uncertain of their significance, then a diagnosis of suspected malignancy is appropriate. If a repeat specimen can be easily obtained, it should be. If additional material cannot be obtained, then consultative assistance should be requested. Although some cases will not be resolved, even by an experienced cytologist, careful application of cytologic criteria usually produces a correct cytologic diagnosis. Tables 1 to 10 summarize useful cytologic criteria.

Bibliography

Bahr GF, Bahr NI: Compendium on Diagnostic Cytology, Sixth Edition. Chicago: Tutorials of Cytology, 1986.
Frost JK: The Cell in Health and Disease, Second Edition. New York: S. Karger, 1986.
Luff RD: The Logic of Cytodiagnosis, unpublished.

Table 1–1. BENIGN CELLULAR FEATURES

NUCLEUS

General	
Location	Centrally located
Shape	Round to oval
Size	Varies by cell type, approximately the size of a neutrophil
Number	Single or multiple
Chromatin	
Appearance	Sharp and crisp
Granularity	Finely granular and evenly distributed
Chromasia	Normal
Nuclear Membrane	Smooth
	Chromatinic rim is of uniform thickness
Nucleoli	Present or absent depending on function and activity of cell. If present, nucleoli are round to oval, single or multiple, generally small in size, and generally have a low nucleolar to nuclear ratio

CYTOPLASM

General	
Shape	Cells generally retain the shape of cell type of origin; this is especially true if cells are mechanically exfoliated
	In a fluid environment, cells can become more rounded
Borders	Well defined
Amount	Scant to abundant cytoplasm depending on cell type and degree of cellular maturation. Cytoplasm of larger, mature cells can fold, making the cells appear smaller

Table continued on following page

Table 1–1. BENIGN CELLULAR FEATURES *Continued*

Differentiation	
Staining Characteristics	Basophilic (blue-green) in metabolically active cells
	Eosinophilic (pink) in metabolically inactive cells
	Orangeophilic (bright orange) in keratinized cells
Density	Thin and transparent in mature or inactive cells
	More dense in immature or metabolically active cells
NUCLEAR TO CYTOPLASMIC RATIO	Low in mature cells
	High in immature cells
CELLULAR ARRANGEMENTS	
Single Cells	Present
Aggregates	Individual cells in close approximation to each other; cell borders maintained
Tissue Fragments	
Sheets	One to two cell layers thick. Cell borders are contiguous and well defined
	Nuclei are uniform in size, shape, and chromatin patterns; polarity is maintained. Nuclear molding can be observed, indicating that cells have exfoliated from the same tissue fragment (this is not a criterion for malignancy)
Pseudosyncytia	Masses of cytoplasm with nuclei exhibiting loss of polarity
	Loss of cell borders
	Not generally present in benign conditions; however, parabasal cells may appear syncytial in smears from post-menopausal women. Nuclei are uniform and possess the bland chromatin patterns characteristic of these cells
SLIDE BACKGROUND	Clean and clear (transparent)
	Inflammatory cells can be present

Table 1–2. INFLAMMATION-ASSOCIATED CELLULAR FEATURES

NUCLEUS	
General	
Location	Centrally located
Shape	Round to oval
Size	Normal or slightly increased; if increased, usually less than three times the size of the nucleus of an intermediate cervical cell; however, occasional larger nuclei can be encountered
	Anisonucleosis can be present
Number	Single or multiple
Chromatin	
Appearance	Sharp and crisp
Granularity	Finely granular and evenly distributed to slightly granular and evenly distributed
Chromasia	Normal to slightly hyperchromatic
Nuclear Membrane	Smooth; undulating or wavy
	Chromatinic rim is of uniform thickness

Table 1–2. INFLAMMATION-ASSOCIATED CELLULAR FEATURES *Continued*

Nucleoli	Can be present in cells where nucleoli are not normally observed (examples: intermediate cervical cells and squamous metaplastic cells)
	If present, nucleoli are round to oval, single or multiple, generally small in size. They generally have a low nucleolar to nuclear ratio
CYTOPLASM	
General	
Shape	Cells generally retain shape of cell type of origin
Borders	Generally well defined
Amount	Scant to abundant cytoplasm depending on degree of maturation of cell
	Cells can increase slightly in size (e.g., squamous metaplastic cells with cellular changes resulting from chlamydial infection or hyperplastic bronchial lining cells)
Differentiation	
Staining Characteristics	Variable staining, including basophilic, eosinophilic, and orangeophilic
	Can see shifts in maturation index and consequent altered staining patterns
Density	Thin and transparent in mature or inactive cells
	More dense in immature or metabolically active cells
Special Features	Perinuclear halos; vacuolization; keratinization
NUCLEAR TO CYTOPLASMIC RATIO	Normal to slightly increased if nuclear enlargement is present
CELLULAR ARRANGEMENTS	
Single cells	Present
Aggregates	Increased number (e.g., aggregates of epithelial cells when a fungal infection is present)
Tissue Fragments	
Sheets	Increased number correlated to host response (e.g., increased number of squamous metaplastic cells in response to inflammation and irritation)
Pseudosyncytia	Not generally present in benign conditions
Three-Dimensional Tissue Fragments	Often difficult to clearly visualize individual cells and cell borders
	Nuclei usually uniform
	Increased number correlated to host response (e.g., increased number of hyperplastic bronchial lining cells in asthma)
Papillary Groups	Three-dimensional tissue fragments with visible fibrovascular stalks or finger-like projections or both
Acinar Structures	Round, three-dimensional tissue fragments with peripherally located nuclei
Slide Background	Acute and chronic inflammatory cells and aggregates of inflammatory cells on epithelial cells ("popcorn balls")
	Cellular debris from degenerated inflammatory and epithelial cells can be present
	This degenerated cellular debris can mimic tumor diathesis but is usually more uniformly granular (e.g., granular material present with trichomonad infections)
	Mucus (generally observed in strands)

Table continued on following page

Table 1–2. INFLAMMATION-ASSOCIATED CELLULAR FEATURES *Continued*

SPECIAL FEATURE	Atypical cellular changes of undetermined significance in the female genital tract: Increased nuclear size; granular, evenly distributed chromatin; hyperchromatic nuclei; slightly increased nuclear to cytoplasmic ratio; and increased incidence of keratinization Cells can resemble low-grade SIL (CIN I or mild dysplasia); however, the degree of atypia and the number of cells are generally less than that observed in low-grade SIL

Table 1–3. DEGENERATIVE CELLULAR FEATURES: CELLULAR CHANGES RESULTING FROM REVERSIBLE CELL INJURY

NUCLEUS

General	
Location	Centrally located
Shape	Round to oval
Size	Enlarged as a result of nuclear swelling
Number	Single or multiple
Chromatin	
Appearance	Hazy and indistinct (smudged or "washed out")
Granularity	Finely granular and evenly distributed but hazy and indistinct
Chromasia	Hypochromatic to hyperchromatic (smudged)
Nuclear Membrane	Smooth
	Chromatinic rim can have even or uneven distribution of chromatin (hazy and indistinct)
Nucleoli	Present or absent, as in cell of origin; if present, hazy and indistinct
	Nucleolar to nuclear ratio can be increased
Special Features	Karyolysis
	Intake of water and consequent swelling

CYTOPLASM

General	
Shape	Cells retain the shape of cell type of origin or become more round
	Disintegration of cytoplasm can occur and is recognized by cytoplasmic fraying ("moth-eaten" appearance); can give rise to naked nuclei
Borders	Not well defined
Amount	Often increased as a result of intake of water, although there is sometimes an apparent decrease in size because of loss of cytoplasm
Differentiation	
Staining Characteristics	Variable staining, including lightly basophilic, eosinophilic, and orangeophilic, depending on degree of maturation or activity of cell before injury
	Increased incidence of eosinophilia
	Increased incidence of amphophilia (both eosinophilic and basophilic staining in the same cell)

Table 1–3 DEGENERATIVE CELLULAR FEATURES: CELLULAR CHANGES RESULTING
FROM REVERSIBLE CELL INJURY *Continued*

Density	Normal or thinner and transparent as a result of intake of water
Special Features	Cytoplasmic vacuolization generally caused by small, diffuse vacuoles that have hazy, indistinct borders
NUCLEAR TO CYTOPLASMIC RATIO	Normal
	Increased because of artifactual nuclear enlargement
	Apparent increase resulting from loss of cytoplasm
CELLULAR ARRANGEMENTS	
Single Cells	Present
Aggregates	Cells can have poorly defined cell borders
Tissue Fragments	
Sheets	Sheets with poorly defined cell borders resulting from degeneration can mimic pseudosyncytial groupings
Pseudosyncytia	Not generally present in benign conditions
SLIDE BACKGROUND	Clean and clear (transparent)
	Material from degenerated inflammatory and epithelial cells; washed out and hazy
AIR DRYING	Can be localized to certain parts of slide
	Enlarged cell size
	Lack of chromatin detail
	Increased eosinophilia

Table 1–4. DEGENERATIVE CELLULAR FEATURES: CELLULAR CHANGES RESULTING FROM
IRREVERSIBLE CELL INJURY

NUCLEUS	
General	
Location	Centrally located
Shape	Round to oval
	Wrinkled
Size	Decreased in size
Number	Single or multiple
Chromatin	
Appearance	Dense, with eventual loss of chromatin pattern
Granularity	Pyknotic, smudged
Chromasia	Hyperchromatic
Nuclear Membrane	Smooth
	Wrinkled; looks like paper crinkled in one's hand
	Concave indentations; angles are not acute and sharp
	Chromatinic rim is not discerned because of dense chromatin
Nucleoli	Not visible, as a result of dense chromatin
Special Features	Karyorrhexis, i.e., condensation and fragmentation of chromatin material; chromatin fragments are round in shape, in contrast to the elongated shape of mitotic figures
CYTOPLASM	
General	
Shape	Cells retain the shape of cell type of origin
	Disintegration of cytoplasm and cytoplasmic fraying can give rise to naked nuclei
Borders	Not well defined
Amount	Often decreased because of cell shrinkage or loss of cytoplasm

Table continued on following page

Table 1–4. DEGENERATIVE CELLULAR FEATURES: CELLULAR CHANGES RESULTING FROM
IRREVERSIBLE CELL INJURY *Continued*

Differentiation	
Staining Characteristics	Variable staining, including basophilic, eosinophilic, and orangeophilic, depending on degree of maturation or activity of cell before injury
	Increased incidence of eosinophilia
	Increased incidence of amphophilia
Density	Normal or dense
NUCLEAR TO CYTOPLASMIC RATIO	Apparent increase resulting from loss of cytoplasm
	Decreased because of decreased nuclear size
CELLULAR ARRANGEMENTS	Same as in degenerative changes resulting from imbibition of water
SLIDE BACKGROUND	Same as in degenerative changes resulting from imbibition of water

Table 1–5. REPAIR

NUCLEUS	
General	
Location	Centrally located
Shape	Round to oval
Size	Uniformly increased (typical repair)
	Anisonucleosis (atypical repair)
Number	Single or multiple
CHROMATIN	
Appearance	Sharp and crisp
Granularity	Finely granular and evenly distributed to granular and evenly distributed (typical repair)
	Increased granularity (atypical repair)
Chromasia	Hypochromatic to hyperchromatic (typical repair)
	Increased hyperchromasia (atypical repair)
Nuclear Membrane	Smooth
	Chromatinic rim is of uniform thickness
Nucleoli	Prominent, single or multiple, round to oval in shape (typical repair)
	Increased variation in size, number, and shape (atypical repair)
Special Feature	Mitotic figures
CYTOPLASM	
General	
Shape	Round to polygonal
Borders	Well defined (typical repair)
	Less well defined (atypical repair)
Amount	Moderate to abundant
Differentiation	
Staining Characteristics	Basophilic
Density	Dense

Table 1–5. REPAIR *Continued*

NUCLEAR TO CYTOPLASMIC RATIO	Generally increased
CELLULAR ARRANGEMENTS	
Single Cells	Not generally present (typical repair)
	Present (atypical repair)
Aggregates	Not generally present (typical repair)
	Present (atypical repair)
Tissue Fragments	
Sheets	Most commonly observed cellular configuration, with well-defined cell borders and well-maintained polarity (typical repair)
	Present, but with some loss of well-defined cell borders; altered nuclear polarity (atypical repair)
Pseudosyncytia	Present more frequently in atypical repair
SLIDE BACKGROUND	Generally inflammatory
	Tumor diathesis not observed
DIFFERENTIAL DIAGNOSES FOR ATYPICAL REPAIR	Poorly differentiated squamous cell carcinoma
	Endocervical adenocarcinoma
DIFFERENTIATING FEATURES	History: previous injury, trauma, therapy, infectious agents, patient's age
	Progression from typical repair to atypical repair
	Majority of cells are cohesive in atypical repair; single, isolated cells are more numerous in carcinoma
	Unidirectional orientation of cytoplasm and nuclei more common in atypical repair than in carcinoma
	Nuclear crowding and overlap are less pronounced in atypical repair than in carcinoma
	At least one feature of typical repair is usually maintained in atypical repair

Table 1-6. THERAPY-INDUCED CELLULAR FEATURES

NUCLEUS

General	
Location	Centrally located
Shape	Round to oval
Size	Increased
Number	Single or multiple
Chromatin	
Appearance	Can exhibit degenerative changes; hazy and smudged; homogeneous; parachromatin clearing; nuclear vacuolization
Granularity	Finely granular and evenly distributed to coarsely granular and evenly distributed
Chromasia	Normal to hyperchromatic
Nuclear Membrane	Smooth or undulating
	Chromatinic rim has even distribution of chromatin or uneven distribution as a result of degenerative changes
Nucleoli	Can be present

CYTOPLASM

General	
Shape	Cell retains shape prior to therapy
Borders	Well or poorly defined
Amount	Normal to abundant
Differentiation	
Staining Characteristics	Basophilic, eosinophilic, or orangeophilic, increased incidence of amphophilia
Density	Same as prior to therapy
	Increased cytoplasmic vacuolization

NUCLEAR TO CYTOPLASMIC RATIO — Normal or slightly increased (can approximate the nuclear to cytoplasmic ratios observed with low-grade SIL in uterine cervix)

CELLULAR ARRANGEMENTS — Cellular configurations same as prior to therapy

SLIDE BACKGROUND
Clean and clear
Inflammatory
Increased number of multinucleated histiocytes
Tumor diathesis if carcinoma is present

Table 1–7. CELLULAR FEATURES OF SQUAMOUS INTRAEPITHELIAL LESIONS OF THE CERVIX

NUCLEUS

General	
Location	Centrally located
Shape	Round to oval
Size	Increased
Number	Single or multiple (generally observe increased incidence of multiple nuclei in low-grade SIL)
Chromatin	
Appearance	Sharp and crisp
Granularity	Finely granular and evenly distributed to coarsely granular and evenly distributed (becomes more granular as the severity of the lesion increases)
Chromasia	Slightly increased to hyperchromatic
Nuclear Membrane	Smooth
	Undulating or wavy
	Slightly angulated, with high-grade SIL (CIN III or CIS)
	Chromatinic rim is of uniform thickness
Nucleoli	Absent or rare and inconspicuous

CYTOPLASM

General	
Shape	Round or polygonal to irregular
Borders	Well defined for single cells of low-grade and high-grade SIL
	Poorly defined in pseudosyncytial groupings of high-grade SIL (CIS)
Amount	Abundant in low-grade SIL (CIN I or mild dysplasia)
	Moderate in high-grade SIL (CIN II or moderate dysplasia)
	Scant in high-grade SIL (CIN III or severe dysplasia and CIS)
Differentiation	
Staining Characteristics	Variable staining, including basophilic, eosinophilic, and orangeophilic
Density	Thin and transparent in low-grade SIL (CIN I or mild dysplasia)
	Dense in high-grade SIL (CIN II and III or moderate and severe dysplasia and CIS)

NUCLEAR TO CYTOPLASMIC RATIO

	Slightly increased in low-grade SIL (CIN I or mild dysplasia)
	Moderately increased in high-grade SIL (CIN II or moderate dysplasia) (approximately 1:3 to 1:2)
	High in high-grade SIL (CIN III or severe dysplasia and CIS)

CELLULAR ARRANGEMENTS

Single Cells	Abundant
Aggregates	Abundant
Tissue Fragments	
Sheets	Can be present (look for cell borders)
Pseudosyncytia	Present in high-grade SIL (CIN III or CIS)

SLIDE BACKGROUND

	Clean and clear or inflammatory
	Tumor diathesis not present

Table 1–8. MALIGNANT CELLULAR FEATURES: GENERAL

NUCLEUS

General	
Location	Centrally or eccentrically located
Shape	Round to oval; irregular, including elongated, triangular, and pleomorphic
Size	Marked variation (anisonucleosis)
Number	Single or multiple

Table continued on following page

Table 1–8. MALIGNANT CELLULAR FEATURES: GENERAL *Continued*

Chromatin	
Appearance	Sharp and crisp
Granularity	Finely granular and evenly distributed to coarsely granular and unevenly distributed
	Granules can be angular and irregular
	Parachromatin clearing
	Extreme variation in the degree and size of clearing can be present
Chromasia	Hypochromatic to hyperchromatic
Nuclear Membrane	Smooth
	Undulating or wavy
	Irregular and sharply angulated
	Chromatinic rim can be of irregular thickness
	Nuclear to cytoplasmic interfaces can be angular and irregular
Nucleoli	Not always present, but if present:
	Round, oval, or irregular (sharp, angular)
	Single or multiple
	Small to large in size
	Nucleolar to nuclear ratio varies
CYTOPLASM	
General	
Shape	Shape of cell type of origin is retained in well-differentiated carcinomas
	Irregular—loss of normal shape; tadpole, caudate, pleomorphic
Borders	Well or poorly defined
Amount	Scant to abundant
Special Feature	Cytoplasmic to nuclear molding:
	Malignant criterion occasionally observed
	Cytoplasm of one cell molds or affects the shape of the nucleus of an adjacent cell
Differentiation	
Staining	Eosinophilic or basophilic
Characteristics	Increased orangeophilia in keratinizing squamous cell carcinoma
Density	Thick and "hard" in squamous cell carcinoma
Vacuolization	Frothy, "granular," finely vacuolated to conspicuous vacuolization in adenocarcinoma
NUCLEAR TO CYTOPLASMIC RATIO	Marked variation
	Increased incidence of high nuclear to cytoplasmic ratios
CELLULAR ARRANGEMENTS	
Single Cells	Present
Aggregates	Present
Tissue Fragments	
Sheets	Present in well-differentiated carcinoma
Pseudosyncytia	Abundant with epithelial tumors
	Loss of cell borders and nuclear polarity
	Atypical nuclei exhibiting nuclear crowding and overlap
Three-Dimensional Tissue Fragments	
Papillary Groups	Present in adenocarcinoma
Acinar Structures	Present in adenocarcinoma
SLIDE BACKGROUND	Clean and clear (exophytic lesions)
	Inflammatory
	Tumor diathesis (dried blood or hemosiderin and necrotic cell debris—appears as a granular precipitate)

Table 1–9. SQUAMOUS CELL CARCINOMA—DIFFERENTIAL FEATURES

NUCLEUS

General	
Location	Centrally or eccentrically located
Shape	Round to oval; irregular
Size	Marked variation (anisonucleosis)
Number	Single or multiple
Chromatin	
Appearance	Sharp and crisp
Granularity	Slightly granular and evenly distributed to coarsely granular and unevenly distributed
Chromasia	Hyperchromatic
Nuclear Membrane	Smooth to irregular
	Chromatinic rim can be of irregular thickness
Nucleoli	Not visualized in well-differentiated squamous cell carcinoma
	Prominent or numerous or both in poorly differentiated squamous cell carcinoma

CYTOPLASM

General	
Shape	Retains squamous shape to highly irregular or pleomorphic
Borders	Well or poorly defined
Amount	Scant to abundant
Differentiation	
Staining	Orangeophilic in well-differentiated squamous cell carcinoma
Characteristics	Basophilic or eosinophilic in poorly differentiated squamous cell carcinoma
Density	Thick and hard

NUCLEAR TO CYTOPLASMIC RATIO	Marked variation

CELLULAR ARRANGEMENTS

Single Cells	Abundant
Aggregates	Abundant
Tissue Fragments	
Sheets	Present in well-differentiated squamous cell carcinoma
Pseudosyncytia	Abundant
Three-Dimensional Tissue Fragments	
Papillary Groups	Not present
Acinar Structures	Not present

SLIDE BACKGROUND	Clean and clear in exophytic lesions
	Tumor diathesis

Table 1–10. ADENOCARCINOMA: DIFFERENTIAL FEATURES

NUCLEUS

General
    Location   Centrally or eccentrically located
    Shape   More round to oval and regular in shape than in squamous cell
                        carcinoma
    Size   Marked variation (anisonucleosis)
    Number   Single or multiple
Chromatin
    Appearance   Sharp and crisp
    Granularity   Less granular than squamous cell carcinoma
    Chromasia   Less hyperchromatic than squamous cell carcinoma
Nuclear Membrane   Smoother than in squamous cell carcinoma
                        Chromatinic rim more uniform than in squamous cell carcinoma
Nucleoli   Often prominent and numerous; can be irregular

CYTOPLASM

General
    Shape   Retains columnar shape or round to oval
    Border   Well or poorly defined
    Amount   Scant to abundant
Differentiation
    Staining   Generally basophilic
      Characteristics
    Density   Light, frothy, "granular;" diffusely vacuolated to conspicuous
                        vacuolization

NUCLEAR TO CYTOPLASMIC RATIO

Marked variation

CELLULAR ARRANGEMENTS

Single Cells   Present
Aggregates   Present
Tissue Fragments
    Sheets   Present in well-differentiated adenocarcinoma
    Pseudosyncytia   Abundant, but nuclei exhibit less crowding and overlap than in
                        squamous cell carcinoma

    Three-Dimensional
    Tissue Fragments
      Papillary Groups   Present
      Acinar Structures   Present

SLIDE BACKGROUND   Tumor diathesis

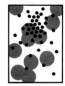

FIGURE 1–1A. Finely Granular, Evenly Distributed Chromatin. Heterochromatin (darkly stained chromatin granules) and euchromatin (lightly stained chromatin material) are evenly distributed. The chromatin granules are small and uniform. The nuclear chromatin is well preserved (sharp and crisp), and the chromasia is baseline normal. Nuclear membranes are smooth, and the chromatinic rims are of uniform thickness along the entire circumference of each nucleus. In addition, nucleoli are conspicuous (easily observed, but not large and prominent) and are round to oval in shape. Nucleolar to nuclear ratios are low. These features are characteristic of benign nuclei. Benign mesothelial cells, peritoneal washing (Papanicolaou stain [throughout unless otherwise indicated] × 1000).

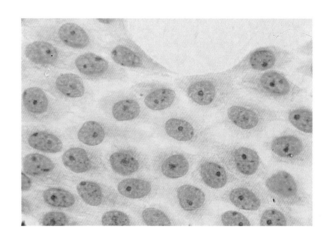

FIGURE 1–1B. Finely Granular, Evenly Distributed Chromatin Compared with Coarsely Granular, Evenly Distributed Chromatin. Nuclei of duodenal mucosal cells containing very finely granular, evenly distributed chromatin are marked by arrows. The nuclei of the epithelial cells are hypochromatic. In contrast, neighboring lymphocytes contain nuclei with coarsely granular, evenly distributed chromatin. The chromatin granules are larger in size but are evenly distributed throughout the nuclei. Nuclei are hyperchromatic. Nuclear membranes are smooth and round, and the chromatinic rims are of uniform thickness. Even though the chromatin granules are larger and the nuclei are hyperchromatic, the remaining features are indicative of benignancy. Duodenal brushing (× 1000).

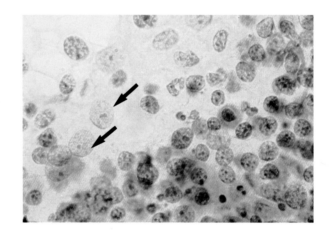

FIGURE 1–1C. Coarsely Granular, Evenly Distributed Chromatin. Moderate-sized to large granules of chromatin are present in the nuclei of these benign granulosa cells aspirated from an ovarian follicular cyst. The chromatin granules are sharp and crisp and are evenly distributed. Nuclear membranes are smooth, and the chromatinic rims are of uniform thickness. The slightly hyperchromatic nuclei and conspicuous nucleoli indicate biosynthetic activity; the uniform appearance and distribution of chromatin indicate a benign state. Ovarian cyst, aspiration (× 1000).

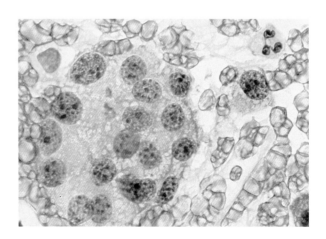

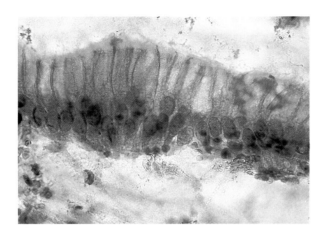

FIGURE 1–2A. Cellular Origin—Benign Columnar Cells. Benign cells in cytologic specimens generally retain the shape they possessed in vivo, especially if mechanically exfoliated. When viewed laterally, benign columnar cells are elongated, with nuclei located at the basal portion of the cell; this arrangement is termed "palisade." Distal esophageal brushing (× 630).

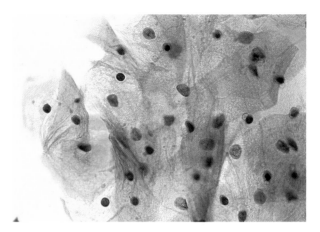

FIGURE 1–2C. Cellular Origin—Benign Stratified Squamous Epithelial Cells. Benign stratified squamous epithelial cells are cytologically characterized by large amounts of transparent cytoplasm in polygonal shapes. These superficial and intermediate cells from the uterine cervix contain pyknotic and vesicular nuclei, respectively. Uterine cervix, Papanicolaou smear (× 630).

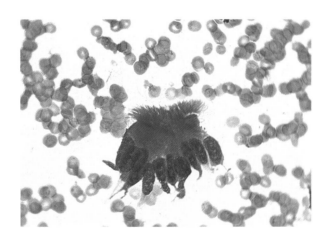

FIGURE 1–2B. Cellular Origin—Benign Columnar Cells. Note the cilia of these benign bronchial epithelial cells. The presence of cilia is indicative of benignancy. Bronchial brushing, Diff-Quik (× 630).

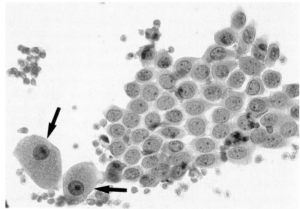

FIGURE 1–2D. Cellular Origin—Hepatocytes and Biliary Ductal Cells. Two distinct cell types are observed in this hepatic aspirate. One type, hepatocytes (at arrows), are polygonal in shape and possess moderate amounts of granular cytoplasm. The adjacent sheet of biliary ductal cells, the second cell type, exhibits well-defined cell borders, an even arrangement and distribution of nuclei (well-maintained polarity), and nuclear uniformity (size, shape, and chromatin pattern). These cells resemble a honeycomb, a configuration that is characteristic of benign glandular cells viewed en face. Liver, fine needle aspiration (× 630).

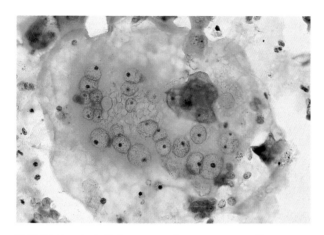

FIGURE 1–3A. Cellular Maturation—Mature Cells. Mature benign cells possess abundant transparent cytoplasm, small nuclei, and low N/C ratios. The cells are usually polygonal in shape, and the nuclei are either pyknotic or vesicular. Even though this transitional cell contains numerous nuclei, the copious volume of the transparent cytoplasm yields a low N/C ratio. Large size, transparent cytoplasm, and low N/C ratio indicate cellular maturity. Urinary bladder washing (× 400).

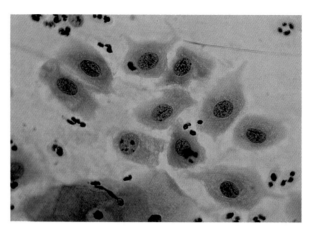

FIGURE 1–4A. Staining Characteristics—Metabolically Active Cells. Metabolically active cells, such as parabasal, mesothelial, and squamous metaplastic cells, stain basophilically (blue-green) with the modified Papanicolaou stain, presumably because of a high concentration of ribosomes in the cytoplasm. Cytoplasm is usually dense, as in these squamous metaplastic cells. Metabolically inactive cells, such as the superficial cells in Figure 1–2C, stain eosinophilically (pink). Uterine cervix, Papanicolaou smear (× 630).

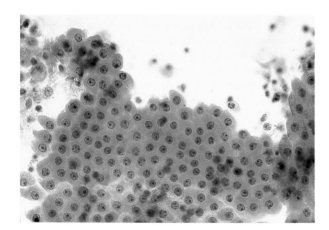

FIGURE 1–3B. Cellular Maturation—Immature Cells. Benign immature cells possess smaller amounts of dense cytoplasm than their mature counterparts. They are more round in shape when exfoliated singly. Their nuclei are vesicular in well-preserved cells and can be the same size or larger than the nuclei of their mature counterparts, yielding a higher N/C ratio. These transitional cells are smaller, have denser cytoplasm, and have higher N/C ratios than the mature transitional cell in Figure 1–3A. Because these cells are cohesively bound in a sheet, they are still polygonal in shape. Urinary bladder washing (× 400).

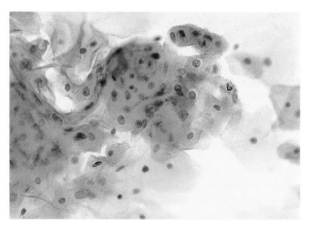

FIGURE 1–4B. Staining Characteristics—Keratinized Cells. Keratinized cells, both benign and malignant, stain orangeophilically. Keratinization is not a normal cellular finding, and its presence indicates the possibility of irritation, infection, a squamous intraepithelial lesion, or malignancy. These dyskeratocytes are indicative of human papilloma virus infection. Uterine cervix, Papanicolaou smear (× 630).

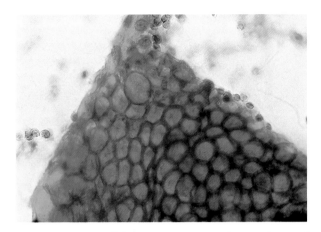

FIGURE 1–5A. Cellular Arrangements—Sheets. Sheets of cells are often one to two cell layers thick. Cell borders are contiguous and well-defined. These gastric mucosal cells have extremely well-defined cell borders. Nuclei in cellular sheets are generally uniform in size, shape, and chromatin pattern; polarity is maintained. Gastric brushing (× 630).

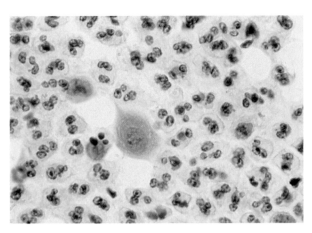

FIGURE 1–6A. Acute Inflammation. Acute inflammatory processes are characterized by polymorphonuclear leukocytes with multilobulated hyperchromatic nuclei. Blood and necrotic debris can also be present. A parabasal cell is present in a background of acute inflammation. Uterine cervix, Papanicolaou smear (× 1000).

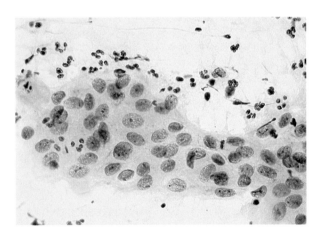

FIGURE 1–5B. Cellular Arrangements—Pseudosyncytia. These cellular configurations are characterized by masses of cytoplasm without visible, intact cell borders. Nuclei exhibit loss of polarity. Although these configurations are not generally present in benign conditions, parabasal cells can be observed in pseudosyntial groupings in the Papanicolaou smears of post-menopausal women. Their nuclei exhibit crowding, overlap, and loss of polarity. Nuclear size, shape, and chromatin patterns, however, are generally uniform. Even though cell borders are not observed and there is some loss of polarity, these nuclei are uniform in size and round to oval in shape, and their chromatin patterns are finely granular and evenly distributed. These features help to distinguish these benign parabasal cells from those of a squamous intraepithelial lesion or malignancy. Uterine cervix, Papanicolaou smear (× 630).

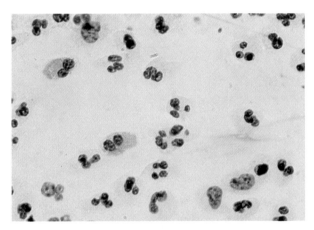

FIGURE 1–6B. Mixed Inflammation. Both acute and chronic inflammatory cells are present in mixed inflammation. The polymorphonuclear leukocytes, including eosinophils, constitute the acute portion of this mixed inflammatory cell picture. Histiocytes (at arrows) constitute the chronic portion. Histiocytes are larger than polymorphonuclear leukocytes and are characterized by round or reniform (bean-shaped) nuclei that are centrally or eccentrically located in the cell. Chromatin patterns can range from finely granular and evenly distributed to coarsely granular and evenly distributed. Nucleoli can be conspicuous. Cytoplasm is round to oval in shape and is diffusely vacuolated or frothy in appearance. Amounts of cytoplasm vary from scant to moderate. Uterine cervix, Papanicolaou smear (× 1000).

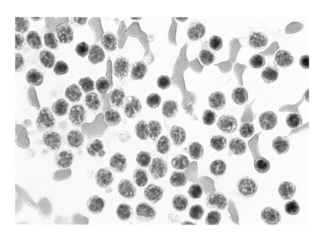

FIGURE 1–6C. Chronic Inflammation. Chronic inflammation is characterized by lymphocytes, histiocytes, and plasma cells. The lymphocytes range from mature to immature. The mature lymphocytes have dense homogeneous nuclei and high N/C ratios. The immature lymphocytes possess vesicular nuclei and often conspicuous or prominent nucleoli; larger amounts of cytoplasm yield slightly lower N/C ratios than do the mature lymphocytes. Pleural fluid (× 1000).

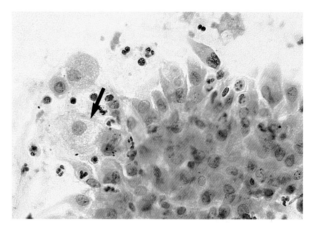

FIGURE 1–6E. Granulomatous Inflammation. Epithelioid histiocytes, indicative of granulomatous inflammation, are usually observed in aggregates or tissue-like fragments. These are sometimes difficult to interpret, especially in fine needle aspirations, where their crowded epithelial appearance can be the cause of a false-positive diagnosis of malignancy. Often, however, more typical histiocytes are in close proximity and can help with the correct interpretation (remember that cells are usually similar to adjacent or neighboring cells). An easily identified histiocyte is marked by the arrow. Adjacent to this cell is a large aggregate of cells that are somewhat elongated in shape and have denser cytoplasm than typical histiocytes. All nuclei, however, are similar in morphology and a progression can be seen from single, round histiocytes to the more "epithelioid" cells in the aggregate. Lung, fine needle aspiration (× 630).

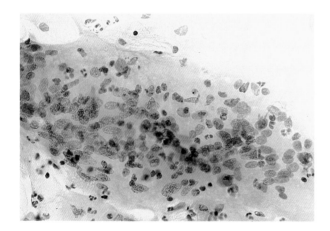

FIGURE 1–6D. Chronic Inflammation. Multinucleated histiocytes are often observed in chronic inflammatory processes. This large cell with randomly arranged nuclei is characteristic of a multinucleated histiocyte. Chromatin patterns are finely granular and evenly distributed but can be more coarse in appearance. The random dispersal of nuclei and chromatin granularity differentiate these cells from the multinucleated cells found in herpes infections. Uterine cervix, Papanicolaou smear (× 400).

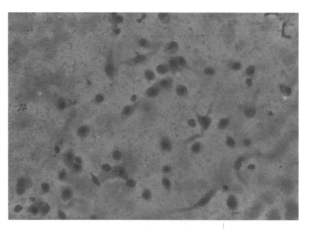

FIGURE 1–6F. Granulomatous Inflammation. Necrosis is a nonspecific finding, the underlying etiology being inflammatory or malignant in nature. Fluffy, granular, necrotic material admixed with abundant leukocytes is usually secondary to an inflammatory process. Hemolyzed or fresh blood admixed with a granular necrotic precipitate is usually indicative of tumor diathesis. The definitive answer, of course, lies with the associated cellular elements. These

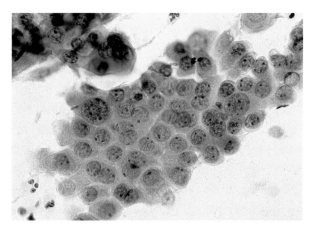

FIGURE 1–7A. Nuclear Enlargement and Anisonucleosis. Nuclear enlargement and anisonucleosis (variation in nuclear size) are often present in epithelial cells from specimens containing inflammatory cells. Nuclear enlargement is usually less than three times the size of the nucleus of an intermediate cervical cell or of a polymorphonuclear leukocyte. These endocervical cells from a Papanicolaou smear exhibit both nuclear enlargement and anisonucleosis. Chromatin is finely granular and evenly distributed, and chromasia is slightly increased. The chromatinic rim is of uniform thickness. Nuclear membranes are smooth (they can be wavy or undulating). Nucleoli are present. Uterine cervix, Papanicolaou smear (× 630).

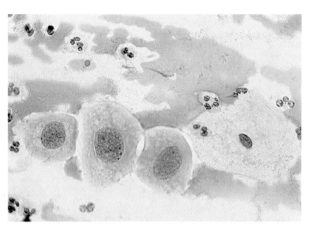

FIGURE 1–7C. Increased Cell Size. Cell size can increase when inflammation is present. These squamous metaplastic cells from a Papanicolaou smear with marked inflammation are enlarged (compare with the adjacent intermediate cell) and possess enlarged nuclei. Although cellular features are reminiscent of a high-grade squamous intraepithelial lesion (CIN II or moderate dysplasia), cellular enlargement is too pronounced; chromatin is finely granular and evenly distributed; and N/C ratios are not quite as increased as would be expected with this intraepithelial lesion. Increased cell size and vacuolation in squamous metaplastic cells are changes that have been described in chlamydial infections. Uterine cervix, Papanicolaou smear (× 630).

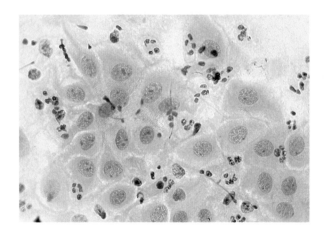

FIGURE 1–7B. Nucleoli. When inflammation is present, nucleoli are often observed in cells in which they are not normally found (e.g., intermediate, parabasal, and squamous metaplastic cells of the uterine cervix). These parabasal cells from an inflammatory atrophic Papanicolaou smear contain multiple, small, round to oval nucleoli. Nucleolar to nuclear ratios are extremely low. Uterine cervix, Papanicolaou smear (× 630).

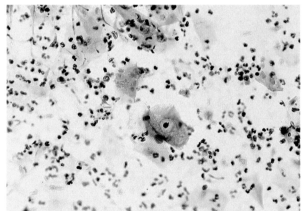

FIGURE 1–7D. Perinuclear Halos. Perinuclear halos are small, evenly circumscribed clearings surrounding the nuclei of epithelial cells in inflammatory smears. They differ from the large, irregular halos of koilocytes by virtue of their small size and round to oval shape. Although perinuclear halos are nonspecific inflammatory cell changes and are observed with many infections, they are often associated with trichomoniasis. Uterine cervix, Papanicolaou smear (× 400).

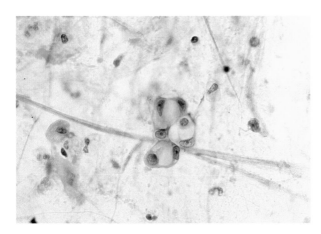

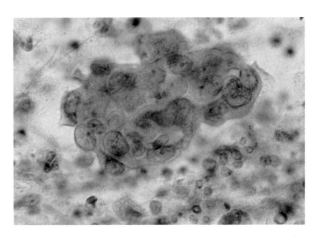

FIGURE 1–7E. Cytoplasmic Vacuolization. These bronchial epithelial cells are present in a sputum sample that contains abundant inflammation and mucin (strands). Hyperdistended vacuoles push benign-appearing nuclei to one side of the cells. Given the slide background, these are most probably mucin-secreting cells; however, degenerative cell changes cannot be excluded. Special stains are needed for the definitive determination of the presence of mucin. Cytoplasmic vacuolization is a feature that is found in both benign and malignant cells. Diffuse vacuolization (numerous small vacuoles) is often associated with inflammation and resulting degenerative cell changes. Likewise, large, distended vacuoles can be degenerative in nature. Large, distended vacuoles can also indicate mucin production, a process associated with infection or irritation and malignancy. The biologic state of the cell can only be assessed by nuclear morphology. Sputum (× 630).

FIGURE 1–7F. Cellular Arrangements—Glandular Groupings. Three-dimensional tissue fragments composed of glandular cells are often present in inflammatory specimens. Although these fragments lack the precise configurations of acini, morulae, or papillary tissue fragments, they still convey a message of stimulated growth, either reactive or malignant. Nuclei must be carefully examined to make a determination of benignancy or malignancy. This fragment of cells is set in a background of marked inflammation in a sputum. The nuclei are very uniform in terms of size, shape, and chromatin patterns. Chromatin is finely granular and evenly distributed, and chromatinic rims are of uniform thickness. Nuclear membranes are smooth. Small nucleoli are present. Although this configuration is an atypical finding in a sputum specimen, nuclear detail indicates benignancy. Sputum (× 1000).

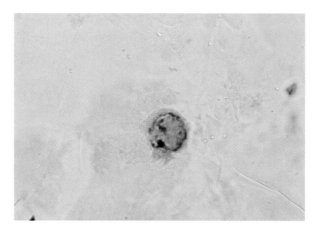

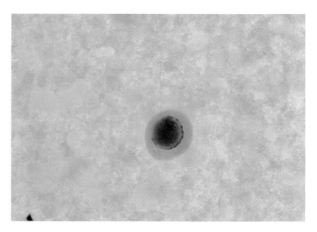

FIGURE 1–8A. Nuclear Degeneration—Chromatin. Cellular degeneration can be a pitfall, either because it imitates malignant cellular changes or because it blurs the structural detail of malignant cells. In general, it is good practice to refrain from interpreting poorly preserved material with features of advanced degeneration. Classic nuclear degeneration is characterized by nuclear enlargement, hyperchromasia, and hazy, indistinct chromatin and chromatinic rims. Heterochromatin and euchromatin are clumped, smudged, and indistinct. Chromatinic rims are not uniform along the entire circumferences of nuclei. They often appear interrupted in some areas and very thick in other areas. Interfaces between heterochromatin and euchromatin and between the chromatinic rims and chromatinic networks are hazy and smudged. This immature transitional cell possesses an enlarged hyperchromatic nucleus and a high N/C ratio. The chromatinic rim is not of uniform thickness. These features are worrisome and suggest the possibility of carcinoma. However, the chromatin is not sharp and crisp—it is clumped, hazy, smudged, and indistinct. The interfaces of the chromatinic rim and nuclear chromatin are similar. These features denote degeneration and preclude a definitive diagnosis on this cell. Urinary bladder washing (× 1000).

FIGURE 1–8B. Nuclear Degeneration—Chromatin. Nuclei sometimes appear exceedingly homogeneous and hyperchromatic when degenerated, with conspicuous lack of chromatin granularity. This transitional cell possesses an enlarged hyperchromatic nucleus that is very smooth and homogeneous in appearance. The chromatinic rim is not of uniform thickness along the entire circumference of the nucleus. In urinary tract specimens, transitional cells such as these are often referred to as "decoy" cells, i.e., decoys for malignancy until the state of cellular preservation is correctly assessed. In addition, a transitional cell such as this can also indicate the possibility of an infection by a human papova virus. Neither degeneration nor infection can be excluded on the basis of this cell. Urine (× 1000).

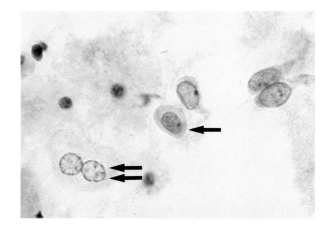

FIGURE 1–8C. Nuclear Degeneration—Chromatin. This urine specimen contains well-preserved and degenerated transitional cells. A well-preserved cell (marked by one arrow) is compared with a degenerated cell (marked by two arrows). The nucleus of the well-preserved cell is round; contains finely granular, evenly distributed chromatin that is sharp and crisp; and has a chromatinic rim of uniform thickness. The nuclear membrane is smooth. Nucleoli are present. The degenerated nuclei are round, contain cleared chromatin, and possess chromatinic rims that are markedly irregular in thickness—chromatin material fluctuates from appearing absent to thick. Chromatin is smudged, denoting degeneration. Urine (× 1000).

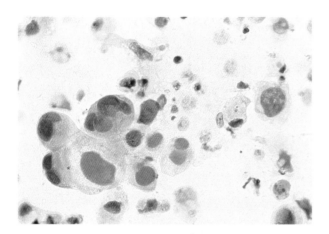

FIGURE 1–8D. Nuclear Degeneration—Chromatin. Degenerative features are superimposed on malignant cells in this voided urine. The majority of cells are enlarged and contain nuclei with extremely homogeneous chromatin, both caused by the imbibition of water. Irregular nuclear shapes, high N/C ratios, and the presence of a tissue fragment in a voided urine sample are suggestive of malignancy. Malignant features are greatly tempered by degenerative features, and caution must be employed when interpreting these cells. Urine (× 630).

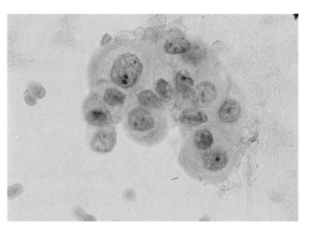

FIGURE 1–9B. Cellular Degeneration—Cytoplasmic Vacuolization. Cytoplasmic vacuolization occurs when ionic and fluid homeostasis is disrupted, resulting in an influx of water. Vacuoles are usually small and diffuse but can be large and hyperdistended. Additionally, nuclear and cytoplasmic swelling caused by imbibition of water often results in lighter-staining cytoplasm and nuclei than encountered in well-preserved cells. Renal pelvic washing (× 1000).

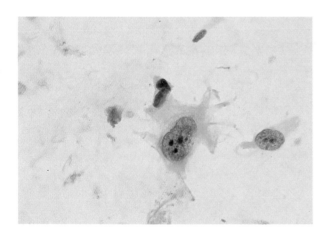

FIGURE 1–9A. Cellular Degeneration—Loss of Cytoplasm. Cellular degeneration often results in the disintegration and eventual loss of cytoplasm. Intact cell borders are not well defined, and cytoplasm is sometimes "motheaten" in appearance. N/C ratios are artifactually higher than normal as a result of the loss of cytoplasm. This cell exhibits both radiation effect (enlargement) and degeneration with loss of cytoplasm. Bronchial washing (× 630).

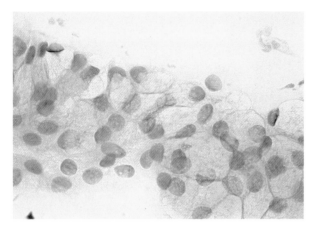

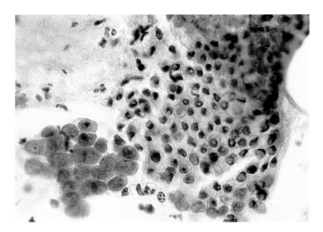

FIGURE 1–10A. Air-Drying Artifact. Air-drying artifact can be diffusely spread across the entire slide or can be localized to certain areas. The affected cells are reminiscent of degenerated cells and are enlarged and very lightly stained. They lack chromatin detail and are very often eosinophilic. Nuclear and cellular details are obscured. Compare these air-dried mucus-producing endocervical cells with the well-preserved mucus-producing endocervical cells in Figure 1–10B. Photomicrographs are the same magnification. Uterine cervix, Papanicolaou smear (× 630).

FIGURE 1–11A. Nuclear Degeneration—Nuclear Membranes. Irreversible cell injury often results in irregular nuclear outlines that are sometimes confused with malignant nuclear changes. Degenerated nuclei are vesicular to pyknotic and possess angular or wrinkled contours. However, they do not possess the acute, sharp angularity characteristic of malignancy. The angles are more concave, round, or "soft" in appearance. Well-preserved cells are adjacent to degenerated cells in this Papanicolaou smear. The cellular arrangement is honeycomb and indicates endocervical origin. The well-preserved cells contain round nuclei with finely granular, evenly distributed chromatin and smooth nuclear membranes. The degenerated cells contain wrinkled nuclei that are becoming hyperchromatic and homogeneous or dense in appearance. Uterine cervix, Papanicolaou smear (× 630).

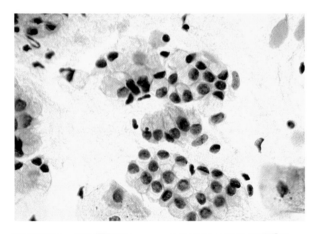

FIGURE 1–10B. Well-Preserved Endocervical Cells. Uterine cervix, Papanicolaou smear (× 630).

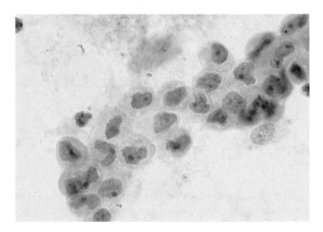

FIGURE 1–11B. Nuclear Degeneration—Nuclear Membranes. These mesothelial cells, from a peritoneal washing, possess irregular nuclear outlines. Nuclear membranes are not round and smooth; they are irregular and angulated. The angles, however, are not as acute, pointed, or sharp, as observed in malignancy. They are softer and rounder. In addition, although chromatin patterns are degenerated, they appear to be finely granular and evenly distributed. These nuclear membranes exhibit the combined effects of reactive and degenerative cellular changes. Peritoneal washing (× 1000).

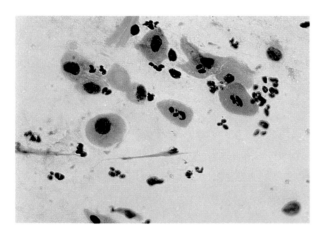

FIGURE 1–12. Nuclear Degeneration—Karyorrhexis. Condensation and fragmentation of chromatin material are degenerative features often seen on inflammatory smears. The final stage of nuclear condensation and fragmentation is karyorrhexis. Large, round chromatin fragments appear where the nucleus of the cell once was. Chromatin fragments in karyorrhexis are often round, whereas they are elongated in mitotic figures. This parabasal cell has lost an intact nucleus and nuclear membrane and retains only round fragments of homogeneous chromatin material. Uterine cervix, Papanicolaou smear (× 1000).

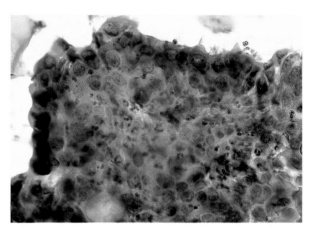

FIGURE 1–13. Staining Characteristics. Staining characteristics are altered by specimen thickness and consequent improper penetration of dye. It would be expected that these well-preserved reactive endocervical cells would stain basophilically; however, it is likely that the orangeophilic staining of these cells is a result of increased specimen thickness and improper dye penetration. Uterine cervix, Papanicolaou smear (× 630).

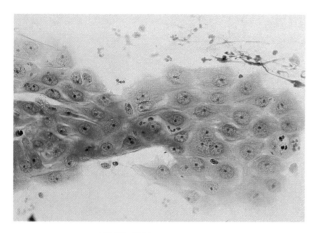

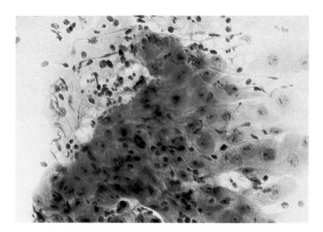

FIGURE 1–14A. Typical Repair. Reparative changes can be seen in conjunction with inflammation; infection; and postirradiation, chemotherapy, or trauma. Typical repair is easily recognized and is distinguished by cohesive sheets of cells with well-defined cell borders; well-maintained nuclear polarity; uniform nuclei in terms of size, shape, and chromatin; finely granular, evenly distributed chromatin; nuclei that are hypochromatic to slightly hyperchromatic; and prominent round nucleoli in almost all nuclei. Uterine cervix, Papanicolaou smear (× 400).

FIGURE 1–14C. Typical Repair. Typical repair is sometimes made more difficult to diagnose because sheets fold on themselves and create the illusion of pseudosyncytial groupings. A comparison of nuclei in all reparative sheets throughout the slide reveals uniformity and reinforces the correct diagnosis of repair. This folded sheet of reparative cells is from the same glass slide as Figure 1–14A. Uterine cervix, Papanicolaou smear (× 400).

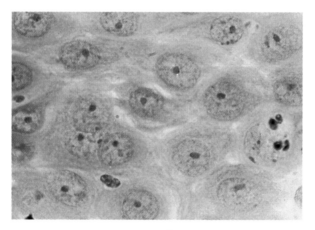

FIGURE 1–14B. Typical Repair. Multinucleation is a feature of typical repair. Uterine cervix, Papanicolaou smear (× 1000).

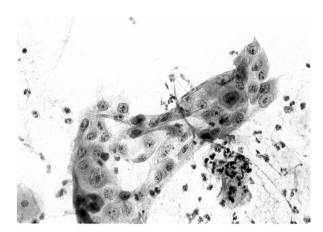

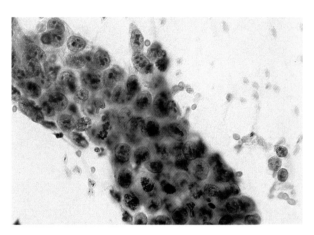

FIGURE 1–15A. Slightly Atypical Repair. Slightly atypical repair retains most of the features of classic repair but can display increased anisonucleosis, increased chromatin granularity, and increased chromasia. Cell borders and nuclear polarity usually remain intact. This reparative sheet of cells has folded on itself. Although marked anisonucleosis, increased chromatin granularity (with an even distribution), and increased chromasia are observed, cell borders are still maintained, cellular polarity is conserved, and, except for size, the morphology of nuclei is similar. Taken together, these features are characteristic of slightly atypical repair. Uterine cervix, Papanicolaou smear (× 400).

FIGURE 1–16. Atypical Repair. Atypical repair can be extremely difficult to distinguish from adenocarcinoma or poorly differentiated squamous cell carcinoma. When dealing with cases such as these, the entire slide must be evaluated; single, isolated fields taken out of context are extremely difficult to diagnose. Some features of typical repair are usually maintained and recognized and aid in rendering the correct interpretation. The cells from this lung aspirate are crowded, have lost polarity, contain prominent nucleoli, and possess mitotic figures. The nuclei, however, are uniform in terms of size, shape, and chromatin patterns. Chromatin is finely granular to slightly granular and evenly distributed. Because of cellular crowding, it is difficult to discern cell borders, but careful focusing with the microscope reveals the presence of some well-maintained cell borders. In addition, these cohesive groups are few in number on the glass slide. At first glance, this group of cells appears to suggest carcinoma, but careful observation reveals features that are more consistent with benignancy, e.g., intact cell borders, bland chromatin patterns, and few cohesive tissue fragments. These latter features are very important in the differential diagnosis of atypical repair. Morphologic characteristics, together with the patient's history of antituberculosis therapy and moderate emphysema, argue for a conservative diagnostic approach. The patient's lung biopsy revealed granulomatous tissue, and the serologic test was positive for coccidioidomycosis. Lung, fine needle aspiration (× 630).

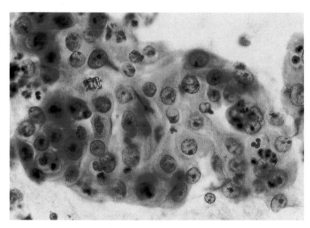

FIGURE 1–15B. Slightly Atypical Repair. Reparative reactions in nongynecologic sites often appear slightly more atypical than those in the female genital tract. These reparative gastric cells from the region of a gastric ulcer possess mitotic figures and an apparent loss of cytoplasmic borders in some areas. Mitotic figures are frequently observed in reparative processes and in exfoliative cytologic studies are present more often in repair than in malignancy. Although the apparent loss of cell borders and nuclear crowding is observed in some areas, well-defined cell borders are evident in other areas. Nuclear morphology is uniform in terms of size, shape, and chromatin pattern. Chromatin patterns are very finely granular and evenly distributed. Regular prominent nucleoli are present. These features support a regenerative or reparative process. Gastric brushing (× 630).

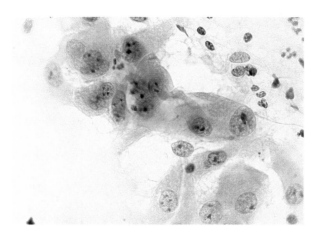

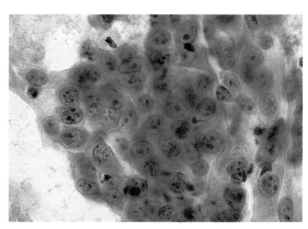

FIGURE 1–17A. Atypical Repair. A small sheet of atypical cells demonstrating cellular and nuclear enlargement. Although the cells exhibit a slight loss of cohesion, loss of nuclear polarity, and variation in size, it can be seen that they exfoliated from the same tissue fragment in vivo. Chromatin is finely granular but somewhat unevenly distributed, and nuclei are hypochromatic. Nucleoli are prominent and irregular. Despite these atypical features, the presence of recognizable cell borders, finely granular chromatin, and hypochromasia points to a benign process. These cells are from the same glass slide as Figures 1–14A and C and follow a progression from classic repair to atypical repair. Uterine cervix, Papanicolaou smear (× 400).

FIGURE 1–18A. Atypical Repair. A two-dimensional tissue fragment is present in this bronchial brushing from a 29-year-old man who is positive for human immunodeficiency virus and has interstitial lung disease. Nuclei appear crowded; polarity is not maintained; and multiple prominent, irregular nucleoli are present. Although these features are atypical, other features characteristic of benignancy are observed and must be considered. Some cell borders are visible. Nuclei are uniform in size and shape, with the majority of nuclei possessing finely granular, evenly distributed chromatin. Chromasia is normal to hypochromatic. Nuclear crowding may in part be artifactual, caused by the two-dimensional configuration of the tissue fragment. Intact cell borders and bland nuclear features favor the diagnosis of atypical repair over carcinoma. Bronchial brushing (× 630).

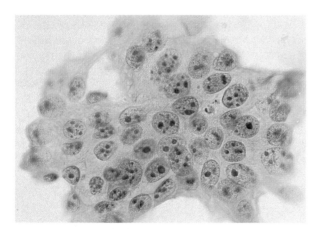

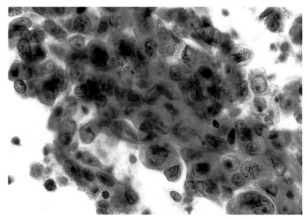

FIGURE 1–17B. Adenocarcinoma. This group of cells is present on an esophageal brushing. Although the nuclei are more uniform in terms of size and shape and the cells are more cohesive than in Figure 1–17A, their chromatin patterns are more granular and they are present in a pseudosyncytial tissue fragment with loss of nuclear polarity and true nuclear crowding. Nucleoli are multiple and prominent and display great variation in size and number. The pseudosyncytial arrangement with loss of cell borders, nuclear crowding, and marked nucleolar variation characterizes these cells as malignant and distinguishes them from atypical repair cells. Esophageal brushing (× 630).

FIGURE 1–18B. Squamous Cell Carcinoma. A multidimensional tissue fragment is present in this lung aspiration. The nuclei vary slightly in size and shape, are crowded, and their polarity is not maintained. The nuclei are hyperchromatic, and chromatin patterns range from granular and unevenly distributed to cleared. Prominent nucleoli are present. Although some cell borders are intact, the overall arrangement of this tissue fragment is very disorganized. These features support the diagnosis of squamous cell carcinoma. Lung, fine needle aspiration (× 630).

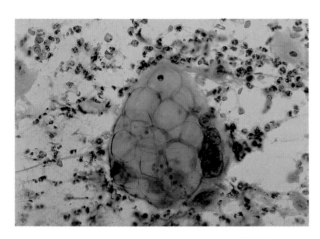

FIGURE 1–19A. Radiation Effect—Cytoplasmic Vacuolization. Radiation can produce marked cellular changes in both benign and malignant cells. These changes affect the nucleus and cytoplasm and can be manifested in benign cells for 20 years or more. Cytoplasmic vacuolization is the first cellular change to occur. This squamous cell is on the Papanicolaou smear of a woman who received radiation therapy for cervical carcinoma. Cellular and nuclear enlargement, multinucleation, and cytoplasmic vacuolization are present. Chromatin is finely granular and evenly distributed, and N/C ratios are within normal limits. Blood and inflammation are present in the slide background. These changes are consistent with radiation effect. Uterine cervix, Papanicolaou smear (× 400).

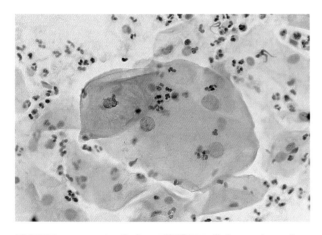

FIGURE 1–19B. Radiation Effect—Cellular and Nuclear Enlargement. These squamous cells are on the Papanicolaou smear of a woman who received radiation therapy for cervical carcinoma, stage IIB. Cellular and nuclear enlargement is present. Nuclei are slightly enlarged (compare with surrounding intermediate cells), but N/C ratios are maintained. Chromatin is bland. Air-drying artifact may also be noted. Uterine cervix, Papanicolaou smear (× 400).

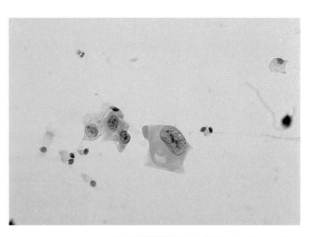

FIGURE 1–19C. Radiation Effect—Cellular and Nuclear Enlargement. This markedly enlarged cell (compare with the small, degenerated columnar cells) is present on the bronchial brushing of an 84-year-old woman who underwent mastectomy and radiation many years ago. The patient now has a pulmonary infiltrate. Cellular and nuclear enlargement is present, with a consequent increase in N/C ratio. Chromatin is finely granular and evenly distributed, and the nucleus is slightly hyperchromatic. Vacuoles are present in both the nucleus and cytoplasm, indicating degeneration. N/C ratios can be significantly altered in radiation effect. If increased N/C ratios are present, bland chromatin patterns and degenerative nuclear features are helpful in reaching a diagnosis of radiation effect rather than squamous intraepithelial lesion or carcinoma. Certain additional features aid in the diagnosis of radiation changes. Low cellularity is helpful, since epithelium exhibiting radiation effect exfoliates fewer cells than carcinomas. In many instances, only single cells or rare, small tissue fragments exhibiting radiation effect are exfoliated. On the other hand, the presence of carcinoma produces numerous malignant cells, observed both singly and in pseudosyncytia. Bland chromatin pattern, cellular and nuclear degeneration, cellularity, and cellular configurations aid in the diagnosis of radiation effect for this cell. Bronchial brushing (× 400).

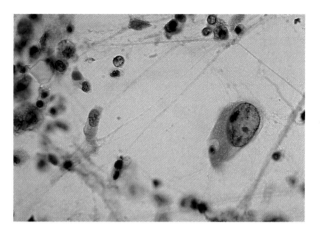

FIGURE 1–20. Radiation and Chemotherapy Effects. This bronchial washing is from a 65-year-old man with small-cell undifferentiated carcinoma who was treated with cytoxan, methotrexate, vincristine, and radiation. An enlarged cell with an enlarged hyperchromatic nucleus is present in a background of benign bronchial cells and inflammation. Nuclear enlargement and chromasia are worrisome, but chromatin is degenerated (smudged and hazy). Only a few single, atypical cells are present on the bronchial washing. Although features are not consistent with a persistent or recurrent small-cell undifferentiated carcinoma, a new or coexisting carcinoma versus radiation and chemotherapy changes must be evaluated. Nuclear and cytoplasmic degeneration, scant cellularity, and cellular configurations favor a diagnosis of radiation and chemotherapy effect in this bronchial washing. Bronchial washing (× 630).

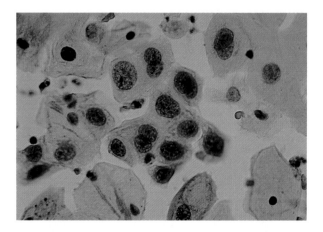

FIGURE 1–21. Radiation Dysplasia. Radiation dysplasia represents cytologic alterations specifically attributable to the effect of ionizing radiation on epithelium, but distinct from residual or recurrent carcinoma. The degree of change resembles that of a high-grade SIL (CIN II or moderate dysplasia), especially in terms of N/C ratios and chromatin patterns. Atypical cells are usually exfoliated in sheets rather than singly. This sheet of atypical cells is on the

Papanicolaou smear of a 49 year old woman who received radiation therapy for invasive squamous cell carcinoma and who subsequently underwent hysterectomy. Nuclei are enlarged and hyperchromatic; N/C ratios are markedly increased. Chromatin patterns are slightly granular and evenly distributed. Although N/C ratios are increased to a degree greater than would be expected in radiation effect, other nuclear and chromatinic features are not markedly atypical. Because N/C ratios are more atypical than those observed with radiation effect, but because other features are not consistent with residual or recurrent carcinoma, the intermediary interpretation of radiation dysplasia is made. Uterine cervix, Papanicolaou smear (× 630).

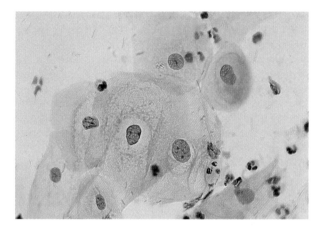

FIGURE 1–22A. Atypical Squamous Cells of Undetermined Significance. Atypical cellular and nuclear enlargement is sometimes observed in squamous cells from the female genital tract. Nuclei can increase to slightly more than three times the size of the nucleus of an intermediate cell, resulting in slightly higher than normal N/C ratios. Chromatin can be granular and nuclei can be hyperchromatic. An increased incidence of keratin is sometimes present. Although the significance of these atypical cells is not always known, they are often present in inflammatory smears and can resemble cells exfoliated from a low-grade SIL. These large intermediate cells contain enlarged nuclei. The nuclei are round to oval, and faint perinuclear halos are present. Nuclear membranes are slightly undulating. Chromatin is finely granular and evenly distributed, and chromatinic rims are of uniform thickness. Chromasia is slightly increased. Although nuclear enlargement and N/C ratios approach those of a low-grade SIL, they are not quite as atypical as would be expected with this lesion. These findings suggest a conservative diagnosis of atypical squamous cells of undetermined significance. Recommendations for clearing the inflammation and a repeat Papanicolaou smear are necessary. Uterine cervix, Papanicolaou smear (× 630).

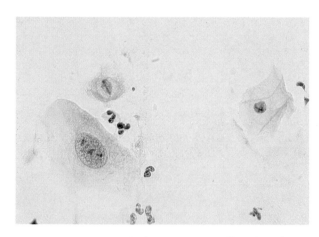

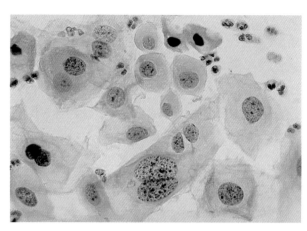

FIGURE 1–22B. Atypical Squamous Cells of Undetermined Significance. Nuclear enlargement and the N/C ratio of this intermediate-type squamous cell are consistent with those of a low-grade SIL. The chromatin, however, is finely granular and evenly distributed, and chromasia is normal. The number of atypical cells on the glass slide is few. These findings prompt caution; therefore, the more conservative diagnosis of atypical squamous cells of undetermined significance is made, but a low-grade SIL cannot be ruled out. Recommendations for clearing the inflammation and a repeat Papanicolaou smear are necessary. Uterine cervix, Papanicolaou smear (× 630).

FIGURE 1–23B. Low-Grade SIL (CIN I or Mild Dysplasia). The largest multinucleated cell contains chromatin that is very granular and evenly distributed, more granular than usually encountered in cells from a low-grade SIL. Nevertheless, abundant transparent cytoplasm still characterizes this cell as mature and consistent with a low-grade SIL. Keratinization and dense opaque nuclei suggest a concurrent human papilloma virus infection. Uterine cervix, Papanicolaou smear (× 630).

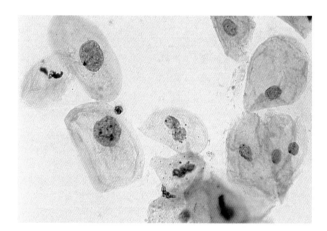

FIGURE 1–23A. Low-Grade SIL (CIN I or Mild Dysplasia). Squamous cells, possessing abundant transparent cytoplasm and enlarged hyperchromatic nuclei, are characteristic of low-grade SIL. Cellular enlargement can be marked; in fact, the largest atypical cells observed in gynecologic material can be from low-grade squamous intraepithelial lesions. Nuclear size is greater than three times the size of the nucleus of an intermediate cervical cell. N/C ratios are increased, although the cytoplasm is abundant. Nuclear membranes can be round, oval, and smooth; slightly undulating; or slightly wrinkled. Chromatin ranges from finely granular and evenly distributed to slightly granular and evenly distributed. Chromatinic rims are of uniform thickness. Chromasia varies from slight to hyperchromatic. Nucleoli are absent. Uterine cervix, Papanicolaou smear (× 630).

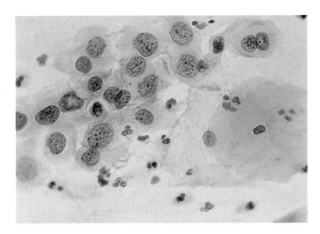

FIGURE 1–24A. High-Grade SIL (CIN II or Moderate Dysplasia). Cells with enlarged nuclei, increased N/C ratios, and slightly granular chromatin patterns are characteristic of high-grade SIL (CIN II or moderate dysplasia). These cells approximate the size of classic squamous metaplastic cells or maturing parabasal cells. Their cytoplasm is dense and can be round or polygonal in shape. N/C ratios range from 1:3 to 1:2. Nuclear membranes can be round and smooth, undulating, or wrinkled. Chromatin is slightly granular and evenly distributed to moderately granular. Chromatinic rims are of uniform thickness. Uterine cervix, Papanicolaou smear (× 630).

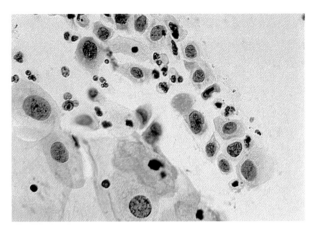

FIGURE 1–25A. High-Grade SIL (CIN III or Severe Dysplasia). Very small cells with enlarged nuclei and extremely high N/C ratios characterize cells from a high-grade SIL (CIN III or severe dysplasia). As with lower grades of SIL, these cells are usually exfoliated singly. Nuclear membranes are round and smooth, undulating, wrinkled, or irregular. Chromatin patterns range from finely granular and evenly distributed to granular and evenly distributed. Nuclei are hyperchromatic. Chromatinic rims are of uniform thickness. Nucleoli are absent. Uterine cervix, Papanicolaou smear (× 630).

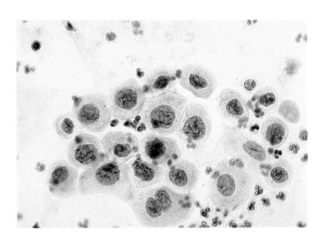

FIGURE 1–24B. High-Grade SIL (CIN II or Moderate Dysplasia). Enlarged hyperchromatic nuclei are present. N/C ratios range from 1:3 to 1:2. Chromatin is slightly granular and evenly distributed, and chromatinic rims are of uniform thickness. Nuclear membranes exhibit irregularities, indentations, and folds. The nuclear morphology is similar to crinkled paper and is most probably degenerative in nature. Uterine cervix, Papanicolaou smear (× 630).

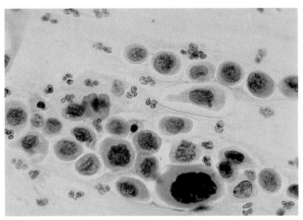

FIGURE 1–25B. High-Grade SIL (CIN III or Severe Dysplasia). Cells with enlarged hyperchromatic nuclei are observed. Irregularities and undulations of the nuclear membranes are striking features, although sharp, acute angles are not. The chromatin is slightly granular and evenly distributed. These features are consistent with high-grade SIL (CIN III or severe dysplasia). Uterine cervix, Papanicolaou smear (× 630).

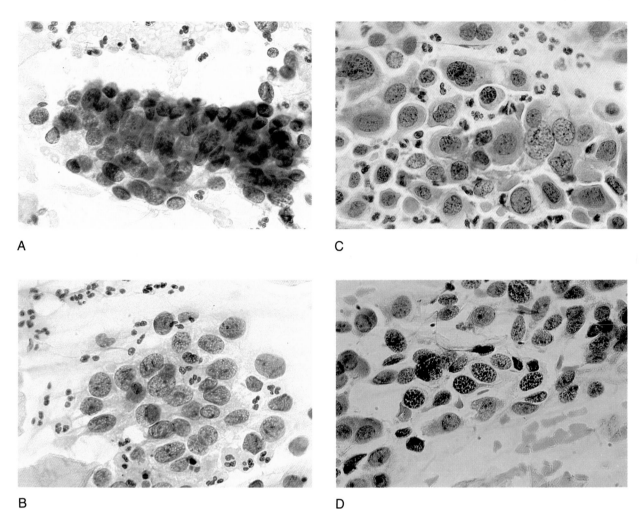

A

C

B

D

FIGURE 1–26A–D. High-Grade SIL (CIN III or CIS).

The presence of pseudosyncytial groupings distinguishes CIS from dysplasia. Tissue fragments from high-grade SIL exhibit loss of cell borders and nuclear polarity. Nuclei are enlarged, hyperchromatic, and crowded. Nuclear membranes can vary, and chromatin patterns range from finely granular and evenly distributed to coarsely granular and evenly distributed. Chromatinic rims are of uniform thickness. Nucleoli are usually not present but can be present in small numbers. This pseudosyncytium possesses enlarged, hyperchromatic, crowded nuclei. Nuclear polarity is not maintained.

A comparison of chromatin granularity is depicted in Figures 1–26A–D. Chromatin is hyperchromatic and dense in Figure 1–26A. Granularity ranges from slightly granular and evenly distributed (Fig. 1–26B) to granular and evenly distributed (Fig. 1–26C) to coarsely granular and evenly distributed ("salt and pepper" chromatin) (Fig. 1–26D). Variations in chromatin patterns are more marked in high-grade SIL (CIN III or CIS) than in lesions of lesser atypia. Uterine cervix, Papanicolaou smear (× 630).

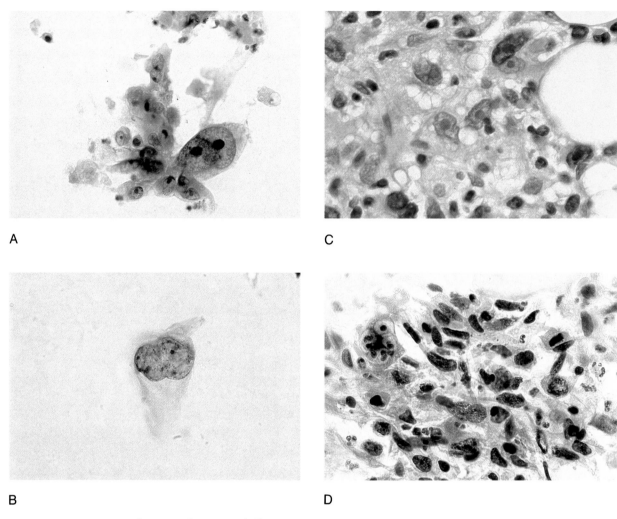

FIGURE 1–27A–D. Nuclear Membranes and Shapes— Malignancy.

Malignant cells classically exhibit great variations in cellular size and shape, nuclear size and shape, N/C ratios, chromatin patterns, the presence or absence of nucleoli, and tissue configurations. Unpredictable changes are present from single cell to single cell and also from cell to cell in the same tissue fragment. No single feature is pathognomonic for malignancy, and multiple features are usually necessary for a definitive diagnosis. Nuclear membranes and shapes vary from smooth and round (Fig. 1–27A) to undulating and scalloped (Fig. 1–27B) to angulated and wrinkled (Fig. 1–27C) to pleomorphic (Fig. 1–27D). N/C ratios vary, as do chromatin patterns and the presence of nucleoli in these cells. Figure 1–27A, bronchial washing; Figure 1–27B, urinary bladder washing; Figure 1–27C, lymph node, fine needle aspirate; Figure 1–27D, uterine cervix, Papanicolaou smear (× 630).

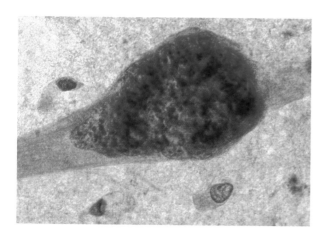

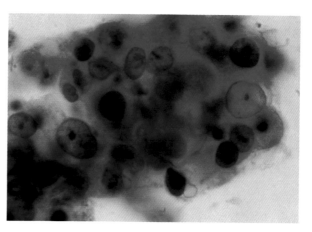

FIGURE 1–28A. Chromatin Pattern—Malignancy. Chromatin patterns in malignancy range from finely granular and evenly distributed to the classic coarsely granular and unevenly distributed. Totally cleared chromatin patterns are also observed. This nucleus possesses coarsely granular, unevenly distributed chromatin that is interspersed with areas of parachromatin clearing. The chromatinic rim where discerned is of uniform thickness. Bronchial washing (× 1000).

FIGURE 1–28C. Chromatin Pattern—Malignancy. The chromatin in this adenocarcinoma is pale and cleared; this makes the nucleoli look particularly prominent. Although this is a nuclear appearance that is common in adenocarcinoma, it may occasionally be found in moderately or poorly differentiated squamous cell carcinoma. Bronchial washing, Diff-Quik (× 1000).

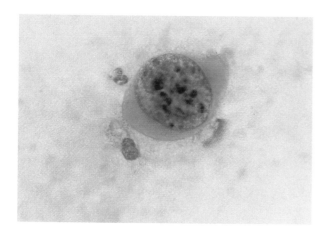

FIGURE 1–28B. Chromatin Pattern—Malignancy. Parachromatin clearing can be a pronounced feature in atypical chromatin patterns. Clumped areas of heterochromatin alternate irregularly with cleared areas of euchromatin. The ratios of chromatin vary and can result in the transcriptionally active euchromatin predominating within the body of the nucleus and the transcriptionally inactive heterochromatin aggregating along the chromatinic rim. Bronchial washing (× 1000).

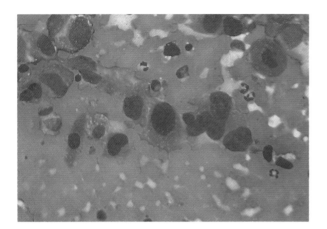

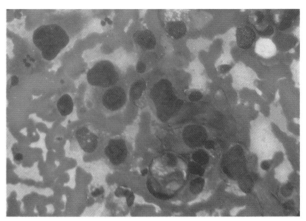

A

B

FIGURE 1–29A–B. Air-Dried Material—Malignancy.

Although chromatin granularity is sometimes obliterated with air-drying fixation, cellular configurations, nuclear shapes, and, to some extent, nuclear polarity and N/C ratios, can still be ascertained. These individual cells exhibit variation in nuclear size and shape. Nuclear shapes are irregular, and N/C ratios are increased. Granular chromatin is maintained despite air drying. Features of malignancy are apparent in this non–small cell carcinoma. Lung, fine needle aspiration, Diff-Quik ($\times$ 600).

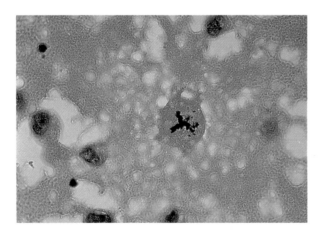

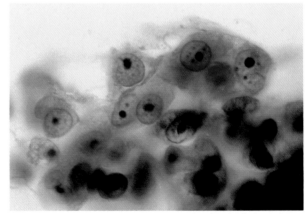

FIGURE 1–30. Atypical Mitoses—Malignancy. Atypical mitotic figures, such as this tripolar mitosis, are indicative of malignancy. Atypical mitotic figures are extremely useful when present in fluid specimens. Pleural fluid ($\times$ 630).

FIGURE 1–31A. Nucleoli—Malignancy. The presence of nucleoli is not part of the criteria for malignancy per se, but, because of abnormal growth and increased protein synthesis, they are often present in malignant cells. Nucleoli are generally larger and possess more irregular shapes in malignant cells than in benign, reactive cells, although this does not always hold true for cell-exhibiting reparative changes. Nucleolar to nuclear ratios can be high in malignant cells. These cells from an adenocarcinoma of ovarian origin possess extremely large, round nucleoli. Their size is larger than generally seen in benign reactive processes. Peritoneal fluid ($\times$ 630).

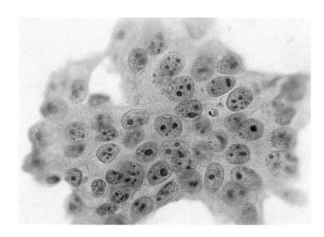

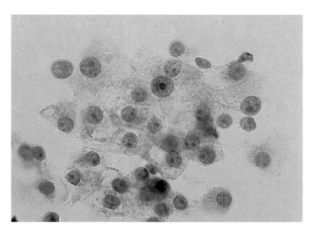

FIGURE 1–31B. Nucleoli. Multiple nucleoli are present in cells from both reactive and malignant processes. In malignancy, variations in nuclear size, shape, and number exist between single malignant cells and those within a tissue fragment. These cells from an adenocarcinoma contain multiple prominent nucleoli. Variations in size and number (1 to 7) are observed. Esophageal brushing (× 630).

FIGURE 1–32B. Cellular Differentiation—Well-Differentiated Carcinoma. These cells from a fine needle aspiration of a liver retain moderate amounts of granular cytoplasm, reminiscent of hepatocytes. Tumor cellularity, loss of cellular cohesion, loss of nuclear polarity, and prominent nucleoli define the aspirate as malignant. Cytoplasmic features characterize the malignant cells as hepatocellular in origin. Liver, fine needle aspiration (× 630).

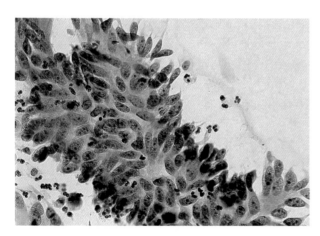

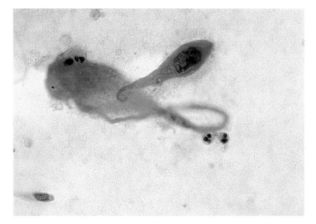

FIGURE 1–32A. Cellular Differentiation—Well-Differentiated Carcinoma. Cell shapes are often retained in well-differentiated carcinomas, aiding in the differential diagnosis of the tumor type. Cells from adenocarcinoma retain their individual columnar shapes or their intercellular relationships. In this specimen, the cells retain their columnar shapes but nuclear crowding, loss of nuclear polarity, chromatin patterns, increased chromasia, and prominent nucleoli indicate their malignant character. Uterine cervix, Papanicolaou smear (× 400).

FIGURE 1–32C. Cellular Differentiation—Poorly Differentiated Carcinoma. Less well-differentiated tumors lose semblance of their origin. Cellular shapes can be lost in pseudosyncytial groupings or can be highly irregular (tadpole, caudate) and pleomorphic. Highly irregular shapes are more often observed in squamous cell carcinomas, as seen here. Sputum preparation (× 630).

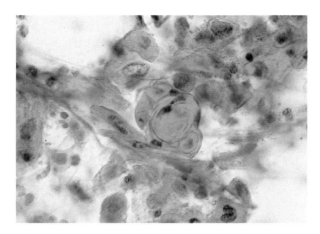

FIGURE 1–33A. Cellular Differentiation—Squamous Carcinoma. In exfoliative cytology, the most common types of malignant differentiation include squamous carcinoma, adenocarcinoma, or small-cell undifferentiated carcinoma. Cytoplasmic and nuclear features aid in the differential diagnoses of these entities. Keratinizing squamous cell carcinoma is characterized by atypical squamous cells with cytoplasm that is keratinized (orange). Cells are often irregular (spindle, tadpole, caudate) in shape; nuclei vary in size and shape and are often pyknotic. Cells wrapping around adjacent cells ("cannibalism") and squamous pearls are sometimes observed. Sputum (× 630).

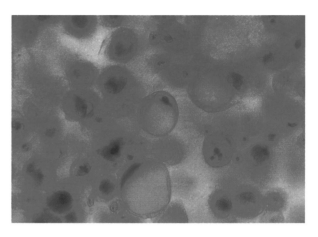

FIGURE 1–33C. Cellular Differentiation—Adenocarcinoma. Secretory vacuoles differentiate adenocarcinoma from squamous cell carcinoma. These classic "signet-ring" cells contain nuclei pushed to the periphery by large secretory vacuoles. Prominent nucleoli are also observed in these cells from a metastatic gastric carcinoma. Peritoneal fluid (× 630).

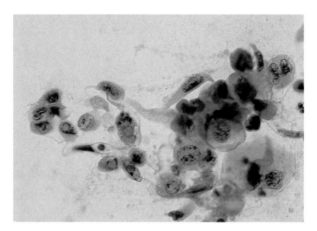

FIGURE 1–33B. Cellular Differentiation—Squamous Carcinoma. Cells that exfoliate from a nonkeratinizing squamous cell carcinoma are usually observed singly and in aggregates. The cells are round to irregular and possess dense, hard, basophilic cytoplasm. Nuclei are enlarged, irregular in shape, and hyperchromatic. Chromatin is granular and unevenly distributed or opaque. Nucleoli can be present or absent. Irregularity of cellular and nuclear shapes, cytoplasmic density, chromatin granularity, and hyperchromasia are more pronounced in squamous cell carcinoma than in adenocarcinoma. These features aid in the differential diagnosis of the two types of tumor. Sputum (× 630).

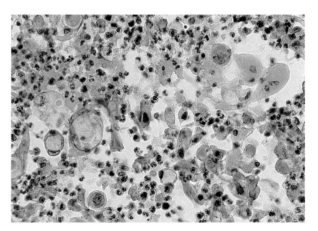

FIGURE 1–33D. Cellular Differentiation—Squamous Carcinoma. Large, hyperdistended vacuoles can be either secretory or degenerative in nature. It is sometimes extremely difficult to ascertain which process is present. This rib aspirate contains cells with large, hyperdistended vacuoles, suggesting the presence of adenocarcinoma. Careful scrutiny, however, reveals squamous cells with hard, dense cytoplasm, more consistent with squamous cell carcinoma. The vacuoles illustrate degenerative changes in squamous carcinoma. Rib, fine needle aspiration (× 400).

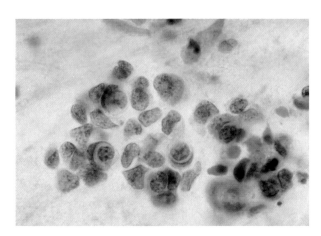

FIGURE 1–34A. Cellular Differentiation—Small-Cell Undifferentiated Carcinoma. Small-cell undifferentiated carcinoma that exfoliates physiologically is characterized by aggregates of small cells with large, round to irregularly shaped nuclei. N/C ratios are extremely high. Chromatin patterns in well-preserved cells are slightly granular to granular and evenly distributed; chromatin patterns in degenerated cells are dense and opaque. Nuclei are hyperchromatic, and nuclear molding is often observed. Nucleoli are absent to inconspicuous. This aggregate of small, atypical cells is from a small-cell undifferentiated carcinoma present in a sputum specimen. Sputum (× 630).

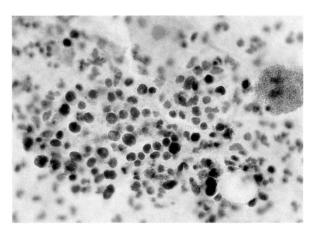

FIGURE 1–34B. Cellular Differentiation—Small-Cell Undifferentiated Carcinoma. Degenerated cells from a small-cell undifferentiated carcinoma are often similar in appearance to lymphocytes. Although chromatin is similar, the malignant epithelial cells usually exhibit nuclear molding and greater variation in nuclear size and shape. Sputum (× 630).

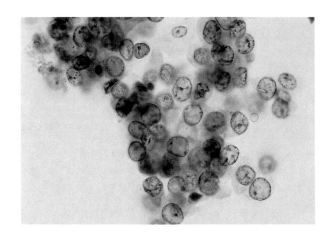

A

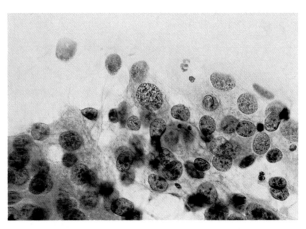

B

FIGURE 1–35A–B. Cellular Differentiation—Poorly Differentiated Malignant Tumors.

Malignant nuclear features are sometimes present without cytoplasmic features to aid in tumor differentiation. If cellular origin cannot be ascertained, the diagnosis of poorly differentiated malignant tumor (or carcinoma, if epithelial features are present) should be made. Pseudosyncytial groupings (Fig. 1–35B) indicating abnormal growth and growth patterns are frequently observed with epithelial tumors. They are characterized by masses of cytoplasm with loss of cell borders and nuclear polarity. Atypical nuclei exhibit enlargement, crowding, overlap, granular chromatin patterns, and hyperchromasia. Figure 1–35A, urinary bladder washing; Figure 1–35B, bronchial brushing (× 630).

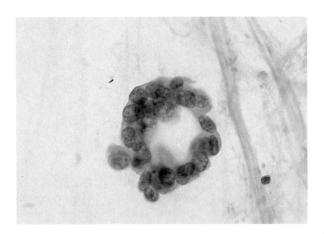

FIGURE 1–36A. Cellular Arrangements—Glandlike Formations. Adenocarcinomas can exfoliate glandular structures that aid in rendering a diagnosis. A gland-like structure with epithelial cells bounding a central lumen is shown. Sputum (× 630).

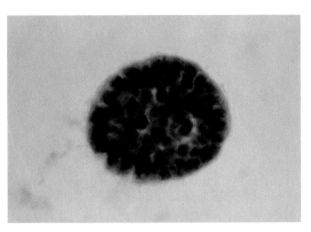

FIGURE 1–36C. Cellular Arrangements—Morulae. Morulae are observed in malignancies of glandular origin but can also be present in mesothelial proliferations and mesotheliomas. These structures are three-dimensional and have smooth outer borders. Focusing up and down with the microscope reveals different planes of cells. These cells in a pleural fluid were consistent with the patient's malignant mesothelioma. Pleural fluid (× 630).

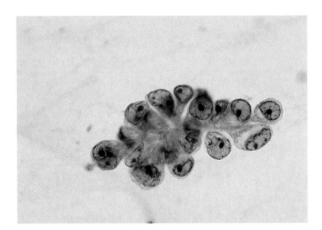

FIGURE 1–36B. Cellular Arrangements—Acinar Formations. Three-dimensional tissue fragments with central lumina bounded by peripherally located nuclei are characteristic of acinar formations. These arrangements, again, are indicative of glandular origin. The lumen in this tissue fragment is observed at its center. Sputum (× 630).

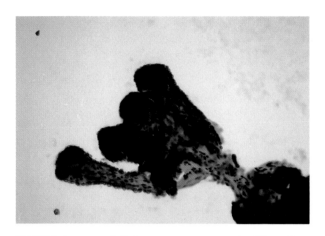

FIGURE 1–37A. Cellular Arrangements—Papillary Formations. Papillary configurations are present in both hyperplastic and malignant processes. Finger-like projections and fibrovascular stalks are cytologically characteristic of this tissue configuration. This tissue fragment is present in a thyroid aspiration. Thyroid, fine needle aspiration (× 160).

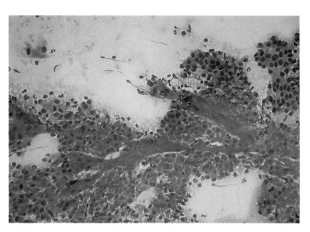

FIGURE 1–37C. Cellular Arrangements—Papillary Formations. The fibrovascular stalk is accentuated in this air-dried preparation. Kidney, fine needle aspiration, Diff-Quik (× 160).

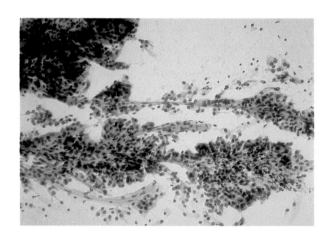

FIGURE 1–37B. Cellular Arrangements—Papillary Formations. This tissue fragment is from a papillary renal cell carcinoma. Kidney, fine needle aspiration (× 160).

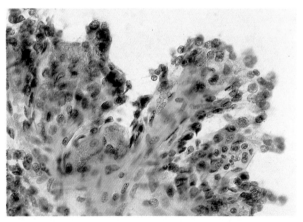

FIGURE 1–37D. Cellular Arrangements—Papillary Formations. The fibrovascular stalk is denoted by elongated stromal cells flowing in one direction throughout the tissue fragment and into the finger-like projections. Red blood cells are sometimes present in the blood vessels in this connective tissue. Thyroid, fine needle aspiration (× 630).

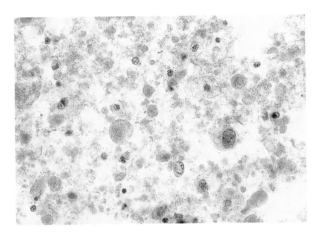

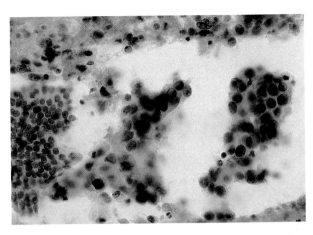

FIGURE 1–38A. Slide Background—Tumor Diathesis. The slide milieu or slide background is often helpful when evaluating smears for the presence or absence of malignancy. Benign smears are classically clean and transparent but can contain inflammatory cells. Cells exfoliated from squamous intraepithelial lesions are also present on slides with clean backgrounds, as are cells exfoliated from exophytic malignant lesions. On the other hand, tumor diathesis is usually associated with infiltrating carcinoma. Fresh or hemolyzed blood (which stains orange or green with the modified Papanicolaou stain) admixed with necrotic cellular debris can be present. The necrotic debris often appears as a nonuniform granular precipitate. Hemolyzed blood and necrotic debris in the form of granular precipitate and dying malignant cells are observed. Lung, fine needle aspiration (× 400).

FIGURE 1–39A. Fine Needle Aspirations—Tumor Cellularity. Malignant nuclear features seen in exfoliative cytology are not always present in fine needle aspirations. If atypical nuclear features are absent, specimen cellularity, cellular configurations, cellular cohesiveness, and the presence of prominent nucleoli are useful diagnostic criteria. Fine needle aspirations of benign tissue usually contain few cells. These cells are normal constituents of the site that has been sampled and are usually observed in cohesive sheets. Malignant aspirates are usually rich in cells. Numerous tumor cells are present in this lung aspirate. A three-dimensional tissue fragment of larger malignant cells is seen adjacent to a sheet of benign columnar cells. A tumor diathesis is also present. Lung, fine needle aspiration (× 400).

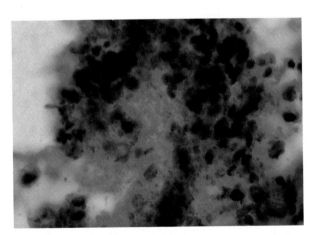

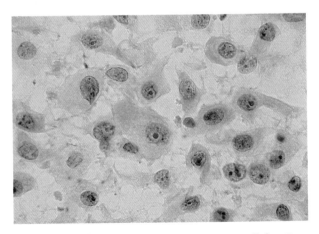

FIGURE 1–38B. Slide Background—Tumor Diathesis. Granular necrotic debris consistent with tumor diathesis is present in this air-dried material. Lung, fine needle aspiration, Diff-Quik (× 600).

FIGURE 1–39B. Fine Needle Aspirations—Cellular Configurations, Cellular Cohesiveness, and Nucleoli. Cellular configurations are instrumental in the diagnosis of fine needle aspirations. In contrast to aspirations of benign tissue, which contain sheets of cells, malignant aspirations contain pseudosyncytia (indicating abnormal growth) and single, isolated cells (indicating loss of cellular cohesion and cell function). Single, isolated cells with numerous prominent nucleoli are observed in this aspiration of a breast adenocarcinoma. Breast, fine needle aspiration (× 630).

C·H·A·P·T·E·R

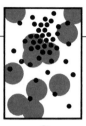

2

GYNECOLOGIC CYTOLOGY

Philip T. Valente

There is no doubt that the institution of widespread Papanicolaou smear screening over the last 4 decades has resulted in a marked reduction in cervical cancer mortality. This has been possible because of this neoplasm's relatively long preinvasive phase and the accessibility of the uterine cervix to cytologic and histologic sampling. Epithelial abnormalities, initially reversible but more apt to progress with increasing severity, have a distinctive morphology and have been classified variously as dysplasia, cervical intraepithelial neoplasia (CIN), and squamous intraepithelial lesions (SIL) (Tables 2–1 and 2–2). Cytologic examination of abnormal cells exfoliated from precursor lesions identifies patients at risk for progression of these lesions to invasive cancer. Referral for colposcopy, which can provide a magnified view of up to 40 times of the cervix, allows for visualization and biopsy to provide histologic confirmation of precancerous lesions. Once the presence of such lesions is confirmed, the diseased epithelium may be ablated by cryosurgery or laser. More extensive lesions may be removed by conization biopsy. The destruction or removal of epithelium destined to become invasive thus aborts the development of frank malignancy.

EVOLUTION OF CERVICAL INTRAEPITHELIAL NEOPLASIA

The morphology of CIN and the time frame of its evolution enable the cytopathologist to identify clinically occult lesions of increasing severity (Figs. 2–109 to 2–140, 2–201C, 2–202A, 2–203C, 2–204A, 2–205A, 2–205B, 2–

209C, and 2–209D). Cytologic changes in the basal layer propagate themselves to the surface through abnormal epithelial maturation (Fig. 2–1). In mild dysplasia (CIN I), markedly abnormal cells are present in the lower third of the epithelium; in moderate dysplasia (CIN II, high-grade SIL), the lower and middle thirds contain such cells; in severe dysplasia and carcinoma in situ (both CIN III, high-grade SIL), such cells reach the upper third and occupy the full thickness of the epithelium, respectively. Cervical intraepithelial neoplasia I (low-grade SIL) frequently regresses, but increasing severity of CIN is associated with increased potential for progression to invasive squamous cell carcinoma, the latter being the common outcome of untreated CIN III. The protracted time frame of the transition from CIN I to carcinoma in situ (CIS) and from CIS to invasive carcinoma is also crucial in that it allows for sufficient lead time to identify precursor lesions. In the 1950s, Reagan et al. (see Patten, 1978, pp 138–145) estimated a 7-year transition time of CIN I to CIS and another 7 years from CIS to invasive cancer because he found the average ages for CIN I, CIS, and invasive cancer to be 34, 41, and 48 years, respectively. There is recent evidence, however, that in some patients, especially younger women, there is a more rapid progression of low-grade CIN to invasion. This, together with the increasing incidence of CIN in the younger population, no doubt related to changing sexual mores, further emphasizes the importance of annual Papanicolaou smear examinations in this younger group. Current recommendations for Papanicolaou smear surveillance agreed on by the American Cancer Society, the American College of Obstetricians and Gynecologists, and the American Medical Association are as follows: that all women who are or who have been sexually active or who have reached the age of 18 years have an annual Papanicolaou test and pelvic examination. After a woman has had three or more consecutive normal annual examinations, the Papanicolaou test may be performed less frequently at the discretion of her physician.

PAPANICOLAOU SMEAR SCREENING

If Papanicolaou smear surveillance is to be effective in the prevention of invasive cervical cancer, standards of Papanicolaou smear adequacy must be maintained. Because the great majority of precancerous lesions arise at or near the squamocolumnar junction, the sample must be taken at the cervical os. In young patients, this epithelial transition is usually located either just outside or at the cervical os but its location may vary. In post-cryosurgery, post-conization, and post-menopausal patients, it is often situated high in the endocervical canal. A process of squamous metaplasia occurs at this epithelial junction in which glandular cells are changed into immature and then mature squamous metaplastic epithelium. It is in this region, known as the transformation zone, that squamous neoplasia tends to arise. The presence of endocervical glandular cells is important, therefore, in order to document that cells from this region have been sampled. Cytologic brushing of the endocervical canal in addition to the traditional spatula specimen has been used increasingly to ensure adequate sampling and has been reported to augment detection of CIN and possibly of glandular abnormalities (see subsequent discussion).

Because sex hormones affect the maturation and glycogen content of squamous epithelium in the vagina and cervix, the Papanicolaou smear may be used for evaluation of a patient's hormonal status. This application of the Papanicolaou smear may be useful in the assessment of ovarian function, pregnancy, infertility, and other abnormal endocrine conditions. Smears for such evaluation should be made from the lateral portion of the middle third of the vaginal wall. In cervical smears, inflammation may obscure or alter the maturation pattern. The maturation index, in which cells are counted and divided by percentage into parabasal, intermediate, and superficial cells, is the most widely used semiquantitative method. For example, maturation induced by estrogen could give a maturation index of 0/10/90. Other indices, including the cornification index, eosinophilic cells index, and folded cell index, may be of some value but are seldom used. Exogenous compounds, such as digitalis, or antibiotics, such as tetracycline, may influence and artificially alter the maturation index. The date of the patient's last menstrual period should be provided in order to judge whether the pattern is compatible with her age and clinical history. Any history of chemotherapy or radiotherapy, which may invalidate hormonal evaluation, is also necessary.

Proper rapid fixation of smears is crucial, since air-drying artifact renders the smears uninterpretable. Obscuring blood, inflammation, or abnormal smear thickness may also preclude interpretation, as may the simple lack of epithelial cells on the slide. Such smears must be reported as unsatisfactory (Figs. 2–39 to 2–48). This point is emphasized in the 1988 Bethesda System (see Table 2–2), which recommends an explicit statement of adequacy at the beginning of every cytology report.

Cytologic Diagnosis in Papanicolaou Smear Screening

The accuracy of cytologic diagnosis in cervicovaginal Papanicolaou smear screening depends on the identification of those morphologic features characteristic of dysplastic or malignant cells. A wide range of reactive, inflammatory, and even physiologic conditions may give rise to cells whose cytomorphology closely mimics that of true precancerous or malignant changes. If inflammatory changes, for example, are overcalled as high-grade SIL, unnecessary surgery, stigma, and psychic trauma may result. On the other hand, if cytologic abnormalities are undervalued, a chance to ablate a precancer and prevent a deadly disease may be missed. This can indeed be a fine line, and no matter what the level of expertise in a cytology laboratory, a certain number of cases are "indeterminate." In the Bethesda System, the word "atypia" is reserved precisely for these indeterminate cases, e.g., squamous atypia of uncertain significance. Cellular abnormalities that are associated with specific conditions with a fair degree of certainty are termed "cellular changes consistent with . . . ." Depending on the clinical setting, such patients may require a repeat Papanicolaou smear, Papanicolaou smear surveillance at closer (3- or 6-month) intervals, or colposcopic or surgical biopsy specimen evaluation.

Premenopause

In premenopausal women, the date of the last menstrual period should always be indicated by the submitting physician. Endometrial cells and the associated background (exodus) are frequently seen up to 10 days after onset of menses (Figs. 2–24 and 2–25). The presence of endometrial cells after 12 days is definitely abnormal and may reflect underlying endometrial disease. If a smear is extensively obscured by menstrual blood or if endometrial cell clusters are difficult to interpret, a repeat smear at midcycle should be requested. Degenerated endometrial cells may mimic endometrial adenocarcinoma, carcinoma in situ (CIS), or small-cell squamous carcinoma.

Pregnancy

Decidual cells (Figs. 2–31, 2–203D, and 2–213D) seen in Papanicolaou smears during pregnancy may be derived from deciduai reaction in cervical stroma or from the endometrium in the postpartum or post-abortal state. They resemble dysplastic cells but have large, distinct nucleoli, whereas CIN cells usually lack nucleoli. Multinucleated cells seen in the first or third trimester may be syncytiotrophoblasts (Figs. 2–30 and 2–218C). These cells may have dozens of overlapping oval nuclei. Their lack of nuclear molding distinguishes them from herpes simplex. Their nuclei are usually hyperchromatic and their cytoplasm hard and solid, in contrast to the delicate chromatin and more finely vacuolated cytoplasm of histiocytes.

Post Partum

In the postpartum state (Figs. 2–20 to 2–23, 2–110, and 2–210A), the smear is often dominated by atypical parabasal or abnormally keratinized cells, which may inappropriately suggest low-grade SIL. These changes will usually have resolved when the smear is repeated in 3 months.

After Menopause

Atrophic smears from post-menopausal women (Figs. 2–32 to 2–37) may pose a number of problems in interpretation. They are often obscured by air drying or inflammation. Atypical parabasal cells may mimic high-grade SIL, or single, atypical orange-straining cells in a degenerated background may simulate malignancy. Sheets of parabasal cells may resemble endometrium. If the smear is repeated after several days of topical estrogen, a clean smear with numerous superficial cells will result (Fig. 2–38). Dysplastic or neoplastic cells do not respond to estrogen and should be evident in the repeat smear.

Reparative Changes

Repair reactions in cervicovaginal smears reflect the proliferation of epithelial cells in response to inflammation, ulceration, or trauma. The cytologic features of these metabolically active cells may be quite striking and, when florid, resemble the features of adenocarcinoma (Figs. 2–79 to 2–83, 2–207B, 2–208A, 2–212B, 2–213B, and 2–213C). Epithelial cells with cytologic features of repair occur in many conditions affecting the uterine cervix. In ectropion, in which the squamocolumnar junction is located on the ectocervix well outside of the external os, the exposed glandular mucosa may become markedly inflamed and exhibit striking epithelial repair. Similar reparative changes may be seen after gynecologic instrumentation, with endocervical polyps, or in the setting of uterine prolapse. Repair cells may be glandular, squamous, or metaplastic. They often appear in large sheets of interlocking cells with long, pseudopod-like extensions. The long axes of the nuclei often have a parallel orientation, giving rise to a "school of fish" appearance. The chromatin is usually finely granular, with prominent round to oval nucleoli. Binucleated and multinucleated cells with nonmolded but overlapping nuclei may be present. Mitoses may also be seen.

INFLAMMATION AND INFECTION

Acute Cervicovaginal Inflammation

Infection is the most common cause of acute cervicovaginal inflammation, although a specific bacterial agent is frequently not identified. Symptomatic cases of acute cervicovaginitis are often associated with the gram-negative rod *Gardnerella vaginalis*. This organism may be apparent in large, confluent sheets, often encrusting the cytoplasm of more mature squamous cells (clue cells) (Fig. 2–50).

Chronic Follicular Cervicitis

In chronic follicular cervicitis (Figs. 2–70 to 2–74, and 2–204B), lymphoid germinal centers are present just below the surface epithelium. A mixed population of small, mature lymphocytes and large, activated lymphoid cells is seen. Tingible body macrophages may also be found. Single lymphoid cells may mimic CIS, but the syncytial aggregates typical of CIS are never identified in follicular cervicitis. Small clusters of degenerated lymphoid cells may resemble the small glandular groups seen in endometrial adenocarcinoma.

Trichomonas Vaginalis

Trichomonas vaginalis is a common, venereally transmitted protozoan. It may be present as an asymptomatic infestation; when tissue invasion occurs, a thin, foamy, foul-smelling discharge results. The flagellated organisms are best seen in wet preparations; in Papanicolaou smears, trichomonads are oval and pear-shaped (Figs. 2–56 to 2–60). The flagellum is not usually visible. An indistinct nucleus must be seen for positive identification, and numerous red cytoplasmic granules may also be seen in well-preserved organisms. Features of inflammatory atypia, including nuclear enlargement, orangeophilia, cytoplasmic vacuolization, and perinuclear halos (*Trichomonas* effect), are usually prominent. Aggregates of polymorphonuclear leukocytes around epithelial cells (the "BB" or "cannon ball" effect) are frequently seen (Fig. 2–61). Nuclear enlargement may mimic low-grade SIL, but in the setting of *Trichomonas* effect it is advisable to repeat the smear after treatment for the *Trichomonas* infection. Care should be taken, however, since high-grade SIL or even invasive cancer often may coexist with *Trichomonas* (Fig. 2–135). In such cases, treatment for *Trichomonas* infection should still be instituted before colposcopic and biopsy evaluation.

Candida albicans

Candida albicans is a saprophytic fungus that may cause a cervicovaginitis, especially in patients with alterations in vaginal flora or pH, as may occur in diabetes mellitus, pregnancy, or oral contraceptive use (Fig. 2–49). To distinguish pathogenic *Candida* organisms from nonpathogens such as the yeast *Torulopsis glabrata*, it is necessary to see both the yeast form and pseudohyphae. Epithelial cells may show inflammatory changes, depending on the degree of concomitant acute inflammation. Cytoplasmic eosinophilia is common.

Chlamydia trachomatis

Chlamydia trachomatis is an obligate intracellular microorganism that is sexually transmitted and known to cause urethritis, cervicitis, and pelvic inflammatory disease. Papanicolaou smear findings that have been associated with *Chlamydia* infection include cytoplasmic vacuolar inclusions with minute reddish dots and larger, targetoid inclusions (Figs. 2–52 to 2–55). Recent studies have shown that these findings are probably nonspecific. *Chlamydia* infection can therefore only be suggested by the Papanicolaou smear. Immunofluorescent antibody testing and culture are the only reliable diagnostic tests. About 25% of cases of chronic follicular cervicitis have been associated with *Chlamydia* infection.

Herpes Simplex Infections

Herpes simplex infections usually present as vesicular lesions on the vulva, vagina, and cervix (Figs. 2–62 to 2–64, 2–196, 2–217A, and 2–217C). Cytologic smears of such lesions reveal multinucleated epithelial cells with characteristically molded nuclei that have ground glass chromatin. Intranuclear inclusions may also be present but are not necessary for diagnosis. Poorly preserved cells with the herpes cytopathic effect described above may resemble squamous cell carcinoma or be mistaken for syncytiotrophoblastic cells in pregnant patients. Proper identification of herpes is essential in order to diagnose this recurrent venereal disease. In pregnant patients, the danger of herpes transmission to the newborn during vaginal delivery may prompt a cesarean section to avoid the devastation of a systemic herpetic infection of the infant. Herpes simplex may also play a role in cervical carcinogenesis, although it appears that human papillomavirus (HPV) either is the major factor or acts as a cocarcinogen with herpes or other factors.

Microglandular Hyperplasia

Microglandular hyperplasia, a change in the endocervical glands associated with the use of oral contraceptive agents, may produce clusters of atypical endocervical cells, mimicking adenocarcinoma (Figs. 2–95 to 2–97). Some cells derived from microglandular hyperplasia may degenerate and resemble parakeratotic cells (Fig. 2–210C). Exogenous progestagens or normal pregnancy may induce an Arias-Stella–like change in endocervical cells (Fig. 2–212C).

INTERPRETIVE PROBLEMS

Radiation Changes

A difficult interpretive problem may be the diagnosis of radiation changes (Figs. 2–88 to 2–94, 2–202, 2–208B, 2–214, and 2–218B) versus post-radiation dysplasia-CIS (Figs. 2–186 and 2–215). Acute radiation changes seen in the first several months following therapy include marked cellular enlargement, nuclear and cytoplasmic vacuolization, acute inflammation, multinucleated giant cells, and epithelial repair. Enlarged cells usually maintain a normal nuclear to cytoplasmic ratio. Chromatin may exhibit a fine wrinkling. Most of these changes regress with time, but abnormal cellular sizes and shapes, polychromasia, and nuclear smudging may persist for many years. In patients with squamous cell carcinoma, the supervention of true CIN, especially within 3 years after treatment for the original tumor, may presage recurrent or metastatic disease, although post-radiation CIN has been documented as occurring as long as 26 years after therapy. Because of the difficulty in distinguishing CIN I from radiation-induced changes, to make a diagnosis of post-radiation dysplasia-CIS cytologic features should suggest at least CIN II. The biologic behavior of such lesions is unpredictable, and some of these CIN lesions may be stable for many years. Close follow-up is required, with periodic biopsy.

Systemic Chemotherapy

Systemic chemotherapy may cause cellular abnormalities that resemble dysplasia (Figs. 2–87 and 2–202D). The latter is especially true with those agents that act as folic acid antagonists (see subsequent discussion). True dysplasia and carcinoma in situ may also occur in chronically immunosuppressed patients.

Intrauterine Devices

The intrauterine device may give rise to atypical glandular cells of endometrial or endocervical origin (Figs. 2–84, 2–85, and 2–208D). Such cells may be vacuolated and mimic endocervical or endometrial adenocarcinoma. They are often ball-like groups of cells with minimal atypia. An intrauterine device may lead to endometrial cell shedding in the second half of the menstrual cycle. *Actinomyces* may also be identified in these patients (Fig. 2–51).

Folic Acid Deficiency

Folic acid deficiency may cause abnormalities in the Papanicolaou smear (Fig. 2–86). These are seen in patients with dietary deficiencies but may also be present in women who are pregnant or in patients on phenytoin (Dilantin) or certain chemotherapeutic agents (folate antagonists). In spite of marked cellular enlargement (4 to 6 ×), there is maintenance of the normal nuclear to cytoplasmic ratio. Multinucleation, cytoplasmic vacuolization, and polychromasia may also be seen. Nuclear membranes are smooth and the chromatin pattern remains finely granular in contrast to that seen in dysplasia, in which chromatin is darker and may be more coarsely granular.

Pemphigus Vulgaris

In pemphigus vulgaris, cellular manifestations may be seen on Papanicolaou smears (Figs. 2–207C, 2–207D, and 2–208C). Even when this bullous disease of the skin is clinically quiescent, subclinical lesions may persist in the cervix or vagina, giving rise to very atypical cells with prominent nucleoli. Loose aggregates of these cells show vesicular nuclei with peculiar, bullet-shaped nucleoli. These cells have been mistaken for adenocarcinoma cells. The clinical history, most important in this context, is often not given, but these cytologic findings should suggest this diagnosis so that additional clinical history can be requested.

Contaminants

A number of unusual contaminants may be present in cervicovaginal smears, including cotton, suture, and talc (Figs. 2–101 to 2–105). Pinworm ova *(Enterobius vermicularis)*, which may resemble certain pollen contaminants, may also be seen. Hematoidin crystals resembling cockleburrs, related to degenerated blood, are observed occasionally (Fig. 2–102). The presence of vegetable matter in an amorphous dirty background may indicate fecal contamination from a rectovaginal fistula (Fig. 2–106).

DIFFERENTIAL DIAGNOSIS

Infection with HPV is quite frequent. Cytologic evidence of HPV, i.e., koilocytotic atypia, is present in 2 to 27% of Papanicolaou smears. They include irregular smudged or pyknotic nuclei, perinuclear clearing, and binucleation or multinucleation. Atypical parakeratotic cells and parakeratotic plaques may also be seen and are related to dyskeratosis in condylomatous epithelium. These latter features are nonspecific and may also be derived from areas of hyperkeratosis or from the surface of high-grade CIN or even invasive carcinoma. Human papilloma virus changes frequently coexist with both low-grade and high-grade CIN. Nuclear enlargement and chromatin granularity indicate associated CIN I, but the line between flat condyloma and CIN I with condyloma may be difficult to draw. In the Bethesda classification, definite condylomatous change and CIN I are grouped together under the rubric of low-grade SIL.

By considering HPV changes a part of the spectrum of low-grade SIL, the Bethesda System reflects current concepts of cervical carcinogenesis. Cervical intraepithelial neoplasia I is very frequently associated with HPV changes, but HPV may also be associated with high-grade SIL. Human papilloma virus DNA has been identified in the great majority of biopsy specimens of condylomas, in CIN lesions, and in many invasive squamous cell carcinomas. Human papilloma virus types 6 and 11 are often associated with benign condylomas and low-grade SIL, whereas HPV types 16, 18, 33, and 35 may be associated with high-grade SIL and invasive squamous carcinoma, although this is not always the case. Human papilloma virus 18 has been identified in adenocarcinoma, adenosquamous carcinoma, and small-cell carcinoma. Incorporation of HPV DNA into the genome of cells of high-grade lesions has been documented. In contrast, HPV DNA is present as episomes in the nuclei of cells of condylomas. These observations suggest a genuine pathogenetic role, although other cofactors (e.g., herpes simplex, cigarette smoking) may be involved. Rapid laboratory methods of HPV typing have been promoted but are of little value in routine patient management at the present time. Newly applied techniques, such as the polymerase chain reaction, may further clarify the role of HPV in cervical carcinogenesis.

Single cells with a higher nuclear to cytoplasmic ratio and more intense hyperchromasia characterize moderate dysplasia (CIN II). Chromatin is more coarsely clumped, and nuclear outlines are more irregular. In severe dysplasia (CIN III), cells are more numerous and many keratinized cells with abnormal hyperchromatic nuclei may be seen. In CIS, syncytial clusters of cells with coarse chromatin become prominent. Cytologic changes ranging from CIN II to CIS are all grouped under the designation of high-grade SIL in the Bethesda classification. Some smears may exhibit the full range of CIN from mild dysplasia to CIS. High-grade lesions are composed of less cohesive cells and tend to exfoliate larger numbers of cells than those of low-grade SIL.

Invasive squamous cell carcinoma (Figs. 2–143 to 2–150, 2–209A, 2–209B, and 2–217D) is usually manifested as large, pleomorphic cells in a dirty background of necrotic debris and inflammation (tumor diathesis). In the absence of such a diathesis, subtle nuclear changes, such as increased nucleolar prominence, may suggest microinvasive squamous cell carcinoma (Figs. 2–141 and 2–142). Paradoxically, as the neoplastic process becomes large, bulky, and necrotic, Papanicolaou smear yield may actually diminish as tumor cells are obscured by blood, inflammation, and necrosis. Keratinizing squamous cell carcinoma is characterized by cell clusters and individual cells varying greatly in size and shape. Enlarged hyperchromatic nuclei are usually angulated. Nucleoli may not be prominent. Cytoplasm is dense and bright orange. Elongated "tadpole" and bizarre spindle cells may be present. Concentric arrangements of keratinized squamous cells may form malignant squamous "pearls." In large-cell nonkeratinizing carcinoma, large, pleomorphic cells have prominent nucleoli but their sheet-like arrangement differs from the overlapping configuration of adenocarcinoma. Smaller cells with less cytoplasm and indistinct nucleoli and a more tightly molded configuration are seen in small-cell squamous carcinoma. Coarsely clumped chromatin gives nuclei a "salt and pepper" appearance. Clusters of small-cell squamous carcinoma may mimic the small, tightly clustered groups of endometrial adenocarcinoma.

Papanicolaou smear surveillance has not been as successful for identifying the precursor lesion of cervical adenocarcinoma as it has been for identifying squamous cell carcinoma precursors. Adenocarcinoma makes up an increasing proportion of invasive cervical cancer. It is not clear if this is a true increase in incidence or only relative to the decreased incidence of invasive squamous cell carcinoma. Difficulties in cytologic detection relate to the origin of some of these tumors high in the endocervical canal or deep in glandular crypts. Furthermore, atypical glandular cells may be very difficult to interpret. It has only been since the 1980s that the cytologic features of the presumed precursor lesions endocervical glandular dysplasia and adenocarcinoma in situ (AIS) have been well described in the cytologic literature. In these precursor lesions, the nuclei show little variation in size and are small, although the nuclear to cytoplasmic ratio is increased (Figs. 2–157 to 2–161, 2–205C, 2–206A, and 2–206B). Chromatin is evenly dispersed, and nucleoli tend to be indistinct and small. Interpretation of these changes is difficult, but tubal metaplasia (Fig. 2–206C) and cervical endometriosis (Fig. 2–206D) are pitfalls in diagnosis. Endocervical brush specimens may increase the sampling in cases of glandular dysplasia-AIS, but the difficulty of interpretation persists. The brush also sometimes removes glandular cells from the lower uterine segment that may be confused with AIS. Strict application of AIS criteria on well-preserved cell clusters should enable the experienced observer to make this diagnosis prospectively.

Invasive adenocarcinoma of the cervix exhibits more striking cytologic features than those seen in AIS (Figs. 2–162, 2–163, 2–207A, and 2–213A). Nuclei show greater pleomorphism, there is margination of chromatin at the nuclear edge, and macronucleoli are present. Rather than having the granular chromatin seen in nuclei of AIS, invasive adenocarcinoma usually has large vesicular nuclei.

Adenoma malignum, also known as minimal deviation adenocarcinoma, is a highly differentiated cervical neoplasm that is fortunately quite rare. Diagnosis may be possible only in a conization or hysterectomy specimen in which glands are seen extending deep into the cervical wall (Figs. 2–164 to 2–166). The diagnosis is quite difficult to make from histologic sections, and Papanicolaou smear diagnosis of the lesion poses even more of a challenge, although subtle cytologic changes have been described. A clinical history of a copious mucinous discharge and the Peutz-Jeghers syndrome (which has been associated with adenoma malignum) should raise the index of suspicion.

Cervicovaginal cytology has been disappointing in its capacity to identify endometrial adenocarcinoma (Figs. 2–171 to 2–175, 2–190, 2–204D, 2–205D, 2–211A, and 2–212A). The routine cervical scrape detects few cases of endometrial neoplasia. Vaginal pool and endocervical aspiration specimens yield suspicious cells in a much larger percentage of cases. More often, the presence of endometrial pathology may be suggested by the inappropriate presence of atypical or degenerated endometrial cells in postmenopausal smears or atypical endometrial cells out of cycle in younger women. Dilation and curettage are usually necessary to determine the cause. Endometrial stromal cells in a postmenopausal smear (Figs. 2–26, 2–28, and 2–216B), often in conjunction with a high estrogen effect, may also be the only evidence of endometrial hyperplasia or adenocarcinoma.

Cytologically well-differentiated endometrial adenocarcinoma is manifested as tight clusters of hyperchromatic cells. Occasional cytoplasmic vacuoles may be present. In moderately and poorly differentiated endometrial adenocarcinoma, cells are more pleomorphic, with larger nucleoli and more abundant cytoplasm. A tumor diathesis is more likely to be present in more poorly differentiated tumors. Small histiocytes, derived from the endometrial stroma, are often present in cases of endometrial hyperplasia and adenocarcinoma. These are usually seen in a nonatrophic (estrogenic) smear pattern and are distinguished from larger, nonspecific macrophages by their small size and their tendency to form loose aggregates on the smear. The presence of atypical squamous cells may indicate benign-appearing squamous differentiation within an adenocarcinoma (adenoacanthoma), or if frankly malignant, adenosquamous carcinoma. However, it should be remembered that the presence of both squamous and glandular cells with abnormal cytologic features could always reflect simultaneous cervical and endometrial tumors or precancerous lesions. Only further clinical investigation and histologic sampling can clarify the nature of the underlying disease. Similarly, although classic presentations of endocervical and endometrial carcinoma differ, localization of the tumor by its cytologic features may be difficult in some cases. Clinical features and fractional curettage may be necessary to determine the site of origin. Less common tumors, such as cervical adenoid cystic carcinoma (Fig. 2–153) and endometrial serous papillary carcinoma (Fig. 2–177), clear cell carcinoma, stromal sarcoma (Fig. 2–180), and malignant mixed mesodermal tumors (Figs. 2–178 and 2–179) may also have unusual cytologic presentations. Endometrial adenocarcinoma may also be mimicked by a number of benign conditions, including atypical repair, atypia associated with microglandular hyperplasia, and parabasal cells in atrophic smears.

TECHNIQUES

Attempts have been made to obtain a direct cytologic sample from the endometrial cavity with devices such as the Endopap sampler (Sherwood, St. Louis, Missouri) for screening post-menopausal women, especially those on hormone therapy. Endometrial polyps and hyperplasia also pose diagnostic difficulties with these techniques. Although the diagnosis of precursor lesions is problematic, some adenocarcinomas can be detected. Furthermore, although the incidence of endometrial adenocarcinoma is high, mortality from endometrial cancer is low, since most cases are Stage I with only superficial myometrial invasion. The cost-effectiveness of mass screening specifically for endometrial adenocarcinoma is therefore questionable. Although useful in individual cases, there is at present no justification for mass screening of asymptomatic women for endometrial cancer using these techniques.

Extrauterine cancer may occasionally be detected with the traditional Papanicolaou smear (Figs. 2–181 to 2–185, 2–216A). Cells may enter the vaginal pool by transtubal migration or may actually exfoliate from metastases to the lower female genital tract. Ovarian carcinoma is the most common tumor type, followed by gastrointestinal (colon), urinary tract (bladder), breast, and melanoma. Malignant lymphoma is rarely seen. Ovarian cancer is usually manifested as small tumor cell clusters in a smear with a clear background. Psammoma bodies may be present, but psammoma bodies by themselves (Fig. 2–107) are not diagnostic of malignancy and may be derived from a variety of benign conditions, including those caused by the intrauterine device, hydrosalpinx or benign epithelial inclusions of pelvic and ovarian surfaces (endosalpingosis). Psammoma bodies are also occasionally seen in primary serous papillary carcinoma of the endometrium.

Cytology has played an important role in following patients exposed in utero to diethylstilbestrol (DES). A large cohort of women were exposed in utero to DES from 1945 to 1971. Many of these patients have vaginal adenosis. One in 2000 develops clear cell carcinoma, which has a good prognosis if detected early. Only a very small percentage of the vaginal clear cell carcinomas in the DES Tumor Registry were detected prospectively in asymptomatic patients. Unfortunately, the great majority of these patients presented with vaginal bleeding and a sizable vaginal mass. Papanicolaou smear surveillance should therefore be emphasized in the management of the DES patient, although cytologic sampling can miss some cases of clear cell carcinoma. In addition, smears from these patients should be evaluated cautiously, since florid, immature squamous metaplasia in areas of vaginal adenosis may give rise to false diagnoses of CIN (Fig. 2–189). Atypical glandular cells can also be detected that may reflect a precursor lesion of clear cell carcinoma or that may resolve spontaneously. Colposcopic biopsy should be performed following the finding of any glandular atypia.

Vaginal cuff cytology of patients who have had hysterectomies may present diagnostic difficulties, especially if glandular cells are paradoxically encountered. When there is a history of adenocarcinoma, recurrent or metastatic adenocarcinoma should be considered. Atypical glandular cells mimicking adenocarcinoma may be seen in rare cases of vaginal endometriosis or may be derived from an inflamed, prolapsed fallopian tube (usually following vaginal hysterectomy) (Figs.

2–191 to 2–194). Pseudoglandular cells derived from endothelial cells in granulation tissue may be seen in patients with vaginal cuff ulcers. Adenosis is seen infrequently in older women.

Vulvar biopsy is easily done, so vulvar cytology has limited applications. It may be useful in the following settings:

1. Rapid diagnosis of herpetic lesions in a woman in labor.
2. Confirmation of a benign clinical diagnosis (fungal infection).
3. Biopsy not possible because of lack of patient cooperation or because of patient's medical status.
4. Follow-up of a previously treated lesion.

Because of the dryness of the vulvar keratinized epithelium, the lesion should be moistened with a wet compress. After removing the crust or dome of any vesicle, the margins of the lesion should be scraped and the cells spread over a small area on a slide that has been moistened with 95% ethyl alcohol. The alcohol evaporates, and the nearly dry slide is immersed in 95% ethyl alcohol.

The lesion most commonly sampled by vulvar scraping is the herpetic vesicle (Fig. 2–196). Herpes simplex and herpes zoster are indistinguishable cytologically, and occasionally zoster may affect the vulva. Fungal infections may also be identified by this method. Although rarely employed, such scrapings may reveal cells suggesting VIN, squamous cell carcinoma, basal cell carcinoma, Paget disease, or melanoma (Figs. 2–197 to 2–200).

In addition to interpretive dilemmas posed by the patient's condition or the clinician's technique in obtaining the cervicovaginal smear, problems may arise in the form of errors in screening and morphologic interpretation. Therefore, quality control is of vital importance. Recent federal regulations limiting the number of slides that may be screened in a 24-hour period and mandating proficiency testing are intended to decrease human error, a factor that can be minimized but not eliminated completely. One quality control technique, the 10% rescreen of healthy patients, is widely practiced but has a low yield of picking up missed cases. Rescreen of previous cases called normal when the most recent smear is positive is a better way to identify screening errors. Despite all efforts, however, there are also some smears that are "true" false negatives, i.e., abnormal cells from a lesion are not present on the slide. Therefore, when an indeterminate diagnosis, e.g., squamous atypia of uncertain significance, is reported, one cannot rely on a single repeat Papanicolaou smear because the repeat may be negative even though the patient still has a lesion. If the first report is assumed to be a laboratory "error," the patient may be lost to follow-up and return years later with an incurable, invasive disease. Rather, serial Papanicolaou smears at 3-month intervals may be indicated. If atypia persists, colposcopy is advisable.

The next important step in Papanicolaou smear surveillance is the communication of an abnormal result to the clinician. In order to standardize and facilitate this communication, a committee of the National Cancer Institute in 1988 proposed the Bethesda System and then revised it in 1991 (see Table 2–2). This system emphasizes that the Papanicolaou class system (Class I–V) is no longer an appropriate method of reporting cytologic diagnoses. It also emphasizes that the cytopathology report is a medical consultation and requires a statement of adequacy in each report. A major innovation in the Bethesda System is the use of the terms "low-grade SIL" for HPV-CIN I and "high-grade SIL" for CIN II or greater. The rationale for this approach is to increase reproducibility, e.g., a high-grade SIL may be called CIN II or CIN III by the same observer at different times but is less likely to be reclassified as low-grade SIL. This distinction is most practical, since it defines those patients (high-grade SIL) who should be referred immediately for colposcopy, since high-grade lesions are more likely to progress than low-grade lesions. Another change in emphasis relates to the use of the word "atypia" only for those cases in which cellular changes are of uncertain significance. This removes the ambiguity associated with this term, which has been quite confusing for clinicians. The Bethesda System seeks to make the diagnosis explicit and suggests that recommendations for follow-up be made. Although often a subjective judgment, the accumulated experience of the cytopathologist must be used in order to make a recommendation to the gynecologist. This is part of the medical consultation and should result in more consistent patient follow-up.

Bibliography

Astarita RW (ed.): Practical Cytopathology. New York: Churchill Livingstone, 1990.

Giuntoli RL, Atkinson BF, Ernst CS, et al.: Atkinson's Correlative Atlas of Colposcopy, Cytology and Histopathology. Philadelphia: J.B. Lippincott Company, 1987.

Koss LG: Diagnostic Cytology and Its Histopathologic Bases, 3rd Edition. Philadelphia: J.B. Lippincott Company, 1979.

Koss LG: The Papanicolaou test for cervical cancer detection: A triumph and a tragedy, JAMA 261:737–743, 1989.

Naib Z: Exfoliative Cytopathology, 3rd Edition. Boston: Little, Brown and Company, 1985.

Patten SF Jr: Diagnostic Cytopathology of the Uterine Cervix. Basel: S. Karger, 1978.

Ramzy I: Clinical Cytopathology and Aspiration Biopsy: Fundamental Principles and Practice. Norwalk, Connecticut: Appleton and Lange, 1990.

Szyfelbein WM, Young RH, Scully RE: Adenoma malignum of the cervix: Cytologic findings. Acta Cytol 28:691–698, 1984.

Table 2–1. COMPARISON OF TRADITIONAL, CIN, AND BETHESDA NOMENCLATURE

	Traditional	Cervical Intraepithelial Neoplasia (CIN)	Bethesda System
R P	HPV (Flat condyloma)	N/A	Low-grade squamous intraepithelial lesion (SIL)
	Mild dysplasia	CIN I	
	Moderate dysplasia	CIN II	High-grade squamous intraepithelial lesion (SIL)
	Severe dysplasia Carcinoma in situ	CIN III	

R = Regression
P = Progression

Table 2-2. THE 1991 BETHESDA SYSTEM FOR REPORTING CERVICAL/VAGINAL CYTOLOGIC DIAGNOSIS

Format of the Report
(a) A statement on **adequacy of the specimen for evaluation**
(b) A **general categorization** which may be used to assist with clerical triage (optional)
(c) The **descriptive diagnosis**
The format and terminology recommended for each of these three elements are presented below.

Adequacy of the Specimen for Evaluation
Satisfactory
Satisfactory for evaluation but limited by . . . (specify reason)
Unsatisfactory for evaluation. . . (specify reason)

General Categorization
Within normal limits
Benign cellular changes: See descriptive diagnosis
Epithelial cell abnormality: See descriptive diagnosis

Descriptive Diagnoses
Benign Cellular Changes
Infection
  Trichomas vaginalis
  Fungal organisms morphologically consistent with *Candida* spp
  Predominance of coccobacilli consistent with shift in vaginal flora
  Bacteria morphologically consistent with *Actinomyces* spp
  Cellular changes associated with herpes simplex virus
  Other

  (Note: for human papillomavirus (HPV) refer to Epithelial Cell Abnormalities, Squamous Cell)

Reactive Changes
  Atrophy with inflammation ("atrophic vaginitis")
  Reactive cellular changes associated with:
    Inflammation (includes typical repair)
    Atrophy with inflammation (atrophic vaginitis)
    Radiation

Table 2–2. THE 1991 BETHESDA SYSTEM FOR REPORTING CERVICAL/VAGINAL CYTOLOGIC DIAGNOSIS

Continued

Intrauterine contraceptive device
Other

Epithelial Cell Abnormalities
Squamous Cell
Atypical squamous cells of undertermined significance: Qualify
Low grade squamous intraepithelial lesion (LSIL), encompassing:
HPV*/Mild dysplasia/CIN I
High grade squamous intraepithelial lesion (HSIL), encompassing:
Moderate dysplasia/CIN II and
Severe dysplasia/CIS/CIN III
Squamous cell carcinoma

Glandular Cell
Endometrial cells, cytologically benign, in a postmenopausal woman
Atypical glandular cells of undetermined significance: Qualify
Adenocarcinoma
Endocervical (includes preinvasive lesions, so-called AIS)
Endometrial
Extrauterine
NOS

Other Malignant Neoplasms: Specify

Hormonal Evaluation (applies to vaginal smears only)
Hormonal pattern compatible with age and history
Hormonal pattern incompatible with age and history: Specify
Hormonal evaluation not possible due to: Specify

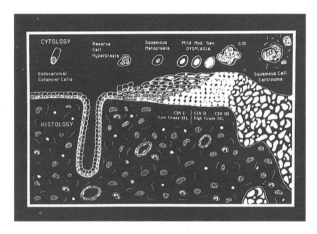

FIGURE 2–1. The correlation between cytology and histology is illustrated schematically; recent studies have suggested a more rapid evolution from CIN I (low-grade SIL) to invasion in some patients, especially younger women (drawing by H. Daniel Schantz).

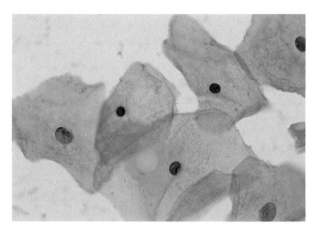

FIGURE 2–3. Normal Squamous Cells. The three squamous cells at the center have the pyknotic, featureless nuclear chromatin of superficial cells; in the nuclei of the three intermediate cells at the periphery, some chromatin granularity can be discerned (× 1000).

NORMAL CELLS

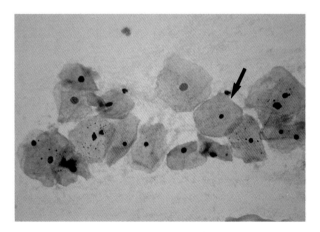

FIGURE 2–2. Normal Squamous Cells. A mixture of superficial and intermediate cells is seen in a clear bacterial background. Superficial cells have pyknotic nuclear chromatin (arrow), whereas intermediate cells have larger nuclei with more open and finely granular chromatin. Cytoplasmic granules are present in several of the cells. The cytoplasm may be eosinophilic or cyanophilic (Papanicolaou stained Papanicolaou smear [throughout unless otherwise indicated] × 400).

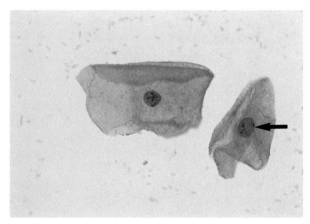

FIGURE 2–4. Normal Squamous Cells. These intermediate cells have an open chromatin pattern with small chromocenters visible; a Barr body is present on the nuclear margin in the cell at the arrow (× 1000).

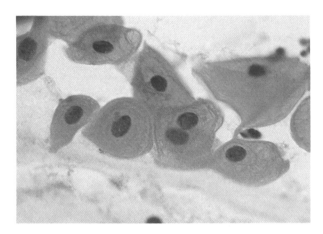

FIGURE 2–5. Normal Squamous Cells. These parabasal cells have a larger nuclear to cytoplasmic ratio than superficial or intermediate cells, but their nuclei are uniform and oval, with a finely granular chromatin pattern. These cells are smaller than intermediate cells. Their smaller oval shape and occasional cytoplasmic vacuolization may lead to their confusion with cells derived from squamous metaplasia. Other factors, such as the patient's condition (e.g., post partum) or the appearance of the rest of the smear (e.g., atrophic), help to identify these cells as parabasal (× 1000).

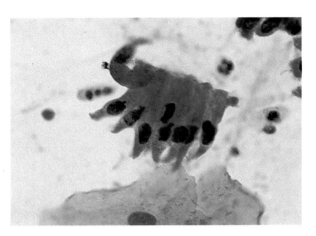

FIGURE 2–7. Normal Endocervical Cells. Short strips of columnar epithelium may exhibit a vertical polarity similar to that seen in histologic sections. Note the triangular cytoplasmic tail at the basal end and the sharp, square surface on the luminal side (× 1000).

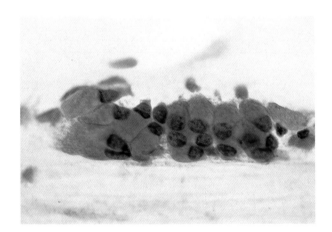

FIGURE 2–6. Normal Endocervical Cells. Endocervical cells are readily identified as columnar cells, with uniform, basally located nuclei and copious, finely vacuolated cytoplasm (× 1000).

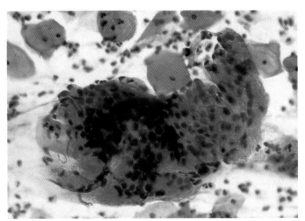

FIGURE 2–8. Normal Endocervical Cells. A benign endocervical group imposed of uniform columnar cells assumes a honeycomb appearance when viewed transversely (× 400).

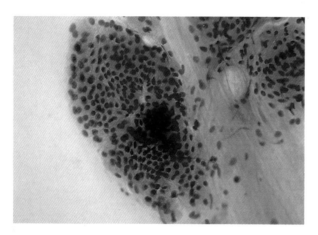

FIGURE 2–9. Normal Endocervical Cells. Larger groups of benign endocervical cells are encountered frequently in endocervical brushing specimens. Note the mucus and bare nuclei of some of the endocervical cells (× 400).

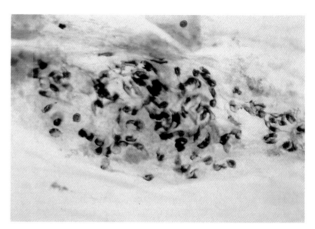

FIGURE 2–11. Degenerated Endocervical Cells. These are frequently manifested as "naked nuclei," often in streams of mucus (× 400).

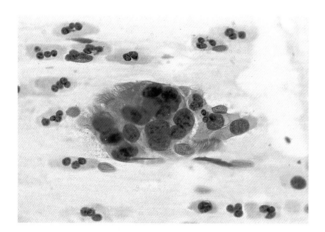

FIGURE 2–10. Ciliated Endocervical Cells. Uncommonly benign ciliated columnar cells may be seen; these correspond to foci of tubal metaplasia, which are sometimes seen in histologic sections (× 1000).

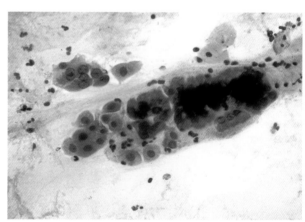

FIGURE 2–12. Squamous Metaplasia. Endocervical cells are closely associated with immature squamous metaplasia. These small cells have uniform oval nuclei and dense, dark cytoplasm (× 400).

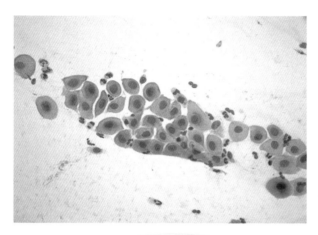

FIGURE 2–13. Squamous Metaplasia. These polygonal cells with dense blue cytoplasm are often seen in loose aggregates. Perinuclear clearing and nuclear polychromasia in several cells represent degenerative changes (× 400).

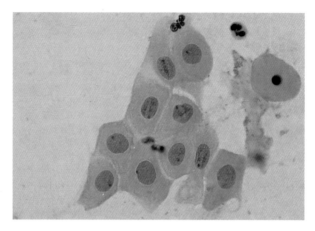

FIGURE 2–14. Squamous Metaplasia. Nuclei in well-preserved cells have uniform oval nuclei with finely granular chromatin and smooth nuclear margins; faint halos may indicate nuclear shrinkage or inflammatory changes (× 1000).

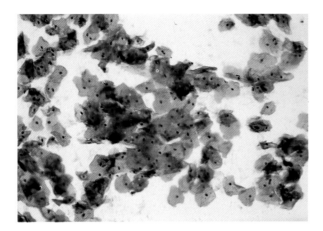

FIGURE 2–15. Normal Squamous Cells, Proliferative Phase. Sampling near peak estrogen levels just prior to ovulation at the middle of the menstrual cycle gives a smear such as this, in which superficial cells predominate in a clear background (× 200).

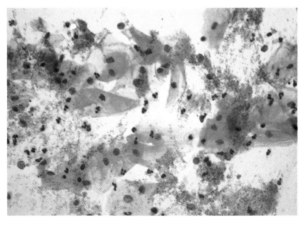

FIGURE 2–16. Normal Squamous Cells, Luteal Phase. In the latter part of the menstrual cycle, intermediate cells predominate. There is folding and fraying of cytoplasm. Bacilli associated with cytolysis result in a dirtier background (× 400).

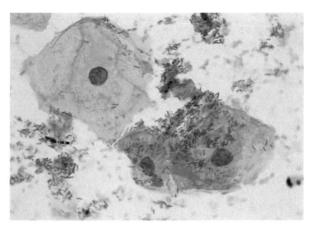

FIGURE 2–17. Normal Squamous Cells, Luteal Phase. Döderlein bacilli are associated with degenerating intermediate cells (× 1000).

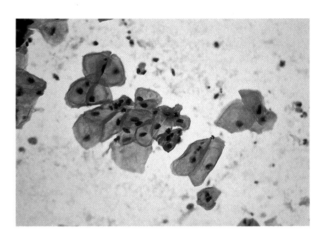

FIGURE 2–18. Normal Squamous Cells, Pregnancy. During pregnancy, intermediate cells develop folded edges ("navicular cells") and aggregate in small clusters. Cells such as these are sometimes seen in nonpregnant patients, particularly women on hormonal therapy (× 400).

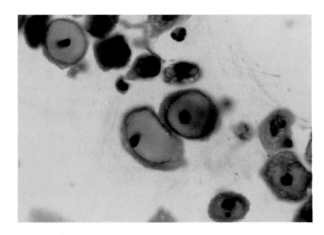

FIGURE 2–19. Normal Squamous Cells, Pregnancy. The clear, granular, intracytoplasmic material in these intermediate cells is glycogen (× 1000).

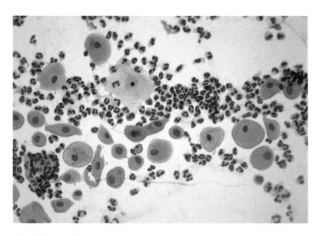

FIGURE 2–20. Normal Squamous Cells, Post Partum. In post partum and lactational smears, parabasal cells predominate. The smear may remain atrophic for a variable period of time but returns gradually to a more mature pattern (× 400).

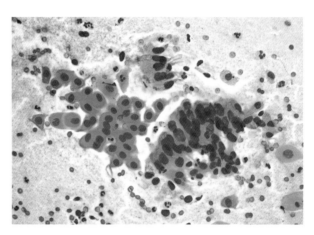

FIGURE 2–22. Squamous and Endocervical Cells, Post Partum. Immature metaplastic and glandular cells may show some atypia as a component of post-partum changes; a repeat test in 3 months may be indicated, since such changes can mask low-grade SIL (× 400).

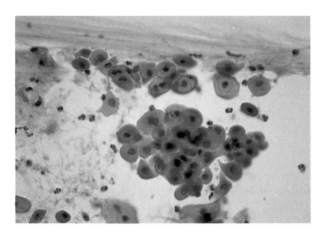

FIGURE 2–21. Normal Squamous Cells, Post Partum. Within several weeks following pregnancy, parabasal cells may show some variation in nuclear size (× 400).

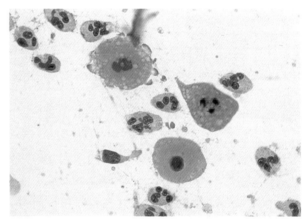

FIGURE 2–23. Degenerated Squamous Cells, Post Partum. Parabasal cells show degenerative changes: karyorrhexis and cytoplasmic vacuolization (× 1000).

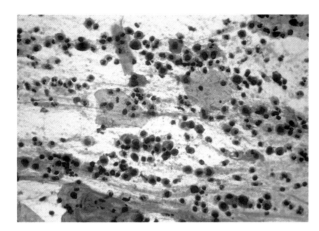

FIGURE 2–24. Menstrual Smear. Numerous histiocytes and polymorphonuclear leukocytes in a dirty background are typical of menstrual shedding (× 400).

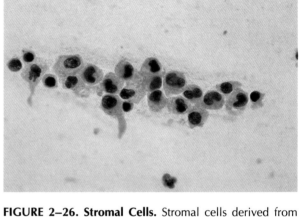

FIGURE 2–26. Stromal Cells. Stromal cells derived from more superficial endometrium closely resemble histiocytes and are best identified when grouped together in clusters (× 400).

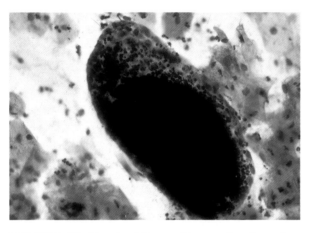

FIGURE 2–25. Menstrual Smear. Menstrual endometrium composed of a central core of densely packed stroma surrounded by degenerated and partially necrotic cells is seen in exodus (× 400).

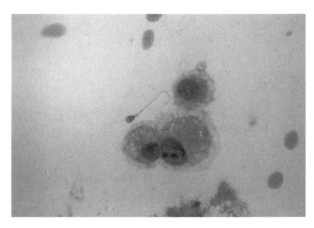

FIGURE 2–27. Histiocytes. These cells have finely vacuolated cytoplasm and uniform, vesicular nuclei. They tend to be rounder than stromal cells, which are smaller and have more hyperchromatic nuclei (× 1000).

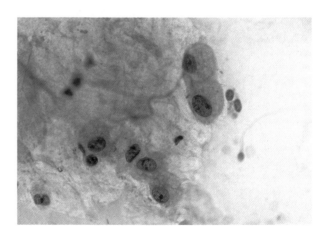

FIGURE 2–28. Stromal Cells. Deep stromal cells are somewhat more spindled and have less cytoplasm; both superficial and deep stromal cells are seen in the menstrual smear (× 1000).

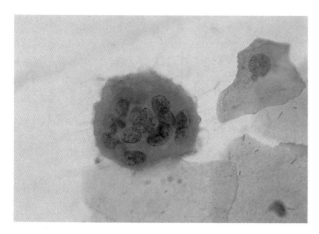

FIGURE 2–29. Multinucleated Histiocyte. A nonspecific finding, these cells may be seen in a wide variety of conditions. Nuclei here are overlapping, with finely granular chromatin (× 1000).

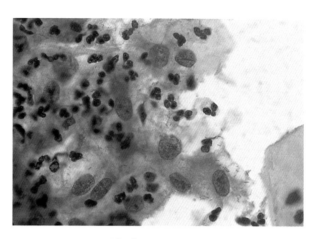

FIGURE 2–31. Decidual Reaction. These cells, which are often of cervical stromal origin, have distinct nucleoli and abundant cytoplasm. Some cytolysis and degeneration is also present in this smear (× 1000).

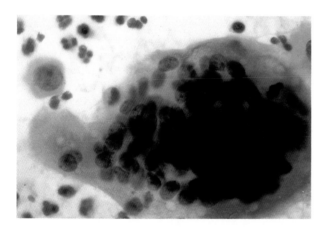

FIGURE 2–30. Syncytiotrophoblast. Multinucleated cells may be seen in Papanicolaou smears, usually in the first or third trimester of pregnancy and sometimes immediately post partum; overlapping hyperchromatic nuclei may be quite numerous (sometimes in excess of 50) (× 1000).

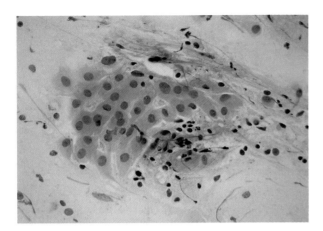

FIGURE 2–32. Atrophic Smear. Numerous parabasal cells may be well preserved in some atrophic smears (× 400).

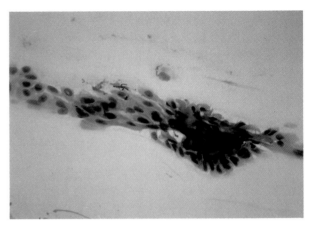

FIGURE 2–34. Atrophic Smear. When air-drying artifact is superimposed on atrophic parabasal fragments, a suspicion of CIN or endometrial carcinoma may be raised (× 400).

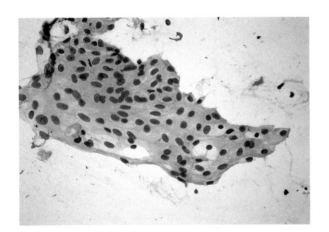

FIGURE 2–33. Atrophic Smear. Small, flat fragments of atrophic epithelium are recognized by uniformity of nuclei and organization of nuclei within the sheet. It is important to distinguish this benign sheet of cells from a syncytium of CIS cells (× 400).

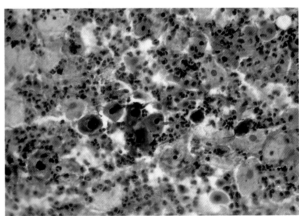

FIGURE 2–35. Atrophic Smear. In atrophic smears, acute inflammation may be prominent (atrophic cervicitis), as seen here; atypical cells with orange to reddish cytoplasm appear to be keratinized and frequently mimic CIN (× 400).

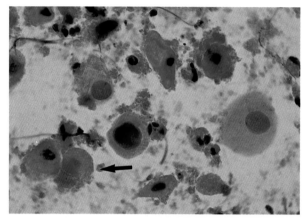

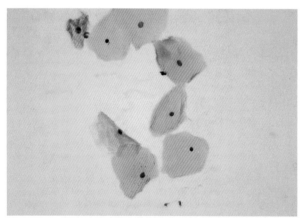

FIGURE 2–36. Atrophic Smear. Atypical parabasal and keratinized cells may strongly suggest CIN II or worse; such changes often disappear after a repeat smear following topical estrogen (× 1000).

FIGURE 2–37B. Atrophic Smear. At this higher magnification of the lower portion of the previous field, the cell with a large nucleus is seen clearly. The chromatin is homogeneous but squamous dysplasia is a consideration. In some degenerated cells, chromatin material condenses to form worrisome "blue blobs." Cytoplasmic fragments (arrow) can mimic *Trichomonas* (× 1000).

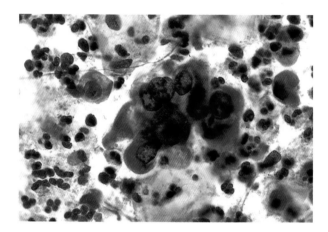

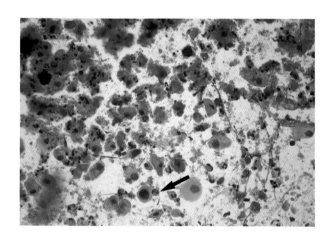

FIGURE 2–37A. Atrophic Smear. Cytolysis may be a prominent feature in some postmenopausal smears; an occasional cell with a large nucleus (arrow) may be seen (× 400).

FIGURE 2–38. Estrogen Test. A repeat smear on the same patient after application of topical estrogen shows that there is now a clean background with a predominance of superficial cells. There are no dysplastic cells (× 400).

SATISFACTORY BUT LIMITED (LESS THAN OPTIMAL) OR UNSATISFACTORY

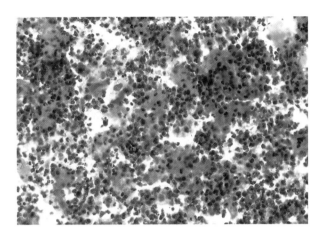

FIGURE 2–39. Satisfactory Smear But Limited. Less than optimal because of obscuring inflammation. Numerous polymorphonuclear leukocytes obscure epithelial cells. If this is representative of the entire slide, the specimen must be classified as unsatisfactory (× 200).

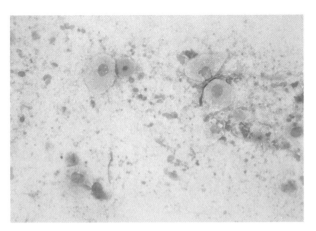

FIGURE 2–41. Unsatisfactory Smear. Unsatisfactory because of air-drying artifact. Nuclei are swollen and have pale and smudged chromatin. Smears with extensive artifact of this type cannot be appropriately evaluated (× 400).

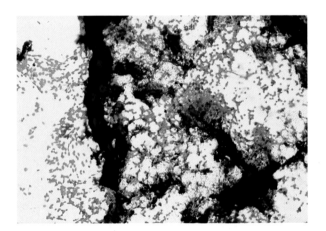

FIGURE 2–40. Unsatisfactory Smear, Menses. Less than optimal as a result of obscuring blood and few epithelial cells. Abundant blood and few epithelial cells are seen in a menstrual smear or a smear from a patient having abnormal vaginal bleeding (× 200).

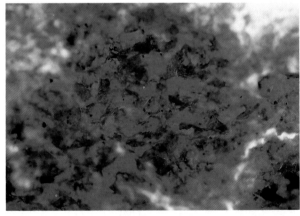

FIGURE 2–42. Unsatisfactory Smear. Unsatisfactory as a result of excessive thickness. If this cell density is present over the majority of the smear, it must be diagnosed as unsatisfactory and a repeat smear must be recommended (× 200).

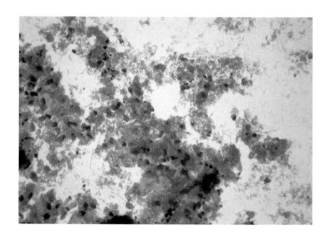

FIGURE 2–43. Unsatisfactory Smear. Excessive cytolysis as seen here with numerous Döderlein bacilli may sometimes obscure a significant diagnosis. In such a case, the correct interpretation is unsatisfactory. If enough cellular detail is intact but there is partial destruction of cells, the smear might be reported as less than optimal (× 200).

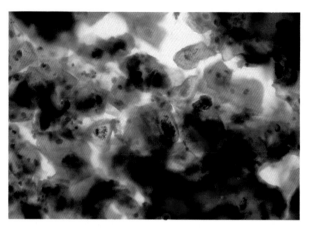

FIGURE 2–45. Unsatisfactory Smear. It is unsatisfactory as a result of excessive thickness and artifact. Epithelial cells are smeared too thick. Some cells show dark yellowish-brown cytoplasmic granules, which appear on a slide when there is inadequate dehydration in processing prior to coverslipping (corn flake artifact) (× 400).

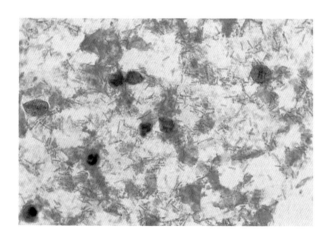

FIGURE 2–44. Unsatisfactory Smear. Excessive cytolysis and associated Döderlein bacilli are seen here; only naked nuclei remain in most areas (× 1000).

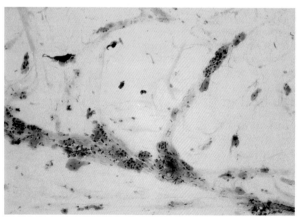

FIGURE 2–46. Unsatisfactory Smear. This is unsatisfactory because of limited squamous component. Occasionally, when the cervical scrape is inadequate, few squames are present in the smear. Abundant endocervical cells and swirled mucus may be present, especially if the cytobrush has been used (× 100).

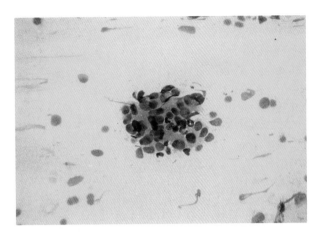

FIGURE 2–47. Unsatisfactory Smear. There is too much air-drying artifact. Large clusters of air-dried endocervical cells are difficult to interpret when a cytobrush specimen has not been properly fixed (× 400).

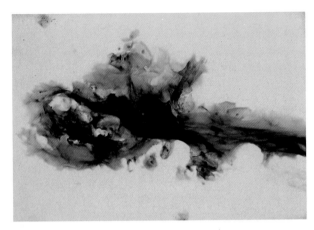

FIGURE 2–48. Unsatisfactory Smear, Lubricant Contaminant. Excessive lubricant is seen here as amorphous blue-gray material that may compromise the quality of the Papanicolaou smear (× 200).

INFECTIONS

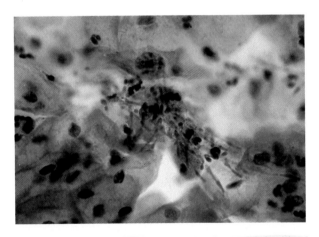

FIGURE 2–49A. *Candida*. Pseudohyphae and budding yeast often form aggregates, as seen here. Note the associated inflammatory atypia of epithelial cells in the background (× 400).

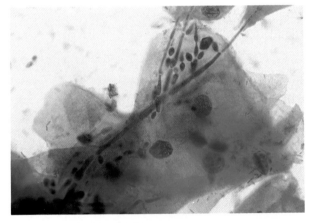

FIGURE 2–49B. *Candida*. At higher magnification, yeast forms are seen budding from pseudohyphae (× 1000).

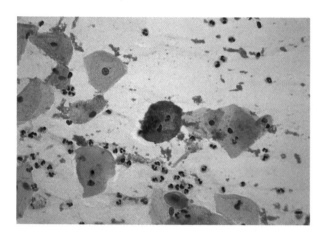

FIGURE 2–50A. *Gardnerella vaginalis*. Squamous cells encrusted with bacteria (clue cells) usually indicate infection with *Gardnerella vaginalis* (× 400).

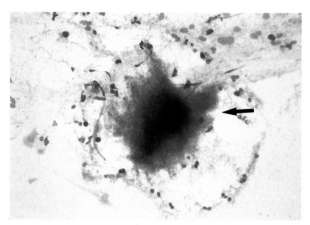

FIGURE 2–51A. *Actinomyces*. These characteristic filamentous organisms form aggregates (arrow) and are seen frequently in users of the intrauterine contraceptive device (× 400).

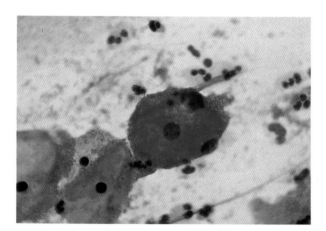

FIGURE 2–50B. *Gardnerella vaginalis*. Higher magnification highlights clue cells formed when bacteria cling to epithelial cell cytoplasm (× 1000).

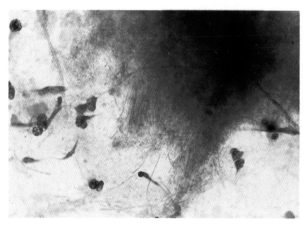

FIGURE 2–51B. *Actinomyces*. At higher magnification, the filamentous architecture of these structures is readily seen (× 1000).

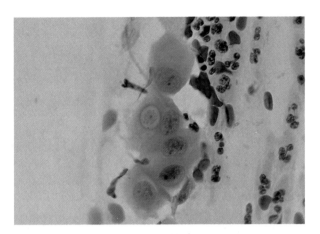

FIGURE 2–52. Cellular Changes Suggestive of *Chlamydia*.
Vacuoles in metaplastic or glandular cells with fine reddish
granules raise the possibility of chlamydia infection. This
finding has not proved to be specific, however (× 1000).

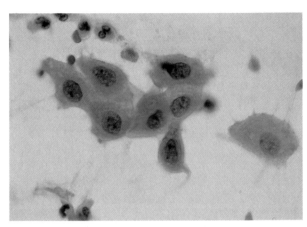

FIGURE 2–54. Cellular Changes Suggestive of *Chlamydia*.
These targetoid inclusions are seen in metaplastic cells
showing inflammatory polychromasia (× 1000).

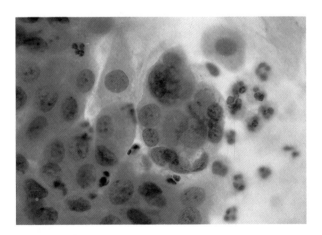

FIGURE 2–53. Cellular Changes Suggestive of *Chlamydia*.
Vacuoles with fine granules; note multinucleated endocervical cell (× 100).

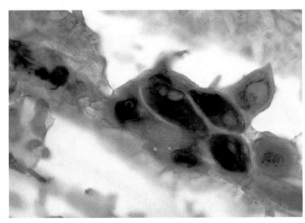

FIGURE 2–55. Cellular Changes Suggestive of *Chlamydia*.
These targetoid inclusions are seen in metaplastic cells
showing inflammatory polychromasia (× 1000).

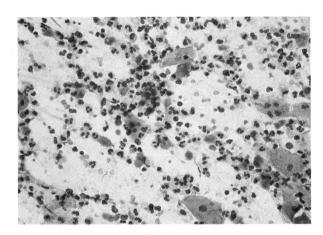

FIGURE 2–56. *Trichomonas*. The marked acute inflammatory exudate in *Trichomonas* infections often obscures the smear. In such cases, a repeat smear after treatment should be recommended (× 200).

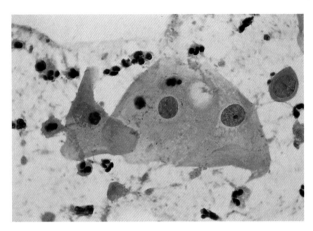

FIGURE 2–58. *Trichomonas* Effect. This refers to the clearing around pyknotic nuclei of superficial cells that is frequently seen in symptomatic infections; note the trichomonads in the upper portion of the field (× 1000).

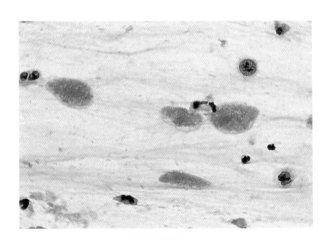

FIGURE 2–57. *Trichomonas*. Well-preserved trichomonads have indistinct nuclei and numerous fine, reddish granules (× 1000).

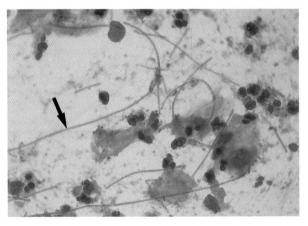

FIGURE 2–59. *Leptothrix*. These fine, filamentous organisms are usually associated with *Trichomonas* (arrow) (× 1000).

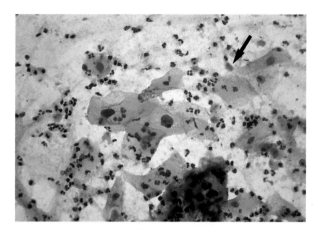

FIGURE 2–60. *Trichomonas* Effect. Acute inflammation and inflammatory atypia together with *Trichomonas* effect (perinuclear clearing) may mimic low-grade SIL and human papilloma virus; a trichomonad is indicated by the arrow. After treatment, a repeat smear should be recommended (× 400).

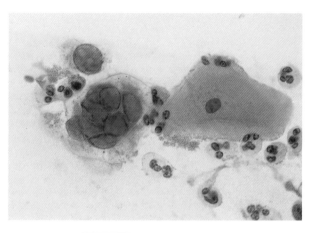

FIGURE 2–62. Herpes Simplex. Air drying may somewhat obscure the infected multinucleated cells, but a cell such as this is still diagnostic (× 1000).

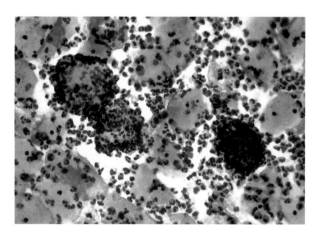

FIGURE 2–61. Acute Inflammation. So-called "BB" shots or "cannon balls" are epithelial cells encased within polymorphs; they are usually associated with *Trichomonas* infection. *Trichomonas* is not visible here. It is generally most productive to hunt for organisms in areas of the slide where the cells are less dense (× 400).

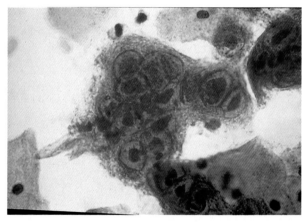

FIGURE 2–63. Herpes Simplex. Molded ground-glass nuclei with intranuclear inclusions are characteristic of herpes cytopathic effect (× 1000).

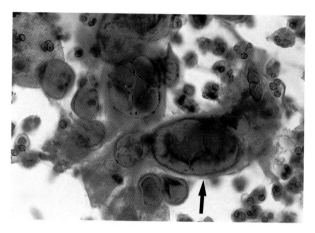

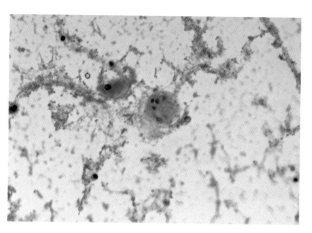

FIGURE 2–64. Herpes Simplex. Molded nuclei may be numerous and impart a bizarre appearance, not to be confused with malignancy. Note the inclusions with a clear halo between the inclusion and the nuclear rim (arrow) (× 1000).

FIGURE 2–65. Amebae. These trophozoites with ingested red cells are consistent with *Entamoeba histolytica*. They are present in the Papanicolaou smear of a 50-year-old woman who reported having a bloody vaginal discharge for 1 year. Ulcerations were seen on the cervix (× 1000). (Courtesy of Edmund S. Cibas, M.D.)

REACTIVE AND INFLAMMATORY CHANGES

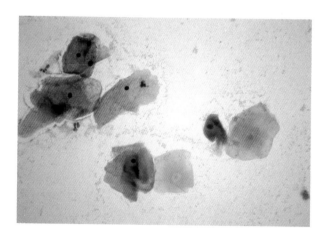

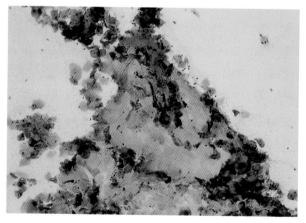

FIGURE 2–66. Anucleate Squames. Anucleate squames may reflect vulvar or skin contamination from touching the spatula to the vulva or the uncovered finger to the slide surface. They may also be seen in a benign reactive process, such as hyperkeratosis in response to uterine prolapse, although plaques of anucleate squames should be seen to suggest hyperkeratosis (× 1000).

FIGURE 2–67. Hyperkeratosis. These plaques of anucleate squames on a smear from a patient with uterine prolapse reflect hyperkeratosis (× 200).

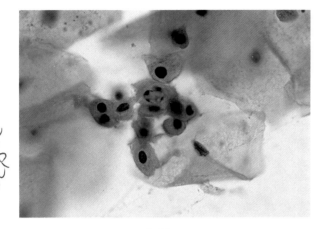

FIGURE 2–68. **Parakeratosis.** Parakeratotic cells without cytologic atypia are usually derived from a benign reparative process resulting from traumatic rubbing of the cervical surface, e.g., uterine prolapse; if there is the slightest atypia, as seen here, they may represent the surface reaction over a flat condyloma or CIN; in such cases, a repeat smear within intervals of less than 1 year may be indicated (× 1000).

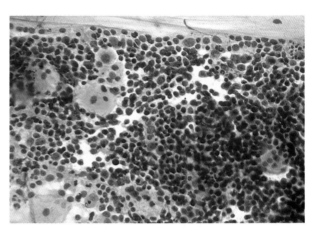

FIGURE 2–70. **Chronic Follicular Cervicitis.** Numerous lymphoid cells suggest this diagnosis, demonstrating the range of reactive lymphoid cell sizes and nuclear features typical of a germinal center (× 400).

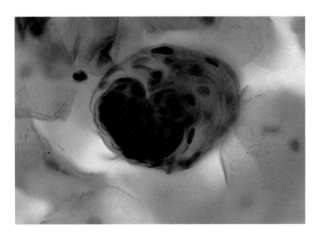

FIGURE 2–69. **Benign Squamous Pearl.** Such whorls of benign cells are nonspecific but may be associated with hyperkeratosis or HPV infection or both (× 1000).

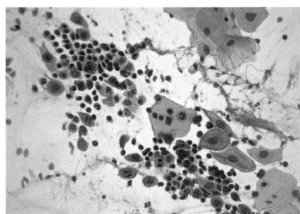

FIGURE 2–71. **Chronic Follicular Cervicitis.** A mixture of small, mature lymph cells and large, immature lymphoid cells is characteristic. The larger lymphoid cells seen here might be mistaken for the single cells of CIS unless the range of lymphoid cell sizes is appreciated (× 400).

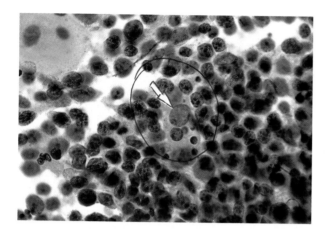

FIGURE 2–72. Chronic Follicular Cervicitis. A tingible body macrophage, as seen here at the arrow, is derived from a germinal center and is diagnostic of follicular cervicitis. Note again how much the nuclei of larger cells resemble CIS (× 1000).

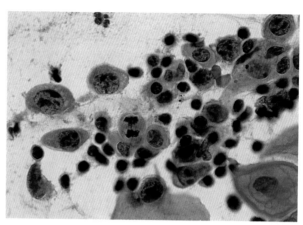

FIGURE 2–74. Chronic Follicular Cervicitis. Large lymphoid cells may suggest adenocarcinoma, but again clusters are lacking; note the mitosis at the center of the field, a feature common in germinal center lymphocytes (× 1000).

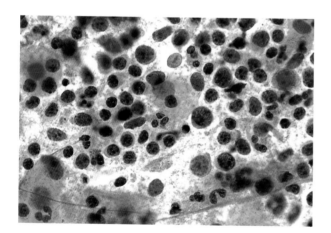

FIGURE 2–73. Chronic Follicular Cervicitis. Individual lymphoid cells closely resemble cells of high-grade SIL, but the syncytial groups seen in CIS are lacking. Small, red nucleoli can be seen in several of the nuclei, not a typical feature of CIS (× 1000).

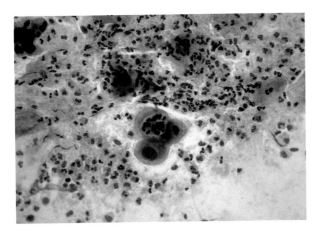

FIGURE 2–75. Inflammatory Changes. Slight nuclear enlargement, polychromasia, and vacuolization are often associated with marked acute inflammation of nonspecific etiology (× 400).

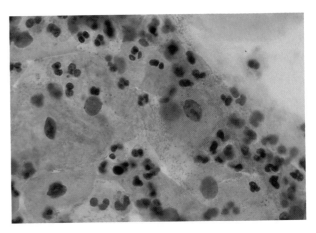

FIGURE 2–77. Inflammatory Changes. Slight nuclear enlargement, indistinct chromatin, and focal eosinophilia are seen in an inflammatory background (× 1000).

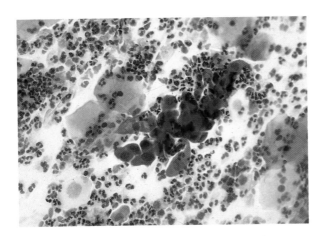

FIGURE 2–76. Inflammatory Changes. Marked eosinophilia and polychromasia of both nucleus and cytoplasm are prominent in this cell group. Eosinophilia and polychromasia are commonly seen in dead or dying cells, air-drying artifact, and radiation effect, as well as in the cell damage associated with inflammatory reactions (× 400).

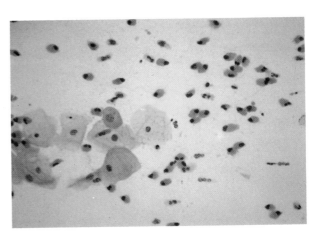

FIGURE 2–78. Eosinophils. A predominance of eosinophils in a Papanicolaou smear is unusual; their presence should raise the suspicion of an allergic reaction (× 400).

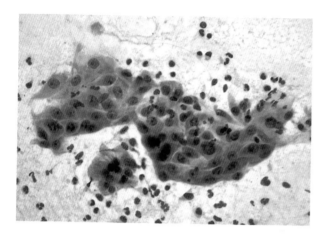

FIGURE 2–79. Repair Reaction. Metaplastic and endocervical cells in this inflammatory smear show features of repair with nuclear enlargement and distinct nucleoli (× 400).

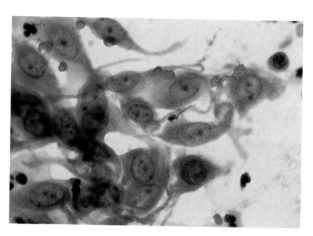

FIGURE 2–80B. Repair Reaction. Higher magnification of these large vesicular nuclei show that they have prominent nucleoli, occasionally multiple, that are usually round; spider-like cytoplasmic processes and a "school of fish" appearance of the entire group of cells are also typical (× 1000).

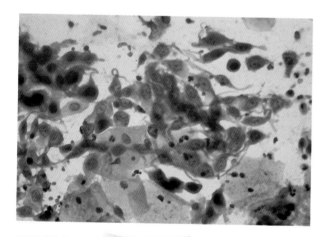

FIGURE 2–80A. Repair Reaction. Classic repair is illustrated here in metaplastic cells. These cells have large vesicular nuclei, cytoplasmic processes, prominent nucleoli, and a sheet-like arrangement. The sheets have a polar organization of nuclei that is continuous and flows from one cell to another (× 400).

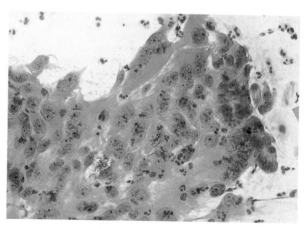

FIGURE 2–81. Repair Reaction. In addition to the classic features of repair described in Figures 2–80A and 2–80B, this sheet of repair cells demonstrates prominent multinucleation (× 400).

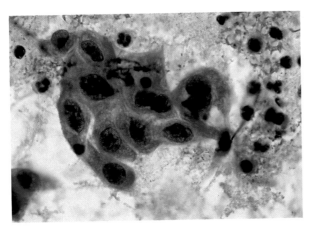

FIGURE 2–82. Atypical Repair Reaction. The nucleoli and nuclear margins here are irregular, and the chromatin is more clumped than in classic repair. Such cases may be very difficult to distinguish from adenocarcinoma. Atypical repair cells tend to form groups with a hint of parallel orientation, whereas an adenocarcinoma usually has numerous pleomorphic single malignant cells as well as groups. The differential diagnostic possibilities here besides atypical repair include polyp, endocervical dysplasia or carcinoma, and endometrial carcinoma (× 1000).

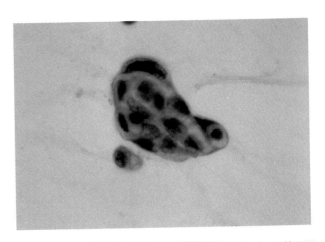

FIGURE 2–84. Intrauterine Contraceptive Device Effect. Atypical, vacuolated glandular cell clusters such as this one may reflect intrauterine contraceptive device effect. This group would be highly suspect for adenocarcinoma in a woman without an intrauterine contraceptive device (× 1000).

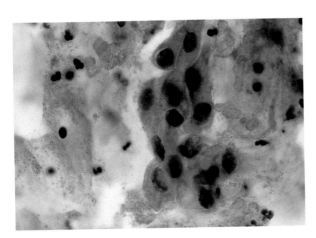

FIGURE 2–83. Endocervical Polyp. Degenerated repair cells from a polyp may cause diagnostic difficulty suggesting CIN or adenocarcinoma; they also tend to shed cohesive groups (× 1000).

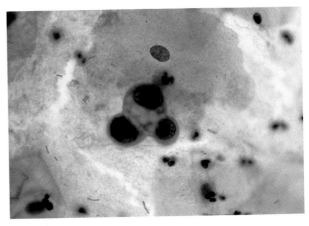

FIGURE 2–85. Intrauterine Contraceptive Device Effect. Atypical glandular or metaplastic cell cluster from a patient with an intrauterine contraceptive device. Cytoplasmic vacuolization may suggest adenocarcinoma, but orientation is still intact and all nuclei are similar to each other (× 1000).

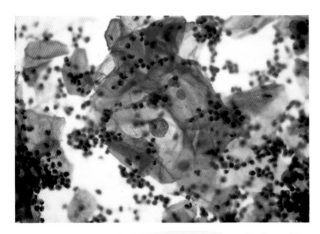

FIGURE 2–86A. Folic Acid Deficiency. Marked nuclear and cytoplasmic enlargement may mimic CIN I (× 400).

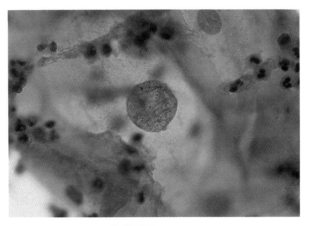

FIGURE 2–86B. Folic Acid Deficiency. In contrast to CIN I, enlarged nuclei appear relatively hypochromatic, with chromatinic wrinkling and folding; multinucleation and cytoplasmic vacuolization may also be seen (× 1000).

RADIATION AND CHEMOTHERAPEUTIC EFFECTS

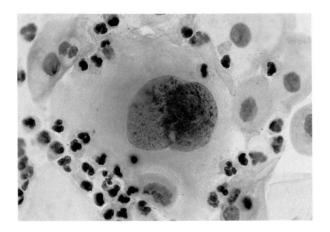

FIGURE 2–87. Chemotherapy Effect. This renal transplant patient had been on azathioprine for several years. Binucleation and chromatinic wrinkling mimic folic acid deficiency somewhat. Chronically immunosuppressed patients may develop high-grade SIL and invasive cancer, so they must be screened periodically (× 1000).

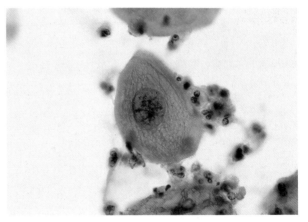

FIGURE 2–88. Radiation Effect. Cellular enlargement with nuclear hyperchromasia and cytoplasmic rills is typical of chronic radiation reaction (× 1000).

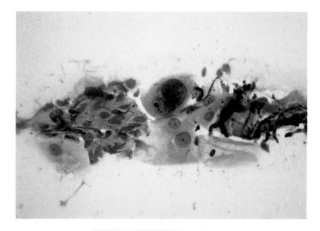

FIGURE 2–89. Radiation Effect. Nuclear enlargement, binucleation, and polychromasia as seen here may be prominent features of radiation effect for many years following cancer therapy (× 400).

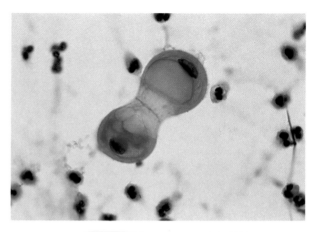

FIGURE 2–91. Radiation Effect. Cytoplasmic vacuolization is often prominent in the acute phase following radiation (× 1000).

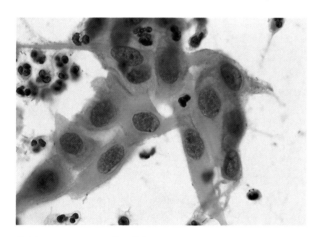

FIGURE 2–90. Radiation Effect. Parabasal cells may be atypical or show repair reaction, as seen here during the acute phase of the radiation reaction (× 1000).

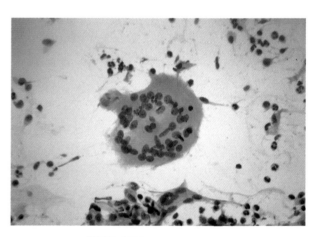

FIGURE 2–92. Radiation Effect. Multinucleated giant cells may appear in the acute phase and persist for years (× 400).

acute effect { vacuolization
polys
(disappear in first few months p̄ radiation)

chronic effect (persist forever)

hyperchromasia
multinucleation
2 tone cytoplasm
chromatin granularity / farrow

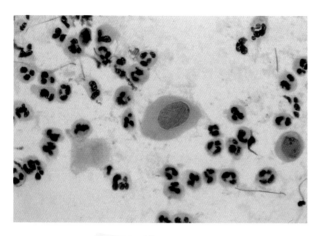

FIGURE 2–93. Radiation Effect. Peculiar chromatin abnormalities, such as the fine granularity and furrows seen here, are common in the chronic radiation reaction (× 1000).

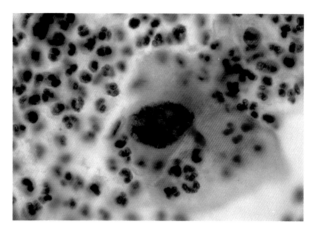

FIGURE 2–94. Radiation Effect. Enlarged epithelial cells may have hyperchromatic nuclei with marked degenerative changes, such as the nuclear vacuoles seen here. Cells with these nuclear abnormalities may be difficult to distinguish from those derived from postradiation dysplasia or recurrent cancer (× 1000).

MISCELLANEOUS FINDINGS

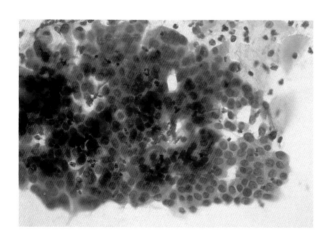

FIGURE 2–95. Microglandular Hyperplasia. This large aggregate of glandular cells has a three-dimensional architecture that resembles microglandular hyperplasia as seen in sections. It is commonly seen in women who are on oral contraceptives (× 400).

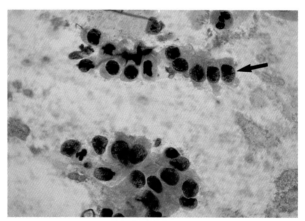

FIGURE 2–96. Microglandular Hyperplasia. These atypical cells are probably derived from the reserve cell proliferation. Columnar orientation is clearly seen in the cells at the arrow. Similar nuclei in adjacent round cells and cell sheets may mimic high-grade SIL (× 1000).

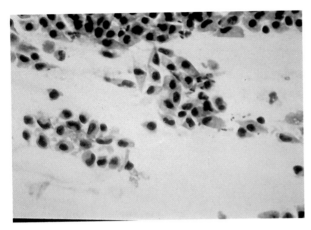

FIGURE 2–97. Microglandular Hyperplasia. Endocervical cells from this reaction may degenerate and mimic atypical parakeratotic cells or high-grade SIL (× 400).

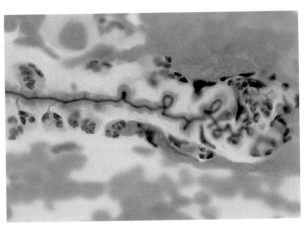

FIGURE 2–100. Curschmann Spirals. These spirals are similar to those seen in the sputum and are a manifestation of inspissated mucus (× 1000).

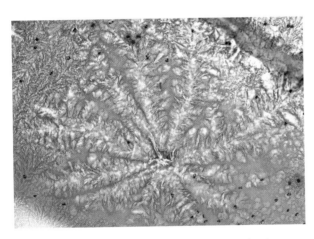

FIGURE 2–98. Ferning. Occasionally, mucus ferning may be apparent in the Papanicolaou smear, especially near peak estrogen levels (× 400).

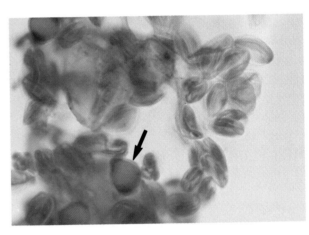

FIGURE 2–101. Pollen. Pollen may occasionally contaminate Papanicolaou smears; this preparation was made from African violet plants, popular in the decor of some cytology laboratories. Notice also the vegetable cells (arrow) (× 1000).

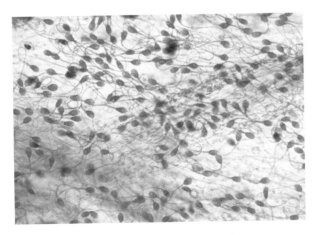

FIGURE 2–99. Spermatozoa. Occasionally, numerous spermatozoa may be seen in the smear; their presence should not be reported unless a rape is under investigation (× 1000).

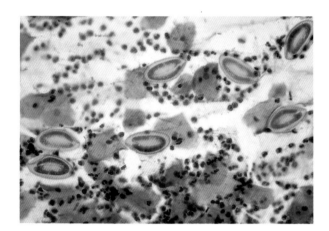

FIGURE 2–102. Pinworm Ova of *Enterobius vermicularis* are readily distinguished from pollen by their refractile outer coats and worm-like internal structure (× 400).

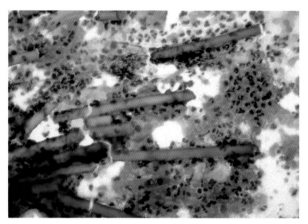

FIGURE 2–104. Foreign Material. Fiber-like structures reminiscent of suture material may occasionally contaminate the Papanicolaou smear. Retained tampon material could result in such a finding (× 400).

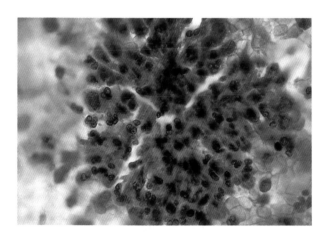

FIGURE 2–103. Hematoidin Crystals. Referred to as "cockleburrs," these rare structures derived from hemoglobin are most often seen in pregnant patients; reddish, crystalline needles are radially arranged and are associated with inflammatory cells (× 1000).

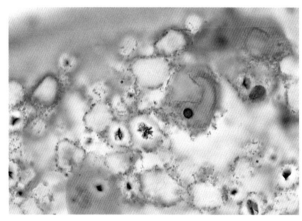

FIGURE 2–105. Starch Talcum Granules. Refractile particles that polarize into Maltese crosses are characteristic of this contaminant (× 1000).

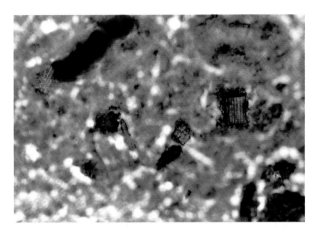

FIGURE 2–106. Fecal Matter. Amorphous debris and vegetable matter may be seen in the presence of a recto-vaginal fistula (× 400).

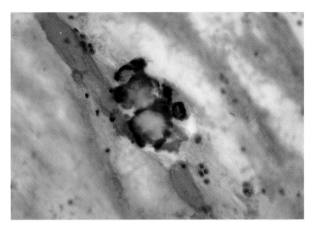

FIGURE 2–107. Psammoma-like Body. Psammoma-like structures without associated malignant cells may be derived from benign endometrial tubal and ovarian conditions, such as ovarian epithelial inclusions (× 400).

ATYPIA AND LOW-GRADE SIL

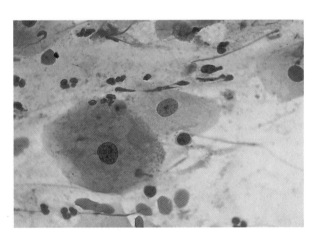

FIGURE 2–108. Squamous Atypia. Occasionally, minimal nuclear enlargement in a number of squamous cells is insufficient for a diagnosis of CIN I; this finding is of uncertain significance (× 1000).

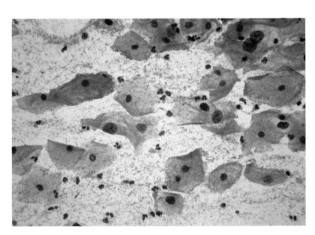

FIGURE 2–109. Cellular Changes Suggestive of Low-Grade SIL (CIN I). Nuclear enlargement is more striking in some of these cells and suggests CIN I; distinction of minimal atypia from trace evidence of CIN I may be difficult in some cases (× 400).

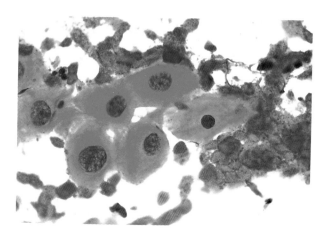

FIGURE 2–110. Squamous Atypia. Atypia in these parabasal cells in a postpartum smear is of uncertain significance; a repeat smear in 3 months is advisable (× 1000).

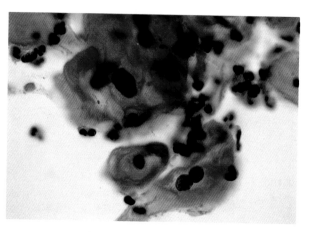

FIGURE 2–112. HPV (Low-Grade SIL). Mild nuclear atypia, binucleation, and cytoplasmic perinuclear clearing (koilocytosis) are major criteria for the diagnosis of HPV (× 1000).

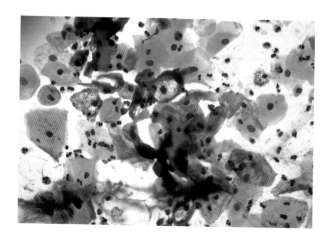

FIGURE 2–111. HPV (Low-Grade SIL). Flat lesions of condyloma are manifested here by koilocytotic cavities around several nuclei and by atypical parakeratosis (× 400).

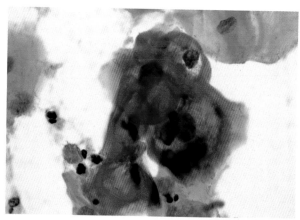

FIGURE 2–113. HPV (Low-Grade SIL). Koilocytotic cells have smudged, and degenerated nuclear chromatin and nuclei are often slightly enlarged (× 1000).

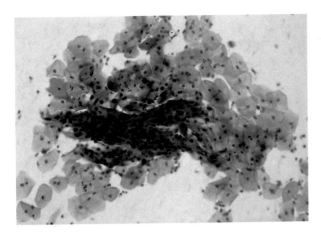

FIGURE 2–114. Low-Grade SIL. Cellular changes suggestive of HPV. Parakeratotic plaques with definite atypia, as seen here in elongated and variable nuclear shapes, may be derived from the surface of a flat condyloma, but they may also be derived from the surface overlying a high-grade SIL (severe keratinizing dysplasia); usually single cells as well as plaques suggesting high-grade SIL are present in a true high-grade SIL. Human papilloma virus and high-grade SIL may also coexist; therefore careful judgment about the rest of the slide may be necessary to reach a decision about whether this is simply HPV, HPV plus SIL, or pure SIL (× 400).

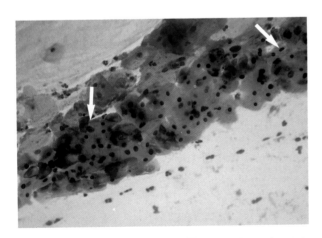

FIGURE 2–115. Low-Grade SIL. Parakeratosis with minimal atypia may be the only evidence of HPV infection, since parakeratosis is more common on the surface of a condyloma than are koilocytotic cells. If it is pure parakeratosis without much nuclear degeneration or size variation, it is not diagnostic of HPV and may represent a trauma-induced type of reactive change. Here, several cells have enlarged nuclei, and two (arrows) have some clearing around the nuclei suggestive of koilocytosis (× 400).

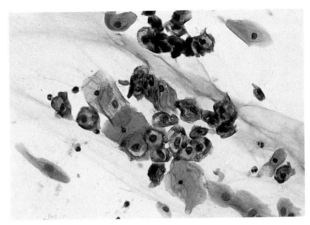

FIGURE 2–116A. Low-Grade SIL (CIN I–HPV). When HPV changes, such as the striking koilocytosis seen here, are accompanied by definite nuclear enlargement and chromatin clumping, coexistent CIN I is likely (× 400).

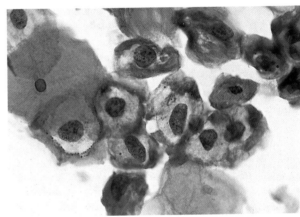

FIGURE 2–116B. Low-Grade SIL (CIN I–HPV). At higher magnification, the chromatin clumping within enlarged nuclei is more apparent and suggests associated CIN I (× 1000).

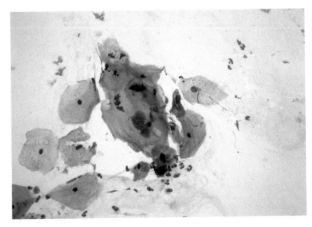

FIGURE 2–117. Low-Grade SIL (CIN I–HPV). Abnormal keratinization and multinucleation, as seen here, suggest CIN I–HPV. Other cytologic features of low-grade SIL are also present in many cases (× 400).

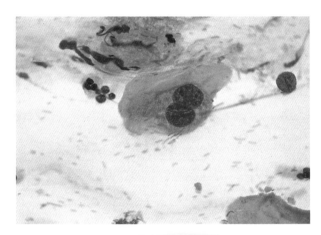

FIGURE 2–118. Low-Grade SIL (CIN I). Nuclear enlargement and granular chromatin in this binucleate cell suggest CIN I (× 1000).

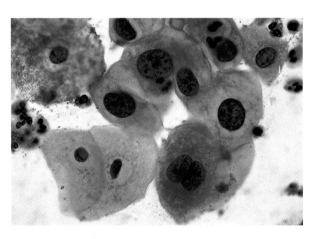

FIGURE 2–120. Low-Grade SIL (CIN I). Nuclear enlargement, chromatin clumping, and binucleation in cells with copious cytoplasm suggest at least CIN I (× 1000).

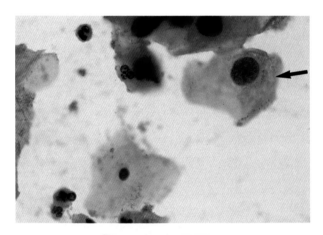

FIGURE 2–119. Low-Grade SIL (CIN I). Contrast the cell (mild dysplasia) at the arrow with the superficial cell in the same field. Nuclear enlargement and chromatin abnormalities are pronounced (× 1000).

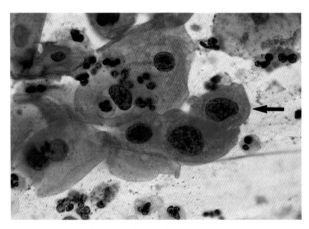

FIGURE 2–121. Low-Grade SIL (CIN I). Nuclear abnormalities again strongly suggest CIN I in metaplastic cells. There is an even more marked increase in the nuclear to cytoplasmic ratio of the cell (at the arrow), which raises the possibility of CIN II; however, the overall picture is that of CIN I (× 1000).

HIGH-GRADE SIL

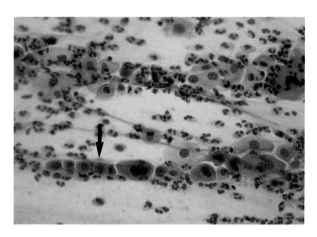

FIGURE 2–122. High-Grade SIL (CIN II). In lesions of high-grade SIL, the dysplastic cells are often oriented in a streaming arrangement. A high nuclear to cytoplasmic ratio and hyperchromatic nuclei with a coarse appearance are present. One of the cells (arrow) even suggests CIS, but the overall picture is that of CIN II (× 200).

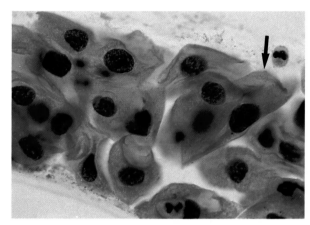

FIGURE 2–124. High-Grade SIL (CIN II). Although some cells with more abundant cytoplasm are consistent with CIN I (arrow), the coarse chromatin clumping and diminished cytoplasm in other cells suggest CIN II (× 1000).

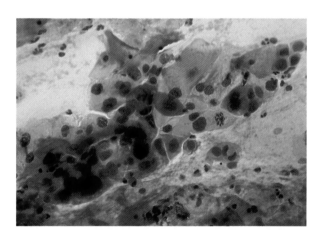

FIGURE 2–123. High-Grade SIL (CIN II). These abnormal cells have features of CIN I and CIN II. A mitosis is seen at center left, but this does not help in the diagnosis of lesions of SIL because mitoses may also be seen in repair reactions (× 400).

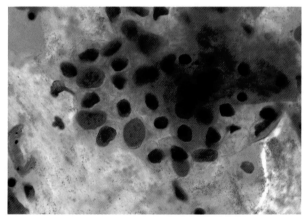

FIGURE 2–125. High-Grade SIL (CIN II). Coarse chromatin clumping is apparent in some nuclei, but in others, the chromatin is pyknotic and obscured by degeneration. Perinuclear halos are prominent and begin to suggest concurrent HPV (× 1000).

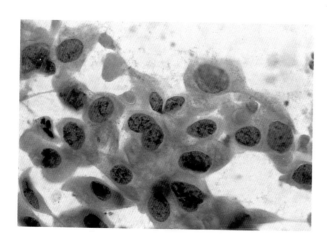

FIGURE 2–126. High-Grade SIL (CIN II). The dense cytoplasm and cell shape suggest that this is a dysplastic process involving metaplastic cells (× 1000).

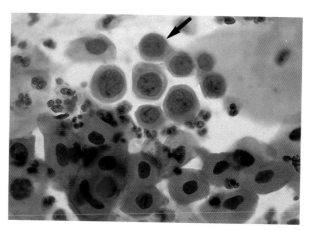

FIGURE 2–128. High-Grade SIL (CIN II–III). Atypical parakeratotic cells may be associated with HPV, but the very high nuclear to cytoplasmic ratios seen in some of the cells (arrow) suggest severe dysplasia or CIS (× 1000).

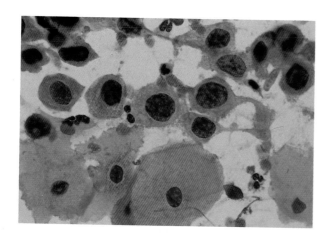

FIGURE 2–127. High-Grade SIL (CIN II). Contrast the high nuclear to cytoplasmic ratio and chromatin clumping in the cells of CIN II with normal intermediate cells in the lower portion of the field (× 1000).

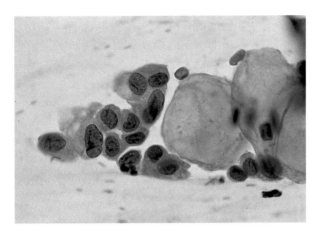

FIGURE 2–129. High-Grade SIL (CIN III). Well-preserved dysplastic cells are probably derived from metaplastic epithelium. Note the lines and ridges in the nuclear chromatin, which are commonly seen in the nuclei of CIS. Cytoplasm is more abundant in these cells than is typical of CIS (× 1000).

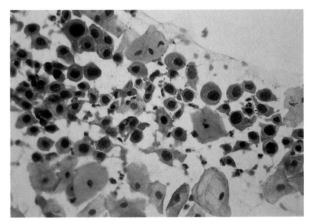

FIGURE 2–131. High-Grade SIL (CIN II–III). Dysplastic cells, including atypical parakeratotic cells, are often numerous in high-grade SIL. They stream out in loose aggregates, as seen here (× 400).

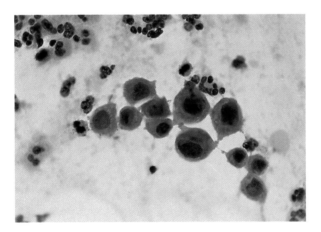

FIGURE 2–130. High-Grade SIL (CIN II). These cells show degenerative changes (chromatin smudging and polychromasia). The nuclear to cytoplasmic ratio and hyperchromasia suggest moderate to severe metaplastic dysplasia. Distinguishing this kind of CIN from degenerative inflammatory changes in benign squamous metaplasia may be difficult. Abnormal nuclear shape and nuclear to cytoplasmic ratios are most important (× 1000).

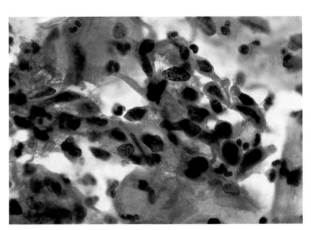

FIGURE 2–132. High-Grade SIL (CIN III). These cells are derived from severe keratinizing dysplasia. They have keratinized orange cytoplasm and angular, elongated, irregular nuclei (× 1000).

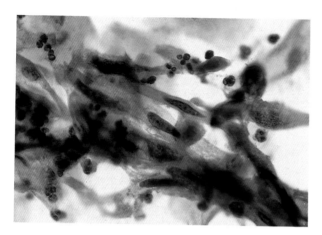

FIGURE 2–133. High-Grade SIL (CIN III). Elongated cells from severe keratinizing dysplasia may raise the suspicion of invasive squamous cell carcinoma. The more pleomorphic in size and shape they are, the higher the probability of invasive cancer (× 1000).

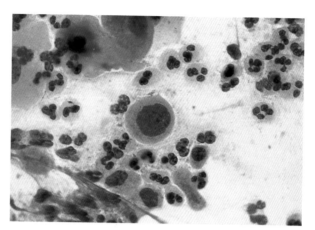

FIGURE 2–135. High-Grade SIL (CIN III). A single cell with coarse but evenly distributed chromatin, irregular nuclear contour, and a high N:C ratio suggests CIN III; note the coexistence of *Trichomonas* in the upper right portion of the field (× 1000).

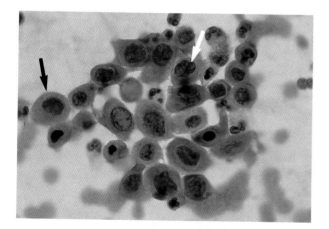

FIGURE 2–134. High-Grade SIL (CIN III). Severe metaplastic dysplasia shows markedly coarse chromatin clumping and irregularity of nuclear outline. Note the nuclear lines and ridges. Some nuclei have a "clover leaf" or tuliplike appearance (arrows) (× 1000).

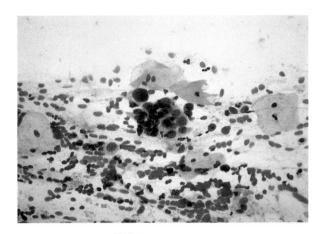

FIGURE 2–136A. High-Grade SIL (CIN III, CIS). The syncytial clusters of cells that are seen here characterize CIS. Scattered groups can resemble endocervical cells at low magnification. Careful screening at higher power is crucial (× 200).

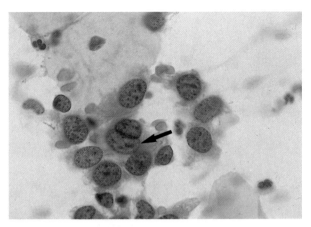

FIGURE 2–137. High-Grade SIL (CIN III, CIS). A somewhat lighter nuclear stain in this case (and in Figs. 2–138, 2–139, and 2–140) highlights chromatin detail. This case shows the nuclear features of the so-called large-cell variant of CIS: both small and coarse chromatin clumps and chromocenters, but even distribution across the nuclei. Small, red nucleoli (arrow) are visible at this high magnification. A high proportion of cells with nucleoli has been thought to suggest microinvasion, but this is a very poor "rule" in actual practice (× 1000).

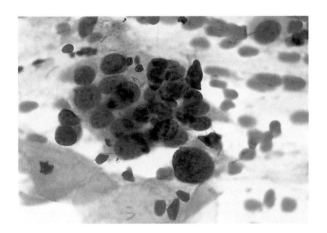

FIGURE 2–136B. High-Grade SIL (CIN III, CIS). At higher magnification, syncytial clusters and single cells of CIS show coarsely granular chromatin. Aggregates of CIS are flat sheets, in contrast to overlapping clusters of endometrial adenocarcinoma, which may be confused with CIS (× 1000).

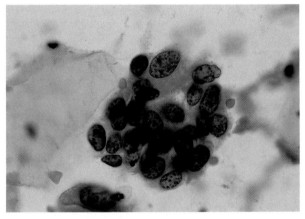

FIGURE 2–138. High-Grade SIL (CIN III, CIS). A combination of individual cell sizes may be seen in any case of CIS; there are small cells and intermediate cells in this one syncytial aggregate. Again, at high magnification, small, red nucleoli are apparent in this noninvasive lesion (× 1000).

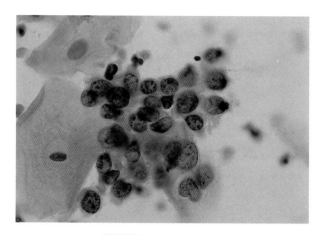

FIGURE 2–139. High-Grade SIL (CIN III, CIS). In this aggregate of CIS, small cells are more numerous than in Figure 2–137, but nucleoli are still visible in some cells (× 1000).

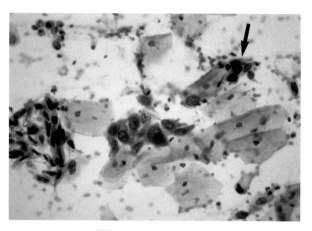

FIGURE 2–140. High-Grade SIL (CIN III, CIS). In this field, aggregates of small-cell CIS (arrow) coexist with severe keratinizing dysplasia (center left), large-cell CIS in the center, and intermediate-cell CIS in various areas of the slide (× 400).

SQUAMOUS CARCINOMA

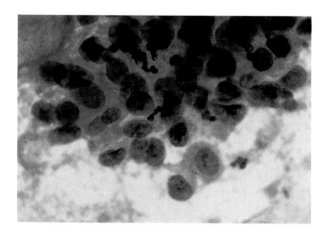

FIGURE 2–141. Microinvasive Squamous Cell Carcinoma. Nucleoli become more prominent in cells shed from early stromal invasion. Nuclear pleomorphism and overlapping may also be increased, as shown here (× 1000).

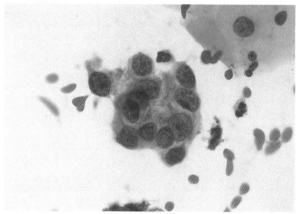

FIGURE 2–142. Microinvasive Squamous Cell Carcinoma. In this case of microinvasive squamous cell carcinoma, chromatin is more open and nucleoli are more prominent than in usual CIS. Note the absence of a tumor diathesis (× 1000).

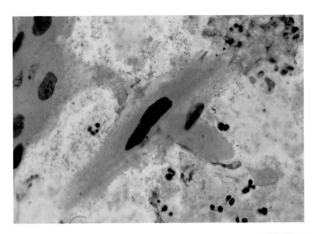

FIGURE 2–143. Squamous Cell Carcinoma, Keratinizing. Malignant keratinized cells are seen in a dirty background of cell necrosis and dried blood. Notice the very large size of these cells as compared with that of the polymorphonuclear leukocytes. The differential diagnosis for large bizarre cells includes invasive carcinoma, radiation effect, keratinizing dysplasia, and, occasionally, HPV infection (× 1000).

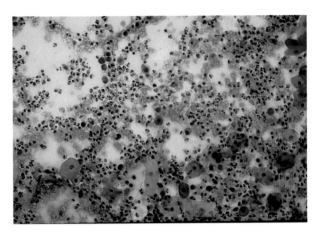

FIGURE 2–145. Squamous Cell Carcinoma, Tumor Diathesis. This lower magnification of the case illustrated in Figure 2–151 shows the bloody, granular background of tumor diathesis (× 200).

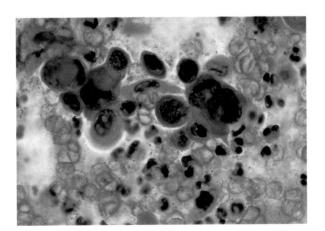

FIGURE 2–144. Squamous Cell Carcinoma, Keratinizing. These pleomorphic cells form a cluster in a dirty background (× 1000).

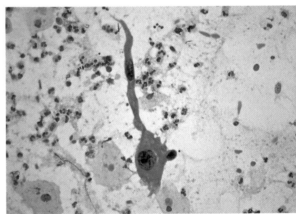

FIGURE 2–146. Squamous Cell Carcinoma, Keratinizing. Large, bizarre, racket-shaped or tadpole cells are often prominent. Again, one may see a few such cells in keratinizing dysplasia or HPV infection (× 400).

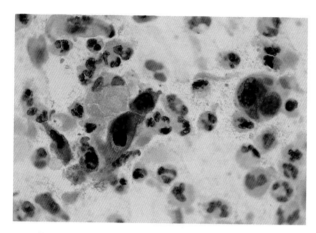

FIGURE 2–147. Squamous Cell Carcinoma, Keratinizing. Some cells may suggest only severe keratinizing dysplasia, but the context of tumor diathesis and the variety of cell shapes are more consistent with invasive squamous cell carcinoma (× 1000).

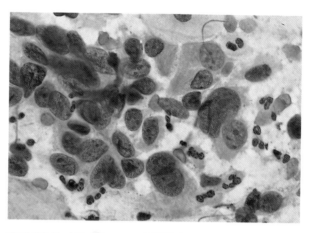

FIGURE 2–149. Squamous Cell Carcinoma, Nonkeratinizing. Large, polygonal cells have prominent nucleoli and overlapping nuclei; these cells may resemble large-cell CIS but are more pleomorphic and have large nucleoli (× 1000).

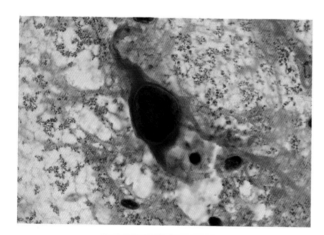

FIGURE 2–148. Squamous Cell Carcinoma, Keratinizing. A single bizarre, keratinized cell is seen here in a necrotic background. Paradoxically, diagnostic malignant cells may become harder to find in smears from patients with large tumors because of the extensive necrosis (× 1000).

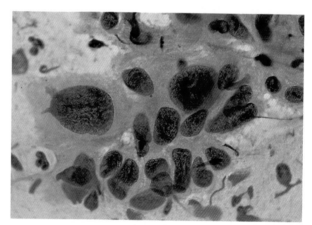

FIGURE 2–150. Squamous Cell Carcinoma, Nonkeratinizing. These pleomorphic cells have less conspicuous nucleoli but do show striking parachromatin clearing (× 1000).

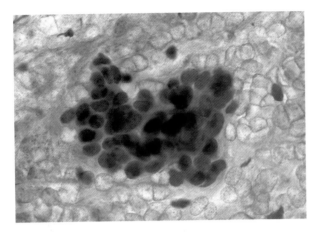

FIGURE 2–151. Small-Cell Carcinoma of the Cervix. Small, hyperchromatic, and molded cells characterize this less common variant of cervical squamous cell carcinoma. As seen here, the cells are slightly degenerated and there is a smudged chromatin pattern that is common in cervical small-cell tumors just as it is in the lung. This may make a group of cells such as this easy to overlook as simply air-dried endocervical or endometrial cells (× 1000).

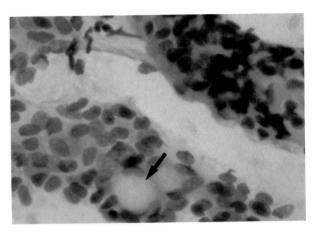

FIGURE 2–153. Adenoid Cystic Carcinoma of the Cervix. This condition is rare in this organ; the cytologic features are similar to those of adenoid cystic carcinoma at other sites; small, relatively uniform cells surround a clear globule (arrow). The cells have a degenerated appearance. These cells could be difficult to distinguish from those of small-cell squamous or neuroendocrine carcinoma, but the presence of characteristic globules should suggest the correct diagnosis (× 1000).

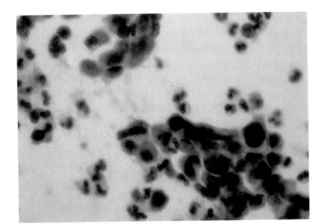

FIGURE 2–152. Neuroendocrine Carcinoma of the Cervix. This tumor resembles small-cell carcinoma closely but may show rosettes; it frequently stains positive by immunoperoxidase for neuroendocrine substances such as chromogranin, serotonin, or adrenocorticotropic hormone. It may exist as a component of a mixed tumor with either an adenocarcinoma or a squamous cell carcinoma of the usual type (× 1000).

GLANDULAR LESIONS

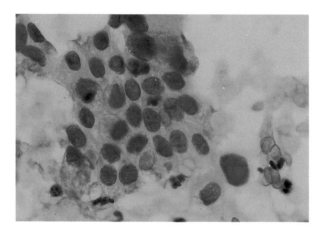

FIGURE 2–154. Atypical Endocervical Cells. A honeycomb arrangement is intact, but there is some variation in nuclear size. Such mild atypia may simply reflect an inflammatory reaction (× 1000).

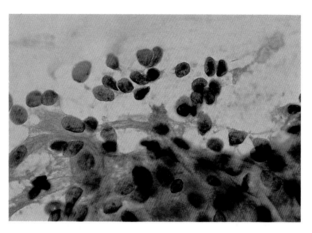

FIGURE 2–156. Degenerated Cells, Probably Endocervical. Size variation of naked nuclei may be a source of concern, but a firm diagnosis cannot be made from this alone. In the sheet seen here, there is some organizational disarray and variation in nuclear size (× 1000).

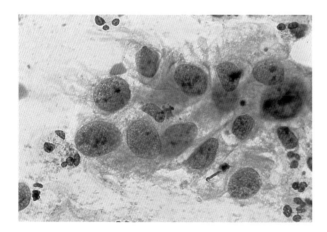

FIGURE 2–155. Atypical Endocervical Cells. These cells are probably shed from atypical repair. These cells are more worrisome than usual repair because of nuclear enlargement, variation in nuclear size, and some prominent nucleoli. Such changes can be seen following instrumentation or hormonal therapy (oral contraceptives, progestogens) or in association with an endocervical polyp (× 1000).

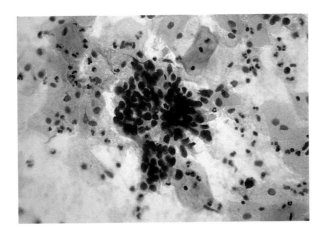

FIGURE 2–157. Adenocarcinoma In Situ, Cervix. Cells with hyperchromatic, elongated nuclei are present in a tight cluster. These findings suggest a glandular arrangement, although the nuclei have features similar to those of CIS (× 400).

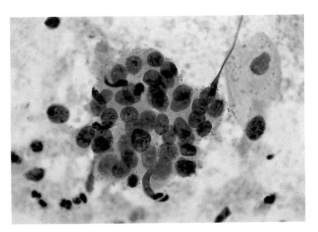

FIGURE 2–159. Adenocarcinoma In Situ, Cervix. Cells are relatively small, with high nuclear to cytoplasmic ratios; coarse chromatin resembles that seen in CIS, but distinct nucleoli are usually present. Some chromatin clumps but no distinct red nucleoli are visible. This is a glandular arrangement demonstrating some nuclear piling and a hint of acinar formation (× 1000).

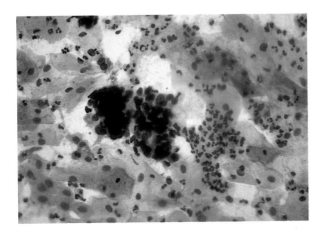

FIGURE 2–158. Adenocarcinoma In Situ, Cervix. This tight cluster of hyperchromatic cells could be mistaken for CIS. Carcinoma in situ involving glands may also have an overlapping glandular arrangement. Other groups on the smear with an elongated, "feathered" appearance, acinar formation, or columnar forms would suggest AIS (× 400).

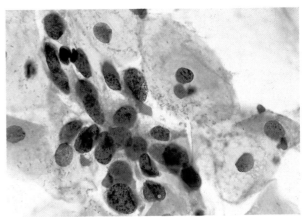

FIGURE 2–160. Adenocarcinoma In Situ, Cervix. Elongated cells and nuclei are present. The cytoplasm has a "feathered" appearance; many cells have coarse chromatin similar to that of CIS, but the flatter syncytial arrangement seen in the usual CIS is lacking (× 1000).

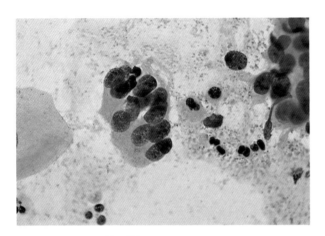

FIGURE 2–161. Adenocarcinoma In Situ, Cervix. These cells with hyperchromatic, irregular nuclei have maintained a columnar configuration. Chromatin clumping is clearly seen in well-preserved nuclei. In contrast, degenerate endocervical cells have smudged nuclei and often lack cytoplasm (× 1000).

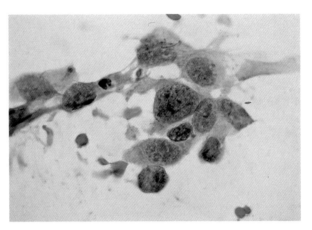

FIGURE 2–163. Adenocarcinoma of the Cervix. Size variation, dyshesion, and large nucleoli are commonly seen. When cytoplasmic vacuolization is not prominent, as in these cells, distinction from large-cell nonkeratinizing squamous cell carcinoma may be difficult. Other groups on the smear should point to one diagnosis or the other (× 1000).

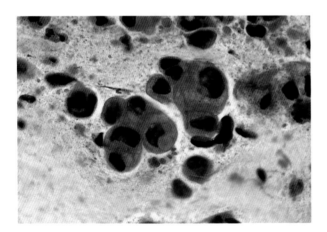

FIGURE 2–162. Adenocarcinoma of the Cervix. This frankly invasive adenocarcinoma demonstrates a mixture of large and small pleomorphic cells. The cytoplasm is vacuolated. There is a tumor diathesis. Nucleoli may be more prominent than is seen here (× 1000).

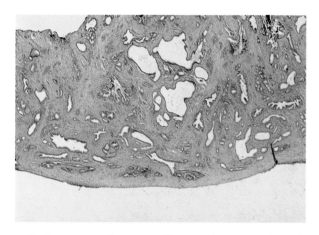

FIGURE 2–164. Adenoma Malignum. This extremely well-differentiated adenocarcinoma is very difficult to diagnose because of its cytologic blandness; here a section of a cervical conization specimen shows stromal permeation by infiltrating glandular structures (hematoxylin and eosin stain). (Courtesy of Edmund S. Cibas, M.D.)

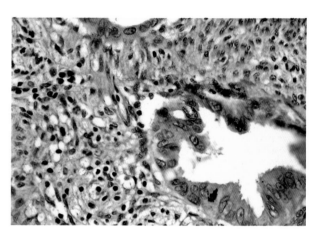

FIGURE 2–166. Adenoma Malignum. A different case of adenoma malignum shows rare foci in which there is more cytologic atypia suggestive of malignancy; such foci may give rise to cells with more striking cytologic features of malignancy, as have been reported by Szyfelbein et al (hematoxylin and eosin stain).

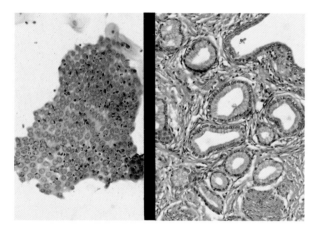

FIGURE 2–165. Adenoma Malignum. Cytologic specimen from a patient with adenoma malignum compared with histologic examination; the bland cytologic appearance usually precludes a cytologic diagnosis of malignancy by Papanicolaou smear (Papanicolaou stain, hematoxylin and eosin stain). (Courtesy of Edmund S. Cibas, M.D.)

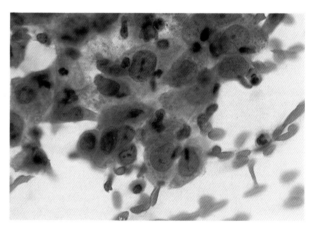

FIGURE 2–167. Clear-Cell Carcinoma of the Cervix. This tumor occurred in an older woman and was not associated with in utero diethylstilbestrol exposure. The same neoplasm arises in the background of vaginal adenosis in women exposed in utero to diethylstilbestrol. Note the copious cytoplasm. In Papanicolaou smears, it may be difficult to distinguish this tumor from the usual adenocarcinoma of endocervical type (× 1000).

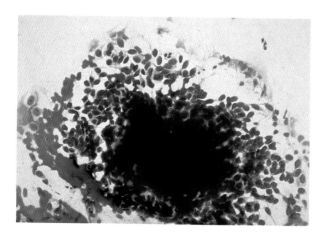

FIGURE 2–168. Dysfunctional Uterine Bleeding. Degenerated endometrial stromal cells and blood reflect endometrial breakdown. Large, dense fragments are opaque centrally and have bland nuclei at the periphery. Endometrial hyperplasia or carcinoma is difficult to exclude if these groups are encountered out of cycle or in postmenopausal smear. Dilation and curettage are necessary to identify the underlying pathologic process (× 400).

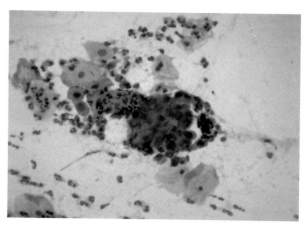

FIGURE 2–170. Endometrial Hyperplasia. This group also suggests adenocarcinoma. Cell clusters derived from atypical hyperplasia, as in this case, often do not result in a firm diagnosis but prompt histologic sampling of the endometrium (× 400).

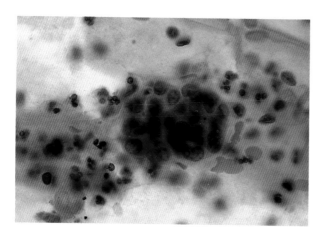

FIGURE 2–169. Endometrial Hyperplasia. This cluster of atypical endometrial cells should raise the suspicion of adenocarcinoma. Further investigation revealed only adenomatous hyperplasia. The differential diagnosis might also include CIS (× 1000).

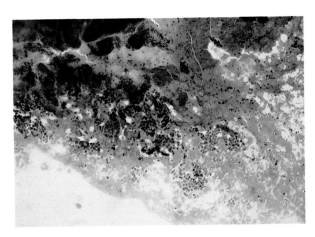

FIGURE 2–171. Endometrial Adenocarcinoma. A bloody background with numerous clusters of atypical glandular cells may be seen, even at low power (× 100).

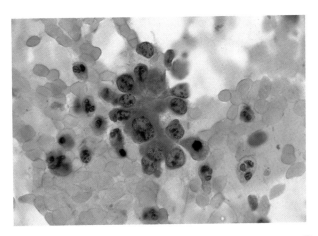

FIGURE 2–173. Endometrial Adenocarcinoma, Well Differentiated. Such tight cell clusters with coarse chromatin are characteristic of endometrial adenocarcinoma; cells are small but have an acinar arrangement, in contrast to the flat syncytium typical of CIS (× 1000).

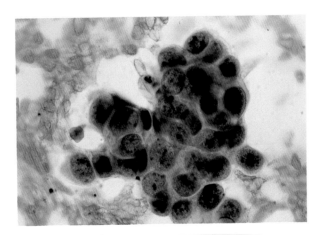

FIGURE 2–172. Endometrial Adenocarcinoma. At higher magnification, these glandular cells are pleomorphic and show hyperchromatic, tightly clustered nuclei (× 1000).

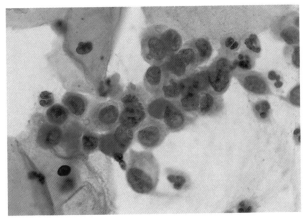

FIGURE 2–174. Endometrial Adenocarcinoma, Moderately Differentiated. These cells are clearly malignant and show cytoplasmic vacuolization (× 1000).

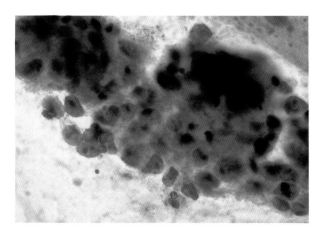

FIGURE 2–175. Endometrial Adenocarcinoma, Poorly Differentiated. Cells are more pleomorphic and show prominent nucleoli (× 1000).

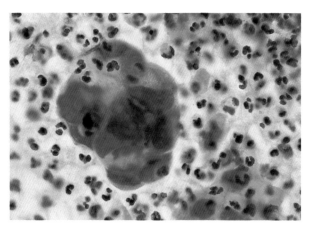

FIGURE 2–177. Endometrial Serous Papillary Adenocarcinoma. Papillary clusters of malignant cells in a tumor diathesis background suggest this tumor variant, which may be primary in the endometrium, since ovarian carcinoma usually presents in a clean background (× 1000).

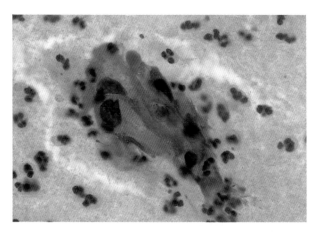

FIGURE 2–176. Endometrial Adenosquamous Carcinoma. A definite malignant squamous component is evident in this case. An endocervical adenosquamous carcinoma would also be difficult to rule out, as would the possibility of separate endometrial glandular and cervical squamous neoplasia (× 1000).

OTHER TUMORS AND LESIONS

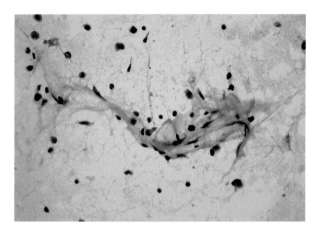

FIGURE 2–178. Malignant, Mixed Mesodermal Tumor of the Uterus. Clusters of spindle cells and individual pleomorphic cells are derived from the sarcomatous component of this neoplasm (× 1000).

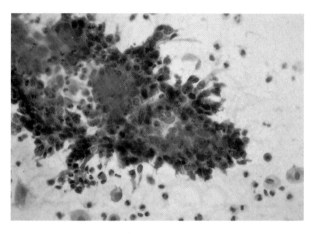

FIGURE 2–180. Endometrial Stromal Sarcoma of the Uterus. These cells, derived from a low-grade stromal sarcoma, resemble the normal deep stromal cells (see Fig. 2–28) but are somewhat larger and have coarser chromatin. High-grade stromal sarcoma sheds many more cells with greater nuclear pleomorphism (× 400).

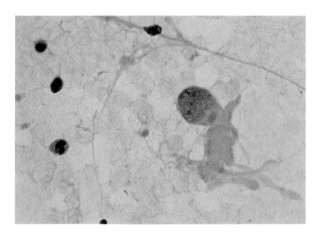

FIGURE 2–179. Malignant Mixed Mesodermal Tumor of the Uterus. In this Papanicolaou smear, a large cell with an eccentric nucleus and copious cytoplasm probably reflects the malignant skeletal muscle component. These cells may sometimes show a hint of cytoplasmic cross striations (× 1000).

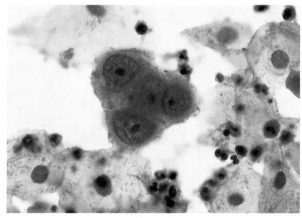

FIGURE 2–181. Metastatic Ovarian Cancer. Papillary groups in a clean background suggest a serous papillary ovarian primary; psammoma bodies may also be seen but are not demonstrated here (× 400).

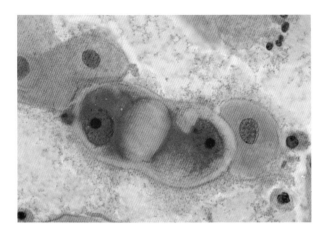

FIGURE 2–182. Metastatic Ovarian Cancer. In this Papanicolaou smear, rare single cells and nonpapillary clusters with prominent nucleoli and cytoplasmic vacuoles were the only evidence of an ovarian primary tumor (× 1000).

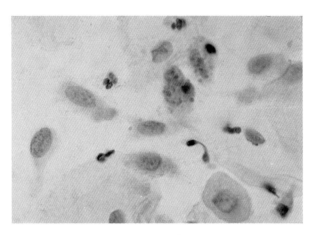

FIGURE 2–184. Metastatic Melanoma. Malignant cells with fine, dusty pigment, together with macrophages having more coarsely clumped melanin pigment, are easily diagnosed; an amelanotic melanoma may prove a greater diagnostic challenge (× 1000).

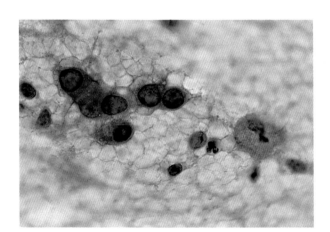

FIGURE 2–183. Metastatic Breast Carcinoma. Because these cells resemble small histiocytes, this diagnosis may be difficult and requires a high index of suspicion. Because of their small size, endometrial carcinoma might also be a consideration in this case (× 1000).

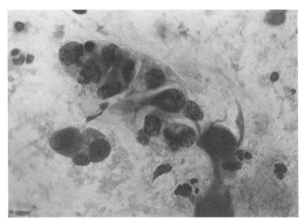

FIGURE 2–185. Metastatic Adenocarcinoma of Colonic Origin. This cluster of malignant cells derived from a metastatic tumor in the vagina shows the classic features of adenocarcinoma: enlarged, vesicular, eccentric nuclei, prominent nucleoli, and vacuolated cytoplasm.

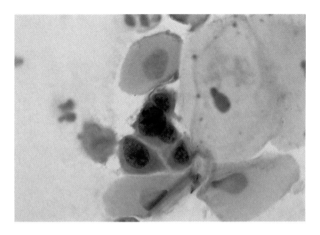

FIGURE 2–186. Postradiation CIS. Chromatin typical of CIS in a postradiation smear is a significant finding that should prompt a colposcopic investigation (× 1000).

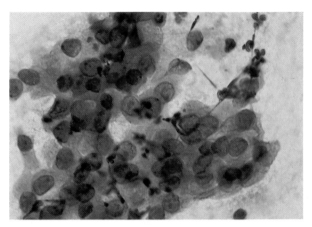

FIGURE 2–188. Adenosis of the Vagina. These reactive glandular cells were obtained from a vaginal scrape in a patient with a history of diethylstilbestrol exposure in utero. Ciliated columnar cells may also be derived from areas of adenosis.

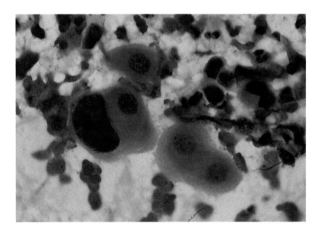

FIGURE 2–187. Postradiation Squamous Cell Carcinoma. The pleomorphic nucleus seen in the smear suggests recurrent invasive carcinoma, and this was subsequently confirmed on biopsy (× 1000).

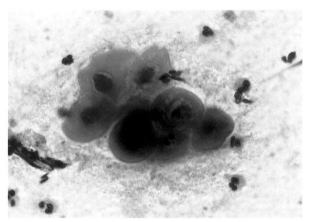

FIGURE 2–189. Atypical Squamous Metaplasia in a Diethylstilbestrol-Exposed Patient. Metaplastic cells from areas of adenosis may show some cytologic atypia, as seen here, and be mistaken for CIN (× 1000).

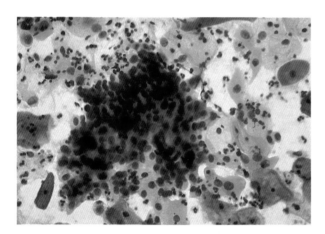

FIGURE 2–190. Recurrent Endometrial Adenocarcinoma of the Vagina. Paradoxic glandular cells from the vaginal cuff in hysterectomized patients should be of concern, especially in patients with a history of adenocarcinoma of the genital tract. This cell cluster, although relatively bland cytologically, is evidence of recurrent endometrial adenocarcinoma. Other sources of glandular cells in posthysterectomy Papanicolaou smear include adenosis, endometriosis, rectovaginal fistulas, and fallopian tube prolapse (× 400).

BENIGN GLANDULAR CELLS

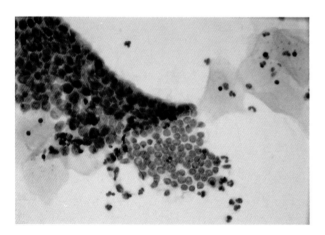

FIGURE 2–191. Fallopian Tube Prolapse in the Vagina. These bland glandular cells are derived from a Fallopian tube that has prolapsed into the vaginal vault following vaginal hysterectomy (× 400).

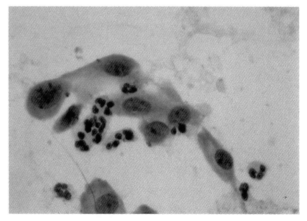

FIGURE 2–192. Fallopian Tube Prolapse in the Vagina. These atypical cells have features of repair and are probably metaplastic. They are derived from an inflamed, prolapsed tube in the vaginal vault (see Figs. 2–192 and 2–193). Such reactive atypia may be mistaken for carcinoma (× 1000).

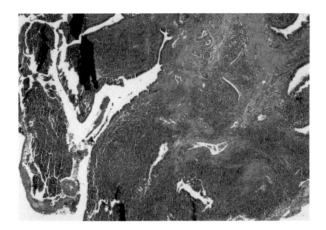

FIGURE 2–193. Fallopian Tube Prolapse in the Vagina. This vaginal vault biopsy, from the patient whose Papanicolaou smear findings are seen in Figure 2–192, shows the papillary structure and marked chronic inflammation in the retained Fallopian tube (hematoxylin and eosin stain, × 100).

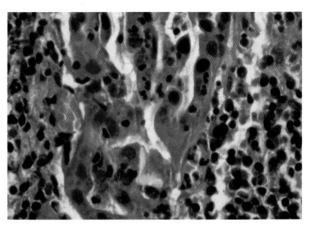

FIGURE 2–194. Fallopian Tube Prolapse in the Vagina. Higher magnification of the tube seen in Figure 2–193 reveals markedly atypical repair. These atypical cells are the source of the cytologic abnormalities seen in Figure 2–192 (hematoxylin and eosin stain, × 400).

VULVAR LESIONS

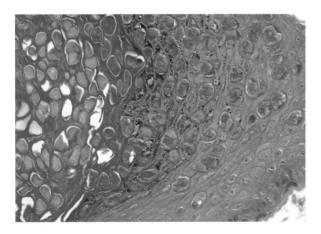

FIGURE 2–195. Molluscum Contagiosum of the Vulva. Characteristic cytoplasm inclusions, seen in this biopsy specimen, may also be seen in vulvar scrape preparations (hematoxylin and eosin stain, × 200).

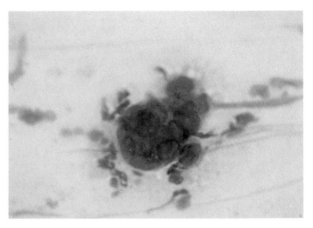

FIGURE 2–196. Herpes, Vulva. Vulvar scrapes are frequently air-dried but may still reveal the diagnostic features of herpes cytopathic effect, as seen here. This smear was obtained from a vulvar lesion in a patient who presented in labor and had had no prenatal care (× 1000).

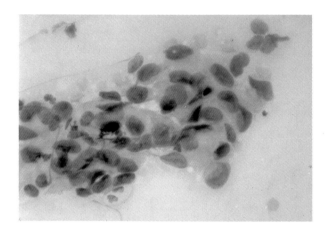

FIGURE 2–197A. Squamous Cell Carcinoma, Vulva. Air-drying artifact is common in vulvar smear. (Courtesy of Patricia Saigo, M.D.)

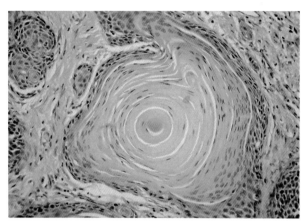

FIGURE 2–197C. Squamous Cell Carcinoma, Vulva. Invasive squamous cell carcinoma of the vulva is frequently characterized by prominent keratinization (hematoxylin and eosin).

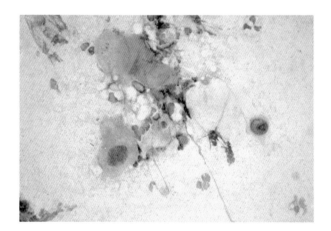

FIGURE 2–197B. Squamous Cell Carcinoma, Vulva. Notice the tumor diathesis as well as the abnormal keratinized cell. (Courtesy of Patricia Saigo, M.D.)

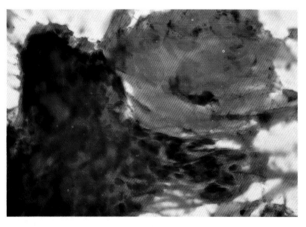

FIGURE 2–198. Squamous Cell Carcinoma, Vulva. In this cytologic preparation from a vulvar tumor, diagnostic malignant cells and anucleate keratin material are present (× 1000).

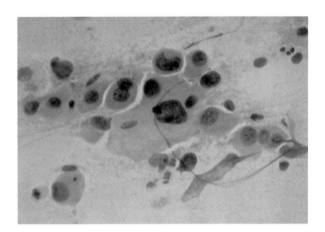

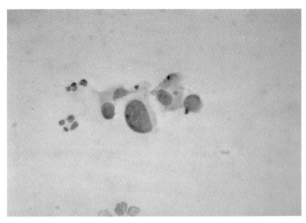

FIGURE 2–199. Paget disease, Vulva. Note the irregular hyperchromatic nuclei. (Courtesy of Patricia Saigo, M.D.)

FIGURE 2–200. Malignant Melanoma, Vulva. Notice that the malignant cell appears unpigmented, but there is pigment in an adjacent cell. Clinical appearance and history must be correlated with the cytologic appearance. (Courtesy of Patricia Saigo, M.D.)

DIFFERENTIAL GROUPING

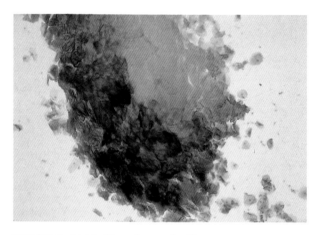

FIGURE 2–201A. Hyperkeratotic Plaque (× 2000).

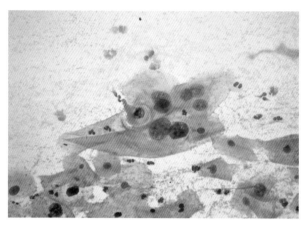

FIGURE 2–201C. Low-Grade SIL (× 400).

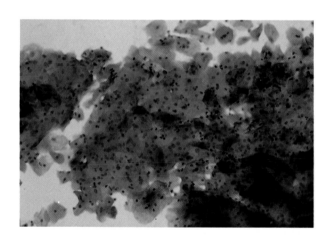

FIGURE 2–201B. Parakeratotic Plaque with Mild Atypia (× 200).

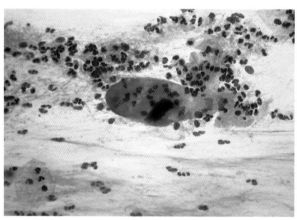

FIGURE 2–201D. Trophoblastic Cell (× 400).

Figure 2–201A shows a bland plaque of anucleate squamous cells. These are usually associated with an underlying hyperkeratosis. Parakeratotic plaques may also reflect a reparative reaction, but the mild atypia seen in Figure 2–201B suggests an origin from the surface of a flat condyloma. A careful search for associated CIN I or high-grade SIL on the smear is necessary. When squamous cells with enlarged, granular nuclei are seen together with atypical parakeratotic cells, a diagnosis of CIN I is justified (Fig. 2–201B). Figure 2–201D shows a large cell with a large, pyknotic nucleus. Seen in a smear from a pregnant patient, it probably represents a degenerated cell of cytotrophoblastic origin rather than CIN I. The large cell size, dark blue cytoplasm, degenerate nucleus, and clinical history favor trophoblastic origin.

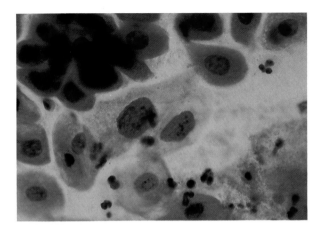

FIGURE 2–202A. Low-Grade SIL (CIN I) (× 1000).

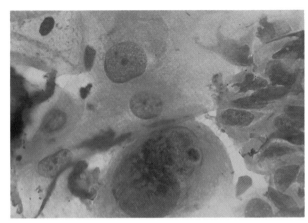

FIGURE 2–202C. Cellular Changes Consistent with Radiation Effect (× 1000).

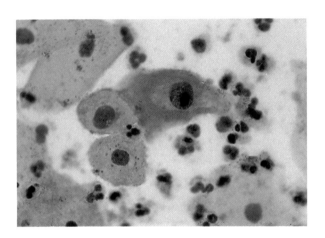

FIGURE 2–202B. Cellular Changes Consistent with Inflammation (× 1000).

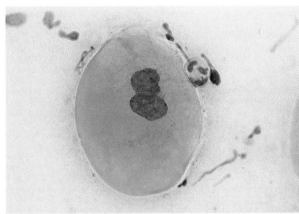

FIGURE 2–202D. Cellular Changes Consistent with Radiation and Chemotherapy Effect (× 1000).

Nuclear hyperchromasia and distinct chromatin clumping characterize CIN I (Fig. 2–202A). Inflammatory changes include polychromasia and degenerative changes within the nucleus (Fig. 2–202B). Radiation and chemotherapy changes (Figs. 2–202C, 2–202D) can closely mimic CIN I, but unusual chromatin abnormalities (wrinkling, vacuolization) and large bizarre cells with abundant cytoplasm together with the clinical history suggest the appropriate diagnosis.

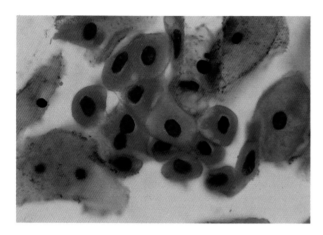

FIGURE 2–203A. Squamous Metaplasia (× 1000).

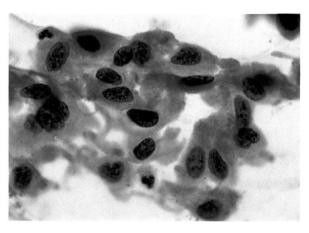

FIGURE 2–203C. High-Grade SIL (CIN II, Metaplastic Dysplasia) (× 1000).

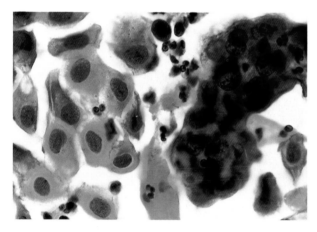

FIGURE 2–203B. Squamous Metaplasia and Repair Atypia. (× 1000).

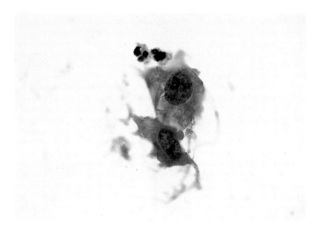

FIGURE 2–203D. Decidual Cells (× 1000).

Figure 2–203A shows squamous metaplasia with some nuclear degeneration. Degenerative changes are more striking in an inflammatory smear (Fig. 2–203B) with associated repair atypia in a cluster of glandular cells. Such glandular atypia may be seen in a patient with an intrauterine contraceptive device or an endocervical polyp. Nuclear abnormalities in these metaplastic cells may mimic CIN II. In true metaplastic dysplasia (Fig. 2–203C), distinct chromatin clumping and clearing are visible in well-preserved nuclei. The oval cell shape, dark blue cytoplasm, and loose cellular aggregation suggest that these dysplastic changes are in metaplastic epithelium. Decidual cells (Fig. 2–203D) in pregnant or postpartum patients have large nuclei, which, if degenerated, could mimic dysplasia. Their discrete nucleoli, delicate cytoplasm, and the appropriate clinical setting suggest a decidual origin.

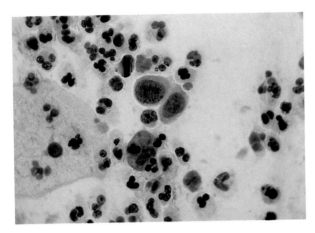

FIGURE 2–204A. High-Grade SIL (CIS) (× 1000).

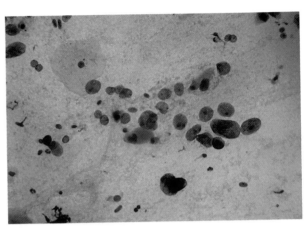

FIGURE 2–204C. Degenerated Cells and Bare Nuclei (× 1000).

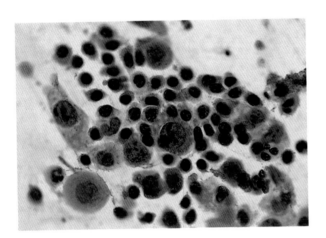

FIGURE 2–204B. Chronic Follicular Cervicitis (× 1000).

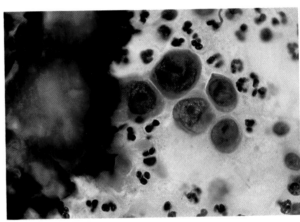

FIGURE 2–204D. Endometrial Adenocarcinoma, Single Cells (× 1000).

Single cells with coarsely granular chromatin and a high nuclear to cytoplasmic ratio may be seen in CIS (Fig. 2–204A). Cells of chronic follicular cervicitis (Fig. 2–204B) are also single and may resemble cells of high-grade SIL. A background of small and large lymphoids and a lack of syncytial groups favor chronic follicular cervicitis. Figure 2–204C illustrates degenerated cells and base nuclei of probable endocervical origin. Although atypical, they are of no diagnostic significance. Larger single cells from a poorly differentiated endometrial adenocarcinoma (Fig. 2–204D) have prominent nucleoli, large chromatin clumps, and irregular, thickened nuclear margins, i.e., features of frankly malignant cells.

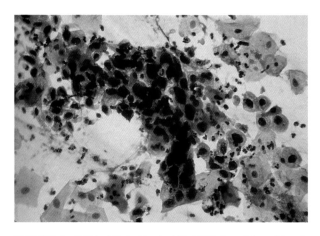

FIGURE 2–205A. High-Grade SIL (CIS) Involving Glands (× 400).

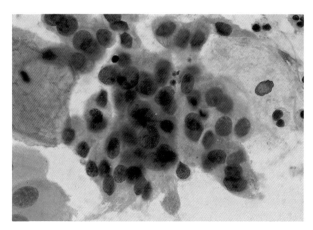

FIGURE 2–205C. Adenocarcinoma In Situ, Cervix (× 1000).

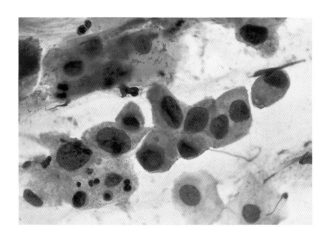

FIGURE 2–205B. High-Grade SIL (CIS) Involving Glands (× 1000).

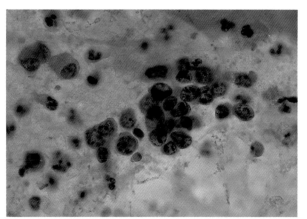

FIGURE 2–205D. Endometrial Adenocarcinoma (× 1000).

When high-grade SIL (CIS) involves glands, hyperchromatic cells have an overlapping, gland-like arrangement rather than the flat, syncytial array of CIS (Fig. 2–205A). Individual cells may also show cytoplasmic vacuolization (Fig. 2–205B). These features may falsely suggest adenocarcinoma. A background with cells more typical of CIN III should point to the correct diagnosis, although CIS may coexist with AIS. True AIS is characterized by hyperchromatic cells with nuclear features of CIS in overlapping glandular groupings (Fig. 2–205C). Cytoplasmic vacuolization is also seen here. The presence of nuclei in groups of AIS cells may correlate with early stromal invasion in some cases. Although nucleoli are seen in this case, no invasion was identified in the subsequent conization biopsy. Endometrial adenocarcinoma cells (Fig. 2–205D) are typically tightly clustered and have less cytoplasm than endocervical primaries, although clinical and histologic localization is necessary in the individual case.

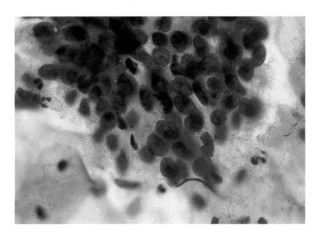

FIGURE 2–206A. Adenocarcinoma In Situ (AIS), Cervix (× 1000).

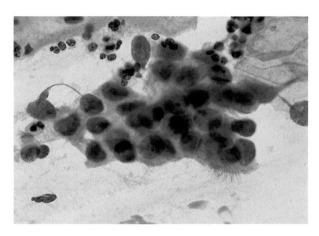

FIGURE 2–206C. Tubal Metaplasia (× 1000).

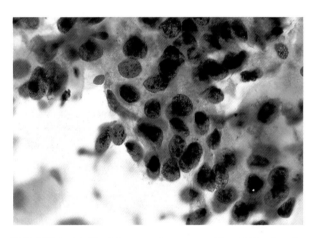

FIGURE 2–206B. Adenocarcinoma In Situ (AIS), Cervix (× 1000).

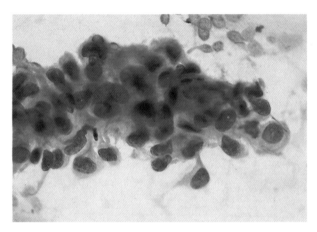

FIGURE 2–206D. Endometriosis, Cervix (× 1000).

Adenocarcinoma in-situ cells (Figs. 2–206A, 2–206B) show coarse, CIS-like chromatin and tightly clustered, overlapping arrangement. Cytoplasmic vacuolization is more prominent in Figure 2–206B. Pitfalls in the cytologic diagnosis of AIS include tubal metaplasia (Fig. 2–206C) and cervical endometriosis (Fig. 2–206D). The cells of tubal metaplasia, although benign, have a relatively high nuclear to cytoplasmic ratio and are tightly clustered. The presence of cilia as seen in this group is helpful in identifying these cells as benign. Atypical glandular cells from cervical endometriosis may also suggest AIS because of similar tight cellular aggregates. Such findings would have to be considered suspicious until the source of these abnormal cells is identified.

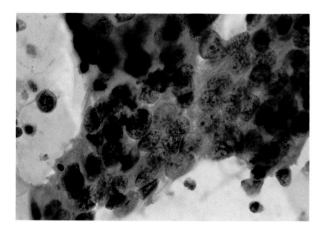

FIGURE 2–207A. Adenocarcinoma, Cervix (× 1000).

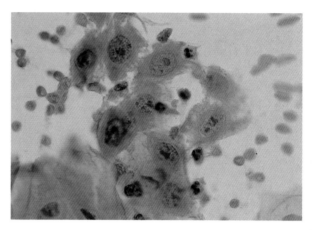

FIGURE 2–207C. Pemphigus Vulgaris (× 1000).

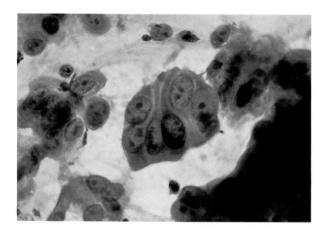

FIGURE 2–207B. Atypical Repair Reaction (× 1000).

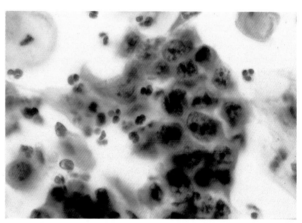

FIGURE 2–207D. Pemphigus Vulgaris (× 1000).

In Figure 2–207A, a large cluster of cells have the cytologic features of adenocarcinoma. The prominent nuclei, vesicular chromatin, and large cell size suggest a cervical primary, and this was subsequently confirmed on a biopsy specimen. A markedly atypical repair reaction (Fig. 2–207B), as seen in this patient with uterine prolapse, may mimic adenocarcinoma closely. Although in retrospect cellular cohesion, i.e., the lack of single malignant cells, may have favored a benign diagnosis in this case, the florid nuclear changes seen here must be classified as suspicious. Cervicovaginal smears from patients with pemphigus vulgaris, even when clinically quiescent, contain cells resembling markedly atypical repair (Fig. 2–207C). Nucleoli are often bullet-shaped. These cells may strongly suggest adenocarcinoma, especially if distorted by degeneration or inflammation (Fig. 2–207D).

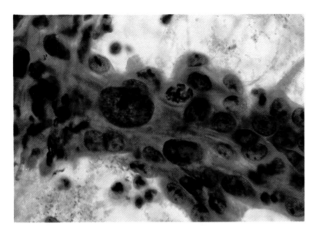

FIGURE 2–208A. Atypical Repair Reaction (× 1000).

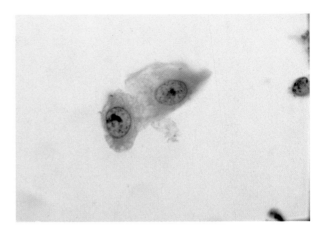

FIGURE 2–208C. Pemphigus Vulgaris (× 1000).

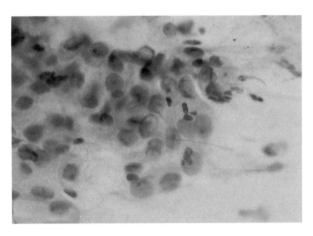

FIGURE 2–208B. Irradiated Endocervical Cells (× 1000).

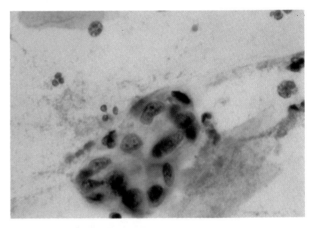

FIGURE 2–208D. Effects of the Intrauterine Contraceptive Device (× 1000).

Clinical history is crucial for the proper interpretation of Papanicolaou smears. The atypical repair reaction seen in Figure 2–208A would definitely raise the suspicion of adenocarcinoma because of the marked variation in nuclear size if the history of endocervical curettage 3 days before had not been given. Similarly, the atypical endocervical cells in Figure 2–208B are explained by a history of cervical irradiation for squamous cell carcinoma. The atypical cells in Fig. 2–208C reflect subclinical pemphigus vulgaris. The atypical glandular group in Fig. 2–208D would be suspicious for malignancy were it not for the history of intrauterine contraceptive device use.

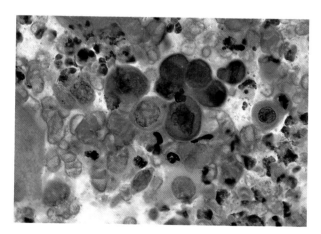

FIGURE 2–209A. Squamous Cell Carcinoma, Cervix (× 400).

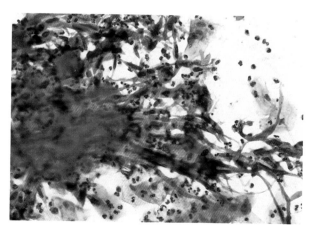

FIGURE 2–209C. Severe Keratinizing Dysplasia (High-Grade SIL) (× 400).

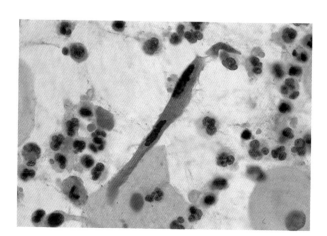

FIGURE 2–209B. Squamous Cell Carcinoma, Cervix (× 1000).

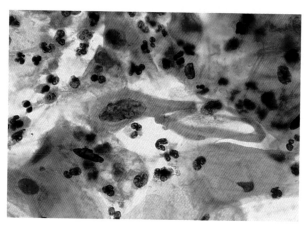

FIGURE 2–209D. Severe Keratinizing Dysplasia (High-Grade SIL) (× 1000).

The distinction between severe keratinizing dysplasia and invasive squamous cell carcinoma can be difficult in some cases. The presence of a tumor diathesis (Fig. 2–209A) is helpful in association with marked nuclear pleomorphism. Individual malignant cells may be elongated and spindle-shaped (Fig. 2–209B). Severe keratinizing dysplasia is often characterized by parakeratotic plaques (Fig. 2–209C). The marked nuclear pleomorphism within the plaque suggests a process more severe than low-grade SIL-HPV–related changes. Individual cells of severe keratinizing dysplasia (Fig. 2–209D) may be sufficiently abnormal to raise the possibility of invasive cancer. The lack of tumor diathesis and associated changes typical of severe dysplasia aid in arriving at the most accurate diagnosis.

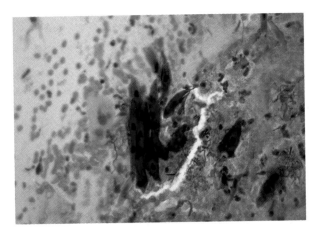

FIGURE 2–210A. Postpartum Changes (× 400).

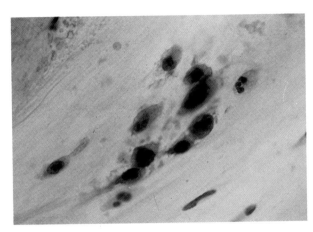

FIGURE 2–210C. Pill Effect (Pseudoparakeratosis) (× 1000).

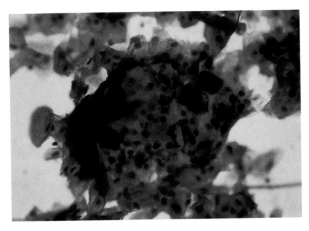

FIGURE 2–210B. Atypical Parakeratotic Plaque (× 400).

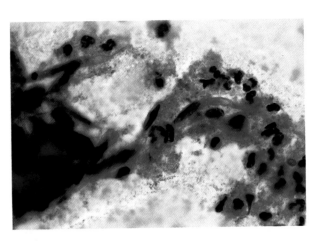

FIGURE 2–210D. Fibroblasts (× 1000).

Abnormal keratinization may be part of a non-neoplastic reactive process. In Figure 2–210A, slightly atypical keratinized cells are seen in a postpartum smear taken 1 day after delivery. Postpartum atypia may persist for several weeks, and when any doubt as to its significance exists, a repeat smear in 3 months should be recommended. Parakeratosis may also reflect a reactive process, but if nuclei are enlarged and slightly atypical, as seen in Figure 2–210B, HPV should be suspected. Careful scrutiny of the remainder of the smear may confirm HPV or SIL or both.

Pseudokeratinization may cause confusion in some smears. In Figure 2–210C, endocervical cells have assumed a pseudoparakeratotic appearance. These cells, seen in patients who are on oral contraceptives, are probably degenerating glandular cells derived from areas of microglandular hyperplasia. Spindle cells, seen in Figure 2–210D, resemble the elongated cells of squamous cell carcinoma. They are actually fibroblasts scraped from the granulation tissue at the site of a conization biopsy performed 13 days earlier.

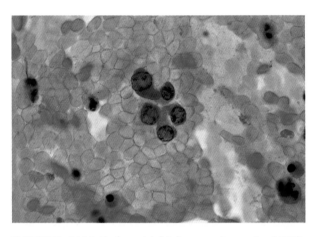

FIGURE 2–211A. Endometrial Adenocarcinoma (× 1000).

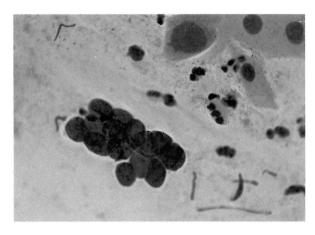

FIGURE 2–211C. Degenerated Cells of Probable Endocervical Origin (× 1000).

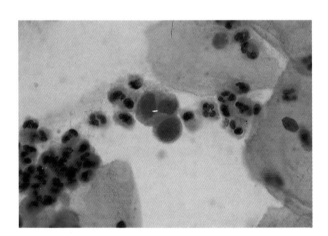

FIGURE 2–211B. Endometrial Adenocarcinoma (× 1000).

Cellular degeneration in both malignant and benign processes may be a source of confusion in some cases. Cell clusters from endometrial adenocarcinoma may be mistaken for degenerated endocervical cells (Fig. 2–211A) or a syncytial group of CIS (Fig. 2–211B). In the latter, nucleoli are still visible despite some nuclear degeneration. Degenerated and bare nuclei of probable endocervical origin, as seen in Figure 2–211C, are nondiagnostic.

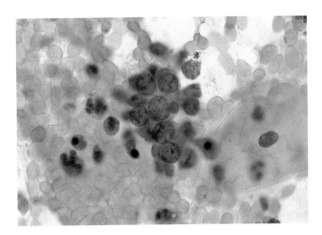

FIGURE 2–212A. Endometrial Adenocarcinoma (× 1000).

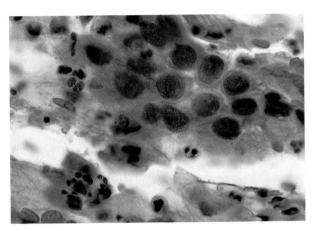

FIGURE 2–212C. Atypical endocervical cells, possibly from an Arias-Stella–like reaction (× 1000).

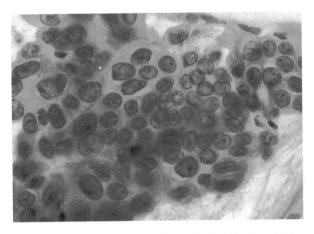

FIGURE 2–212B. Atypical Endocervical Cells, Repair Reaction (× 1000).

Atypical glandular cells may be a source of diagnostic confusion. In endometrial adenocarcinoma (Fig. 2–212A), overlapping, tightly clustered cells show cytologic features of malignancy, with chromatin clumping and distinct nucleoli. In atypical repair (Fig. 2–212B), variation in nuclear size and some irregularities of nuclear contours may suggest adenocarcinoma, but the conservation of some polarity of the group and lack of single cells favor atypical repair. With a history of recent biopsy or instrumentation, one should be cautious in suggesting a malignant diagnosis. Glandular atypia may be induced iatrogenically, as seen in Figure 2–212C. This patient was 50 years old and on progestational agent therapy for some irregular bleeding. The uniformly enlarged glandular cells contrast with the smaller columnar cells (arrow). The larger cells probably reflect a hormonally mediated Arias-Stella–like reaction.

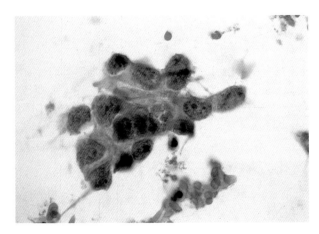

FIGURE 2–213A. Adenocarcinoma, Cervix (× 1000).

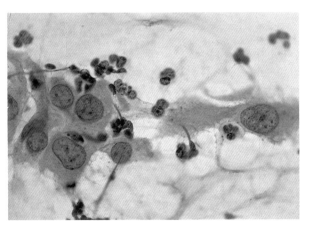

FIGURE 2–213C. Atypical Repair Reaction (× 1000).

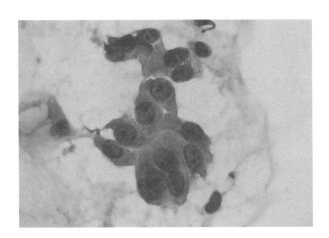

FIGURE 2–213B. Atypical Repair Reaction (× 1000).

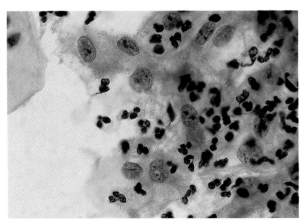

FIGURE 2–213D. Decidual Cells (× 1000).

The diagnosis of adenocarcinoma in Papanicolaou smears may be complicated by florid repair reactions in metaplastic or glandular epithelial cells. Figure 2–213A shows cells diagnostic of adenocarcinoma with coarse chromatin clumps and large nucleoli. The large cell size, nucleolar prominence, and copious cytoplasm suggest an endocervical adenocarcinoma. The cells in Figure 2–213B have similar features and would have to be considered suspect for adenocarcinoma. However, they were derived from a florid repair reaction associated with uterine prolapse. In retrospect, the flat cellular arrangement and finely granular chromatin might suggest a repair process. Some chromatin clumping and irregularities of nuclear outlines are worrisome. Figure 2–213C shows cytologic features more characteristic of repair, with a sheet-like arrangement, elongated, abundant cytoplasm, finely granular chromatin, and smooth nuclear contours. Other cells with nucleoli, such as the decidual cells seen in Figure 2–213D, lack a glandular configuration and require the appropriate clinical context.

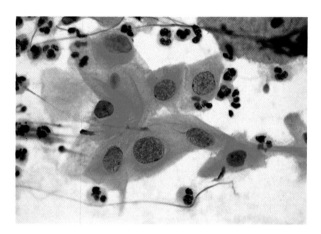

FIGURE 2–214A. Radiation Effect (× 1000).

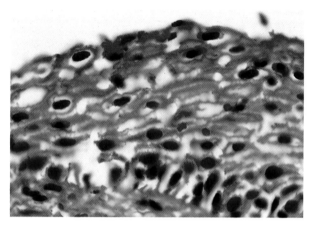

FIGURE 2–214C. Radiation Effect, Hematoxylin and Eosin Stain (× 400).

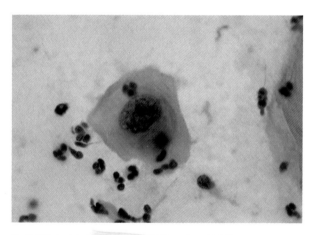

FIGURE 2–214B. Radiation Effect (× 1000).

Cellular changes following radiation therapy for cervical cancer are a source of diagnostic difficulty. Nuclear and cytoplasmic enlargement frequently mimics low-grade SIL (Fig. 2–214A). Degenerative changes, such as the nuclear vacuoles seen in Figure 2–214B, may be striking. Cytologic features suggesting at least CIN II are required for a firm diagnosis of post-radiation dysplasia. Figure 2–214C illustrates the histologic correlate of these changes in a cervical biopsy. Nuclear hyperchromasia is apparent, but there is no significant loss of polarity, nuclear pleomorphism, or mitotic activity.

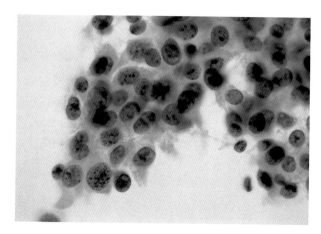

FIGURE 2–215A. Post-Radiation Dysplasia.

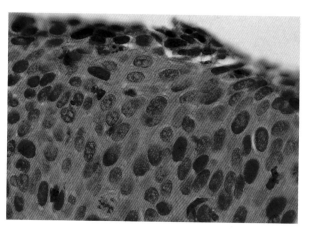

FIGURE 2–215C. Post-Radiation CIS, Hematoxylin and Eosin Stain (× 1000).

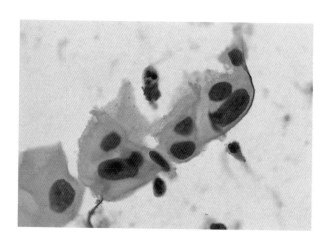

FIGURE 2–215B. Post-Radiation Dysplasia.

In true post-radiation dysplasia (Fig. 2–215A), coarsely granular chromatin and a syncytial arrangement of cells suggest CIS. In Figure 2–215B, hyperchromatic nuclei and relatively copious cytoplasm are consistent with CIN II. Colposcopic biopsy of a CIN III equivalent lesion shows a loss of polarity, nuclear pleomorphism, and mitotic activity (Fig. 2–215C).

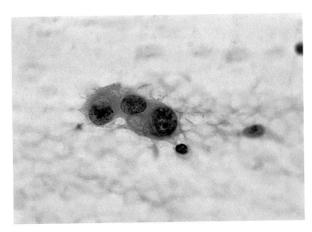

FIGURE 2–216A. Metastatic Breast Carcinoma (× 1000).

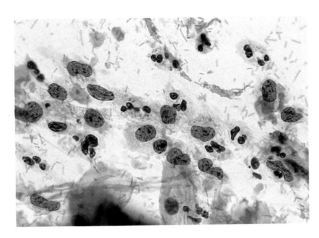

FIGURE 2–216C. Histiocytes (× 1000).

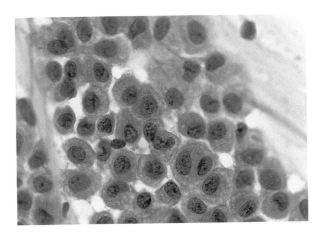

FIGURE 2–216B. Superficial Stromal Cells, Cervicovaginal Smear (× 1000).

Cells derived from metastatic breast carcinoma may be seen in Papanicolaou smears but may present some diagnostic difficulty. They may be single or in small clusters (Fig. 2–216A). Their relatively small, eccentric nuclei may suggest endometrial stromal cells (Fig. 2–216B) or histiocytes (Fig. 2–216C). Some nuclei, however, should retain malignant features, such as chromatin coarseness or a prominent nucleus. Even if recognized as malignant, these cells may be mistaken for endometrial carcinoma. A clean background and, most important, a clinical history of breast carcinoma should raise the index of suspicion.

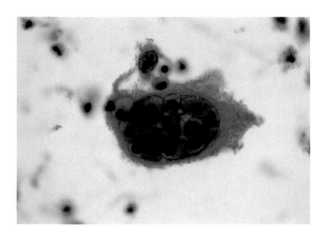

FIGURE 2–217A. Herpes Effect (× 1000).

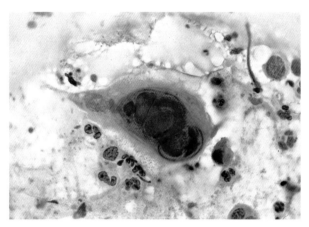

FIGURE 2–217C. Herpes Effect (× 1000).

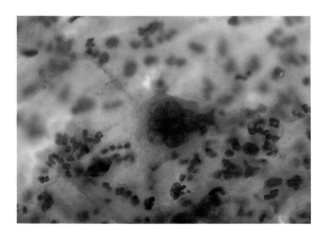

FIGURE 2–217B. Inflammatory Changes (× 1000).

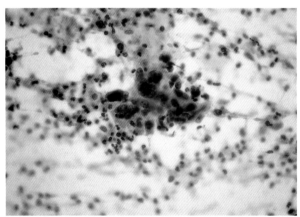

FIGURE 2–217D. Squamous Cell Carcinoma, Cervix (× 400).

Changes characteristic of herpes cytopathic effect are usually easily recognized. Molded, "ground-glass" nuclei may have intranuclear inclusions (Figs. 2–217A, 2–217C); these changes are sufficiently apparent for a firm diagnosis. Occasionally, epithelial cells in inflammatory smears may become multinucleated and mimic herpes (Fig. 2–217B). The lack of distinct molding and internal structure within nuclei, such as discrete nuclei, aids in distinguishing these reactive cells from those of herpes infection. Degenerated, multinucleated cells from cervical squamous cell carcinoma may also resemble herpes effect (Fig. 2–217D), but the remainder of the smear should provide sufficient evidence for the appropriate diagnosis.

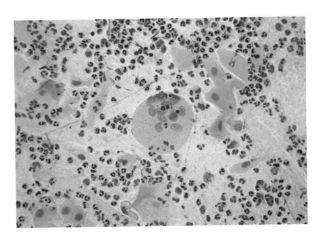

FIGURE 2–218A. Multinucleated Histiocyte, Tuberculous Endometritis (× 400).

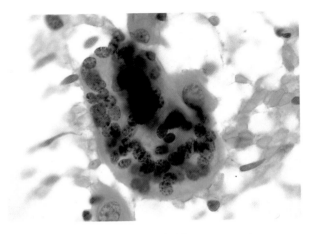

FIGURE 2–218C. Syncytiotrophoblast (× 1000).

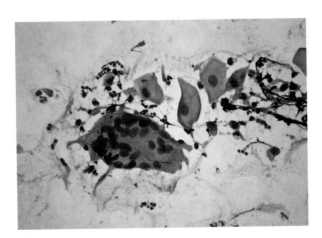

FIGURE 2–218B. Multinucleated Histiocyte, Radiation Reaction (× 400).

Multinucleated histiocytes may be seen in many Papanicolaou smears and are a nonspecific finding. The multinucleated cell seen in the inflammatory background of Figure 2–218A, however, was from a documented case of tuberculous endometritis. Large, multinucleated histiocytes with many nonmolded nuclei are characteristic of the radiation reaction (Fig. 2–218B). The cytoplasm of these histiocytes is usually delicate, light blue, or even finely vacuolated. In contrast, the syncytiotrophoblast (Fig. 2–218C) has a dark blue, denser cytoplasm and numerous overlapping nuclei, which tend to be hyperchromatic.

C·H·A·P·T·E·R

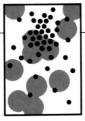

3

RESPIRATORY CYTOLOGY

Jan F. Silverman
Barbara F. Atkinson

SECTION I: STANDARD PULMONARY CYTOLOGY

Respiratory cytopathology involves the evaluation of a variety of specimens, including sputum specimens, bronchial brush and wash, bronchial lavage, transbronchial needle aspiration, and percutaneous pulmonary fine needle aspiration. This chapter is divided into two sections: standard pulmonary cytology is discussed first, followed by needle aspiration cytology. Each of these specimen types has advantages in certain conditions. Pulmonary specimens in general are used to evaluate the following: a lung mass, a suspicious infiltrate, a post-infectious infiltrate that has not resolved, cough with sputum production, presumptive infection in an immunosuppressed patient, and patients with laryngeal tumors. Sputum and bronchoscopy specimens are generally obtained first in the work-up for a central lung mass, and a fine needle aspiration (FNA) is performed when the diagnosis cannot be made by bronchoscopy. However, in peripheral lesions or possible metastases, FNA may be the initial procedure of choice.

The diagnostic yield for each of the specimen types has been variously reported. A very large study reported by Kato and colleagues (1983) found that the success rate for diagnosis of lung cancer was as follows: sputum, 64.5%; bronchial brush, 81.1%; transbronchial biopsy, 84.2%; transbronchial aspiration, 84.2%; and percutaneous FNA, 88.9%. The diagnostic rate from bronchial biopsy specimens was 81.7%. The total percentage of tumors that were diagnosed before treatment was 95.7%. In general, the sensitivity is increased dramatically by the use of multiple specimens.

Each specimen type has specific value and usefulness. Sputum cytology has been used much less frequently in recent years because of the speed with which lung cancer patients undergo a work-up. If the patient is hospitalized, there is generally not enough time to wait for three consecutive morning sputum specimens. However, sputum cytology is easily done on an outpatient basis. At least one sputum sample may be of value, since it may save the time and cost of an extensive diagnostic work-up. Three consecutive sputum samples obtained first thing in the morning have been traditionally considered the ideal procedure. The yield of diagnosing a tumor increases with the number of sputum samples examined (as well as the care taken to examine each specimen). The sputum sample having the best diagnostic yield is one taken after bronchoscopy, and this should be requested after each bronchoscopy. Spontaneous sputum specimens are most effective, although induced sputum specimens can be diagnostic if carefully performed. Abundant sputum production is occasionally a sign of bronchorrhea associated with bronchioloalveolar cell carcinoma. The pneumonic form of bronchioloalveolar cell carcinoma is sometimes readily diagnosed with sputum cytology.

Bronchial brush and wash cytologic procedures are generally done together during bronchoscopy. Bronchial brush has the highest yield for diagnosis of bronchogenic lung cancer whenever there is visualization of the tumor and a direct brush of the lesion. The lesions that are not diagnosed as well by bronchial brushing are peripheral, metastatic, submucosal, and mass lesions extrinsic to the bronchus. Bronchial wash specimens, while generally having a lower diagnostic yield than brushings, are important for diagnosis of peripheral lesions, infections, and bronchioloalveolar cell carcinoma.

Bronchial lavage differs from bronchial wash in that about 100 ml of fluid is used to rinse a lobe of the lung and then aspirated back, whereas in bronchial wash only 25 ml of fluid is used. Bronchial lavage is done for the diagnosis of infections, particularly *Pneumocystis carinii*, the work-up of interstitial lung disease and sarcoidosis, and the treatment of alveolar proteinosis.

In pulmonary specimens, as for all specimen types, optimal preparation is important. Sputum may be prepared in either of two ways. A direct smear can be made and fixed with alcohol. The essential factor in this technique is that the individual preparing the specimen must carefully examine the entire sputum specimen and then pick the most suspicious particles for spreading on the slide. If this is done carefully, the yield is excellent; on the other hand, if there is no selection or evaluation of the mucus, the yield is poor. An alternative method is to put the sputum specimen into Saccomanno's carbowax fixative, which is a cell fixative and also a mucolytic agent. After blenderizing and centrifugation, a portion of the specimen is used to make cytospin preparations. This is the procedure of choice in some laboratories because it is safer for the person doing the preparation and there is sampling of the entire specimen.

Bronchial brushes are smeared directly on the slide and fixed immediately in alcohol. It is important that the brush be smeared quickly on only a small area of the slide and then fixed. Bronchial wash and lavage specimens are sent to the laboratory fresh and may be fixed in carbowax or alcohol and treated in the same way as a sputum specimen. If special stains are needed, additional cytospins can be prepared. Ancillary studies, such as flow cytometry and electron microscopy, can be performed on lavage and wash specimens. Fine needle aspirations are discussed in Section II.

NORMAL COMPONENTS OF PULMONARY CYTOLOGY

An essential assessment for all pulmonary specimens is whether there has been an adequate sampling of the lung (Fig. 3–1). The criterion generally used for sputum cytology is the presence of alveolar macrophages (Fig. 3–2). For bronchial brush and wash specimens, ciliated columnar and mucous goblet cells and alveolar macrophages should be identified. If these cells are not found, the specimen should be categorized as unsatisfactory because of the absence of sufficient pulmonary material.

The normal cell population includes ciliated columnar cells, mucous goblet cells, basal reserve cells, macrophages, and inflammatory cells. Ciliated columnar cells have a columnar shape, cilia, and a terminal bar (Fig. 3–1). The nucleus is eccentrically located with a small, triangular, basally placed tail of cytoplasm. Goblet cells have eccentrically oriented nuclei and either clear cytoplasm or pinkish mucinous vacuoles. Basal reserve cells are seen either attached to a strip of ciliated columnar cells or as a honeycomb group of small cells with scant cytoplasm (Fig. 3–4). Occasionally, these cells may resemble those of small-cell anaplastic carcinoma but maintain a honeycomb arrangement with no loss of polarity (see Fig. 3–38E). Although basal reserve cells have a relatively high nuclear to cytoplasmic ratio, there is no evidence of nuclear molding. Alveolar macrophages characteristically have one or more small nuclei and abundant cytoplasm. Pulmonary macrophages are more easily identified with anthracotic pigment, as seen in the cytoplasm. A variety of inflammatory cells are common, including polymorphonuclear leukocytes, eosinophils, lymphocytes, and monocytes. Occasionally, Type II cells can be recognized in bronchial wash or lavage specimens (Fig. 3–5). These cells are generally round and have a dense or foamy cytoplasm, medium-sized nucleus, and prominent nucleoli. They generally have a very benign appearance and are single. Squamous cells are often seen in sputum specimens and are occasionally seen in other bronchial specimens. If single superficial or intermediate cells are present, they generally represent oral contamination. Squamous metaplasia of the bronchus is characterized by groups of squamous cells having a higher nuclear to cytoplasmic ratio than in mature squamous cells. The cells are similar in size to squamous metaplasia in the cervix (Figs. 2–13 and 3–3).

INFLAMMATORY AND INFECTIOUS CONDITIONS

A variety of changes can be identified in association with inflammatory conditions. Curschmann spirals are mucous casts of bronchioles and may be seen in a variety of conditions, including chronic bronchitis and asthma (Fig. 3–6B). Eosinophils and Charcot-Leyden crystals may be seen in the sputum of patients with asthma (Fig. 3–7). Asbestos (ferruginous) bodies may be seen in patients who have been exposed to asbestos (Fig. 3–6A). Occasionally, an individual who has had only an environmental exposure will have an asbestos body in a pulmonary specimen. Asbestos bodies should be noted in the cytology report because of the increased incidence of pulmonary tumors and mesothelioma in occupationally exposed individuals. A detailed environmental and occupational history should also be obtained.

Specimens from patients with aspiration pneumonia may contain fragments of vegetable material or skeletal muscle (Fig. 3–8). In a sputum sample, this indicates oral contamination, but in a bronchial wash specimen, it requires additional history, since it may represent aspiration.

Pulmonary infarction is a frequent cause of false-positive pulmonary cytology readings. The specimens may contain necrotic debris with degenerating and regenerative cells. Cytologic features of repair include sheets of cells having prominent nucleoli, vesicular chromatin pattern, and abundant cytoplasm.

Peribronchial granuloma is a feature of sarcoidosis. Occasionally, bronchial brush specimens contain epithelioid cells and multinucleated giant cells (Fig. 3–15). Bronchial lavage specimens for sarcoidosis generally demonstrate numerous macrophages and an increased number of lymphocytes. Flow cytometry may be useful on these lavage specimens to measure the ratio of T-helper lymphocytes to T-suppressor cells and the ratio of lymphocytes to alveolar macrophages.

Bronchoalveolar lavage specimens from patients with alveolar proteinosis reveal relatively few cells, some macrophages, and an occasional Type II cell. The surfactant-like material that fills the alveolar space looks pinkish and foamy and may mimic the appearance of the alveolar exudate associated with *Pneumocystis* pneumonia.

Chemotherapy and radiation cause changes in the lung similar to those at other sites. Chemotherapeutic atypia is most commonly seen in patients who have been treated with busulfan (Myleran) or bleomycin. Usually single cells, which are increased in size, are shed (Fig. 3–37B). They often have a slightly higher than normal nuclear to cytoplasmic ratio and a hyperchromatic degenerative nuclear chromatin associated with abundant cytoplasm. Because atypical cells from treatment are rarely in groups, this is a helpful feature in distinguishing them from carcinoma. Radiation therapy causes repair-like sheets and atypical cells to appear (Fig. 3–36B). Follow-up bronchial brushing of patients irradiated for small-cell anaplastic carcinoma is common in cytology specimens. Irradiation effects include cell enlargement, pleomorphism, degeneration, and repair reaction. Although these changes may be worrisome, the cells and groups resemble a large-cell tumor rather than a small-cell carcinoma. However, a large-cell carcinoma can be excluded since intact, nondegenerate cells with malignant criteria are not appreciated.

Pneumocystis carinii pneumonia (PCP) has become a prevalent infection in persons with AIDS and other immunosuppressed patients. Induced sputums may be attempted for a diagnosis of *Pneumocystis*, but the authors have had relatively poor success with this specimen type. Bronchoalveolar lavage is preferred to diagnose PCP. If numerous organisms are present, they can be recognized in the Papanicolaou-stained smears (Fig. 3–9A). The characteristic alveolar exudate is present, and outlines of the cyst can be seen within the exudate. A silver stain such as Grocott can be used to confirm the diagnosis and identify the cysts if only a few are present (Fig. 3–9B). Alternatively, Giemsa or toluidine blue stain is used in some laboratories because they are faster than silver stains and can identify the trophozoites of PCP.

Bacterial infections are generally not diagnosed by cytology. Tuberculosis can only be recognized if acid-fast stains for mycobacteria are used (Fig. 3–15A, B, C). The clinician must suggest the possibility of tuberculosis so the stain can be ordered. Legionnaires' disease can occasionally be diagnosed by Dieterle stain, but this stain is not sensitive and is difficult to read. Immunofluorescent tests are more appropriate. *Nocardia* and *Actinomyces* can be identified, but clinical correlation is important.

Viral diseases with characteristic cellular findings in the lung include cytomegalovirus (CMV) and herpes. CMV is characterized by a very large cell with a single eosinophilic or basophilic inclusion in the nucleus. The large intranuclear inclusion is surrounded by a clear halo, and the nuclear membrane appears dense (Fig. 3–14A). Each cell has only one nucleus (rarely binucleated). The cytopathic effect of herpes is characterized by large multinucleated cells with nuclear molding, a chromatin pattern with an opaque or ground-glass smudged appearance (Fig. 3–14B), and occasionally red intranuclear inclusions. Respiratory syncytial virus may occasionally be identified in specimens from children. This virus produces very large cells with multiple nuclei. Adenovirus does not have a characteristic cytologic appearance but might be suspected when there are normal-sized bronchial epithelial cells with a nucleus that has either a ground-glass appearance or small red reticular inclusions.

Viral pneumonia is associated with a variety of atypical cell changes. "Ciliocytophthoria" is a term used to describe ciliated columnar cells that have split into two parts, the basal portion of the cell with the nucleus and the luminal portion of the cell with the cilia. This is a nonspecific viral change. Patients with viral atypia often shed clusters of partially degenerate ciliated columnar cells that form tight, almost papillary-like, cell balls, known as Creola bodies (Fig. 3–16). These are sometimes suspicious for adenocarcinoma. It is important to look at any ball-like arrangement of cells to see if cilia or a terminal bar can be identified on any cells at the edge of the group (Figs. 3–17, 3–35A). If they are present on one cell, then the entire atypical group is considered reactive but not malignant. Specific viral changes are discussed later.

A variety of fungi are identified in pulmonary specimens. *Aspergillus* has hyphae that are septate and characterized by 45-degree angle branching away from the septation (Fig. 3–10). *Aspergillus* is normally present in the environment, so its presence in a pulmonary specimen does not always indicate infection. Most often, its presence represents an infection that has several forms. Allergic bronchopulmonary aspergillosis is characterized by *Aspergillus* within mucous plugs in the bronchi. *Aspergillus* may grow within a preexisting lung cavity and develop into a fungus ball. Invasive aspergillosis is an extremely serious disease in immunosuppressed patients in whom the organism directly invades tissue. Each type of Aspergillus disease is associated with a different clinical situation and has a different significance; therefore, clinical correlation is important.

Aspergillus infections, particularly fungus balls and allergic broncopulmonary aspergillosis, may be associated with marked bronchial atypia of both glandular and squamous types (Figs. 3–36C, 3–36D). If hyphal fragments are identified or if the patient has a history of aspergillosis, the atypia should be conservatively evaluated so that a false-positive diagnosis of malignancy can be avoided.

The hyphae of *Phycomycetes* are nonseptated and larger than *Aspergillus* and have wavy contours, in contrast to those of *Aspergillus*, which generally are straight with regular cell walls. *Candida* is commonly seen in pulmonary specimens (Figs. 3–11A, 3–11B). It is part of the normal oral flora, so its presence in sputum may not indicate an infection. In immunosuppressed patients, thrush is common, and abundant *Candida* may be observed. This may mask an invasive candidiasis of the lower respiratory tract. The finding of *Candida* in a brush or wash specimen should be reported. *Candida* is usually present as both yeast and pseudohyphae or conidiophores. It occasionally needs to be differentiated from *Aspergillus*. The pseudohyphae of *Candida* are not septated but form several elongated budding structures that mimic septations (Fig. 3–11B). The yeast is seen budding from the septation-like spot on the pseudohyphae (Fig. 3–12A), and this distinguishes *Candida* from *Aspergillus*.

Three other organisms may be identified in the lung as budding yeast. *Histoplasma* is generally smaller than *Candida*, and *Cryptococcus* is usually slightly larger. *Cryptococcus* is characterized by a mucoid capsule, which is sometimes suggested on Papanicolaou smear by a clear zone around the stained organism. A periodic acid–Schiff (PAS) or mucicarmine stain is used to demonstrate the capsule (Fig. 3–13). North American *Blastomyces* has a wide base in contrast to the pinched-off narrow base of *Cryptococcus, Histoplasma,* and *Candida.* Silver stain, such as Grocott, should be used for confirmation.

Coccidioidomycosis is caused by *Coccidioides immitis.* The characteristic structure is a spherule that is much larger than other yeast, measuring approximately 30μ in diameter versus 7 to 10 μ for most yeast. Within the spherule are numerous endospores that become extruded from the spherule (Fig. 3–12B). Silver stain is also appropriate for documenting the morphology of this organism (Fig. 3–12C).

NEOPLASIA OF THE LUNG

Bronchiogenic lung carcinomas and other pulmonary tumors are discussed in detail in Section II. Illustrations of the appearance of the bronchogenic carcinomas as seen in bronchial brush and wash specimens are as follows: squamous cell carcinoma Figures 3–18 to 3–21, adenocarcinoma including bronchioloalveolar cell type, Figures 3–22 to 3–25, large-cell undifferentiated carcinoma, Figures 3–26 to 3–27, and small-cell carcinoma, Figures 3–28 to 3–29. In general, the diagnostic cytologic features of lung carcinoma are the same in exfoliative pulmonary specimens and FNA, but there are a few differences. Squamous cell carcinoma sheds more single cells, and generally the nuclei are more pyknotic and degenerate in sputum and bronchial brush specimens than those seen from needle aspirations (Fig. 3–38C). The tumors tend to appear more highly keratinized. Cells of small-cell anaplastic carcinoma may be smaller and more degenerate in sputum specimens and bronchial washings than in FNA and bronchial brush samples. They may also be more dispersed and therefore more difficult to identify. All cells tend to round up more in sputum so that squamous cell carcinoma may be more easily mistaken for adenocarcinoma in sputum and bronchial lavage or wash specimens.

Two diagnoses that can sometimes be made by brush but not by FNA are squamous cell dysplasia and carcinoma in situ, which must be differentiated from squamous metaplasia and from invasive squamous cell carcinoma. Squamous cell dysplasia and carcinoma in situ are often present as single cells with enlarged, irregular, and atypical nuclei. Progressive degrees of atypia, from minimal dysplasia to marked dysplasia and carcinoma in situ, may be seen similar to the progression seen with cervical intraepithelial neoplasia, but it is less important to identify progressive separations because all are significant and deserve additional work-up. Cells of precursor lesions of the bronchus are usually keratinized. The nuclei are usually quite hyperchromatic and irregular and the nuclear to cytoplasmic ratio is increased. Sheets of abnormal keratinized cells are sometimes seen, but the nuclear abnormalities and pleomorphism are less than that seen in squamous cell carcinoma (Fig. 3–18). Individuals who have been heavy smokers often have multiple squamous lesions of various stages throughout their tracheobronchial tract; therefore, an in situ squamous lesion may be present in one area and a tumor of another type may be present in a different focus.

The bronchial adenoma tumors are sometimes diagnosed by bronchial brushes. These tumors are all malignant but usually are clinically less aggressive than bronchogenic carcinomas. This group includes carcinoid tumor (Figure 3–30), mucoepedermoid carcinoma (Figure 3–31A and 3–31B), and adenoid, cystic carcinoma. These tumors are discussed in Section II.

Metastatic carcinoma should be suspected whenever there is a history of a previous malignancy or multiple lesions are present on the chest radiograph. Needle aspiration is generally the diagnostic method of choice because most metastases to the lung do not penetrate a bronchus and are not diagnosed well by standard specimen types. Intrabronchial metastases may occur from a variety of primary tumors. The most common include renal cell carcinoma (Fig. 3–35C), breast carcinoma, and malignant melanoma (Fig. 3–32). If large tissue fragments are present, the possibility of metastatic tumor should be suspected (Figs. 3–33A, 3–33B). Occasionally, the clue that a malignancy is metastatic is that it does not look like any of the usual primary bronchogenic carcinomas. In general, most metastases to the bronchus are adenocarcinomas and cytologically identical to bronchogenic adenocarcinoma, so a metastasis may not be suspected unless clinical history indicates a previous primary tumor or presentation suggests this possibility. Occasionally metastatic adenocarcinoma, such as from the breast, may not be as pleomorphic as a usual bronchogenic carcinoma.

SECTION II: RESPIRATORY FINE NEEDLE ASPIRATION CYTOLOGY

Although percutaneous needle aspiration of the lung was first utilized in the nineteenth century to diagnose pneumonia, it was not until the recent improvement in radiologic techniques and the fine needle aspiration (FNA) biopsy procedure that it became a popular tool to diagnose neoplastic, infectious, and inflammatory pulmonary diseases. The FNA lung procedure consists of positioning the patient so that the lesion closest to the chest wall is facing upward. The effect of respiration on the nodule's movement can be seen by fluoroscopic examination. The depth needed for the needle's penetration is estimated, and this measurement is transferred to the biopsy needle, at which point the needle is clasped with a rubber-tipped forceps. A cradle x-ray tabletop or biplane fluoroscopy facilitates accurate needle placement. The skin surface is cleansed with povidone-iodine (Betadine), and local anesthesia is injected into the skin, followed by a small skin stab wound.

A 22-gauge (0.6-mm) biopsy needle held by the rubber-tipped forceps at the estimated depth is then guided into the lesion in a direction parallel to the x-ray beam. The needle is positioned so that its tip and hub are superimposed on each other and on the target. Occasionally, the needle must be angled to avoid skeletal interference. If possible, a puncture is performed above the rib in order to avoid the intercostal artery. There is less chance of pneumothorax if both pleural surfaces are penetrated with one motion and the fissures are not crossed. Often, a gritty sensation is transposed to the needle tip when the nodule is entered. One can usually prove accurate placement if the needle tip stays with the nodule on rotation of the cradle top or if the nodule moves when the needle hub is moved. Sometimes a lateral projection film is necessary to document the needle tip position.

When the needle point has been placed in the desired position, the stylet is removed, a 20-ml syringe is attached, and the needle is moved to-and-fro, with suction applied while keeping the needle within the lesion. The vacuum is released before the removal of the needle, and both the needle and syringe are withdrawn. The syringe is then detached from the needle, filled with air, and reattached, and the needle contents are expressed onto the center of a sterile frosted-end glass slide. An assistant usually helps prepare the slides.

The aspirated material is expressed onto slides and pressed with another slide, in a manner similar to the preparation of a bone marrow aspirate. Approximately half the smears are immediately wet-fixed by spraying with 95% ethyl alcohol or placed in alcohol-filled Coplin jars for subsequent Papanicolaou staining. The remaining smears are air-dried and stained by a modified rapid Wright stain (Diff-Quik, available from Harleco, Gibbstown, NJ). From each separate pass, two air-dried smears are chosen for rapid Diff-Quik staining, which can be performed within 30 seconds and therefore lends itself to a "quick read" of the material. Immediate interpretation of the FNA biopsy determines the adequacy of the specimen and can often give an accurate assessment similar to a frozen-section diagnosis in most cases. In addition, if an unusual pulmonary lesion is encountered, additional specimens can be obtained for adjunct studies such as electron microscopy (EM), immunocytochemistry, flow cytometry (FCM), cytogenetics, and microbiologic examination. Immediate interpretation can also decrease the pneumothorax rate since unnecessary additional aspirates can be avoided if diagnostic material is appreciated in the initial specimens with the quick-read cytopathologic evaluation.

A number of needles are available for pulmonary FNA biopsy, including 22- or 23-gauge Chiba needles measuring 15 or 20 cm in length. A coaxial system using an outer 19-gauge Greene needle with an inner 22- or 23-gauge aspirating needle is preferred by some, since multiple specimens can be obtained with only one puncture of the pleura. The Rotex biopsy screw needle has also been employed by some investigators. Transbronchial FNA biopsy (Wang biopsy) is used to evaluate submucosal lesions and peribronchial and/or tracheal lymph nodes. Fine needle aspiration biopsy can also be done using other types of radiologic imaging including computed tomography (CT) and ultrasound. The latter procedure is best for pleural-based lesions.

The main indication for transthoracic FNA biopsy is evaluation of a localized pulmonary nodule undiagnosed by conventional exfoliative respiratory cytologic procedures. Fine needle aspiration biopsy is especially useful in specific clinical situations including the following:

1. Preoperative diagnosis of a small peripheral lung nodule.
2. Diagnosis of inoperable or metastatic malignancies.
3. Diagnosis of small-cell carcinoma, best treated with chemotherapy and/or irradiation.
4. Diagnosis of infectious processes, especially in immunocompromised patients.
5. Diagnosis of complex diffuse pulmonary diseases of unknown etiology not diagnosed by other techniques.

Contraindications to FNA include uncooperative patients; those with severe recent hemoptysis, bleeding diathesis, severe pulmonary hypertension, or vascular lesions (e.g., aneurysm, pulmonary arteriovenous malformation, or pulmonary varix); severely debilitated patients, especially those having chronic obstructive pulmonary disease (COPD) with Po_2 under 60 mm Hg or less than 50% predicted outflow; and patients with large bullae or only one functioning lung and pulmonary hydatid cyst (e.g., from *Echinococcus*) because of the possible release of antigenic cyst fluid that could result in anaphylaxis.

Complications of pulmonary FNA biopsy include pneumothorax, pulmonary hemorrhage with hemoptysis, air embolism, needle tract seeding of tumor cells, and death. Except for pneumothorax and hemoptysis, the other complications are quite rare. Pneumothorax is the most common complication of percutaneous transthoracic FNA biopsy, occurring in 5 to 50% or more of patients; its average incidence is approximately 25%. Fortunately, most pneumothoraces are minor and require no treatment. However, in 4 to 10% of lung FNAs, chest tube insertion is needed to treat a symptomatic or large pneumothorax. The incidence of pneumothorax decreases with the experience of the operator and the necessity of fewer passes, accomplished by immediate assessment of each pass, as discussed above. However, some current reports note a higher pneumothorax rate during the aspiration of smaller and more challenging lesions that may require more needle passes for successful sampling.

The main value of pulmonary FNA biopsy is in the diagnosis of malignancy. It has an accuracy rate of 80 to 95% in most series. The procedure has a false-negative rate of between 7 and 10% and a false-positive rate between 1 and 2%. Conflicting results on the accuracy of tumor classification based on correlating the cytology with the surgical pathology have been reported. However, small-cell undifferentiated carcinoma is most accurately identified in most series. Recently, there has been renewed interest in the diagnosis of infectious and inflammatory pulmonary diseases by FNA biopsy, coinciding with the AIDS epidemic and an increased number of immunosuppressed patients having opportunistic infections secondary to chemotherapy or irradiation.

NORMAL CYTOLOGY

The normal cytologic elements seen in pulmonary FNA biopsies are identical to those described in detail in the section on exfoliative respiratory cytology. The cellular elements include benign bronchial epithelial cells consisting of columnar, goblet, and reserve cells, along with alveolar macrophages and occasional benign hematopoietic cells (Fig. 3–39). Benign mesothelial cells are often seen in FNA biopsies. Mesothelial cells are usually arranged in sheet-like groupings and consist of cells having uniform nuclei with small nucleoli and occasional nuclear grooves and surrounding pale, well-defined cytoplasm (Fig. 3–40). In rare instances, mesenchymal cells such as smooth muscle cells, fibroblasts, adipocytes, mesothelial cells, and chondrocytes can be seen in FNA biopsies.

NON-NEOPLASTIC CONDITIONS

Fine needle aspiration of the lung was first utilized by Leyden in 1883 to diagnose pneumonia. Table 3–1 lists the infectious and inflammatory pulmonary lesions that can be sampled by FNA biopsy. Lung abscesses consist of tannish yellow or green, semisolid purulent material that cytologically demonstrates sheets of neutrophils, many of which are undergoing liquefactive necrosis, along with necrotic cells, cell debris, fibrin, and histiocytes. In some cases, bacteria are identified in the Diff-Quik–stained smears, both within the cytoplasm of histiocytes and occasional neutrophils and in the background (Fig. 3–41). The major differential diagnosis to be considered is squamous cell carcinoma of the lung undergoing cavitation with extensive necrosis and acute inflammation, which can both radiologically and cytologically simulate a lung abscess. The smears of "carcinomatous abscess" demonstrate an intense acute inflammatory cell exudate with an occasional foreign body reaction to the keratinous material. In some cases of squamous cell carcinoma of the lung associated with extensive acute inflammation, only a few diagnostic dysplastic or malignant cells are present. Subtle clues for the presence of squamous cell carcinoma include keratinous fragments and ghost cells. The diagnosis is much more challenging in the Diff-Quik–stained smears because the cytoplasmic orangophilia seen in Papanicolaou-stained smears is not present (Fig. 3–43). The diagnosis should be suspected when irregular cells having pyknotic nuclei and dense cytoplasm with sharp borders are found.

Fine needle aspiration cytology of granulomatous lesions demonstrates clusters of epithelioid histiocytes with elongated or bent nuclei and surrounding amphophilic cytoplasm (Figs. 3–44 and 3–45). Diagnostic considerations include sarcoid, tuberculosis, and fungal diseases. Multinucleated histiocytes may be present, which by itself is a nonspecific feature. Morphologic features of a number of fungi appreciated in FNA biopsy have been detailed in an earlier section of this chapter. Cryptococcosis, histoplasmosis, aspergillosis, coccidioidomycosis, and phycomycosis are the most common pulmonary fungal infections (Figs. 3–45 and 3–46) (Table 3–2). Tuberculosis and some fungal infections, such as histoplasmosis, may cytologically have a background of caseating necrosis consisting of finely grained necrotic material with a few scattered epithelioid cells, multinucleated Langhans giant cells, and occasional small calcified fragments (Figs. 3–47 to 3–49). Special stains for organisms, such as Gomori methenamine silver (GMS) for fungi and acid-fast bacilli (AFB) stain for mycobacterium, are crucial, along with culture of the aspirated material (Fig. 3–50).

Although bronchoalveolar lavage is the procedure of choice for the diagnosis of PCP, occasional cases have an atypical presentation with cavitary or nodular lesions. The cysts of *P. carinii* can be identified by cyst wall stains, including GMS, Gram-Weigert, Grocott, PAS, and toluidine blue. Trophozoites are best seen with cresyl violet, Diff-Quik, Giemsa, May-Grunwald-Giemsa, PAS, and Wright-Giemsa stains. Recently, immunofluorescence and immunoperoxidase stains or hybridization probes have been used to diagnose PCP.

Other organisms appreciated in FNA biopsy include parasites such as *Echinococcus*, amoeba, lung flukes, and such viruses as herpes simplex and cytomegalovirus. Differential diagnosis of viral infections includes reactive alveolar cells, drug reactions, repair, or malignancy due to the misinterpretation of the intranuclear viral inclusions for large nucleoli of reactive or neoplastic cells. In any infectious or inflammatory process, inflammatory atypia of epithelial cells, fibroblasts, and histiocytes can be a potential source of a false-positive diagnosis of malignancy. Diagnostic features in favor of an inflammatory or infectious process include cytologic evidence of inflammation or specific organisms and the presence of only a limited number of atypical cells suggesting "malignant" cytologic features. In general, the atypical cells are also poorly preserved or degenerating. Metaplastic cells in cavitary lesions (e.g., tuberculosis or aspergilloma) can also be mistaken for malignant cells. However, the squamous metaplastic cells should maintain a low nuclear cytoplasmic ratio even though there may be nuclear atypia including irregular, clumped chromatin and occasionally large nucleoli. Regeneration and repair found in aspirated material show features similar to those seen in exfoliative respiratory cytology (Fig. 3–51). Degenerating histiocytes may have atypical features, including nuclear hyperchromasia and nucleoli. An important differential diagnosis includes adenocarcinoma due to the vacuolated pale foamy nature of the histiocyte's cytoplasm. Diagnostic histiocytic features include eccentric, reniform nuclei with a lower nuclear to cytoplasmic ratio than in adenocarcinoma. Bronchioloalveolar cell carcinoma is the most common malignancy confused with atypical degenerating histiocytes.

Frequently, patients who have had prior irradiation and/or chemotherapy have a lung aspiration performed to evaluate a new lesion. A false-positive diagnosis of malignancy is possible in these patients because of the presence of atypical cells either of pulmonary epithelial origin or from the mesothelium. Helpful features to suggest a correct diagnosis of chemotherapeutic or irradiation changes include atypical cells having large hyperchromatic irregular nuclei that show a degenerative or smudged quality to the chromatin (Figs. 3–52 to 3–54). Pulmonary infarct is another uncommonly aspirated lesion that may be a potential cause for a false-positive diagnosis of malignancy because of the presence of atypical benign bronchioloalveolar cells arranged in clusters and squamous metaplastic cells. Differences between epithelial repair and carcinoma are noted in Table 3–3.

Noncellular material that has been seen in FNA biopsies includes ferruginous bodies, corpora amylacea, calcospherites, hemosiderin, silicate crystals (e.g., talc), and amyloid (Fig. 3–55). Cytologic features of aspiration pneumonia have also been described in which abundant foreign material consistent with vegetable matter was appreciated. The plant origin of these structures was suggested from the angulated shape and thick refractile cell wall with numerous internal basophilic round bodies consistent with storage vacuoles. Differential diagnosis of vegetable material includes fungi and malignant cells. The cytologic features of primary pulmonary neoplasms are shown in Table 3–4.

LUNG TUMORS

Squamous Cell Carcinoma

Squamous cell carcinoma consists of occasional aggregates and sheets of malignant cells along with numerous single cells (Figs. 3–56 and 3–57). In moderately or well-differentiated squamous cell carcinoma, the malignant cells are pleomorphic and show evidence of cytoplasmic keratinization (orangophilia) or Herxheimer spirals (Fig. 3–58). The nuclei and cytoplasm show considerable variation in size and shape, and spindle and tadpole cells are present. Pearl formation and intercellular bridges along with concentric cytoplasmic keratin rings may be seen in some of the cells. In more poorly differentiated carcinomas, the cells have a cyanophilic cytoplasm (Fig. 3–59). The major differential diagnosis in these cases includes the intermediate type of small-cell carcinoma and large-cell carcinoma. Syncytial groups of malignant cells with spindle-shaped malignant cells at the periphery are a feature of squamous cell carcinoma (Fig. 3–60). Although prominent nucleoli are not a feature of small cell carcinoma, they are present in poorly differentiated squamous cell carcinoma and large-cell carcinoma. In general, squamous cell carcinoma has coarsely granular, irregularly distributed chromatin along with other nuclei taking on a opaque India ink appearance. A prominent tumor diathesis is usually present (Fig. 3–61). Some cases of squamous cell carcinoma have associated acute inflammation and foreign body reaction, as previously discussed (Fig. 3–62). Lastly, regeneration and repair may also enter into the differential diagnosis. A repair reaction is characterized by a sheet-like arrangement of cells that have enlarged nuclei with a vesicular chromatin pattern and prominent nucleoli. There is no loss of polarity in a repair reaction, and the cells are not arranged in a syncytial fashion.

Adenocarcinoma

The malignant cells are generally arranged in three-dimensional ball-like clusters, acinar groupings, or side-by-side (Figs. 3–63 to 3–67). The cells can have a columnar, cuboidal, or round shape, and intracytoplasmic vacuoles or nuclear molding may be present. Occasionally, the cells are aligned to form a luminal border. In more poorly differentiated adenocarcinomas, the malignant cells have a syncytial arrangement (Figs. 3–68 and 3–69). The cells demonstrate an increased nuclear to cytoplasmic ratio with nuclei having an oval to round shape with irregularly distributed, finely granular chromatin and prominent nucleoli. Basophilic cytoplasm with fine or coarse vacuolization may be seen. A necrotic or clear background may be present in adenocarcinoma. Bronchioloalveolar cell carcinoma, a subtype of adenocarcinoma, demonstrates papillary groupings that generally show uniform malignant cells having prominent depth of focus with a lack of significant nuclear molding (Fig. 3–70). Other features of bronchioloalveolar cell carcinoma include cells showing features of atypical alveolar macrophages and bronchial lining cells (Fig. 3–71). Occasionally, malignant cells are arranged along alveolar septae and possess hobnail-shaped nuclei (Figs. 3–72 and 3–73). These septal arrangements are only seen in aspirates and not in bronchoscopy specimens. Although psammoma bodies or optically clear nuclei are occasionally present in conventional adenocarcinoma, they are more characteristic of this subtype of adenocarcinoma (Figs. 3–74 and 3–75). Examination by electron microscopy (EM) usually demonstrates ultrastructural features of Clara cells or, rarely, Type II cells (Fig. 3–76). The differential diagnosis of pulmonary adenocarcinoma includes entities previously mentioned, including chemotherapy and irradiation effects, viral pneumonitis, pulmonary infarct, and metastatic adenocarcinoma.

Large-Cell Carcinoma

Large-cell carcinoma consists of numerous malignant cells arranged individually and in syncytial groupings (Figs. 3–77 to 3–82). The tumor cells have a markedly increased nuclear to cytoplasmic ratio, with the nuclei having finely to coarsely granular, irregularly distributed chromatin and one or more prominent irregular nucleoli. There is considerable variation in nuclear size and shape, with many very large malignant cells present. Basophilic cytoplasm is seen, but not cytoplasmic keratinization, gland formation, or histochemical evidence of cytoplasmic mucin. Giant cell carcinoma, a subtype of large-cell carcinoma, consists of predominantly individually scattered malignant cells that are multinucleated and often show evidence of neutrophilic cytophagocytosis (see Fig. 3–80). Large-cell carcinoma usually contains abundant necrotic debris in the background. The differential diagnosis of large-cell carcinoma includes poorly differentiated adenocarcinoma, small-cell carcinoma of the intermediate type, and squamous cell carcinoma. In fact, some cases initially classified as large-cell carcinoma from the FNA biopsy or bronchial specimen subsequently are reclassified as another cell type when a more complete examination of the resected tumor is performed. Other diagnostic considerations include metastatic carcinoma, malignant melanoma, and sarcoma. Pertinent clinical information and ancillary studies are often needed to arrive at a correct diagnosis. Immunocytochemistry and EM may be extremely beneficial in making a correct diagnosis of sarcoma and certain metastatic carcinomas, including amelanotic malignant melanoma.

Small-Cell Carcinoma

Small-cell undifferentiated carcinoma consists of numerous small single cells and syncytial groupings of cells with nuclear molding (Figs. 3–83 to 3–88). The nuclei vary from round or oval to irregular shapes. The tumor cells have an extremely high nuclear to cytoplasmic ratio, with a scant amount of indistinct surrounding cytoplasm (see Figs. 3–83 and 3–84). Nuclear chromatin is finely granular, with some clumping and parachromatin clearing. In general, nucleoli are inconspicuous or small. The intermediate type of small-cell carcinoma has slightly larger nuclei with a finely granular chromatin and more cytoplasm. Occasional cases of small-cell carcinoma demonstrate a few scattered larger malignant cells with more abundant cytoplasm and more prominent nucleoli (see Fig. 3–85). Small foci of squamous or glandular differentiation may also be found. When a large-cell component is found in addition to a small-cell carcinoma, both should be diagnosed. The tumor is generally treated as a small-cell carcinoma, but the prognosis is not as good. The background of small-cell carcinoma shows extensive necrotic debris and strands of basophilic material representing extravasated smudged nuclear material (Fig. 3–86). This "crush artifact" is best seen in aspirates.

The differential diagnosis includes benign and malignant lymphoid processes, which in general do not aggregate or demonstrate nuclear molding (Fig. 3–87). Lymphoid lesions also show bluish cytoplasmic fragments called "lymphoglandular bodies" in the background of the Diff-Quik–stained smears. The Diff-Quik stain is also quite useful in demonstrating the hematopoietic nature of these lymphoid cells. However, occasional cases require immunocytochemical or EM studies in order to make a correct diagnosis (Fig. 3–88). Small-cell carcinoma shows cytoplasmic positivity with neuroendocrine markers, including neuron-specific enolase (NSE), whereas non-Hodgkin lymphoma is positive with common hematopoietic markers such as leukocyte common antigen (LCA) and specific B- or T-cell markers. Electron microscopy can demonstrate neurosecretory granules in many cases of small-cell carcinoma.

Other neoplasms entering into the differential diagnosis include poorly differentiated non–small-cell carcinoma and carcinoid tumor. Poorly differentiated non–small-cell carcinomas may occasionally have cells in the size range of small-cell carcinoma, but the nuclear features are diagnostic. Non–small-cell carcinomas have a more vesicular chromatin pattern, with the presence of prominent nucleoli, in contrast to small-cell carcinoma. Generally, at least some of the cells have more cytoplasm than a typical small-cell carcinoma. Carcinoid tumors share similar histogenetic and cytologic features with small-cell carcinomas but consist of a population of neoplastic cells having a more uniform appearance with a lower nuclear to cytoplasmic ratio and more cytoplasm. They lack nuclear molding, significant atypia, and background necrosis.

Carcinoid Tumor

The neoplastic cells are predominantly single, although occasional small sheets and groups can be seen, along with some aggregates demonstrating acinar formation (Fig. 3–89). The tumor cells have uniform round to oval nuclei with evenly distributed, finely granular chromatin and inconspicuous nucleoli. The nuclear to cytoplasmic ratio is relatively high, with a moderate amount of surrounding granular amphophilic to basophilic cytoplasm. In the Diff-Quik stain, the cells of carcinoid tumor take on a somewhat plasmacytoid appearance but lack a perinuclear hof. Immunocytochemical demonstration of neuroendocrine differentiation (e.g., NSE and chromogranin) and ultrastructural evidence of neurosecretory granules are confirmatory but seldom needed. Other unusual bronchial gland tumors that have been diagnosed by pulmonary FNA biopsy include adenoid cystic carcinoma, mucoepidermoid carcinoma, and pleomorphic adenoma.

Pulmonary Hamartoma

Pulmonary hamartoma consists of fibromyxoid fragments having fibroblasts embedded in a fibrillary background, along with fragments of hyaline cartilage, adipocytes, and epithelial cells (Figs. 3–90 and 3–91).

Metastatic Carcinoma

Metastatic carcinoma to the lung is extremely common and must be differentiated from primary lung carcinoma. A known extrapulmonary malignancy and radiologic evidence of multiple nodules are helpful but not always available or definitive. Occasional metastatic carcinomas present as a single lung lesion, and some primary lung malignancies, such as bronchioloalveolar carcinoma, can be multifocal. The cytomorphologic features of certain metastatic carcinomas may suggest the correct diagnosis. Metastatic malignant melanoma is characterized by the presence of numerous bizarre cells arranged individually or in loose aggregates (Figs. 3–92 to 3–95). Tumor cells often have macronucleoli and nuclear cytoplasmic inclusions. Binucleated or multinucleated tumor cells are also seen, along with polygonal and spindle-shaped cells. Intracytoplasmic melanin pigment is diagnostic when present, although malignant melanoma can be suspected when the other cytomorphologic features are appreciated in the absence of melanin. Immunocytochemical staining for S-100 and/or HMB-45 with negative staining for epithelial markers such as cytokeratin (AE1/3) is supportive evidence, as is ultrastructural demonstration of premelanosomes and/or melanosomes. Metastatic renal cell carcinoma consists of loose aggregates of tumor cells, which often demonstrate abundant pale cytoplasm that contains intracytoplasmic glycogen or lipid (Figs. 3–96 and 3–97). In the better-differentiated lesions, the chromatin is finely granular with small nucleoli, whereas poorly differentiated metastatic renal cell carcinoma shows a greater degree of nuclear pleomorphism, hyperchromasia, and prominence of nucleoli.

Tumor cells are often associated and attached to vascularized fragments. Metastatic well-differentiated prostatic carcinoma shows uniform cells arranged in small acinar groupings or individually scattered. Immunoperoxidase stains for prostatic acid phosphatase and prostatic specific antigen can be a helpful adjunctive study. Metastatic breast carcinoma shows varying patterns based on the histologic differentiation of the malignancy or specific subtype (Fig. 3–98). Metastatic ductal carcinomas consist of sheets and clusters of malignant cells that share cytologic features with adenocarcinoma of the lung. Occasional cases of metastatic ductal and lobular carcinoma of the breast have subtle bland cytologic features. Although not specific, immunocytochemical studies for estrogen receptor protein can support the diagnosis of metastatic breast carcinoma from those primary tumors positive for this antigen. Adenocarcinomas from many other sites may share similar cytologic features with lung carcinomas (Figs. 3–99 and 3–100). Comparison with the surgical pathology specimen of the primary tumors is essential for a correct diagnosis. Squamous cell and transitional cell carcinomas of, for example, the cervix, bladder, or esophagus may be indistinguishable from primary lung carcinomas.

Sarcomas

Primary and metastatic sarcoma can involve the lung. Cytologic features are quite variable, depending on the histogenesis of the sarcoma and differentiation of the malignancy. Diagnostic features that suggest a sarcoma include the presence of malignant spindle cells arranged singly or in small groups. Spindle cell sarcomas have cells with hyperchromatic nuclei and surrounding basophilic wispy cytoplasm. Such an appearance can be seen in leiomyosarcoma, fibrosarcoma, malignant schwannoma, and synovial sarcoma (Figs. 3–101 and 3–102). Cytologic clues that may suggest the correct classification include the presence of medium-sized oval or spindle-shaped cells with more pointed nuclei in fibrosarcoma and round epithelioid cells arranged in small clusters or cords in synovial sarcoma. Long spindle-shaped oval cells with blunt cigar-shaped nuclei suggest leiomyosarcoma, and thin, elongated, wavy spindle cells are present in malignant schwannoma. Malignant fibrous histiocytoma can demonstrate a variety of cell types, including spindle-shaped cells, multinucleated pleomorphic giant cells, and undifferentiated mesenchymal cells (Fig. 3–103). Specific cytologic features, such as evidence of lipoblasts, can suggest a correct diagnosis of liposarcoma. Vascular patterns may be seen in angiosarcoma, and the presence of extracellular matrix material such as osteoid in osteosarcoma and cartilage in chondrosarcoma is also a useful finding. Lastly, immunocytochemical and/or EM studies can be quite beneficial in making the correct diagnosis of sarcoma and often allow subclassification when specific diagnostic features are found.

Carcinosarcoma is an unusual neoplasm containing both epithelial groups and bizarre spindle-shaped cells arranged in loose groups and microtissue fragments along with single cells in a dissociative fashion (Fig. 3–104). The malignant cells show dual immunocytochemical staining for cytokeratin and vimentin, which, although typical of this neoplasm, does not allow differentiation from other malignancies, such as large-cell carcinoma, which can also show dual staining (Fig. 3–105).

Lymphoma

Aspirates from non-Hodgkin lymphoma are generally hypercellular and show a uniform population of disassociated, atypical lymphoid cells (Fig. 3–106). The presence of lymphoglandular bodies, a feature of both benign and malignant lymphoid processes, is helpful to distinguish lymphoma and benign lymphoid processes from small-cell carcinoma. In non-Hodgkin's lymphoma, the cytologic features of the malignant lymphoid cells vary depending on the type of lymphoma. Well-differentiated lymphocytic lymphoma consists of a uniform population of small, round lymphocytes, and poorly differentiated lymphocytic lymphoma shows small lymphocytes having irregular nuclear folds or cleavage with the lack of prominent nucleoli. Large-cell lymphoma can be either cleaved or noncleaved. Noncleaved lymphomas often possess prominent nucleoli. Immunoblastic lymphomas have more abundant amphophilic cytoplasm with plasmacytoid features. Lymphoblastic lymphomas consist of a uniform population of intermediate-size cells with irregular or oval nuclei, a finely granular chromatin pattern, and inconspicuous nucleoli.

Hodgkin lymphoma has a polymorphic population of cells, including a variable number of small lymphocytes, eosinophils, neutrophils, histiocytes, and plasma cells. Associated granulomatous fragments may be present. The diagnosis is based on finding diagnostic Reed-Sternberg cells, although mononuclear variant Hodgkin cells may be present.

Mesothelioma

An FNA of mesothelioma arising from the visceral pleura can generate differential diagnoses that include primary lung adenocarcinoma and metastatic malignancy. Radiologic findings of a pleural-based lesion diffusely involving the pleural surface are more supportive of mesothelioma than of lung carcinoma. Epithelial and mixed epithelial-fibrous mesothelioma share cytologic features with metastatic adenocarcinomas of the pleura and peripheral adenocarcinoma of the lung (Fig. 3–107). Immunocytochemistry and EM studies can be helpful in making a correct diagnosis. A panel of immunoperoxidase stains is recommended, with positive staining for CEA, EMA, Leu-M1, and/or B72.3 favoring adenocarcinoma (Fig. 3–108). Both adenocarcinoma and mesotheliomas are AEI/3 positive, and occasional cases of mesothelioma also demonstrate EMA positivity. Ultrastructural evidence of long microvilli would favor a mesothelioma. Often the correct diagnosis is based on the gross involvement of the pleura and more extensive histologic examination.

Bibliography

Bedrossian CWM, Acetta PA, Kelly LV: Cytopathology of non-neoplastic pulmonary disease. Lab Medicine 14:86–95, 1983.

Bonfiglio TA: Cytopathologic Interpretation of Transthoracic Fine Needle Biopsies. New York; Masson Publishing, 1983.

Frable WJ: Thin Needle Aspiration Cytology. Philadelphia: W.B. Saunders, 1983.

Johnston WW, Frable WJ: Diagnostic Respiratory Cytopathology. New York: Masson Publishing, 1979.

Kato H, Konako C, Ono J, et al.: Cytology of the Lung: Techniques and Interpretation. New York: Igaku-Shoin, 1983.

Rosenthal DL: Cytopathology of pulmonary disease. In Wied GL (ed.): Monographs in Clinical Cytology, vol. 11. Basel, Karger, 1988.

Saccomano G: Diagnostic Pulmonary Cytology. Chicago: American Society of Clinical Pathologists, 1978.

Strigle SM, Gal AA: A review of pulmonary cytopathology in the acquired immunodeficiency syndrome. Diagn Cytopathol 5:44–54, 1989.

Tao L-C: Guides to Clinical Aspiration Biopsy: Lung, Pleura and Mediastinum. New York; Igaku-Shoin, 1988.

Young J: Pulmonary Cytopathology. New York; Oxford University Press, 1985.

Table 3–1. NON-NEOPLASTIC PULMONARY LESIONS THAT MIGHT BE SAMPLED BY FNA BIOPSY

Abscess
Granulomatous processes, such as sarcoid and fungi
Pneumocystis carinii (pneumocystoma)
Irradiation- and/or chemotherapy-related abnormalities
Viral infections
Other parasites
Pulmonary infarction
Pseudolymphoma and other inflammatory pseudotumors
Amyloid
Pneumoconiosis
Aspiration pneumonia
Wegener granulomatosis

Table 3–2. CYTOLOGY OF FUNGI

Organism	Features
Blastomyces	8–15 μ; thick refractile walls; single, broad-based budding
Cryptococcus	5–20 μ; narrow-based budding ("tear drop"); mucicarmine positive capsule; crystalloid artifact
Coccidioides immitis	Spherules (>100 μ); endspores (2–5 μ)
Histoplasma	1–5 μ; budding in macrophages, GMS stain needed
Aspergillus	45° branching hyphae; septate; calcium oxalate crystals
Phycomycetes	Nonseptate ribbon-like hyphae with varying width (6–50 μ)

Table 3–3. CYTOLOGIC DIFFERENTIAL DIAGNOSTIC FEATURES
OF EPITHELIAL REPAIR VERSUS MALIGNANCY

Epithelial Repair	Pulmonary Malignancy
Groups of cells	Groups of cells
Few single cells	Many single cells
Flat metaplastic sheets	Syncytial arrangement of cells
Distinct cell borders	Variable cytoplasmic borders
Cellular polarity maintained	Loss of polarity
Enlarged nuclei	Enlarged nuclei
Round or oval nuclei with smooth nuclear membrane	Irregular nuclear borders
Uniform nuclei	Variable nuclei
Vesicular, hypochromatic nuclei, with even chromatin distribution	Opaque to hyperchromatic nuclei with irregular chromatin distribution
Nucleoli	Nucleoli
Normal mitotic figures	Abnormal mitotic figures
No diathesis seen	Clean background or diathesis present

Table 3–4. CYTOLOGIC FEATURES OF PRIMARY PULMONARY NEOPLASMS

Feature	Squamous Cell Carcinoma	Adenocarcinoma	Bronchioloalveolar Cell Carcinoma	Large-Cell Carcinoma	Small-Cell Carcinoma	Carcinoid
Cellular pattern	Sheets, syncytial, isolated cells; little nuclear overlapping	3-D cell balls; acinar or side-by-side septae; single cells, syncytial—poorly differentiated	3-D cell balls or single cells; side-by-side septae	Isolated single cells, syncytial	Single and syncytial, nuclear molding; vertebrae pattern	Single, acini, or sheets; loosely cohesive and isolated cells
Slide background	Necrotic—diathesis, neutrophilic exudate	Clean or diathesis	Clean or diathesis	Diathesis	Diathesis; DNA strands; necrotic cells	Clean
Cytoplasm	Pleomorphic orangeophilic to cyanophilic; dense, glassy, refractile; sharp cytoplasmic borders; keratin rings; spindle shape	Basophilic; lacy, finely and coarsely vacuolated; columnar, cuboidal, or round cells; eccentric nucleus	Basophilic; finely vacuolated; vacuoles increased with Diff-Quik; psammoma bodies	Cyanophilic—poorly defined; can be finely vacuolated; cytophagocytosis	Scant	Oval to cuboidal; basophilic to amphophilic; granular
Nucleus	Coarsely granular and/or opaque chromatin; nucleoli are poorly differentiated; irregular and bizarre shapes	Finely granular irregular chromatin distribution; prominent nucleoli—one or more; nuclear moldings	Round—oval to slightly irregular; lack of cellular and nuclear molding; uniform size and shape; eccentric nuclei; optically clear nuclei	Round to oval shape; finely to coarsely granular chromatin; multinucleated; large prominent nucleoli	Oval to angulated molding; variable size; no large nucleoli or very tiny micronucleoli; dense chromasia	Regular, round to oval; finely granular, even chromatin; small nucleoli

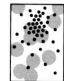

NORMAL CELLS

FIGURE 3–1. Normal Bronchial Cells. In this wash specimen, ciliated columnar cells, mucous goblet cells, and alveolar macrophages can be identified. The cilia and terminal bar are not visible in every columnar cell, but the eccentric nucleus with the cytoplasmic tail is characteristic. The mucous goblet cell has foamy cytoplasm. A large, multinucleated giant cell as well as several smaller alveolar macrophages with pigmented cytoplasm are seen. Bronchial wash, Papanicolaou stain (× 400).

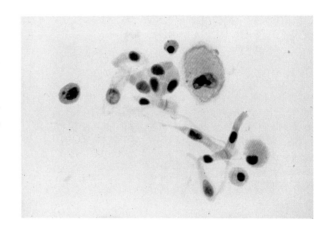

FIGURE 3–2. Satisfactory Sputum. Several squamous cells are present. Even at this low magnification, alveolar macrophages (arrow) can be identified. Sputum and Papanicolaou stain (× 225).

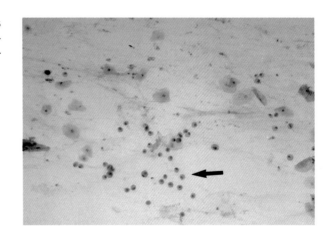

FIGURE 3–3. Squamous Metaplasia. Squamous metaplasia can be recognized when it is in a group such as this. The nuclear to cytoplasmic ratio is greater than for more differentiated squamous cells. The cellular organization and cytoplasm is that of squamous epithelium. Bronchial brush, Papanicolaou stain (× 400).

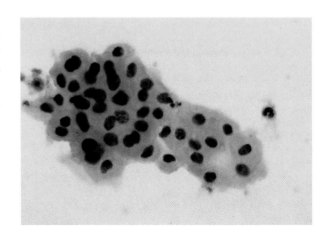

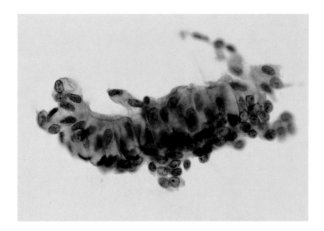

FIGURE 3–4. Columnar Epithelium With Basal Reserve Cells. The organization of the ciliated columnar cells is apparent. The basal reserve cells are the small cells attached at the bottom of the strip. Bronchial brush, Papanicolaou stain (× 400).

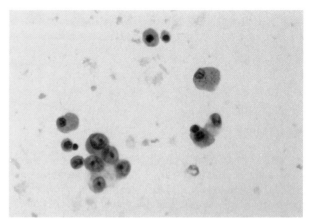

FIGURE 3–5. Alveolar Type II Cell. The cells in the cluster are reactive Type II cells. These were seen in sputum from a 21 year old man with adult respiratory disease syndrome after traumatic injuries in a car accident. These cells can be recognized best when they are clustered. Whenever they are seen, a clinical history must be correlated because in a different clinical situation cells such as this would be suspect for an adenocarcinoma. Sputum, Papanicolaou stain (× 250).

MISCELLANEOUS FINDINGS

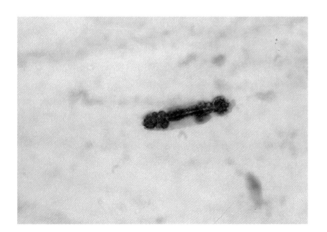

FIGURE 3–6A. Asbestos (Ferruginous) Body. This characteristic coated fiber has been phagocitized by a macrophage. Note the greenish-yellow color of the coating and the knob-like precipitation at the ends of the fiber. Bronchial wash, Papanicolaou stain (× 400).

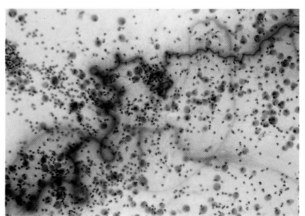

FIGURE 3–6B. Curschmann Spiral. A Curschmann spiral is a mucous cast of a bronchiole. They may be quite large, as seen here, or much smaller. The curly structure is common. They are normal but are seen commonly with asthma and chronic bronchitis. Sputum, Papanicolaou stain (× 160).

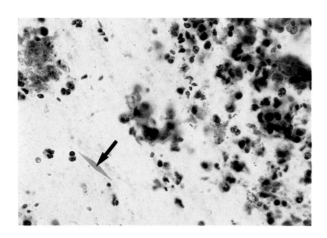

FIGURE 3–7. Charcot-Leyden Crystal. The crystal (arrow) is seen in a background of necrotic debris and inflammatory infiltrate. Degenerate eosinophils are seen. The crystal is precipitated eosinophil granular material. This patient had severe asthma. Bronchial brush, Papanicolaou stain (× 160). (Figure courtesy of Douglas King, C.T. (A.S.C.P.)

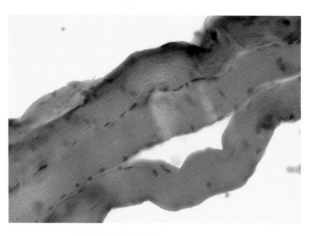

FIGURE 3–8. Striated Muscle. Numerous large fragments of striated muscle are seen here. These were identified in a bronchial wash specimen from a patient with an infiltrate on radiograph. After obtaining a detailed clinical history, it was interpreted as representing an aspirated material, which led to a diagnosis of aspiration pneumonia. Bronchial wash, Papanicolaou stain (× 160).

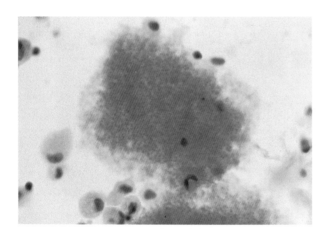

FIGURE 3–9A. Pneumocystis. The foamy alveolar exudate characteristic of massive pneumocystis infection is seen here on a Papanicolaou stain. The pinkish, foamy material is the nonstaining cyst and cell walls. The trophozoites are seen as tiny dots within cystic clear zones. Bronchoalveolar lavage, Papanicolaou stain (× 400). (Courtesy of Carolyn Leach, M.D.)

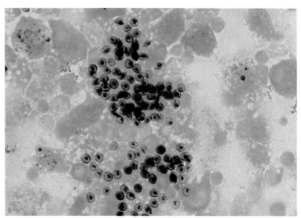

FIGURE 3–9B. Pneumocystis. This is a Grocott silver stain demonstrating the staining of the cyst wall. The intracystic bodies show well in this case and distinguish this specimen from that of a yeast. These are not always seen so well, in which case the cup-like forms and indented shapes are distinctive; a yeast is always round to oval in shape. Bronchoalveolar lavage, Grocott silver stain (× 400).

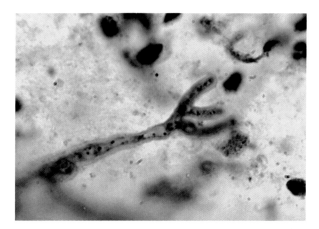

FIGURE 3–10. Aspergillus. Characteristic 45-degree angle budding is present. In the Papanicolaou stain, the speculations do not always show clearly. The cell wall stains greenish blue, and the fungal cell body is well demonstrated, whereas in silver stain the cell wall is stained and the cell body is not seen. Bronchial brush, Papanicolaou stain (× 630).

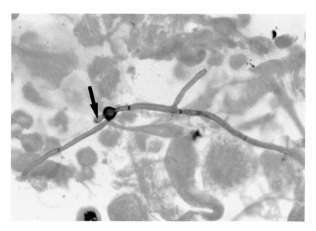

FIGURE 3–11B. Candida. This is a Grocott silver stain of *Candida*. Notice that the organism looks septate but a yeast is seen (arrow). There are pseudohyphae budding from the yeast. The pseudohyphae of *Candida* are subtly smaller than the true hyphal fragments of aspergillus. Bronchial wash, Grocott silver stain (× 400).

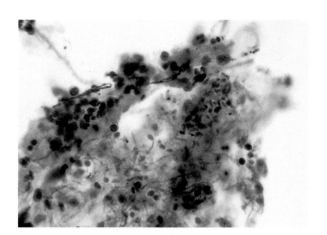

FIGURE 3–11A. Candida. Notice the combination of yeast and pseudohyphal (conidiospore) fragments. This kind of clustering of organisms is typical. Bronchial brush, Papanicolaou stain (× 225).

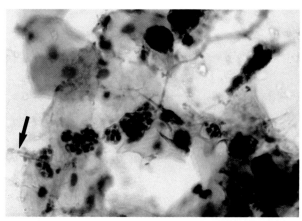

FIGURE 3–12A. Candida. This Papanicolaou stained-smear shows yeast in clusters overlying epithelial cells. The appearance of each cluster mimics a spherule of *Coccidioides immitis*. This artifact is seen when mucous traps the yeast over the surface of epithelial cells; Some pseudohyphal yeast budding is seen (arrow) that distinguishes this specimen from that of Coccidioides. Sputum, Papanicolaou stain (× 225).

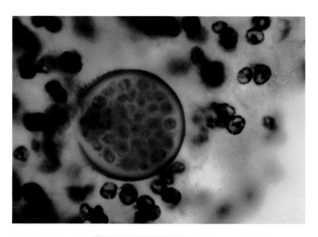

FIGURE 3–12B. Coccidioides immitis. This is a high-power magnification of a spherule of *C. immitis* demonstrating endospores within the spherule. Bronchial wash, Papanicolaou stain (× 1000). (Courtesy of Phillip White, C.T. (A.S.C.P.)

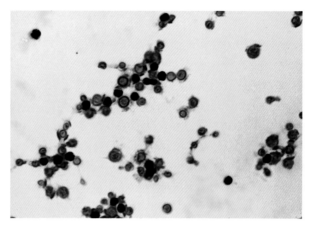

FIGURE 3–13. Cryptococcus. Papanicolaou smear containing *Cryptococcus* with a capsule shrunken against the cell wall of the organism. The organism has a deep eosinophilic color. A few lymphocytes are seen in the background. A mucicarmine or Periodic acid-Schiff stain demonstrates the capsule and differentiates this organism from the other yeast. Bronchial wash, Papanicolaou stain (× 225).

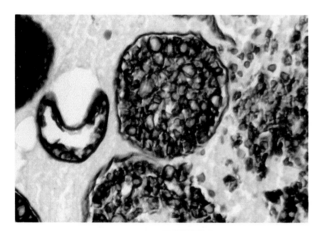

FIGURE 3–12C. Coccidioides immitis. This silver stain demonstrates spherules and endospores. Some spherules have ruptured with release of endospores. Bronchial wash, Grocott stain (× 1000). (Courtesy of Phillip White, C.T. (A.S.C.P.)

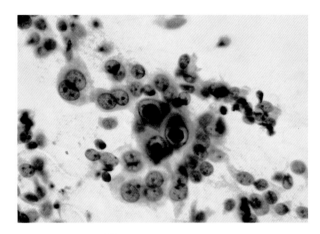

FIGURE 3–14A. Cytomegalovirus. Three cells infected with cytomegalovirus are seen in the center of the field. They each have large, intranuclear basophilic inclusions surrounded by a clear halo. Individually, each of these cells is much larger than the surrounding columnar epithelial cells. Bronchial brush, Papanicolaou stain (× 400).

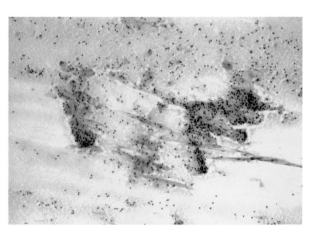

FIGURE 3–15A. Granuloma. This a low-power view of a brush specimen of a granuloma. Even at low magnification, there is a cellular cohesion suggestive of a granuloma. Bronchial brush, Papanicolaou stain (× 160).

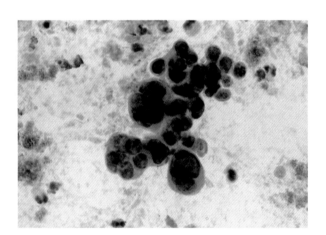

FIGURE 3–14B. Herpes. Several multinucleated giant cells are seen. There is marked nuclear molding and an opaque to ground glass appearance of the nuclear chromatin. Bronchial brush, Papanicolaou stain (× 400).

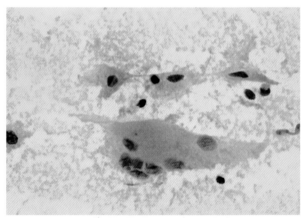

FIGURE 3–15B. Granuloma. This higher-power view of cells from the granuloma shows a multinucleated giant cell as well as several epitheloid cells. The presence of multinucleated cells does not indicate that a granuloma is present, since they may be macrophages, which are common in the lung. Bronchial brush, Papanicolaou stain (× 400).

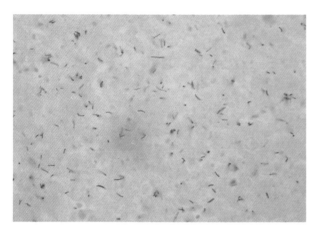

FIGURE 3–15C. This acid-fast stain demonstrates abundant **Mycobacteria**. The organism's size is characteristic, and there is usually a slightly beaded staining quality. Bronchial brush, Ziehl-Nelson stain (× 1000).

ATYPICAL GLANDULAR CELLS

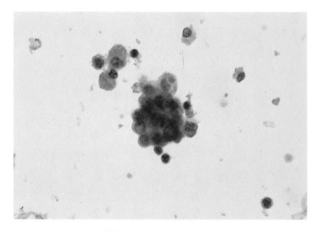

FIGURE 3–16. Creola Body. Tight cellular balls of glandular epithelium can be shed in a variety of benign conditions, such as asthma, chronic bronchitis, and viral pneumonia. These must not be mistaken for adenocarcinoma. If cilia are present at the edges of the group, then the group should be considered benign. Sputum, Papanicolaou stain (× 225).

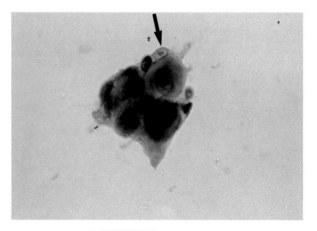

FIGURE 3–17. Atypia from Viral Pneumonia. Notice that within this cell grouping there is marked variation in the size of the nuclei and cells. The clue that this is a benign reactive process is that there is at least one relatively normal columnar cell at an edge (arrow) and that there are very sharp, smooth borders to the larger cells. The cytoplasm is dense, which might represent reactive cytoplasm or squamous metaplasia, but can also be seen in neoplasms. Bronchial brush, Papanicolaou stain (× 400).

SQUAMOUS CARCINOMA

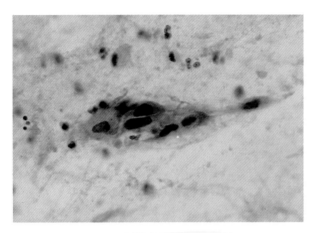

FIGURE 3–18. Squamous Cell Carcinoma. This sheet of highly abnormal keratinized cells indicates (at a minimum) a marked squamous atypia but might have been shed from an invasive squamous cell carcinoma. If cells and groups such as this are the worst seen in this specimen, then the best diagnosis would be cells consistent with either squamous carcinoma in situ or invasive squamous cell carcinoma. Bronchial brush, Papanicolaou stain (× 225).

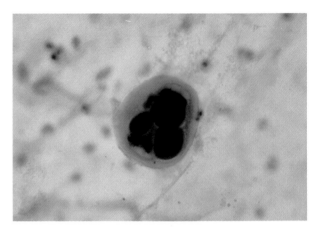

FIGURE 3–20. Squamous Pearl from Squamous Cell Carcinoma. The pearl-like arrangement of one cell surrounding other cells is seen here. All the cells are keratinized, although those in the center have an orangeophilic cytoplasm. The nuclei are highly abnormal, irregular, and hyperchromatic, indicating that this is a malignant pearl. Bronchial brush, Papanicolaou stain (× 400).

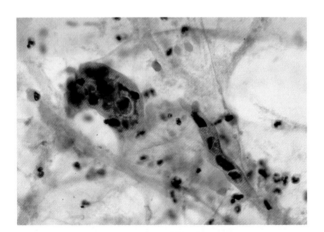

FIGURE 3–19. Squamous Cell Carcinoma. Note the highly keratinized squamous pearl and abnormal squamous cell. The nuclei are very irregular in shape and have a dense, hyperchromatic chromatin pattern. There is necrotic debris in the background, a common feature of keratinized squamous carcinomas. Bronchial brush, Papanicolaou stain (× 225).

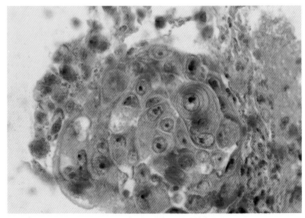

FIGURE 3–21. Squamous Cell Carcinoma. This is a cell block preparation demonstrating intercellular bridges and some pearl formation. Notice that the nuclear chromatin is more vesicular and nucleoli are quite prominent. This type of nucleus is more typical of that in an adenocarcinoma but can be seen in moderately and poorly differentiated squamous cell carcinomas. Bronchial wash cell block, hematoxylin and eosin stain (× 400).

ADENOCARCINOMA

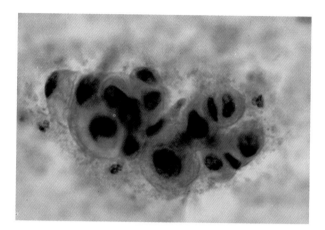

FIGURE 3–22. Adenocarcinoma. This demonstrates a glandular cell grouping. There are nuclei at several planes of focus, and there is vacuolization of the cytoplasm in some of the cells. Bronchial brush, Papanicolaou stain (× 400).

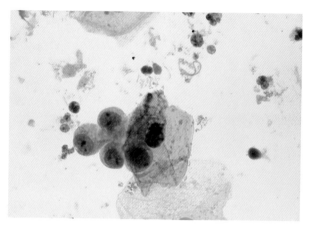

FIGURE 3–24. Bronchioloalveolar Cell Carcinoma. This is a sputum specimen showing a cluster of malignant cells together with normal inflammatory and squamous cells. The malignant cells have a rather bland appearance, which is typical of many bronchioloalveolar cell carcinomas. All the malignant cells are similar to each other. The nuclear to cytoplasmic ratio is not very high, and the nuclear chromatin is not very abnormal. One reason these can be recognized as malignant is that a group such as this does not belong in a sputum specimen. If cells such as these are in a bronchial wash specimen, they might be alveolar Type II cells; however, alveolar Type II cells rarely exfoliate. If they do, they are seen as single cells and not as clusters. A process associated with many reactive Type II cells, such as desquamative interstitial pneumonitis, could be a consideration here, but with an appropriate history of mass or infiltrate, a diagnosis of malignancy can be made. Sputum, Papanicolaou stain (× 400).

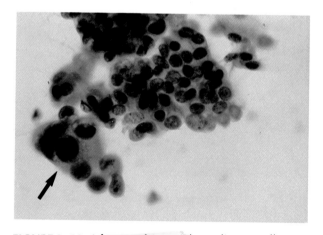

FIGURE 3–23. Adenocarcinoma. The malignant cells seen at the arrow are much larger than the cells in the normal columnar sheet, and the nuclei are several times larger than that of normal cells. The malignant nuclei are also irregularly spaced within their group, and several of the cells have an abnormally high nuclear to cytoplasmic ratio. Bronchial brush, Papanicolaou stain (× 400).

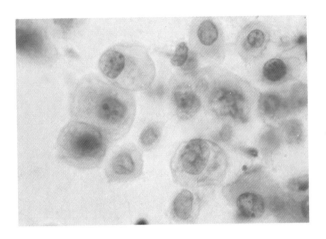

FIGURE 3–25. Bronchioloalveolar Cell Carcinoma. These cells are from a bronchioloalveolar cell carcinoma in a bronchial wash. Notice again how delicate and bland the cells are. In this field the cells are predominately single; however, clusters were also identified elsewhere. There is some variation in the size and shape of the cells and nuclei, and these cells are larger than normal columnar cells. The nuclei are relatively bland, and the nuclear to cytoplasmic ratio is that of normal cells, which often makes the diagnosis of malignancy difficult. A specific diagnosis of bronchioloalveolar cell carcinoma versus adenocarcinoma usually cannot be made without tissue sampling to document alveolar septal growth, but bland uniform cells may suggest this possibility. Bronchial wash, Papanicolaou stain (× 630).

LARGE-CELL CARCINOMA

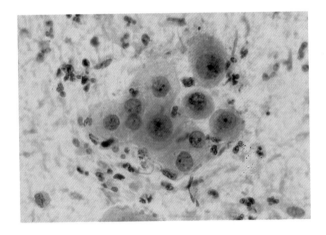

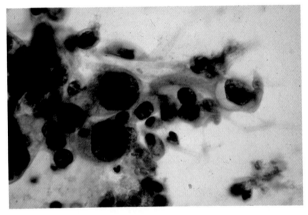

FIGURE 3–26. Large-Cell Undifferentiated Carcinoma. This tumor has no evidence of cytoplasmic differentiation. The cells are arranged in a flat sheet, and the cytoplasm is relatively delicate. The cells have uniform nuclear to cytoplasmic ratios but vary considerably in cell size. They are quite large compared with the polymorphonuclear leukocytes. This raises the possibility that this tumor could be a bronchioloalveolar cell carcinoma; however, without evidence of glandular grouping or mucin, it is not possible to even make a diagnosis of adenocarcinoma. These cells are malignant because of their huge size, as compared with the background benign cellular element. Bronchial brush, Papanicolaou stain (× 400).

FIGURE 3–27. Large-Cell Undifferentiated Carcinoma. These cells have many features of malignancy in contrast to the previous figure. There is marked pleomorphism of cell and nuclear size and abnormal nuclear hyperchromatism. The major difficulty here is classifying these cells appropriately as to tumor type. The dense cytoplasm suggests a squamous carcinoma. There is a hint of a vacuole around one nucleus, which might raise a consideration of an adenocarcinoma, but a flat sheet-like group of cells makes an adenocarcinoma less likely. If there is no definite evidence of keratinization, acinar groupings, or vacuoles, then the malignancy is best classified as a large-cell undifferentiated carcinoma. Bronchial brush, Papanicolaou stain (× 400).

SMALL-CELL CARCINOMA

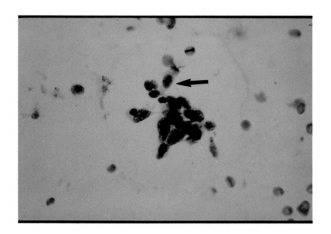

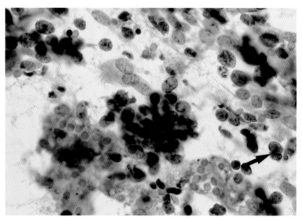

FIGURE 3–28. Small-Cell Anaplastic Carcinoma. A ciliated columnar cell (arrow) can be identified and can be used as a comparison for the other cells in the field. The nuclei of the tumor cells are slightly bigger than the nucleus of this ciliated columnar cell. There is very scant cytoplasm around each of the nuclei, but a definite faint greenish rim can be seen around all of the cells. There is very prominent nuclear molding between cells. This molding is characteristic of the cell groupings of small-cell carcinoma. It can be seen in other epithelial tumors but does not occur in lymphocytes. Bronchial brush, Papanicolaou stain (× 400).

FIGURE 3–29. Small-Cell Carcinoma. Ciliated columnar cells are seen adjacent to a group of tumor cells. The chromatin of the normal ciliated cells is pale and finely granular compared with the hyperchromatic nuclei of the small-cell carcinoma. Again notice the faint rim of cytoplasm around each of the nuclei and the prominent nuclear molding (arrow). A cluster of lymphocytes does not show this type of nuclear molding. Bronchial brush, Papanicolaou stain (× 400).

OTHER TUMORS

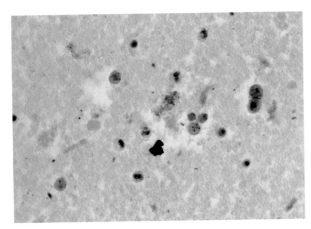

FIGURE 3–30. Carcinoid Tumor. These cells are also relatively small but generally slightly larger than small-cell anaplastic carcinoma. The nuclei are round and without molding, and there are nucleoli present. Nucleoli are not a feature of nuclei of small-cell anaplastic carcinoma, although rarely micronucleoli are seen. Some cells have scant cytoplasm but others have slightly more abundant cytoplasm than do small-cell carcinomas. Carcinoid tumor should always be considered when there are similarities to small-cell anaplastic carcinoma but nucleoli are present and cytoplasm is distinct. Bronchial wash, Papanicolaou stain (× 400).

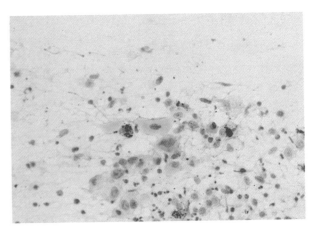

FIGURE 3–31B. Mucoepidermoid Carcinoma. Several highly abnormal squamous cells are seen. In light of the glandular component of A, mucoepidermoid carcinoma or mixed adenosquamous carcinoma are the major considerations. Clinical history, presentation, and correlation with bronchoscopic findings are necessary to arrive at the correct decision between these entities. The components depicted here are both well-differentiated, which is more common with mucoepidermoid tumors. Adenosquamous carcinomas generally are more poorly differentiated. Bronchial brush, Papanicolaou stain (× 225). (Courtesy of Linda Green, M.D.)

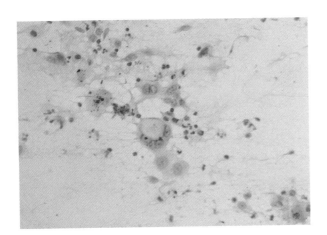

FIGURE 3–31A. Mucoepidermoid Carcinoma. A large, vacuolated cell is visible along with several other atypical cells. Adenocarcinoma would be a consideration but a squamous component is seen in B. Bronchial brush, Papanicolaou stain (× 225). (Figure courtesy of Linda Green, M.D.)

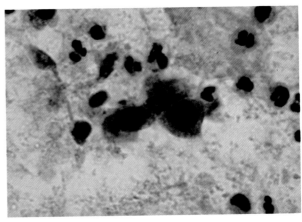

FIGURE 3–32. Malignant Melanoma. Several large, malignant cells can be identified by their highly abnormal nuclei. Pigment in the cytoplasm is very prominent in these cells. The nuclei have very large red nucleoli. This patient presented with pneumonia, and her sputum specimen demonstrated melanoma although she had not had prior history of malignant melanoma. Sputum, Papanicolaou stain (× 225).

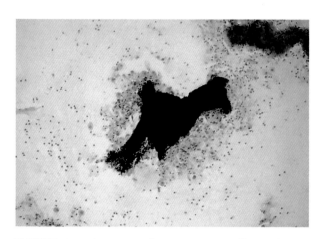

FIGURE 3–33A. Metastatic Squamous Cell Carcinoma from the Cervix. This is a low-power view of a tissue fragment found in a bronchial wash specimen. It is unusual to see whole tissue fragments from a washed or brushed bronchogenic carcinoma. See the next figure for a higher magnification view of the edge of the fragment. Bronchial wash, Papanicolaou stain (× 160).

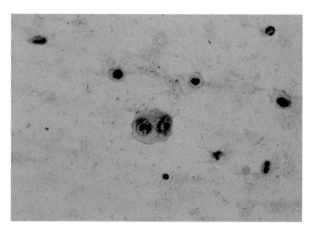

FIGURE 3–34. Hodgkin Lymphoma. This Reed-Sternberg cell was found in a bronchial brush specimen. The differential includes cytomegalovirus infection and adenocarcinoma. Cells of cytomegalovirus are rarely binucleate, therefore, careful examination is necessary to determine whether this is a binucleate single cell or two cells. This cell alone is not enough to diagnose a lymphoma or carcinoma. The next figure includes another cell from this case. Bronchial brush, Papanicolaou stain (× 225).

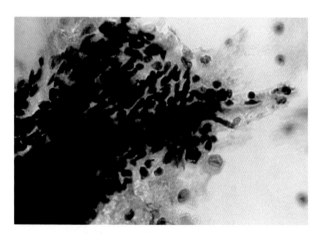

FIGURE 3–33B. Metastatic Squamous Cell Carcinoma from Cervix. This is a higher-power view of the edge of the tissue fragment seen in the previous figure. Notice the elongated spindled nature of many of the nuclei. The chromatin is very hyperchromatic. Nuclear shapes are very abnormal, and cytoplasm is scant. The differential diagnosis includes small-cell anaplastic carcinoma, bronchogenic squamous carcinoma, or other metastatic tumor. This patient had a small-cell carcinoma of the cervix diagnosed 2 years previously, and, on review, the cells were identical to those of the primary tumor. Bronchial wash, Papanicolaou stain (× 225).

DIFFERENTIAL GROUPING

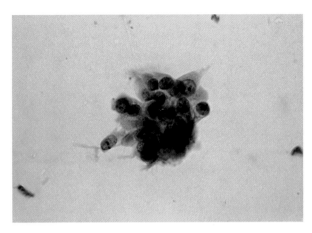

FIGURE 3–35A. Reactive Glandular Atypia from Viral Pneumonia. Notice that the arrangement of cells is glandular, with nuclei overlying each other at different planes of focus. Notice the variation in size of the nuclei within the group and the nuclear hyperchromatism. As you follow the border of the group, it is possible to see a terminal bar, a suggestion of cilia on one of the cells (arrow), and a sharp, flat, outer border on one cell on the opposite edge of the group. These are characteristic of a reactive grouping. A group of cells having any evidence of cilia or a terminal bar should not be diagnosed as malignant. This patient was recovering from a viral pneumonia and had a persistent cough. These symptoms resolved, and the patient had no further evidence of disease. Bronchial brush, Papanicolaou stain (× 225).

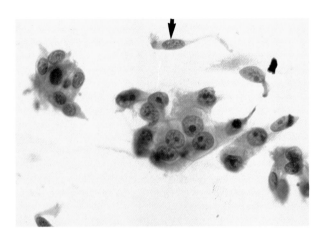

FIGURE 3–35C. Metastatic Renal Cell Carcinoma. The malignant cells are much larger than the normal ciliated cells (arrow). These cells can be readily identified as malignant because of their size, nucleoli, and lack of meaningful organization within the group. Without knowledge of the patient's prior history of renal cell carcinoma, this cell would probably be classified as representing a large-cell undifferentiated carcinoma of the bronchus because there is no evidence of glandular grouping or cytoplasmic vacuolization. Comparison with a patient's previous malignancy is essential, and in this case, comparison revealed similar cells. Bronchial brush (× 400).

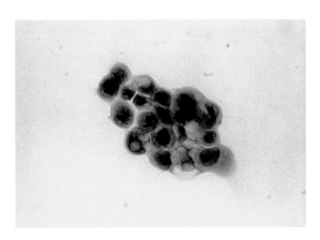

FIGURE 3–35B. Lung Adenocarcinoma. In comparison with the previous figure, there is no evidence of cilia in any of these cells. There is some nuclear crowding and a hint of an acinar arrangement of the cells. Cytoplasmic vacuolization indicates that this is an adenocarcinoma. Bronchial brush, Papanicolaou stain (× 225).

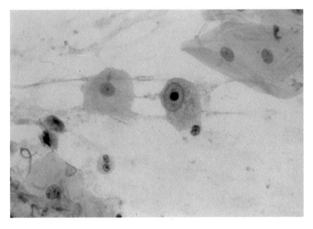

FIGURE 3–35D. Hodgkin Lymphoma. This Reed-Sternberg variant cell has a single nucleus. This cell closely mimics both cytomegalovirus infection and adenocarcinoma. It is not typical for cytomegalovirus because its "inclusion" does not have a surrounding halo. Many similar single cells were present in the smear. They were suspected of being adenocarcinoma because of the nuclear chromatin feature and prominent nucleoli and the delicate, almost foamy cytoplasm. After an extensive search, Reed-Sternberg cells similar to those seen in the previous figure were found. The clinical history supported lymphoma, followed by tissue confirmation. Bronchial wash, brush (× 400).

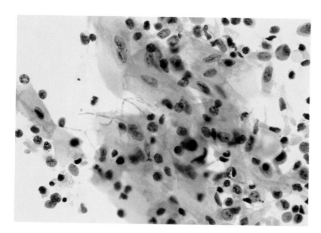

FIGURE 3–36A. Squamous Atypia from Candida. This plaque-like group of squamous cells has degenerated but slightly atypical nuclei. It is important to notice that pseudohyphae of *Candida* are present. As in the cervix, this organism in the mouth or upper airways may be associated with squamous atypia. It is usually not of a degree that the cells are suspect for carcinoma. Bronchial wash, Papanicolaou stain (× 225).

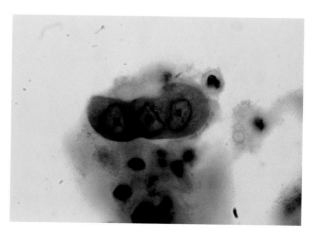

FIGURE 3–36C. Squamous Atypia from Aspergillus. This sheet of highly abnormal cells was obtained from a patient with an aspergillus fungus ball in a cavity. This brush specimen was taken from a bronchus leading to the cavity. The cells here have irregular nuclear shape, very prominent nucleoli, and clear chromatin. If these cells were found on a routine bronchial brush of a patient without a history of aspergillus, the differential would include squamous cell carcinoma, either in situ or invasive. If the patient has a history of a fungus ball, these cells can be diagnosed as representing marked squamous atypia. A biopsy is indicated, since sometimes squamous cell carcinoma is associated with cavitary aspergillus. This cavity was resected, and the bronchus and cavity lining confirmed marked squamous atypia without invasive carcinoma. Bronchial brush, Papanicolaou stain (× 630).

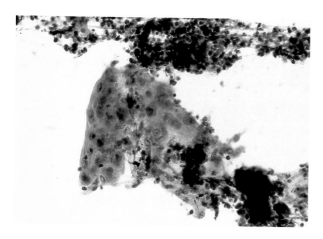

FIGURE 3–36B. Radiation Effect in a Patient Treated for Small-Cell Carcinoma. Note the repair-like appearance of these cells and the necrotic debris in the background. The group is tightly cohesive and has maintained polarity. Individual cells have abundant cytoplasm. This kind of grouping might be suspect for a squamous or large-cell carcinoma but certainly is not compatible with persistent small-cell carcinoma. This is acute radiation atypia and repair. It is important to examine the necrotic debris under high magnification to be sure that small-cell carcinoma is not present. Bronchial brush, Papanicolaou stain (× 225).

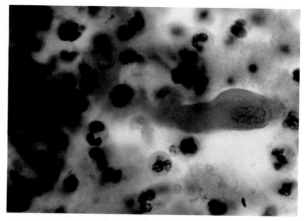

FIGURE 3–36D. Marked Squamous Atypia from Aspergillus. This single cell is suspect for squamous cell carcinoma. It has highly keratinized cytoplasm and a very abnormal nucleus. However, the nucleus does not have the dense hyperchromatism that is usually characteristic of a keratinized squamous cell carcinoma. Again, if appropriate history is not available, a false-positive diagnosis could occur. Bronchial brush, Papanicolaou stain (× 630).

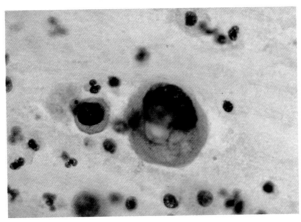

FIGURE 3–37A. Large-Cell Carcinoma with Giant Cells. There is a marked size variation between the two malignant cells seen here. Numerous malignant giant cells were noted throughout the smear. The largest one here has cytoplasmic vacuolization, which may indicate that it is an adenocarcinoma. The nuclear hyperchromasia is not typical of adenocarcinoma. The rest of the specimen did not have evidence of glandular groupings; therefore, this malignancy was classified as a large-cell undifferentiated carcinoma with giant cells. Bronchial brush, Papanicolaou stain (× 400).

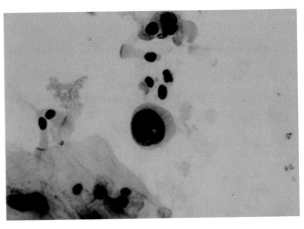

FIGURE 3–37C. Large-Cell Undifferentiated Carcinoma. This sputum specimen has normal ciliated columnar cells to compare with the very large malignant cell. Note that the malignant cell has a regular round nucleus but a very high nuclear to cytoplasmic ratio. If the patient had a history of chemotherapy or radiation, a cell such as this might only represent an atypia; however, this patient had a large mass and previously had had no treatment for malignancy. Bronchial wash, Papanicolaou stain (× 400). (Courtesy of Richard H. Ochs, M.D.)

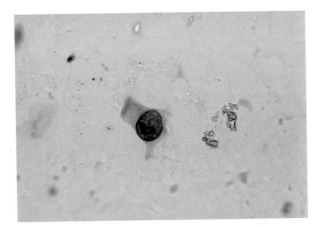

FIGURE 3–37B. Chemotherapy Effect. Notice that, in contrast to the cell in the next figure, this cell has maintained a columnar shape and still retains a sharp, luminal, flat border suggesting a terminal bar. The nucleus is large but the nuclear to cytoplasmic ratio is normal, since abundant cytoplasm is present. The chromatin is hyperchromatic, but finely granular. Nucleoli are prominent and irregular, but, relative to the scale of the entire cell, they are not out of proportion. This patient had been treated for chronic myelogenous leukemia. Bronchial wash, Papanicolaou stain (× 400).

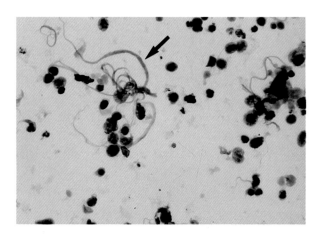

FIGURE 3–38A. Small-Cell Carcinoma. This is a needle aspiration of a small-cell carcinoma showing "crush artifact" (arrow). This feature is much more prominent on an aspirate specimen than on brushings or washings. The diagnostic cells are the ones that demonstrate nuclear molding. Lung, fine needle aspiration, Papanicolaou stain (× 400).

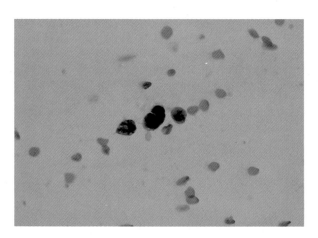

FIGURE 3–38B. Small-Cell Carcinoma. This brush specimen demonstrates several malignant cells that have scant cytoplasm and nuclear molding typical of small-cell carcinoma. Bronchial brush, Papanicolaou stain (× 400).

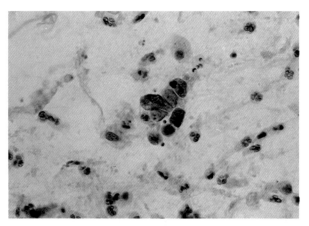

FIGURE 3–38C. Squamous Cell Carcinoma Mimicking Small-Cell Carcinoma. These cells are approximately the same size as the intermediate type of small-cell carcinoma. A macrophage and some polymorphonuclear leukocytes are present to use as a size comparison. The nuclei are slightly larger than in the previous figure, and the cytoplasm appears slightly more abundant; however, it is still scant. Nuclear molding is present. One nucleus is significantly larger than is usually seen in a small-cell carcinoma. Because of the variation in nuclear chromatin and the size of the cells, we were not certain whether this was an intermediate type of small-cell carcinoma, a poorly differentiated squamous cell carcinoma composed of small cells, or a mixed small-cell carcinoma having a squamous or adenocarcinoma component. When the tumor was resected, it was found to be a squamous cell carcinoma in which the individual cells looked very similar to those seen here. A few cells demonstrated definite keratinization, and the final diagnoses was poorly differentiated squamous carcinoma. It is important to recognize cases in which cells are not typical of small-cell carcinoma because the treatment and prognosis is different for non–small-cell carcinomas. A biopsy or resection specimen is necessary whenever there is a question about the cytologic diagnosis. Bronchial brush, Papanicolaou stain (× 400).

Illustration continued on following page

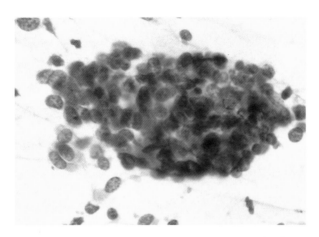

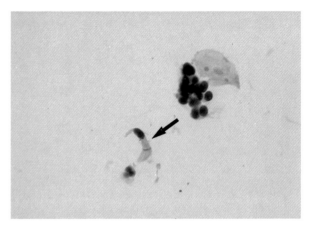

FIGURE 3–38D. *Continued* **Poorly Differentiated Adenocarcinoma Mimicking Small-Cell Carcinoma.** As in the previous figure, this was a very difficult cytologic specimen. There are some normal ciliated columnar cells to compare the size of the abnormal cells. The abnormal nuclei are slightly larger than the ciliated columnar cells, and the chromatin is more hyperchromatic. Some nuclear molding is present, and the cytoplasm is very scant. The feature that is unusual for small-cell carcinoma is the piking up of cells and the overlapping of nuclei. The typical small-cell carcinoma is arranged in sheets and not in three-dimensional groupings, as seen here. The differential in this case is small-cell carcinoma versus a mixed small-cell carcinoma and adenocarcinoma versus an adenocarcinoma composed of small cells. Because the predominate cell population was in grouped arrangements, we suggested adenocarcinoma but requested a biopsy or resection for a definitive diagnosis. This tumor was found to be a poorly differentiated bronchogenic adenocarcinoma. Bronchial brush, Papanicolaou stain (× 400).

FIGURE 3–38E. *Continued* **Bronchial Reserve Cells Mimicking Small-Cell Carcinoma.** Notice the ciliated columnar cells (arrow). The impressive feature is the over-staining of the nuclear chromatin in the normal cells, which gives an opaque quality to the nucleus. The chromatin of the nuclei in the abnormal group looks exactly the same, but the abnormal cells only have scant cytoplasm around the nuclei. The cellular organization is regular. These are normal bronchial reserve cells; the reason that they look abnormal is a result of overstaining the smears. This bronchial wash specimen was fixed in Saccomanno carbowax fixative, and the carbowax was not adequately rinsed from the cells. This makes these normal reserve cells resemble small-cell anaplastic carcinoma. The key to a correct diagnosis is to recognize that the nuclei of the normal cells do not have normal chromatin appearance. Bronchial brush, Papanicolaou stain (× 400).

NEEDLE ASPIRATIONS, NORMAL CELLS

FIGURE 3–39. Normal Bronchial Cells. A few scattered bronchial epithelial cells having columnar shape with basally placed nuclei are seen along with some alveolar macrophages with vacuolated cytoplasm. Lung FNA, Diff-Quik stain (× 200).

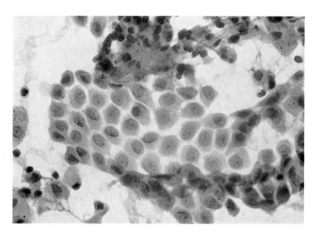

FIGURE 3–40B. Mesothelial Cells. Arranged in a sheet-like grouping, having uniform-appearing nuclei with small nucleoli and occasional nuclear grooves. Lung FNA, Papanicolaou stain (× 400).

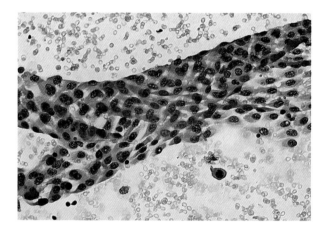

FIGURE 3–40A. Reactive Mesothelial Cells. Strip of mesothelial cells arranged in a two-dimensional sheet with folding. Lung FNA, Diff-Quik stain (× 200).

MISCELLANEOUS FINDINGS

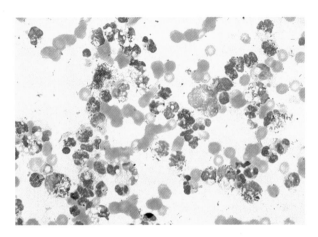

FIGURE 3–41. Lung Abscess. Fine needle aspirate of lung abscess showing numerous neutrophils, with bacteria in background. Lung FNA, Diff-Quik stain (× 200).

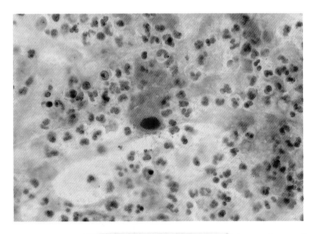

FIGURE 3–42. Squamous Cell Carcinoma. An aspirate of "carcinomatous abscess" showing intense acute inflammatory cell exudate with rare keratinized malignant squamous cells. If atypical keratinized squamous cells are not appreciated, a false-negative diagnosis of lung abscess is quite possible. Lung FNA, Papanicolaou stain (× 200).

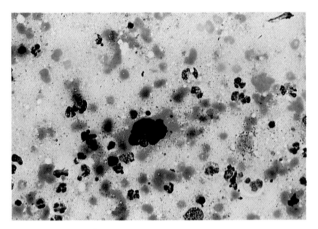

FIGURE 3–43. Squamous Cell Carcinoma. Fine needle aspirate of keratinizing squamous cell carcinoma with associated acute inflammatory cell reaction showing rare malignant keratinized squamous cell with enlarged and irregular hyperchromatic to opaque nuclei and surrounding dense cytoplasm. If there is predominance of neutrophils with only a very rare keratinized squamous cell, a false-negative diagnosis of abscess is possible. Some benign cavitary lesions of the lung can occasionally show a lining of squamous metaplastic cells with inflammatory atypia. Therefore, a false-positive diagnosis of malignancy is possible in this setting. Assessment of the degree of nuclear atypicality is important in order to differentiate a keratinized squamous cell carcinoma associated with acute inflammation from atypical squamous metaplasia lining a benign cavitary lesion, i.e., a tuberculous or fungal cavity. Lung FNA, Diff-Quik stain (× 200).

INFECTIONS

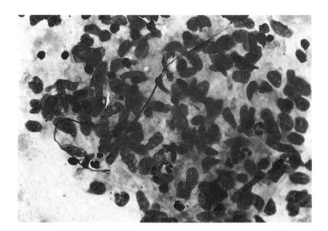

FIGURE 3–44. Granuloma. Aspirate of granulomatous lesion of lung consisting of loose aggregate of epithelioid histiocytes, some having elongated to bent nuclei with surrounding amphophilic cytoplasm. Some associated acute inflammation is also present. The elongated nuclei of epithelioid histiocytes can potentially be confused with the mesenchymal cells seen in benign and malignant stromal tumors. The bent nuclei and cohesive nature of the aggregate, along with a moderate amount of amphophilic cytoplasm, suggests the correct diagnosis of a granuloma. Lung FNA, Diff-Quik stain (× 400).

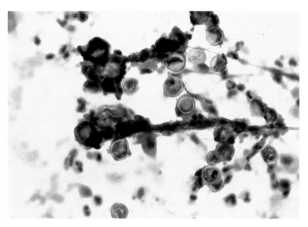

FIGURE 3–45B. Blastomycosis. Aspirate consisting of fungal yeast forms with well-defined cell walls and internal structures. The differential features of fungi are outlined in Table 3–2. In general, *Cryptococcus* shows narrow-based budding with a capsule, whereas the yeast cells of histoplasmosis are smaller and lack the well-defined cell wall and internal structure of *Blastomyces*. Lung FNA, Papanicolaou stain (× 400).

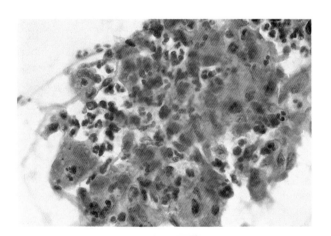

FIGURE 3–45A. Blastomycosis. Fine needle aspirate of granulomatous inflammation associated with blastomycosis. Note loose aggregate of epithelioid histiocytes associated with neutrophils. Lung FNA, Papanicolaou stain (× 400).

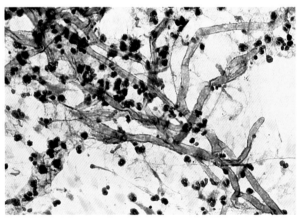

FIGURE 3–46. Aspergillosis. Aspirate of aspergillosis showing organisms that have acute angle branching and septation. Acute inflammation is prominent in the background. *Phycomycetes*-type fungi are nonseptated, with ribbon-like hyphae with varying widths. Lung FNA, Papanicolaou stain (× 200).

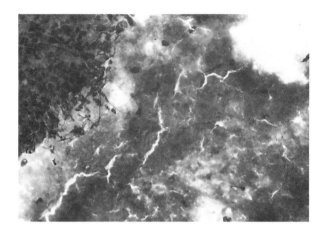

FIGURE 3–47. Tuberculosis. An aspirate from the center of an active granuloma of tuberculosis has a smear pattern demonstrating granular fluffy necrotic material consistent with caseation-type necrosis. Differential diagnosis includes the caseation-type necrosis seen in fungal granulomas and tumor necrosis. In tumor necrosis, the faint outline of the necrotic tumor cells are present. Lung FNA, Diff-Quik stain (× 100).

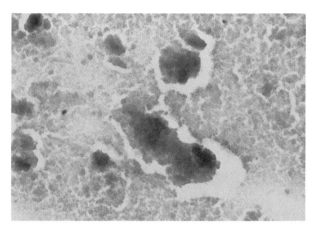

FIGURE 3–49. Tuberculosis. In the Papanicolaou-stained smears, clumps of granular to fluffy necrotic material consistent with caseation-type necrosis is seen. Lung FNA, Papanicolaou stain (× 200).

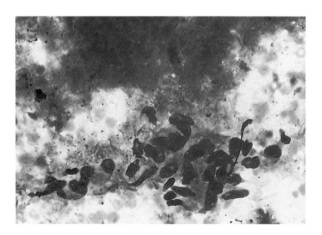

FIGURE 3–48. Tuberculosis. An aspirate of tuberculous granuloma shows a loose aggregate of epithelioid histiocytes consistent with granulomatous inflammation and with clumps of necrotic material consistent with caseation necrosis. Differential diagnosis includes other types of granuloma, which can show a similar pattern. Special stains and cultures are needed for a definitive diagnosis. Lung FNA, Diff-Quik stain (× 400).

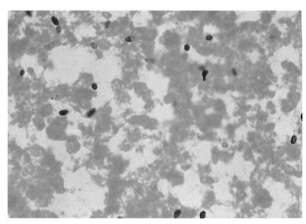

FIGURE 3–50. Histoplasmosis. An aspirate of a necrotic lesion in which fungi consistent with histoplasmosis were appreciated with a special stain. Differential diagnosis includes a *Candida* infection, which has yeast that are somewhat larger and associated pseudohyphae. *Blastomyces* are in general larger, with well-defined cell walls, internal structures, and broad-based budding. Lung FNA, Methenamine silver stain (× 200).

MISCELLANEOUS FINDINGS

FIGURE 3–51. Pulmonary Infarct. Fine needle aspirate of lung showing epithelial cells that demonstrate features of regeneration and repair. This is characterized by the sheet-like arrangement of cells that have an unremarkable nuclear to cytoplasmic ratio, although the nuclei are mildly enlarged, with a vesicular chromatin pattern and prominent nucleoli. There is no loss of polarity. The differential diagnosis includes adenocarcinoma, which consists of syncytial groupings of cells and single cells. There is a greater degree of nuclear atypicality, with higher nuclear to cytoplasmic ratios and loss of polarity of the cells in carcinoma. Lung FNA, Papanicolaou stain (× 400).

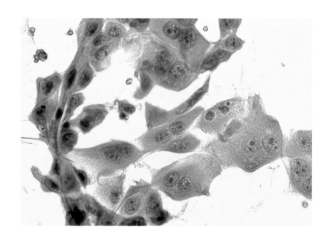

FIGURE 3–52. Chemotherapeutic Effect. Fine needle aspirate specimen of ill-defined lesion in patient with Hodgkin disease of the lung and mediastinum treated with chemotherapy. Fine needle aspiration cytology shows mildly atypical epithelial cells, most likely reflecting changes secondary to chemotherapy, including repair-type arrangement with binucleation. Differential diagnosis includes carcinoma, which has cells arranged in a more syncytial fashion, with a greater degree of nuclear atypicality and higher nuclear to cytoplasmic ratio. Degenerative features, including cytoplasmic and nuclear vacuolization and bichromasia, favor chemotherapy-irradiation effect. Lung FNA, Diff-Quik stain (× 200).

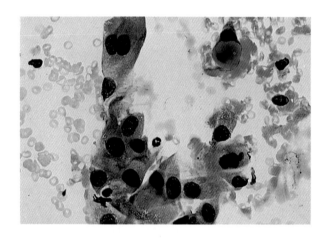

FIGURE 3–53. Chemotherapeutic Effect. Fine needle aspirate of atypical epithelial cells secondary to chemotherapy. The cells are arranged in a sheet-like fashion and show slightly enlarged nuclei with smudged nuclear chromatin pattern. Lung FNA, Diff-Quik stain (× 400).

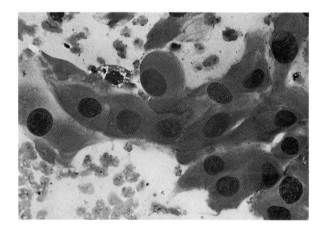

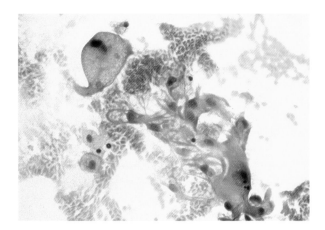

FIGURE 3–54. Irradiation Effect. Fine needle aspirate of atypical cells secondary to irradiation. Note degenerative smudged quality of nuclei and bichromasia of cytoplasm. Differential diagnosis includes carcinoma, although the sheet-like pattern, degenerative quality of the cells, and low nuclear to cytoplasmic ratio favor irradiation effect. Lung FNA, Papanicolaou stain (× 200).

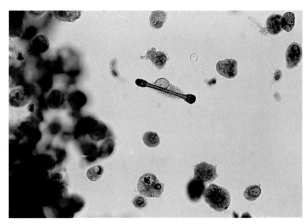

FIGURE 3–55. Asbestosis. Fine needle aspirate biopsy specimen of lung showing benign alveolar macrophages with a single ferruginous body characterized by its dumbbell shape and yellow-brown color. Lung FNA, Papanicolaou stain (× 200).

SQUAMOUS CARCINOMA

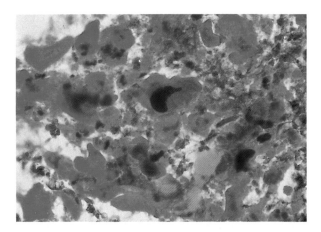

FIGURE 3–56. Squamous Cell Carcinoma. Fine needle aspirate of keratinized squamous cell carcinoma of the lung consisting of scattered malignant keratinized cells, some of which have orangeophilic cytoplasm and irregular, opaque nuclei. Note the necrotic debris, which makes a very "dirty" background. Lung FNA, Papanicolaou stain (× 400).

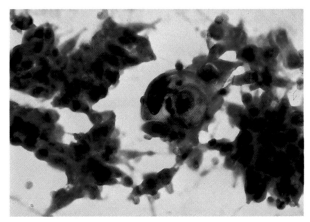

FIGURE 3–57. Squamous Cell Carcinoma. A malignant squamous pearl is seen in the center of the field. The remaining cells probably represent dysplastic-appearing squamous cells that show no evidence of intracytoplasmic keratinization. Lung FNA, Papanicolaou stain (× 200).

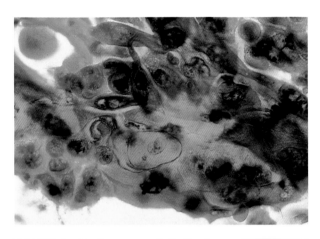

FIGURE 3–58. Squamous Cell Carcinoma. Keratinizing squamous cell carcinoma showing malignant cells with pleomorphic nuclei and extensive cytoplasmic keratinization (orangeophilia). Lung FNA, Papanicolaou stain (× 600).

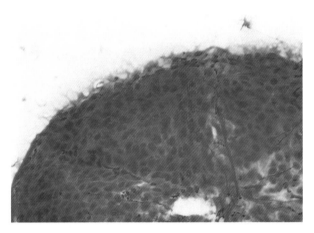

FIGURE 3–60A. Squamous Cell Carcinoma. Microtissue fragment of poorly differentiated squamous cell carcinoma showing surface flattening and spindling of malignant cells. Differential diagnosis includes a microtissue fragment of adenocarcinoma, although the surface spindling is more typical of squamous cell carcinoma. A benign fragment of squamous epithelium representing a skin plug is also considered in the differential, although the nuclear atypicality and the lack of an hyperkeratinized layer is against that diagnosis. Lung FNA, Diff-Quik stain (× 400).

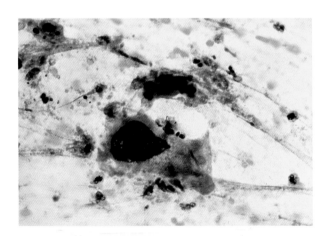

FIGURE 3–59. Squamous Cell Carcinoma. A poorly differentiated keratinizing squamous cell carcinoma consisting of malignant cells that have hyperchromatic, enlarged, irregular nuclei with surrounding amphophilic cytoplasm and well-defined cell membrane. Note the necrotic-type cellular background. Differential diagnosis includes adenocarcinoma and large-cell carcinoma. The presence of individual cells with more opaque cytoplasm and well-defined cell borders favors a poorly differentiated squamous cell carcinoma over an adenocarcinoma. Individually scattered malignant cells can be seen in both large-cell carcinoma and squamous cell carcinoma, although the nuclear and cytoplasmic features in this case favor a squamous cell carcinoma. Lung FNA, Papanicolaou stain (× 400).

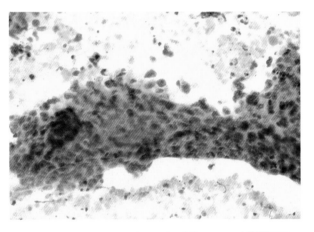

FIGURE 3–60B. Sheet of poorly differentiated **Squamous Cell Carcinoma** demonstrating surface flattening of malignant cells. Note necrotic debris in the background. In this photomicrograph, there is clearly more pleomorphism and lack of cohesion of the cells at the edge of the fragment. Differential diagnosis includes intermediate-type small-cell carcinoma, which can also have cells with elongated shapes. However, the more abundant cytoplasm and large microtissue fragment is indicative of a squamous cell carcinoma. Lung FNA, Papanicolaou stain (× 400).

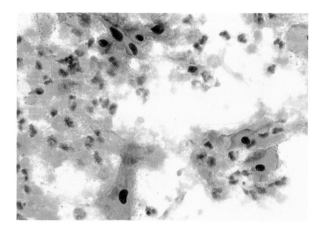

FIGURE 3–61. Squamous Cell Carcinoma. An aspirate of keratinizing squamous cell carcinoma showing extensive tumor diathesis and some acute inflammation in the background. Differential diagnosis includes lung abscess. Lung FNA, Papanicolaou stain (× 200).

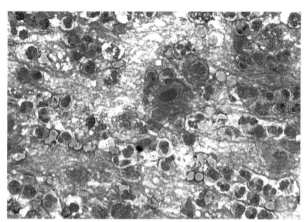

FIGURE 3–62. Squamous Cell Carcinoma. Fine needle aspirate of keratinizing squamous cell carcinoma associated with extensive tumor diathesis. The presence of only a single atypical cell in the center of the field is suggested but not diagnostic of keratinizing squamous cell carcinoma associated with extensive tumor necrosis. A search for other malignant cells should be performed. Lung FNA, Diff-Quik stain (× 200).

ADENOCARCINOMA

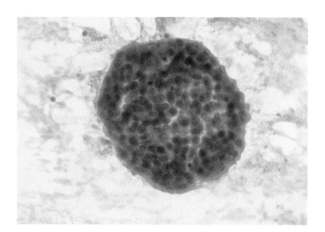

FIGURE 3–63. Adenocarcinoma. Fine needle aspiration biopsy specimen of an adenocarcinoma of the lung demonstrating neoplastic cells arranged in a three-dimensional, ball-like cluster. Tumor cells are relatively uniform, with high nuclear to cytoplasmic ratios. Differential diagnosis includes metastatic adenocarcinoma. Lung FNA, Papanicolaou stain (× 200).

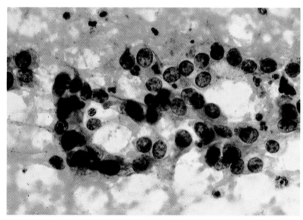

FIGURE 3–64. Adenocarcinoma. Fine needle aspirate of adenocarcinoma of the lung demonstrating neoplastic cells arranged in acinar groupings, with lumen formation. Differential diagnosis includes metastatic adenocarcinoma. Lung FNA, Papanicolaou stain (× 400).

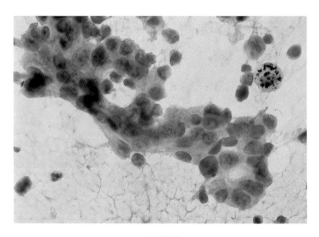

FIGURE 3–65. Adenocarcinoma. Aspiration of adenocarcinoma of the lung showing some abortive gland formation. Lung FNA, Papanicolaou stain (× 400).

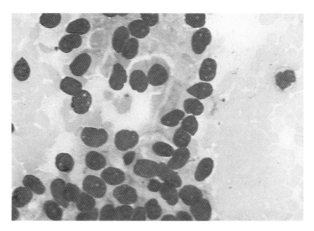

FIGURE 3–67. Adenocarcinoma. Fine needle aspirate of adenocarcinoma of the lung demonstrating neoplastic cells aligned side-by-side. Differential diagnosis includes a repair reaction, which would consist of cells arranged in a sheet-like pattern with well-defined cell borders and no loss of polarity. The cytologic features of this case are indistinguishable from those of metastatic adenocarcinoma. Lung FNA, Diff-Quik stain (× 600).

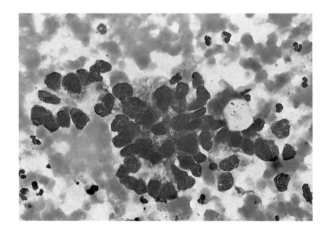

FIGURE 3–66. Adenocarcinoma. Fine needle aspirate of adenocarcinoma of the lung demonstrating clusters of neoplastic cells in which there is some attempt at gland formation. The cells have basally placed, hyperchromatic, irregular nuclei. Lung FNA, Diff-Quik stain (× 400).

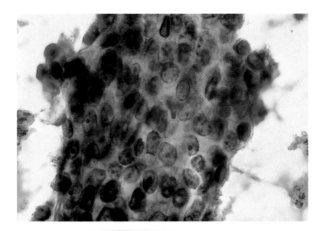

FIGURE 3–68. Adenocarcinoma. Adenocarcinoma of the lung characterized by three-dimensional cluster of neoplastic cells, with loss of polarity. Note hyperchromatic to vesicular nuclei with prominent nucleoli. Lung FNA, Papanicolaou stain (× 600).

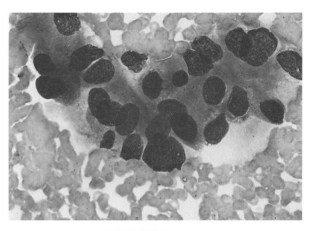

FIGURE 3–69. Adenocarcinoma. Cluster of poorly differentiated malignant cells that have enlarged and irregular, hyperchromatic nuclei with loss of polarity. A moderate amount of surrounding amphophilic cytoplasm is present. Lung FNA, Diff-Quik stain (× 600).

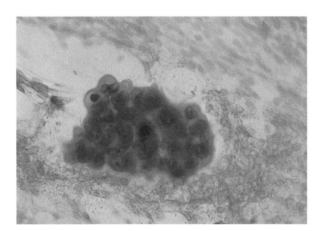

FIGURE 3–70. Bronchioloalveolar Cell Carcinoma. Aspirate consisting of clusters of uniform malignant cells showing prominent depth of focus with lack of significant nuclear molding. Differential diagnosis includes Creola bodies, which share similar features, although the cells may have a more vacuolated appearance and a few cells should demonstrate terminal bars and cilia. Lung FNA, Papanicolaou stain (× 400).

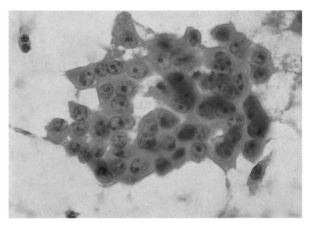

FIGURE 3–71. Bronchioloalveolar Cell Carcinoma. Loose cluster of neoplastic epithelial cells suggesting bronchioloalveolar cell carcinoma characterized by uniform appearance of the tumor cells, including some having a cuboidal to columnar shape; this suggests atypical bronchial lining cells. Differential diagnosis includes repair reaction, which consists of sheet-like groups of cells having vesicular nuclei with prominent nucleoli. The features, which are more consistent with a bronchioloalveolar cell carcinoma, include higher nuclear to cytoplasmic ratio, with some loss of polarity of the cells and individually scattered atypical cells. Lung FNA, Papanicolaou stain (× 400).

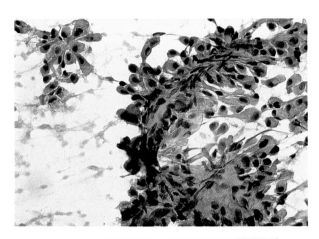

FIGURE 3–72. Bronchioloalveolar Cell Carcinoma. Low power view of aspirate of bronchioloalveolar cell carcinoma demonstrating neoplastic cells arranged along alveolar septae. Differential diagnosis includes the usual type of adenocarcinoma of the lung and metastatic adenocarcinoma. Lung FNA, Papanicolaou stain (× 200).

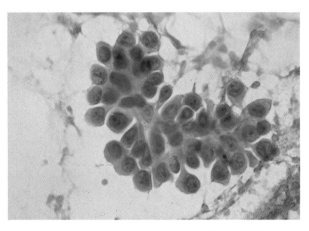

FIGURE 3–73B. Bronchioloalveolar Cell Carcinoma consisting of a loose cluster of neoplastic cells with hobnail-shaped nuclei. Malignant features include a high nuclear to cytoplasmic ratio, with the presence of small to prominent nucleoli and nuclear irregularity. Lung FNA, Papanicolaou stain (× 400).

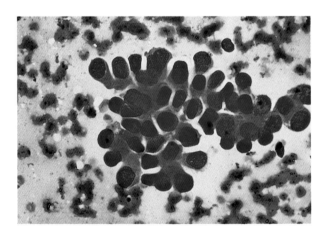

FIGURE 3–73A. Bronchioloalveolar Cell Carcinoma. Diff-Quik stain of bronchioloalveolar carcinoma demonstrating neoplastic cells, which appear to be aligned along alveolar septae, and possessing hobnail-shaped nuclei. Lung FNA, Diff-Quik stain (× 400).

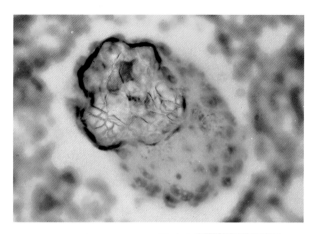

FIGURE 3–74. Bronchioloalveolar Cell Carcinoma. Aspirate of bronchioloalveolar cell carcinoma consisting of neoplastic cells in which a large psammoma body is present, staining in a bas-relief fashion. Differential diagnosis of papillary groupings with psammoma bodies includes metastatic papillary adenocarcinoma of many origins including thyroid and ovary. Lung FNA, Diff-Quik stain (× 400).

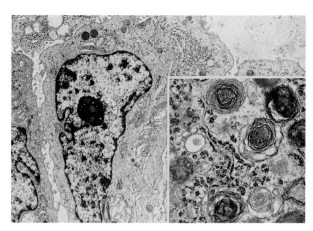

FIGURE 3–76. Bronchioloalveolar Cell Carcinoma. Electron microscopic examination of aspirated material from bronchioloalveolar cell carcinoma demonstrating neoplastic cells with enlarged hyperchromatic to vesicular nuclei and prominent nucleoli. Inset shows presence of intracytoplasmic laminated surfactant-type granules typical of normal alveolar type II cells and seen in some cases of bronchioloalveolar cell carcinoma.

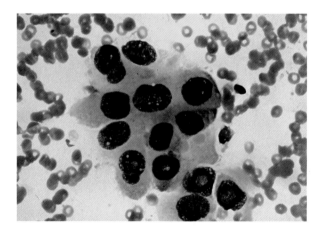

FIGURE 3–75. Bronchioloalveolar Cell Carcinoma. Cluster of neoplastic cells from bronchioloalveolar cell carcinoma, with optically clear nuclei. Optically clear nuclei can be seen in the usual type of adenocarcinoma, although it is a feature of bronchioloalveolar cell carcinoma. Differential diagnosis includes metastatic carcinomas from the thyroid, kidney, or metastatic malignant melanoma. Lung FNA, Diff-Quik stain (× 400).

LARGE-CELL CARCINOMA

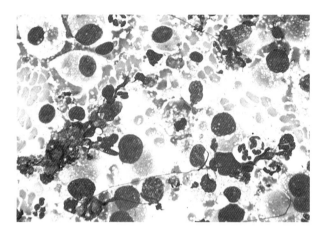

FIGURE 3–77. Large-Cell Carcinoma. FNA biopsy of large-cell carcinoma of the lung consisting of individually scattered neoplastic cells that have enlarged hyperchromatic nuclei with prominent nucleoli and surrounding pale to amphophilic cytoplasm. Differential diagnosis includes poorly differentiated adenocarcinoma or poorly differentiated metastatic carcinoma from a number of sites, including the kidney (in this case because of the somewhat clear nature of the cytoplasm). If the cells demonstrate intracytoplasmic mucinous material with special stains, then the diagnosis of poorly differentiated adenocarcinoma would be more appropriate. Lung FNA, Diff-Quik stain (× 200).

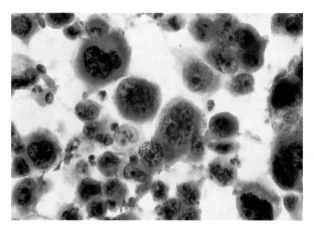

FIGURE 3–79. Giant Cell Carcinoma. High-power view of giant cell carcinoma of the lung consisting of individually scattered neoplastic cells with multiple nuclei. The differential diagnosis includes sarcoma and malignant melanoma. Ancillary studies, including immunohistochemistry and electron microscopy, can be beneficial in establishing a correct diagnosis. Lung FNA, Papanicolaou stain (× 600).

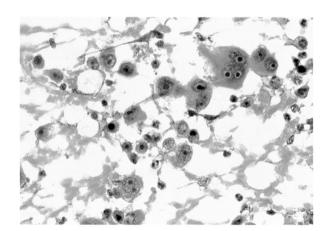

FIGURE 3–78. Large-Cell Carcinoma. Fine needle aspiration biopsy specimen of large-cell carcinoma in which there are individually scattered large cells showing extensive pleomorphism and increased nuclear to cytoplasmic ratio. A few multinucleated tumor giant cells are present. Differential diagnosis includes a primary or metastatic sarcoma involving the lung. Lung FNA, Papanicolaou stain (× 200).

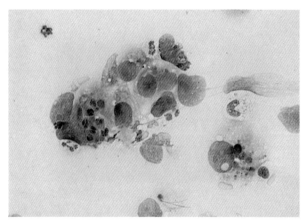

FIGURE 3–80. Giant Cell Carcinoma. Aspirate of giant cell carcinoma of the lung showing a few scattered malignant cells that demonstrate neutrophilic phagocytosis. Differential diagnosis includes metastatic giant cell carcinoma or sarcoma. Lung FNA, Papanicolaou stain (× 200).

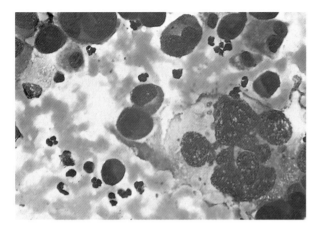

FIGURE 3–81. Large-Cell Carcinoma of the lung consisting of individually scattered neoplastic cells, including some that are quite bizarre and multinucleated. Differential diagnosis includes poorly differentiated adenocarcinoma of the lung, sarcoma, and metastatic malignant melanoma. Intracytoplasmic mucin positivity indicates a poorly differentiated adenocarcinoma. Immunohistochemistry and electron microscopy can be occasionally helpful in the definitive diagnosis of a sarcoma or metastatic malignant melanoma. Lung FNA, Diff-Quik stain (× 400).

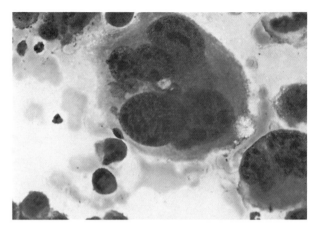

FIGURE 3–82. Giant Cell Carcinoma. High-power view of malignant cells from giant cell carcinoma of the lung showing multinucleated tumor giant cells, including some cells that are quite bizarre. There is pleomorphism of the nuclei with one very bizarre multinucleated malignant giant cell. Lung FNA, Diff-Quik stain (× 600).

SMALL-CELL CARCINOMA

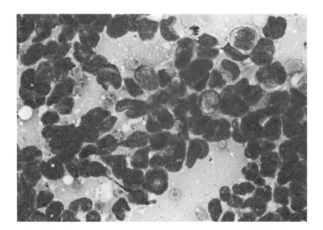

FIGURE 3–83. Small-Cell Carcinoma. Fine needle aspiration of small-cell carcinoma of the lung showing neoplastic cells that have a very high nuclear to cytoplasmic ratio. The nuclei have irregular shapes, but evenly dispersed chromatin patterns and lack prominent nucleoli. Lung FNA, Diff-Quik stain (× 400).

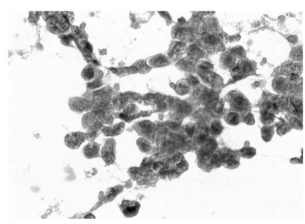

FIGURE 3–84. Small-Cell Carcinoma. Small-cell carcinoma of the lung arranged in loose clusters in which prominent nuclear molding is present. Note hyperchromatic nuclei without presence of prominent nucleoli. Lung FNA, Papanicolaou stain (× 400).

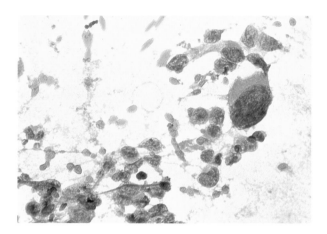

FIGURE 3–85. Small-Cell Carcinoma. Aspirate of small-cell carcinoma of the lung in which a rare larger malignant cell is present. This cell has an enlarged hyperchromatic nucleus with a prominent nucleolus and a moderate amount of cytoplasm. Differential diagnosis includes a mixed small-cell and large-cell carcinoma. However, if only a rare large malignant cell is present, the malignancy should be classified as a small-cell carcinoma. Lung FNA, Papanicolaou stain (× 400).

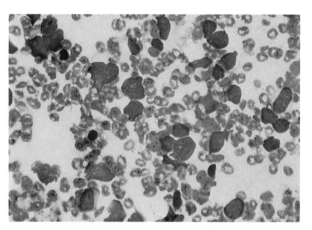

FIGURE 3–87. Small-Cell Carcinoma. An aspirate of a case of small-cell carcinoma having a less common presentation consisting predominantly of dissociated cells with a high nuclear to cytoplasmic ratio and a thin rim of surrounding cytoplasm. Such cases may be confused with lymphoma, although the background lacks lymphoglandular bodies (cytoplasmic fragments). Moreover, in general, small-cell carcinoma of the lung does not possess prominent nucleoli or evidence of significant nuclear cleavage, features commonly seen in some cases of non-Hodgkin lymphoma. Lung FNA, Diff-Quik stain (× 400).

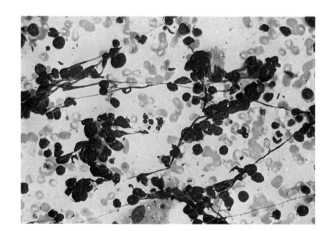

FIGURE 3–86. Small-Cell Carcinoma. Aspirate of small-cell carcinoma showing extensive tumor debris and strands of basophilic material representing extravasated, smudged nuclear material comparable to the "crush" artifact seen in histologic section. Lung FNA, Diff-Quik stain (× 200).

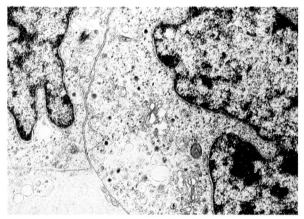

FIGURE 3–88. Small-Cell Carcinoma. Ultrastructural examination of aspirated material demonstrating features of small-cell carcinoma of the lung, including the presence of several neurosecretory-type granules in the cytoplasm.

OTHER TUMORS

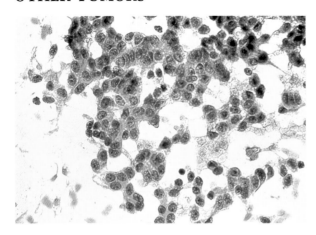

FIGURE 3–89. Carcinoid Tumor. An aspirate of a carcinoid tumor of the lung consisting of neoplastic cells arranged predominately in a dissociated fashion, although some loose clusters are present. Tumor cells have round to oval nuclei with evenly dispersed granular chromatin and inconspicuous nuclei. Differential diagnosis includes clusters of bronchial lining cells and alveolar pneumocytes. The lack of terminal bar and cilia excludes bronchial lining cells. The dissociative nature of the cells having round to oval nuclei and granular cytoplasm are features of a carcinoid tumor and are not present in alveolar pneumocytes. Lung FNA, Papanicolaou stain (× 200).

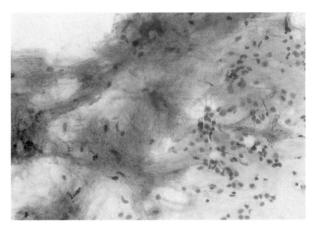

FIGURE 3–91. Hamartoma. An aspirate of hamartoma of the lung demonstrating fibromyxoid background stroma and a few scattered benign epithelial cells. Differential diagnosis would include extracellular mucinous material or necrotic debris. The material does not stain for mucin and has a more stringy fibrillary quality consistent with fibromyxoid stroma of a pulmonary hamartoma. Lung FNA, Papanicolaou stain (× 200).

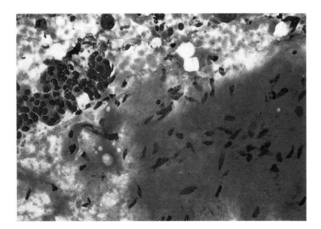

FIGURE 3–90. Hamartoma. Fine needle aspiration biopsy specimen of hamartoma of lung showing clusters of metachromatically stained stromal material in which interspersed spindle-shaped cells are present. Adjacent is a group of bland-appearing epithelial cells. This finding should be correlated with the radiologic appearance of the lesion before a definitive diagnosis of hamartoma is made. Lung FNA, Diff-Quik stain (× 200).

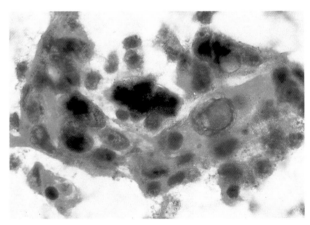

FIGURE 3–92. Metastatic Malignant Melanoma. An aspirate of malignant melanoma metastatic to the lung demonstrating loose clusters of malignant cells, some of which possess prominent intranuclear cytoplasmic inclusions. Note extensive intracytoplasmic pigmentation. Lung FNA, Papanicolaou stain (× 600).

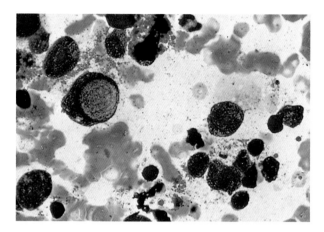

FIGURE 3–93. Metastatic Malignant Melanoma. An aspirate of metastatic malignant melanoma of the lung demonstrating individually scattered neoplastic cells, some of which have a high nuclear to cytoplasmic ratio and prominent intranuclear cytoplasmic inclusions. Note brownish-black cytoplasmic pigmentation. Lung FNA, Diff-Quik stain (× 600).

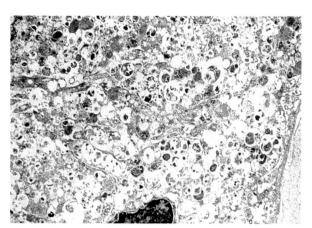

FIGURE 3–95. Metastatic Malignant Melanoma. Electron microscopic examination performed on aspirated material from a lung nodule in a patient with no prior primary carcinoma. Ultrastructural examination shows numerous intracytoplasmic melanosomes confirming a cytologic impression of malignant melanoma.

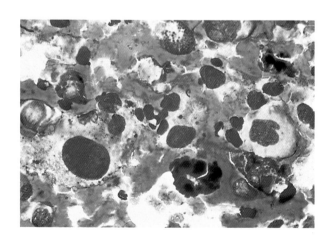

FIGURE 3–94. Metastatic Malignant Melanoma. Fine needle aspiration biopsy specimen of metastatic malignant melanoma of the lung demonstrating neoplastic cells that show considerable variation in nuclear size and shape. Also note dense intracytoplasmic pigmentation. Lung FNA, Diff-Quik stain (× 600).

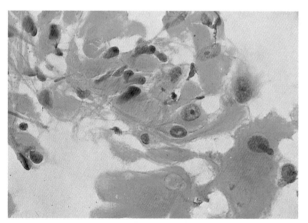

FIGURE 3–96. Metastatic Renal Cell Carcinoma. Fine needle aspirate of metastatic renal cell carcinoma of the lung consisting of loose clusters of neoplastic cells with abundant, pale cytoplasm. The patient had a prior history of resection of renal cell carcinoma, clear cell type. Differential diagnosis of this lesion would include a large cell carcinoma of the lung or other clear cell carcinomas (primary or metastatic). Lung FNA, Papanicolaou stain (× 400).

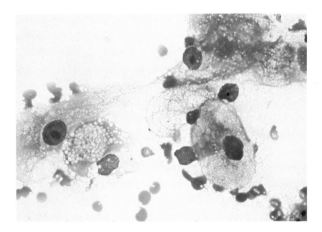

FIGURE 3–97. Metastatic Renal Cell Carcinoma. An aspirate of metastatic renal cell carcinoma, clear cell type, demonstrating individually scattered neoplastic cells with abundant, finely vacuolated, pale cytoplasm. Although the nuclear to cytoplasmic ratio is relatively low for malignant cells, note the round nuclei with very prominent nucleoli. Macrophages usually have reniform-shaped nuclei, with less atypia. Lung FNA, Diff-Quik stain (× 400).

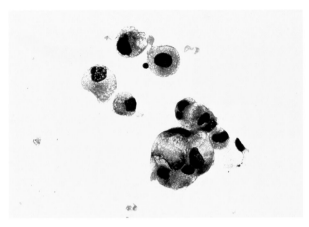

FIGURE 3–99. Metastatic Gastric Carcinoma. Metastatic adenocarcinoma of the stomach to the lung. Note malignant signet cells having hyperchromatic irregular nuclei, with coarse cytoplasmic vacuolization and displacement of the nuclei to the periphery. Differential diagnosis includes signet cell carcinoma of gastrointestinal, breast or ovarian origin. Lung FNA, Papanicolaou stain (× 400).

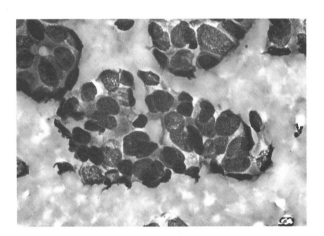

FIGURE 3–98. Metastatic Breast Carcinoma. Fine needle aspiration biopsy of metastatic carcinoma of the breast consisting of malignant cells arranged in loose clusters. Differential diagnosis includes other metastatic adenocarcinomas or a primary adenocarcinoma of the lung. Lung FNA, Diff-Quik stain (× 400).

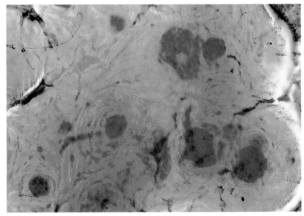

FIGURE 3–100. Metastatic Breast Carcinoma. Metastatic mucinous (colloid) carcinoma of the breast to the lung. Note uniform clusters of neoplastic cells lacking cellular detail, with abundant surrounding extracellular mucinous material. Lung FNA, Papanicolaou stain (× 200).

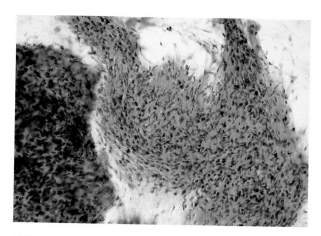

FIGURE 3–101. Metastatic Malignant Synovial Sarcoma. Low-power view of metastatic malignant synovial sarcoma to the lung demonstrating microtissue fragments of spindle-shaped cells with hypercellularity. Differential diagnosis includes other spindle-shaped sarcomas. Lung FNA, Papanicolaou stain (× 200).

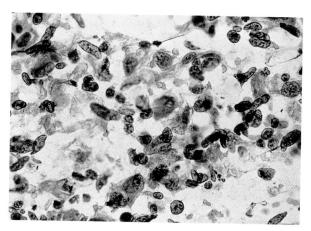

FIGURE 3–103. Metastatic Malignant Fibrous Histiocytoma. Fine needle aspiration of metastatic malignant fibrous histiocytoma consisting of spindle to polygonal-shaped neoplastic cells arranged in a dissociative fashion. Differential diagnosis includes giant cell carcinoma of the lung, metastatic malignant melanoma, and other primary and metastatic sarcomas. Lung FNA, Papanicolaou stain (× 400).

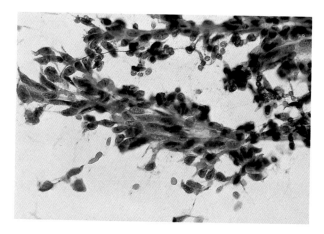

FIGURE 3–102. Metastatic Synovial Sarcoma. High-power view of synovial sarcoma metastatic to the lung consisting of a loose ·cluster of spindle-shaped neoplastic cells that have hyperchromatic and irregular nuclei with surrounding amphophilic spindle-shaped cytoplasm. Differential diagnosis includes primary sarcomas of the lung or metastatic sarcoma. Although mesenchymal repair is considered in the differential, the hypercellularity with a greater degree of nuclear atypicality would favor a malignant process. Lung FNA, Papanicolaou stain (× 400).

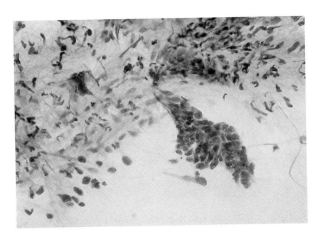

FIGURE 3–104A. Carcinosarcoma of the Lung. Fine needle aspiration of primary carcinosarcoma of the lung consisting of clusters of neoplastic cells that have high nuclear to cytoplasmic ratios and associated with moderately cellular stromal fragments. Lung FNA, Papanicolaou stain (× 250).

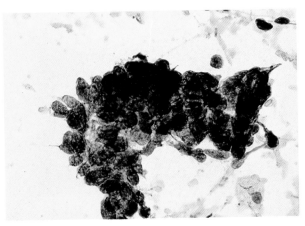

FIGURE 3–105. Carcinosarcoma of the Lung. Immunocytochemical stain for cytokeratin performed on an aspirate of carcinosarcoma showing intense cytoplasmic staining of the primitive neoplastic cells. Lung FNA, immunoperoxidase stain (× 400).

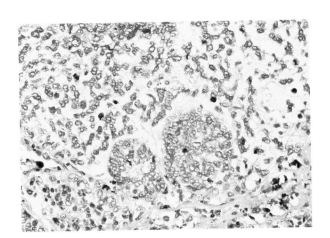

FIGURE 3–104B. Corresponding histologic specimen showing a neoplastic epithelial cluster surrounded by small, neoplastic cells set in a myxoid stroma. Lung FNA, hematoxylin and eosin stain (× 400).

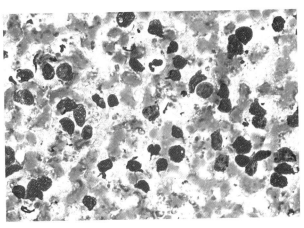

FIGURE 3–106. Lymphoma. Note nuclear irregularity of the malignant cells along with the presence of lymphoglandular bodies (cytoplasmic fragments) in the background. Lung FNA, Diff-Quik stain (× 250).

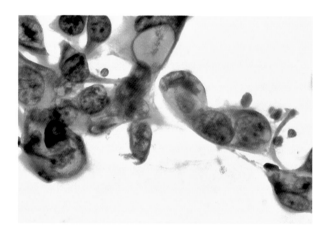

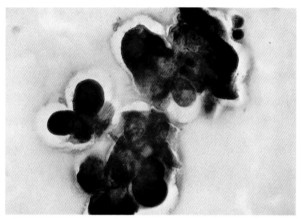

FIGURE 3–107. Adenocarcinoma. Fine needle aspiration of a pleural-based lesion showing neoplastic cells that have hyperchromatic and irregular nuclei, with occasional cells demonstrating coarse cytoplasmic vacuolization. Differential diagnosis includes metastatic adenocarcinoma and mesothelioma, epithelial type. Ancillary studies are needed in order to make a definitive diagnosis. Lung FNA, Papanicolaou stain (× 600).

FIGURE 3–108. Adenocarcinoma. Immunoperoxidase stains for carcinoembryonic antigen demonstrating intense cytoplasmic staining of the neoplastic cells. This finding along with a positive stain for epithelial membrane antigen, Leu-M1, and B72.3 favor the diagnosis of adenocarcinoma rather than mesothelioma. Lung FNA, immunoperoxidase stain (× 600).

C·H·A·P·T·E·R

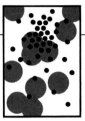

4

EFFUSIONS (PLEURAL, PERICARDIAL, AND PERITONEAL) AND PERITONEAL WASHINGS

Edmund S. Cibas

GENERAL PRINCIPLES

The serous cavities (pleural, pericardial, and peritoneal) are lined by a single layer of mesothelial cells with underlying connective tissue. These spaces normally contain only a small amount of fluid, just enough to lubricate the opposing surfaces as they move against each other, and, as such, are not really cavities at all. In a variety of disease states, however, a greater collection of fluid (effusion) accumulates. Effusions occur either as a result of direct injury to the mesothelium or because hemodynamic disorders such as congestive heart failure or portal hypertension (as seen in liver disease) upset the normal balance of fluid flowing into and out of the serous cavities. Although a variety of agents and conditions—bacteria, viruses, fungi, trauma, irradiation, pulmonary infarcts, uremia, and autoimmune disorders like rheumatoid arthritis and systemic lupus erythematosus—may damage the mesothelium, the serosal surfaces, most importantly, are common sites of metastasis for many tumors.

The evaluation of effusions is usually straightforward, given a properly prepared specimen and the appropriate clinical history. Fluid is collected in heparinized containers to prevent clotting, and the specimen is sent unfixed to the laboratory. If the laboratory is closed, the specimen can be stored in a refrigerator without fixative for several days; the cells are relatively stable in their own milieu. If any greater delay is anticipated, specimens can be fixed by adding an equal volume of 50% ethanol. The author's routine preparation includes cytospins (or occasionally smears) and a cell block, which are prepared by centrifuging 200 ml of the fluid (or the entire specimen if less is received). Any leftover fluid is saved in the refrigerator in case additional slides are needed, or it may be used for other studies such as flow cytometry. The supernatant is discarded, and cytospin preparations (or smears) are made from several drops of the sediment. These slides are alcohol-fixed and Papanicolaou-stained.

If a hematologic malignancy is suspected, an additional set of air-dried cytospins are Wright-stained, and the immunoperoxidase method for lymphocyte surface markers is used. The remainder of the sediment is resuspended in 10% formalin. The specimen is later recentrifuged, and the pellet is wrapped in filter paper, placed in a cassette, and processed for paraffin embedding and hematoxylin and eosin sections. Most immunocytochemical stains, with the exception of many lymphoid surface markers, can be done on sections from this cell block.

Essential clinical information includes the patient's age and sex and any known history of malignancy or other predisposing factors to the development of an effusion. If available, biopsies of any previous malignancies should be reviewed and compared with the effusion at hand. The cell blocks are especially useful here, as they provide the best morphologic comparison to biopsy material.

Benign Elements

The most important (and problematic) cell encountered is the mesothelial cell. In effusions, the reactive mesothelial cells are round to oval, and if well preserved, some display a characteristic outer halo or "brush border," which corresponds to their long, branching microvilli (Fig. 4–1). Inside this clear halo, the cytoplasm is rather dense owing to the arrangement of tonofilaments around the nucleus; this is sometimes appreciated as a ring of dense cytoplasm around the nucleus. Adjacent mesothelial cells are often separated by a narrow space or "window," and cell-in-cell arrangements are sometimes seen. The nucleus is usually centrally placed, round to oval, and has a prominent, smooth nuclear membrane. The chromatin may be pale or rather dark and clumped, and one or more prominent nucleoli are usually present.

Binucleation and even multinucleation are common (Fig. 4–2), and mitoses may be seen in very reactive fluids (Fig. 4–3). Mesothelial cells may be vacuolated (Fig. 4–4), making their distinction from histiocytes, another common cell in these fluids, somewhat difficult. The latter typically have smaller, more irregular nuclei and less prominent nucleoli and nuclear membranes (Fig. 4–5). Mesothelial cells, unlike histiocytes, are strongly keratin-positive with immunohistochemical techniques (Fig. 4–6).

Reactive mesothelial cells appear most commonly as single cells and less commonly as small clusters (Fig. 4–7). Large clusters of mesothelial cells, although they may occur in some rare benign mesothelial proliferations, are extremely uncommon in benign fluids and are best regarded with a high degree of suspicion. Glandular or acinar arrangements are also very uncommon.

Reactive mesothelial cells in some benign conditions may be extremely atypical; this is especially true of pericardial fluids.

Non-neoplastic Conditions

Acute inflammation (mostly neutrophils) is usually caused by pyogenic bacteria (Figs. 4–8A and 4–8B). Pulmonary tuberculosis, by contrast, typically produces a characteristic picture of numerous lymphocytes with very few mesothelial cells, and it may be difficult to distinguish from lymphoma or leukemia (see Figs. 4–49 and 4–50). Effusions with numerous eosinophils (Figs. 4–9A and 4–9B) present a very striking picture but are somewhat mysterious: although some patients may have a history of an allergic disorder, trauma, malignancy, or hypersensitivity to drugs, the cause of the effusion remains obscure in many cases. Pericardial tamponade in the absence of malignancy, as expected, shows blood elements only (Figs. 4–10A and 4–10B).

Patients with rheumatoid arthritis whose disease involves the pleura show a characteristic effusion composed of clumps of amorphous material along with histiocytes, multinucleated giant cells, and a few mesothelial cells (Fig. 4–11).

Malignant Effusions

Malignant cells, in most cases, are easily identified in fluids because they make up a second population of cells morphologically distinct from the mesothelial cells. It is important to note that the malignant cells are not necessarily larger, more pleomorphic, and more hyperchromatic than the mesothelial cells. They may, in fact, occasionally be the same size as or smaller than mesothelial cells, and they may be more monomorphous than the reactive mesothelial cells surrounding them. Some combination of features, however, such as a high nuclear to cytoplasmic ratio, a prominent nucleolus, abnormal chromatin texture, or an irregular nuclear contour, usually betrays their malignant nature. Most commonly, the malignant cells can be distinguished from benign mesothelial cells by virtue of their tendency to form large clusters. However, some malignant tumors, most notably lymphomas but also some adenocarcinomas of the breast and stomach and melanoma, exfoliate as single cells, so careful attention to cellular detail is crucial for an accurate diagnosis.

The most common cause of a malignant pleural effusion in men is lung cancer and in women breast cancer. A malignant peritoneal effusion is most commonly caused by a gastrointestinal malignancy in men and ovarian cancer in women. In most cases of a malignant effusion, there is a previously documented tumor, and the task is simply to acknowledge that the malignant cells, for example, are "consistent with metastasis from the patient's known breast cancer." In some cases, however, there is no previous history of malignancy. In this situation, the most common source of a positive pleural fluid for both men and women is lung cancer, inasmuch as it is extremely uncommon for breast cancer to present as a positive effusion. In the absence of a known malignancy, the most common sources of a positive peritoneal fluid are cancer of the gastrointestinal tract (especially the stomach or pancreas) for men and ovarian cancer for women. A malignant mesothelioma should always be considered in this situation (discussed later). Some patients with lymphoma also may present with a positive effusion.

Adenocarcinomas are by far the most common tumors found in effusions, and some adenocarcinomas have characteristic features that help confirm their site of origin. Many infiltrating ductal carcinomas of the breast exfoliate as large clusters of cells resembling microscopic cannonballs (Figs. 4–12A and B), because of the relatively smooth outer contour of these groups. The typical colorectal carcinoma produces elongated, hyperchromatic cells in acinar arrangements. Some gastric adenocarcinomas have a characteristic signet ring cell appearance, and clear cell carcinomas of the kidney (Figs. 4–15A and 4–15B) and female reproductive tract are composed of cells with prominent nucleoli and abundant fragile-appearing vacuolated cytoplasm.

Some mucinous tumors of the ovary and appendix cause a distinctive syndrome known as pseudomyxoma peritonei in which abundant extracellular mucin produced by the tumor dissects through connective tissues and seeds the peritoneal cavity (Figs. 4–16A and 4–16B). Fluid obtained from such patients is gelatinous and composed principally of extracellular mucin with occasional vacuolated histiocytes (whose valiant but impossible task it is to rid the peritoneum of the offending substance). Tumor cells may be few and far between in this abundant mucinous background.

Psammoma bodies are encountered in a variety of tumors, most typically in carcinoma of the ovary (Fig. 4–17A) and papillary carcinoma of the thyroid, but also in some adenocarcinomas of the lung and in mesothelioma (Fig. 4–17B). By themselves, they should not be taken to indicate primary malignancy of any specific organ, and they may not even be associated with malignancy. Some reactive mesothelial proliferations, most notably in the peritoneum, produce psammoma bodies. If, however, the specimen is a spontaneous pleural or peritoneal effusion (as opposed to a peritoneal washing specimen) and psammoma bodies are present, the likelihood is very high that there is a malignancy.

In addition to the morphologic features, some histochemical and immunocytochemical stains may help identify the primary site of a metastatic adenocarcinoma. Mucin stains and immunocytochemical studies for carcinoembryonic antigen (CEA) are typically negative in clear cell carcinoma of the kidney, hepatocellular carcinoma, and most adenocarcinomas of the prostate. Specific markers for prostate cancer (prostate-specific antigen) and thyroid cancer (thyroglobulin) can be very useful in establishing the diagnosis of a metastasis from these sites. It cannot be stressed enough, however, that if available, previous biopsies should be reviewed and compared to the positive fluid to help establish the likely site of origin.

Melanomas may be pigmented or not. If there is no pigment, the tumor cells with their prominent nucleoli are easily mistaken for adenocarcinoma. Squamous cell carcinoma—most commonly metastatic from lung, head and neck, or uterine cervix—is uncommon in fluids but occasionally may be seen (Figs. 4–18A and 4–18B). Spindle cell sarcomas may also rarely involve serous cavities (Figs. 4–19 and 4–20). Small-cell undifferentiated carcinomas, most commonly of the lung, have a characteristic appearance and are discussed in the differential diagnosis of lymphomas (discussed later).

The cells of malignant lymphoma and leukemia are dyshesive and give a characteristic picture of numerous atypical single cells, often with few mesothelial cells in the background (Figs. 4–21 to 4–23). Irregular nuclear contours with nuclear budding, prominent nucleoli, and nuclear fragmentation are all common in lymphomas, but the specific features in an individual case depend on the type of lymphoma in question (large-cell or small-cell, cleaved or noncleaved, etc.) (Figs. 4–22A to 4–22B). A diagnosis of involvement by Hodgkin disease can be made if Reed-Sternberg cells are identified in a background of mixed inflammatory cells and atypical mononuclear cells (Figs. 4–24A to 4–24C). The cells of multiple myeloma retain features of plasma cells, showing eccentric nuclei, a coarse peripheral ("clock-face") chromatin distribution, and prominent nucleoli (Figs. 4–25A and 4–25B).

The blasts of acute leukemia can also be recognized in effusions. These cells are round, about two to three times the size of lymphocytes, and have a pale dispersed chromatin pattern and occasional nucleoli (Fig. 4–23). It is not usually possible to distinguish lymphoblasts from myeloblasts on Papanicolaou-stained smears, but this does not create a problem because usually the type of leukemia is already known. The granules of myeloblasts may be identified on air-dried Wright-stained preparations. In patients with circulating blasts, the possibility that the fluid was contaminated by peripheral blood during a traumatic tap should always be excluded before a definite diagnosis of serosal involvement is rendered.

Malignant mesothelioma presents one of the great challenges in effusion cytology. When well differentiated, the malignant cells may be difficult to distinguish from reactive mesothelial cells, and when less well differentiated, they may mimic a metastatic adenocarcinoma. The classic description of a very cellular sample containing large groups of cells with scalloped borders (so-called mulberry clusters) is perhaps the most commonly encountered pattern and corresponds to tumors of the epithelial type of mesothelioma (Figs. 4–26A and 4–26B), but other patterns exist that may not be so easy to recognize.

Some mesotheliomas exfoliate as single cells with no tendency to form clusters and may be accompanied by an intense lymphohistiocytic response (Fig. 4–27). These may be impossible to distinguish from a reactive fluid with inflammation. Those mesotheliomas with a prominent or exclusively sarcomatoid pattern exfoliate less commonly; when they do, the malignant cells often cannot be recognized as mesothelial in origin. Unusual patterns are occasionally encountered. Thus it is important to keep in mind that mesothelioma has many faces and should be considered in the differential diagnosis of any unexplained effusion. Histochemical and immunocytochemical studies as well as electron microscopy are often helpful and are discussed below.

Peritoneal Washings

Peritoneal washings are now commonly performed during any exploratory laparotomy for gynecologic disease. Peritoneal involvement by tumor can be undetectable by visual inspection alone, and inasmuch as the presence of peritoneal tumor indicates a worse prognosis, the results of peritoneal washing cytology (PWC) are included in the staging systems for ovarian and endometrial cancer. Although the independent prognostic value of PWC, particularly in the evaluation of cancer of the endometrium, is somewhat controversial, the result of this examination is often considered when the treatment decision is made.

Immediately after entering the peritoneal cavity, the surgeon instills 50 to 100 ml of a balanced salt solution into the pelvis, cul-de-sac, and the two paracolic gutters. Because the diaphragm may be a hidden site of metastasis, its undersurface is often washed as well, or alternatively, it may be scraped and the specimen smeared onto a glass slide.

Peritoneal washings differ from peritoneal fluid in several ways. Most importantly, the washing procedure mechanically strips large sheets of mesothelium from its underlying connective tissue. This produces a very cellular sample containing flat sheets that may be quite large (Fig. 4–28A). The mesothelial cells are typically arranged in a honeycomb pattern with benign nuclear features, although some variation in nuclear size, shape, and chromatin distribution is normal (Fig. 4–28B). If large, these sheets are often folded or rolled. In cell block sections the sheets appear as long, thin strips of mesothelial cells (Fig. 4–28C). Sometimes the sheets may be squeezed together so that the nuclear to cytoplasmic ratio is artifactually increased. Single cells with both flattened and rounded contours are also encountered.

Unlike peritoneal fluid, washings often contain fragments of skeletal muscle (Fig. 4–29) and adipose tissue. Occasional clusters of benign ciliated cells most likely represent detached fragments of epithelium from the tubal fimbriae. Endometriosis of the peritoneum cannot be diagnosed reliably by this technique, because peritoneal washings rarely provide both the endometrial-like epithelium and stroma needed for this diagnosis. Hemosiderin-laden macrophages are a nonspecific indication of prior hemorrhage. Washings done in the setting of colonic perforation may show strips of colonic epithelium and vegetable matter (Fig. 4–30).

Inflammation of the peritoneum caused by previous surgery, pelvic inflammatory disease, tubo-ovarian abscess, ruptured ectopic pregnancy or ruptured cyst, endometriosis, or other disorders may result in reactive mesothelial proliferation and adhesions. The reactive mesothelial proliferation may show significant atypia. Psammoma bodies can result from such benign hyperplasias and should not be equated with a malignancy in this specimen type.

Some tumors identified in peritoneal washings are illustrated in Figures 4–31 to 4–36. It is always wise to compare the peritoneal washing specimen with the concurrent resection specimen in order to arrive at an accurate diagnosis (Figs. 4–35A to 4–35C). This helps to avoid mistakes in diagnosis such as the misinterpretation of reactive mesothelium, endometriosis, or endosalpingiosis as a malignant tumor. Such a side-by-side comparison may be especially helpful in resolving equivocal cases, inasmuch as an "atypical" or "suspicious" diagnosis can be confusing to the physicians treating the patient. Patients who are examined a second time after initial treatment may show marked mesothelial atypia due to treatment effect. This should not be confused with recurrent disease; comparison of the atypical cells with the previous diagnostic material is crucial for appropriate evaluation.

DIFFERENTIAL DIAGNOSIS

Reactive Mesothelial Cells Versus Metastatic Tumor

Mesothelial atypia, as mentioned before, can be striking. Two things may be helpful to identify the atypical cells as mesothelial and exclude metastatic cancer. First, a knowledge of the clinical history may reveal an explanation for the mesothelial atypia, such as anemia, cirrhosis, systemic lupus erythematosus, pulmonary infarct, renal failure, or any other condition that may result in a long-standing fluid accumulation. In such a situation, it is wise to be conservative in diagnosis. Second, in reactive fluids one generally finds a spectrum of changes from bland mesothelial cells to markedly atypical mesothelial cells; some features, such as a brush border or the characteristic dense cytoplasm, help identify all these cells as belonging to the same cell type.

In metastatic carcinomas, two distinct cell populations can often be identified on careful examination and separated (Fig. 4–37). As previously mentioned, however, some tumors, especially adenocarcinomas of the breast or stomach, and even melanoma may mimic mesothelial cells, and a two-cell population is not readily apparent. Special stains for mucin and CEA should be considered in patients with a history of breast cancer and equivocal findings on cytology. A positive mucin stain or immunoreactivity for CEA helps confirm a diagnosis of malignancy. Melanomas can also be treacherous because they do not tend to form cell clusters (Fig. 4–38A). A careful search for the characteristic finely granular dark pigmentation should be made (Fig. 4–38B), but some melanomas contain no visible pigment. The malignant cells may be identified by a positive result with the Fontana stain or with antibodies to HMB-45, a marker of melanocytic differentiation (Fig. 4–38C). On rare occasions, false-positive results for one or another antibody may occur; a correct interpretation is facilitated by the use of several markers and ultimately depends on the sum of clinical information and morphologic examination.

Vacuolated Cells

Cells in effusions that have large intracytoplasmic vacuoles may be either benign or malignant. Not every cell with a vacuole represents an adenocarcinoma: the two most common benign elements—mesothelial cells and histiocytes—are frequently vacuolated (Figs. 4–39A and 4–39B). Most adenocarcinomas with cytoplasmic vacuoles are easily identified when contrasted with a population of mesothelial cells in the background (Fig. 4–39C), but some may show little cytologic atypia and may be confused with vacuolated mesothelial cells. In such cases, stains for mucin or CEA may be helpful.

Some mesotheliomas contain a large population of vacuolated cells (Fig. 4–39D). Their characteristic staining patterns are discussed later. In addition, there is a rare type of lymphoma that produces signet ring cells; the nuclei of these cells are displaced by a massive intracellular accumulation of immunoglobulin (Figs. 4–39E to 4–39G). Immunoperoxidase studies for kappa and lambda light chains may be performed on the cytologic preparations, and if malignant, the cells show monotypic staining for one or the other light chain. Liposarcoma rarely involves the body cavities; if it does, large atypical vacuolated cells are found in the fluid. If air-dried slides are available (or if they can be prepared from a residual, unfixed, refrigerated specimen), a fat stain such as oil red O demonstrates intracellular lipid.

Reactive Mesothelial Cells Versus Mesothelioma

Reactive mesothelial cells rarely form large groups of cells in effusions (Fig. 4–40A). Therefore, a cellular sample composed of large clusters of cells with features of mesothelial cells, especially in the absence of any explanation for the effusion, should arouse a high suspicion of mesothelioma (Fig. 4–40B). Clustering alone is enough to arouse suspicion because the most common "epithelial" type of mesothelioma is usually well differentiated and its cells may show only slight enlargement and pleomorphism. Given how atypical reactive mesothelial cells can look, the cells of these well-differentiated tumors may strike one at first as very unimpressive indeed. For this reason, it is particularly important to pay attention to the architectural features.

Unfortunately, some well-differentiated malignant mesotheliomas show no clustering at all (Fig. 4–41B) and may result in a false-negative diagnosis. There are no reliable antigenic markers to distinguish reactive mesothelial cells from mesothelioma, but in some cases flow cytometry may detect DNA abnormalities characteristic of malignant tumors. However, at least half of the malignant mesotheliomas may have no detectable DNA abnormality by this technique. Perhaps most importantly, good correlation of cytologic findings with clinical information is essential. Any accumulation of fluid in these cavities is abnormal and needs to be explained. The absence of a benign explanation for fluid accumulation is worrisome. In addition, if fluid is pleural and unilateral, if it is large, and if a careful occupational history reveals that the patient or any family member has been exposed to asbestos, it is very likely that the fluid is malignant.

Mesothelioma Versus Adenocarcinoma

Diffuse malignant mesothelioma is so called because of the tendency of small plaques of tumor to coalesce into larger nodules, which then spread to form a thick mat of tumor surrounding the lungs, intestines, or heart, depending on the site of origin. This picture can be mimicked radiographically by metastatic tumors, particularly by adenocarcinoma of the lung, breast, and ovary. The mimicking does not stop there. In cytologic preparations, adenocarcinomas often exfoliate as three-dimensional clusters that resemble the clusters of mesothelioma (Figs. 4–42 and 4–43). Cellular features more typical of mesothelioma include a scalloped peripheral outline to the cell clusters (many adenocarcinomas have smooth round contours), papillary clusters with connective tissue cores, dense cytoplasm with a light peripheral halo, and intercellular windows. None of these is diagnostic of mesothelial derivation, and all can occasionally be seen in adenocarcinomas. Again, a search for two distinct cell populations may identify cells that are distinctly nonmesothelial.

Although an intelligent guess may be made on the basis of morphologic features, a reliable distinction between adenocarcinoma and mesothelioma often depends on histochemical and immunocytochemical stains. There are three histochemical tests that can aid in this distinction. The periodic acid–Schiff diastase (PAS-D) and mucicarmine stains detect neutral mucosubstances. With these tests, mesotheliomas are generally negative, whereas about 50% of adenocarcinomas are positive. Of these, the PAS-D is perhaps the most useful.

With the mucicarmine method, false-positive reactions reported by a number of investigators have damaged the credibility of the test, but with proper tissue fixation and adherence to standard histochemical methods the technique can be quite specific. In the PAS-D–stained sections, care must be taken not to confuse fine positive-staining granules and interposed positive-staining basement membrane material for true secretory vacuoles, which typically show a dark central zone surrounded by a pale zone and a dense outer border (Fig. 4–44). Alcian blue (pH 2.5) or colloidal iron stains reveal the acid mucopolysaccharides present in both adenocarcinomas and mesotheliomas, but the staining is diminished only in mesothelioma when the sections are pretreated with hyaluronidase. This diminution of staining constitutes a positive reaction and excludes adenocarcinoma as a diagnostic possibility, but only a minority of mesotheliomas are positive.

Immunocytochemical studies provide additional discriminatory ability inasmuch as several antibodies now available stain adenocarcinomas and not mesotheliomas. Although early studies reported positive staining of some mesotheliomas for CEA, methodologic improvements, such as adsorption of antisera with splenic tissue to remove cross-reacting substances, have improved the specificity of the technique. With these improvements, mesotheliomas are generally negative for CEA (Fig. 4–45), whereas more than half of all adenocarcinomas are positive (Fig. 4–47). (Adenocarcinomas of the kidney and prostate are usually CEA-negative.)

Other markers that stain adenocarcinomas and not mesotheliomas are Leu-M1 and Ca19-9 (Fig. 4–48). Keratin antibodies stain both mesotheliomas and adenocarcinomas, but the staining patterns are different: adenocarcinomas often show staining that accentuates the periphery of the cell, whereas this is never the predominant pattern in mesotheliomas, in which a perinuclear accentuation is common (Fig. 4–46).

Table 4–1 summarizes the commonly employed studies used in this differential diagnosis. The combined use of mucin stains and immunoperoxidase for CEA can positively identify approximately 80% of adenocarcinomas in effusions. Unfortunately, this still leaves a number of cases that cannot be distinguished from mesothelioma by these techniques. In such cases, electron microscopy may be helpful if it identifies the characteristic long branching microvilli of mesothelioma.

Tuberculous Effusion Versus Chronic Lymphocytic Leukemia or Well-Differentiated Lymphocytic Lymphoma

Effusions in these conditions are remarkably similar in their cellular composition, namely, a predominance of small round mature lymphocytes and few mesothelial cells (Figs. 4–49 and 4–50). In fact, a distinction is virtually impossible on morphologic grounds. Since most chronic lymphocytic leukemias and well-differentiated lymphocytic lymphomas are B-cell neoplasms, a diagnosis of malignancy can be established by demonstrating monotypic staining for light chains on air-dried cytospins. The possibility of contamination of the effusion by peripheral blood during a traumatic tap should be excluded before a definitive diagnosis of malignancy is rendered. Even a small amount of blood containing leukemic blasts may confound the interpretation and give a false-positive result. Knowledge of the peripheral blood count at the time the tap was performed and careful examination of the specimen for fresh blood are essential for accurate diagnosis. If the possibility of contamination by leukemic blood is suspected, discretion in diagnosis is advised.

Lymphoma Versus Reactive Nonspecific Lymphocytosis

In some settings benign inflammatory reactions composed of lymphoid cells may raise the suspicion of lymphoma (Figs. 4–51 and 4–52). Reactive lymphoid infiltrates, however, are composed predominantly of T lymphocytes, whereas most lymphomas are B-cell neoplasms. (The T-cell lymphomas are usually very pleomorphic and are rarely confused with reactive lymphocytes.) Evaluation for a pan–B-cell marker and a pan–T-cell marker can be done on air-dried cytospins. A positive staining reaction of most cells for the T-cell marker supports a reactive process and makes lymphoma much less likely.

Lymphoma Versus Other Small-Cell Tumors

A host of small-cell tumors (Figs. 4–53 to 4–57) are composed of cells in roughly the same size range as many lymphomas: small-cell carcinoma of the lung (and other sites such as the uterine cervix and prostate), lobular carcinoma of the breast, embryonal and alveolar rhabdomyosarcoma, neuroblastoma, Ewing sarcoma, and others. Some of these can be distinguished from lymphoma by their tendency to form cell clusters. Lymphomas, by contrast, are typically composed of numerous dispersed single cells and show no true cluster formation. If there is any doubt, immunohistochemical studies may help identify the cells in question: lymphoma is positive for leukocyte common antigen; lobular carcinoma and small-cell carcinoma for keratin and epithelial membrane antigen; rhabdomyosarcoma for desmin and myoglobin; neuroblastoma for neuron-specific enolase; and Ewing sarcoma for vimentin. Because none of these markers is reliable by itself as a discriminant in all instances, it is recommended that immunoperoxidase studies with the appropriate panel of antibodies be performed and the results correlated with the clinical setting before a diagnosis is reached in a difficult case.

Pleomorphic Neoplasms

When an effusion contains large pleomorphic malignant cells, the differential diagnosis includes poorly differentiated carcinoma (Fig. 4–58), metastatic sarcoma (Fig. 4–59), sarcomatoid mesothelioma (Figs. 4–60A and 4–60B), and metastatic nonseminomatous germ cell tumor (Fig. 4–61). The cells of these tumors may be arranged as single cells or as cell groups, but because of their lack of differentiation, they provide no clue to their cell of origin. A history that includes any previous tumor diagnosis is of utmost importance and must lead to a comparison of the cells in the effusion to the available biopsy material.

Sarcomas rarely manifest themselves initially as a positive effusion, but primary sarcoma of the chest wall, although very rare, may mimic a sarcomatoid mesothelioma in its clinical presentation and cytologic appearance in pleural fluids. Likewise, nonseminomatous germ cell tumors (embryonal cell carcinoma, endodermal sinus tumor, immature teratoma, choriocarcinoma, or any combination of these) rarely present with a positive fluid. Unfortunately, in some cases clinical information may not be forthcoming or there might not be access to previous biopsy material. For this differential diagnosis, immunohistochemical studies are of limited value. All these tumors, including some sarcomas, may be positive for keratin proteins. The poorly differentiated carcinomas may be CEA-positive, whereas sarcomas, mesotheliomas, and germ cell tumors (except for teratomas) are typically negative. Strong reactivity for human chorionic gonadotropin and alphafetoprotein may be seen in some germ cell tumors but also in a proportion of poorly differentiated carcinomas. For this differential diagnosis, there is no substitute for a good clinical history and a review of prior biopsy material.

Peritoneal Washings: Tumor Versus Treatment Effect

Chemotherapy and radiotherapy to the abdomen and pelvis for peritoneal involvement by tumors of the female reproductive tract may induce marked mesothelial atypia. A "second-look" laparotomy is often done to evaluate the effect of therapy and plan further treatment. Peritoneal washings taken at this time should be compared with any positive specimens obtained prior to therapy so that the treatment-induced mesothelial atypia can be distinguished from recurrent tumor. Chemotherapy and radiotherapy cause cell enlargement, with a proportional increase in the diameter of both nucleus and cytoplasm (Fig. 4–62A). Nuclei may become hyperchromatic, and chromatin detail may become somewhat obscured or "smudged" (Fig. 4–62B). Although the nuclei are enlarged, there is overall preservation of the nuclear to cytoplasmic ratio. Distinguishing treatment atypia from tumor is facilitated when the specimen is contrasted with previous positive material (Fig. 4–63).

Bibliography

Cibas ES, Corson JM, Pinkus GS: The distinction of adenocarcinoma from malignant mesothelioma in cell blocks of effusions: The role of routine mucin histochemistry and immunohistochemical assessment of carcinoembryonic antigen, keratin proteins, epithelial membrane antigen, and milk fat globule-derived antigen. Hum Pathol 18:67–74, 1987.

Ernst CS, Atkinson B, Chianese D, et al.: Differential diagnosis between mesotheliomas and metastatic adenocarcinomas using monoclonal antibodies against gastrointestinal carcinoma antigen and stage-specific embryonic antigen. Appl Pathol 4:115–124, 1986.

Johnston WW: The malignant pleural effusion: A review of cytopathologic diagnoses of 584 specimens from 472 consecutive patients. Cancer 56:905–909, 1985.

Koss LG: Diagnostic Cytology and Its Histopathologic Bases, 3rd Ed. Philadelphia: Lippincott, 1979.

Martin SE, Zhang H-Z, Magyarosy E, et al.: Immunologic methods in cytology: Definitive diagnosis of non-Hodgkin's lymphoma using immunologic markers for T- and B-cells. Am J Clin Pathol 82:666–673, 1984.

Ravinsky E: Cytology of peritoneal washings in gynecologic patients: Diagnostic criteria and pitfalls. Acta Cytol 30:8–16, 1986.

Ziselman EM, Harkavy SE, Hogan M, et al.: Peritoneal washing cytology: Uses and diagnostic criteria in gynecologic neoplasms. Acta Cytol 28:105–110, 1984.

ACKNOWLEDGMENTS

The author would like to thank Geraldine S. Pinkus, M.D., of the Brigham and Women's Hospital for performing the immunoperoxidase studies and Barbara Atkinson, M.D., for kindly providing Figure 4–17B. Special thanks go to Ms. Robin Lee and Ms. Bea Mooar, whose expert assistance was invaluable.

Table 4–1. HISTOCHEMICAL AND IMMUNOCYTOCHEMICAL REACTIONS OF ADENOCARCINOMAS AND MESOTHELIOMAS

Reaction	Adenocarcinoma	Mesothelioma
Periodic acid–Schiff diastase	+	−
Mucicarmine	+	−
Hyaluronidase-alcian blue (colloidal iron)	−	+
Carcinoembryonic antigen	+	−
Leu-M1	+	−
Ca19-9	+	−
Keratin proteins	+*	+†

*Peripheral predominant.
†Perinuclear predominant.

NORMAL CELLS

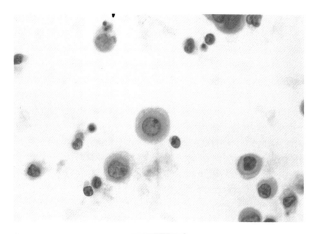

FIGURE 4–1. Reactive Mesothelial Cells, Peritoneal Fluid. The mesothelial cell in the center has a characteristic peripheral cytoplasmic halo representing the brush border; the cytoplasm within the halo is, in contrast, rather dense. There is a small nucleolus, and the chromatin pattern is finely granular. Compare the size of the mesothelial cell with the adjacent small lymphocyte (Papanicolaou-stained cytospin, × 250).

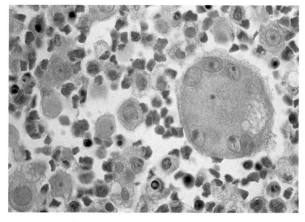

FIGURE 4–2. Reactive Mesothelial Cells, Pleural Fluid. The cytoplasmic halo can also be appreciated in cell block preparations. In this field, there is a large, multinucleated mesothelial cell. It is identified as a mesothelial cell by virtue of its cytoplasmic halo and the similarity of its nuclei to those of adjacent mesothelial cells (hematoxylin- and eosin-stained cell block, × 250).

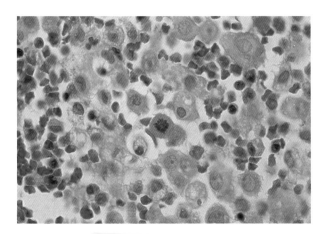

FIGURE 4–3. Reactive Mesothelial Cells, Pleural Fluid. Mitoses are sometimes seen in reactive mesothelial cells (hematoxylin- and eosin-stained cell block, × 250).

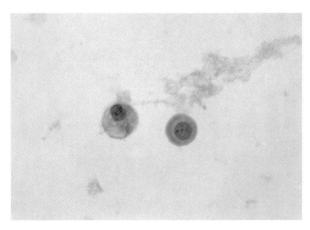

FIGURE 4–5. Histiocyte and Mesothelial Cell, Pleural Fluid. Histiocytes are common in effusions and may occasionally be difficult to distinguish from mesothelial cells. The histiocyte on the left has a smaller, more irregular nucleus and more abundant cytoplasm, as compared with the nearby mesothelial cell (Papanicolaou-stained cytospin, × 250).

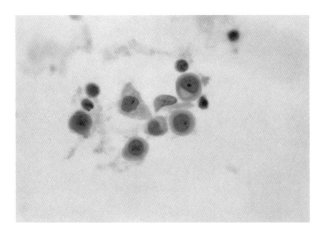

FIGURE 4–4. Reactive Mesothelial Cells, Pleural Fluid. One of the mesothelial cells has a well-defined cytoplasmic vacuole. The similarity of its nucleus to those of adjacent mesothelial cells identifies it as a mesothelial cell (Papanicolaou-stained cytospin, × 250).

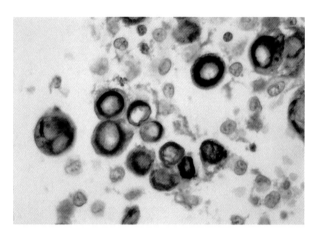

FIGURE 4–6. Reactive Mesothelial Cells, Pleural Fluid. Mesothelial cells are strongly positive for keratin proteins, and many show a characteristic perinuclear distribution of the keratin filaments (immunoperoxidase method for keratin proteins AE1/AE3, × 250).

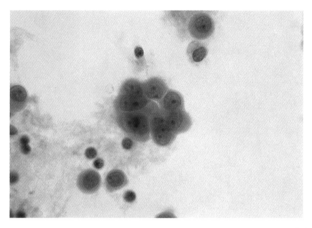

FIGURE 4–7. Reactive Mesothelial Cells, Pleural Fluid. Mesothelial cells in benign fluids, such as this one from a patient with congestive heart failure, may occasionally aggregate into small clusters. A prominent "window" is apparent (Papanicolaou-stained cytospin, × 250).

NON-NEOPLASTIC CONDITIONS

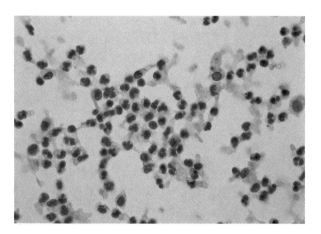

FIGURE 4–8A. Spontaneous Bacterial Peritonitis, Peritoneal Fluid. Acute inflammation of pleura, pericardium, and peritoneum is characterized by numerous polymorphonuclear leukocytes (Papanicolaou-stained cytospin, × 150).

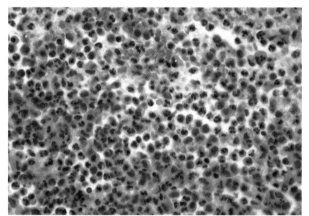

FIGURE 4–8B. Spontaneous Bacterial Peritonitis, Peritoneal Fluid, same specimen as Figure 4–8A (hematoxylin- and eosin-cell block, × 150).

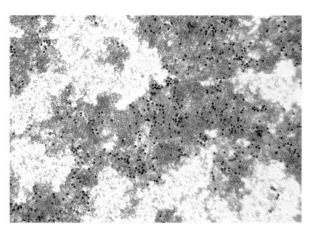

FIGURE 4–9A. Eosinophilic Pleural Effusion. This pleural fluid contained numerous eosinophils. The cause was never elucidated, as is common for many of these patients (Papanicolaou-stained cytospin, × 150).

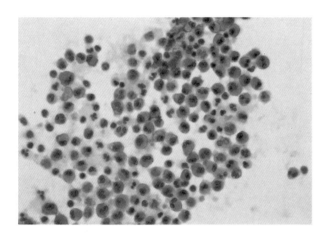

FIGURE 4–10A. Pericardial Tamponade. Although bleeding into the pericardium may be caused by metastatic tumor, many cases are unrelated to cancer; such cases show blood elements only. Note that on this alcohol-fixed cytospin the red cells have lysed, leaving only a granular background (Papanicolaou-stained cytospin, × 50).

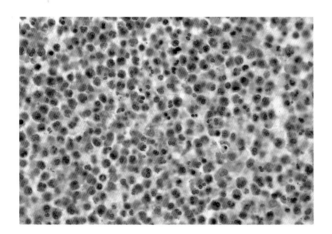

FIGURE 4–9B. Eosinophilic Pleural Effusion, same specimen as Figure 4–9A (hematoxylin- and eosin-cell block, × 150).

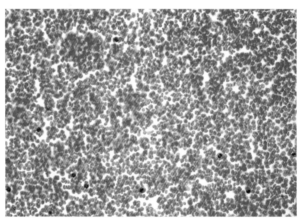

FIGURE 4–10B. Pericardial Tamponade, same specimen as Figure 4–10A (hematoxylin- and eosin-stained cell block, × 100).

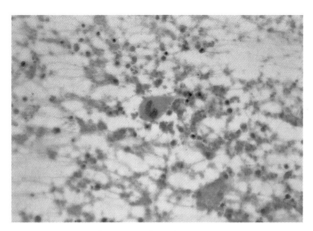

FIGURE 4–11. Rheumatoid Arthritis, Pleural Fluid. Effusions from patients whose rheumatoid disease involves the pleura contain abundant amorphous granular material and histiocytes. The latter are often multinucleated (as seen here) or elongated in shape. Mesothelial cells are typically few in number. This constellation of findings is quite characteristic of rheumatoid arthritis (Papanicolaou-stained smear, × 100).

MALIGNANT TUMORS

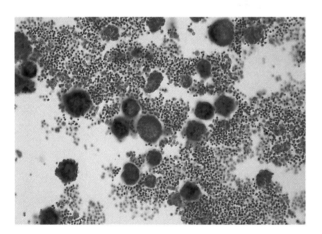

FIGURE 4–12A. Ductal Carcinoma of the Breast, Pleural Fluid. The most common cytologic pattern of infiltrating ductal carcinoma of the breast in effusions is that of well-circumscribed round masses of cells, as seen here. Also encountered are acinar structures (see Figs. 4–12B and 4–47) and tandem or linear arrangements (not illustrated) (Papanicolaou stain, × 50).

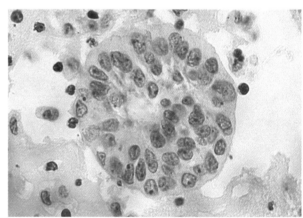

FIGURE 4–12B. Ductal Carcinoma of the Breast, Pleural Fluid. The cells of ductal carcinoma may be small and uniform or large and pleomorphic. In this specimen, the cells are rather uniform and nucleoli are not especially prominent. The chromatin pattern is granular and the nuclear membranes are irregular, however; these features, along with the arrangement in a large spherical aggregate with smooth contours, establish a diagnosis of malignancy (hematoxylin- and eosin-stained cell block, × 150).

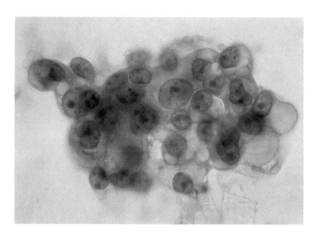

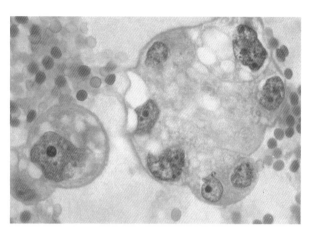

FIGURE 4–13A. Adenocarcinoma of the Ovary, Peritoneal Fluid. These large cells are identified as malignant because of the marked variation in nuclear size and shape, the prominent nucleoli, and the abundant cytoplasmic vacuoles. This tumor was a papillary serous adenocarcinoma, the most common malignant tumor of the ovary, and also the one that most frequently spreads to the peritoneum (and pleura) (Papanicolaou-stained smear, × 250).

FIGURE 4–14. Adenocarcinoma of the Lung, Pleural Fluid. The tumor cells show marked variation in size and shape, prominent nucleoli, and numerous cytoplasmic vacuoles, features that identify them as malignant. These cells cannot be distinguished from other adenocarcinomas, such as the ovarian cancer in Figure 4–13B (hematoxylin- and eosin-stained cell block, × 250).

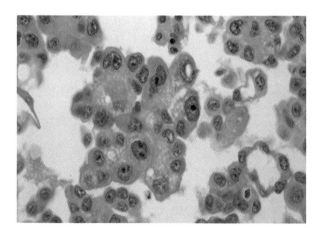

FIGURE 4–13B. Adenocarcinoma of the Ovary, Peritoneal Fluid. The cell block preparation of this papillary serous adenocarcinoma also shows the marked variation in nuclear size and shape characteristic of these tumors (hematoxylin- and eosin-stained cell block, × 150).

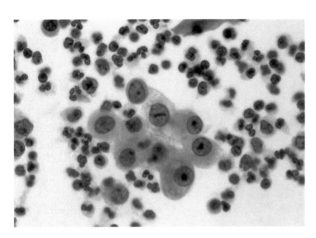

FIGURE 4–15A. Clear Cell Carcinoma of the Kidney, Pleural Fluid. The cells of clear cell carcinoma of the kidney may be difficult to distinguish from reactive mesothelial cells. The tumor cells, as seen here, have abundant, vacuolated cytoplasm that in areas is almost transparent, quite unlike the typically dense cytoplasm of mesothelial cells. The cells also typically have more prominent nucleoli than mesothelial cells (Papanicolaou-stained cytospin, × 250).

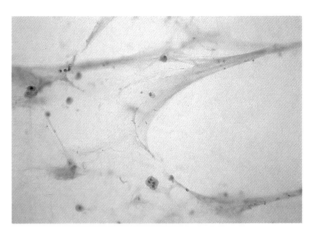

FIGURE 4–16A. Pseudomyxoma Peritonei, Peritoneal Fluid. The specimen is composed of a translucent film of mucoid material in which occasional macrophages, some in clusters, are suspended. Malignant cells are either very infrequent or absent; in this case, they were identified only on a subsequent peritoneal washing specimen (see Figs. 4–32A and 4–32B) (Papanicolaou-stained smear, × 50).

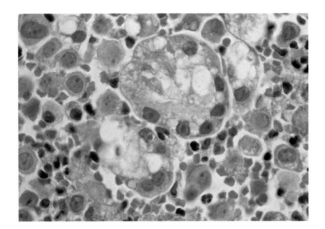

FIGURE 4–15B. Clear Cell Carcinoma of the Kidney, same specimen as Figure 4–15A. Careful attention to the presence of cell groups with rounded contours, the characteristic abundant vacuolated cytoplasm, and the prominent nucleoli lead to a correct diagnosis of malignancy (hematoxylin- and eosin-stained cell block, × 150).

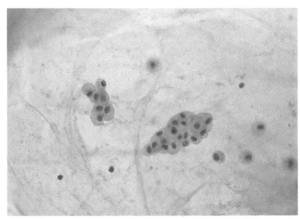

FIGURE 4–16B. Pseudomyxoma Peritonei, Peritoneal Fluid, same specimen as Figure 4–16A. A higher-power view shows two clusters of histiocytes suspended in mucus (Papanicolaou-stained smear, × 100).

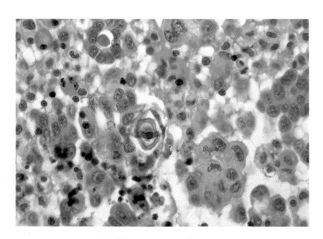

FIGURE 4–17A. Psammoma Body, Adenocarcinoma of the Ovary, Peritoneal Fluid, same specimen as Figure 4–13B. These concentric lamellar structures composed of calcium may be seen in a variety of malignancies (see Fig. 4–17B) as well as in reactive mesothelial proliferations. A diagnosis of malignancy, therefore, should be based on the surrounding cells and not just on the presence of psammoma bodies (hematoxylin- and eosin-stained cell block, × 250).

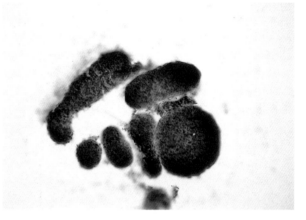

FIGURE 4–18A. Squamous Cell Carcinoma of the Uterine Cervix, Pericardial Fluid. This nonkeratinizing squamous cell carcinoma is exfoliated in the form of large round to oval balls of pleomorphic cells with granular chromatin. Its appearance was strikingly unchanged from that of the primary tumor resected 9 years earlier. The arrangement of tumor cells into spherical aggregates with round contours can be seen in squamous cell carcinoma (predominantly nonkeratinizing tumors) as well as in many breast cancers (see Figs. 4–12A and 4–12B). The orangeophilia of the clusters is an artifact of staining and does not represent keratinization (Papanicolaou-stained cytospin, × 25).

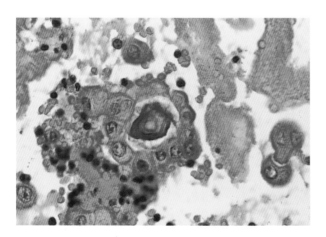

FIGURE 4–17B. Psammoma Body, Malignant Mesothelioma, Pleural Fluid (hematoxylin- and eosin-stained cell block, × 250). (Courtesy of Barbara Atkinson, M.D.)

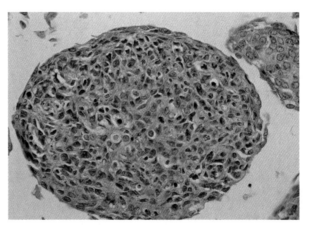

FIGURE 4–18B. Squamous Cell Carcinoma of the Uterine Cervix, Pericardial Fluid, same specimen as Figure 4–18A. A high-power view of the cell block preparation shows the marked pleomorphism of the cells in these large aggregates (hematoxylin- and eosin-stained cell block, × 100).

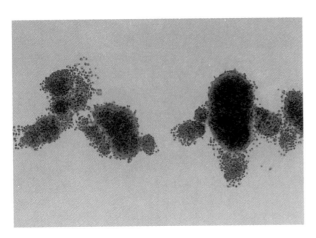

FIGURE 4–19A. Malignant Schwannoma (Malignant Peripheral Nerve Sheath Tumor), Pleural Fluid. On low power, the large balls of this metastatic sarcoma bear a striking resemblance to the previous case of squamous cell carcinoma (Papanicolaou-stained smear, × 25).

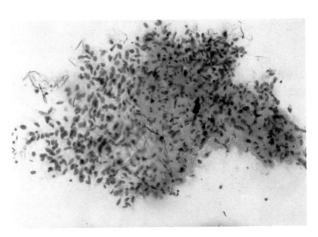

FIGURE 4–20A. Leiomyosarcoma of the Uterus, Peritoneal Fluid. Spindle cell sarcomas often exfoliate as large sheets of elongated (or spindle-like) tumor cells. As with the malignant schwannoma, the cells show peripheral detachment from the large aggregates on the smear preparation. Such large aggregates of atypical cells are not seen in benign fluids (Papanicolaou-stained smear, × 50).

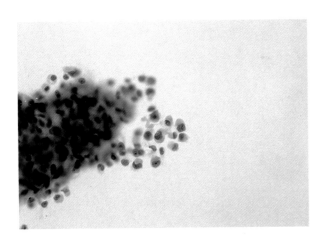

FIGURE 4–19B. Malignant Schwannoma (Malignant Peripheral Nerve Sheath Tumor), Pleural Fluid, same specimen as Figure 4–19A. A higher-power view reveals that the cells of the metastatic sarcoma are less cohesive around the periphery of the clusters than the cells of the squamous cell carcinoma in Figures 4–18A and 4–18B. A diagnosis as to cell type in both cases was made by comparing the fluids with the previous biopsy specimens (Papanicolaou-stained smear, × 100).

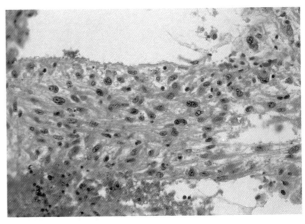

FIGURE 4–20B. Leiomyosarcoma of the Uterus, Peritoneal Fluid. The marked variation in nuclear size and shape and the arrangement of the cells in fascicles in the cell block preparations was similar to that seen in the original tumor (hematoxylin- and eosin-stained cell block, × 75).

FIGURE 4–21. Malignant Lymphoma, Pleural Fluid. The cells are single and dispersed, as is characteristic of lymphomas. Like the cells of many lymphomas, these cells show marked nuclear irregularity, with folds, blebs, and creases, as well as prominent nucleoli (Papanicolaou-stained smear, × 250).

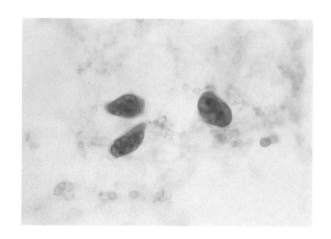

FIGURE 4–22A. Malignant Lymphoma, Lymphoblastic Type, Pleural Fluid. Not all lymphoma cells are as atypical as in Figure 4–21. The cells of lymphoblastic lymphoma are only slightly larger than normal lymphocytes, and nuclear irregularity may be mild. The chromatin pattern is paler than that of normal lymphocytes, and small nucleoli are present. These cells may be difficult to distinguish from normal lymphocytes, especially in alcohol-fixed, Papanicolaou-stained specimens (Papanicolaou-stained cytospin, × 250).

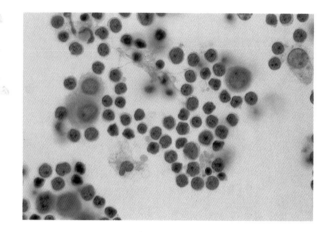

FIGURE 4–22B. Malignant Lymphoma, Lymphoblastic Type, Pleural Fluid, same specimen as Figure 4–22A. The cells of lymphoblastic lymphoma in the cell block may also be difficult to distinguish from mature lymphocytes (hematoxylin- and eosin-stained cell block, × 250).

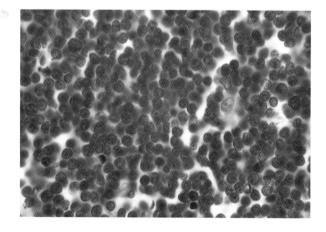

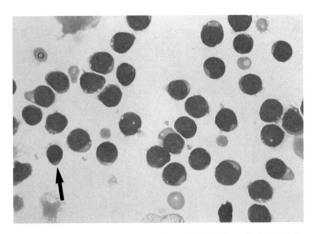

FIGURE 4–22C. Malignant Lymphoma, Lymphoblastic Type, Pleural Fluid, same specimen as in Figures 4–22A and 4–22B. This air-dried Wright stain allows better appreciation of the dispersed chromatin pattern of the lymphoblasts. The chromatin of an adjacent normal lymphocyte (arrow) is darker and more clumped (Wright-stained smear, × 250).

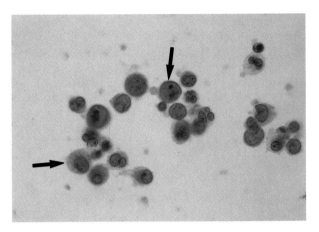

FIGURE 4–23. Acute Myelogenous Leukemia, Pleural Fluid. Leukemic blasts (long arrows) have a finely dispersed chromatin pattern, prominent nucleoli, and scant cytoplasm. They are approximately the same size as mesothelial cells (short arrow). More mature myeloid cells, including neutrophils, are also present (Papanicolaou-stained cytospin, × 250).

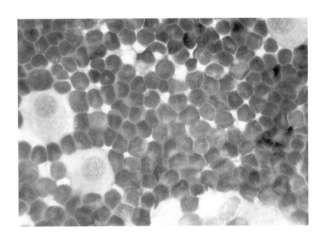

FIGURE 4–22D. Malignant Lymphoma, Lymphoblastic Type, Pleural Fluid, same specimen as in Figures 4–22A through 4–22C. The majority of the small cells are positive for terminal deoxytransferase, a marker of lymphoblastic differentiation and therefore not found in normal lymphocytes (the large, nonreactive cells are mesothelial cells). The malignant cells of lymphoblastic lymphoma, seen here, are indistinguishable from the cells of acute lymphoblastic leukemia (the distinction between these two neoplasms is made clinically and not pathologically). Note that a correct diagnosis of lymphoma in fluids depends on a knowledge of the patient's precise histologic diagnosis as well as on judicious use of appropriate marker studies (immunoperoxidase method for terminal deoxytransferase, cytospin, × 250).

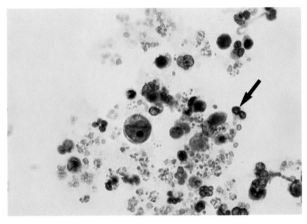

FIGURE 4–24A. Hodgkin Disease, Pleural Fluid. The background is composed of a mixture of lymphocytes, neutrophils, and an occasional eosinophil (arrow). In the center is a highly atypical mononuclear cell with a prominent nucleolus. Without a prior history of Hodgkin disease or diagnostic Reed-Sternberg cells, these findings are also compatible with a diagnosis of non-Hodgkin lymphoma (Papanicolaou-stained cytospin, × 250).

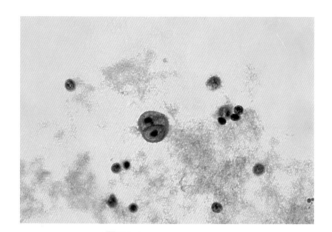

FIGURE 4–24B. Hodgkin Disease, Pleural Fluid. A diagnostic Reed-Sternberg cell with mirror-image nuclei containing large, "inclusion-like" nucleoli is present. A diagnosis of Hodgkin disease can be made on cytologic specimens if cells like this are identified in the typical background (see Fig. 4–24A). (Papanicolaou-stained cytospin, × 250).

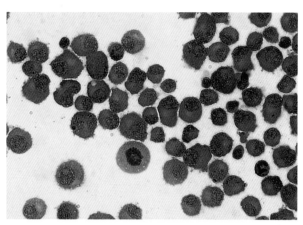

FIGURE 4–25A. Multiple Myeloma, Pleural Fluid. This specimen is identified as malignant on the basis of its monomorphous population of atypical cells. They have retained the eccentric nuclei, the clumped chromatin pattern, and the prominent perinuclear hof, or clear zone, characteristic of plasma cells (Wright-stained smear, × 100).

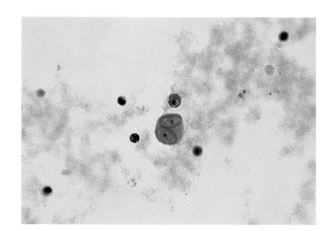

FIGURE 4–24C. Binucleate Mesothelial Cell, same specimen as Figures 4–24A and 4–24B. Mesothelial cells can be distinguished from Reed-Sternberg cells on the basis of their smaller nucleoli and their characteristic cytoplasm (Papanicolaou-stained cytospin, × 250).

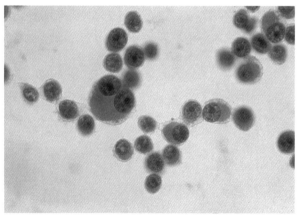

FIGURE 4–25B. Multiple Myeloma, Pleural Fluid. Binucleation and even multinucleation are common in this tumor (Papanicolaou-stained smear, × 250).

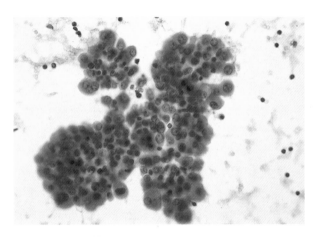

FIGURE 4–26A. Malignant Mesothelioma, Epithelial Type, Pleural Fluid. One of the most common patterns of exfoliation by mesothelioma is the cellular sample containing numerous large clusters of cells with features of mesothelial cells, i.e., abundant dense cytoplasm, round to oval nuclei, and frequent multinucleation. It is not uncommon for the cells of these tumors to show only minimal deviation from benign reactive mesothelial cells. In this case they are enlarged, but the nuclear to cytoplasmic ratio is not as strikingly increased as it often is in other tumors. The clue to the diagnosis of malignancy is the size of the cell clusters (Papanicolaou-stained smear, × 100).

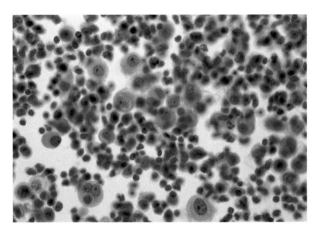

FIGURE 4–27. Malignant Mesothelioma with Prominent Lymphocytic-Histiocytic Response, Pleural Fluid. The cells of this malignant mesothelioma are only mildly atypical and are partially obscured by an intense chronic inflammatory response. Marked inflammation was a prominent component of the biopsy specimen as well. Such cases are easily misinterpreted as reactive; ancillary techniques, such as DNA content measurements or cytogenetic analysis, may be necessary to help establish a diagnosis of malignancy (Papanicolaou-stained cytospin, × 150).

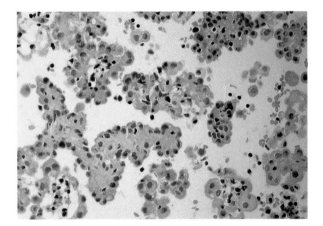

FIGURE 4–26B. Malignant Mesothelioma, Epithelial Type, Pleural Fluid, same specimen as Figure 4–26A (hematoxylin- and eosin-stained cell block, × 50).

PERITONEAL WASHINGS

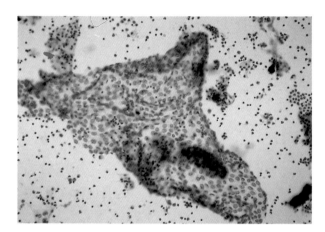

FIGURE 4–28A. Benign Mesothelial Cells, peritoneal washing specimen. Mesothelial cells obtained from washing the peritoneum are pulled off in the form of thin sheets that may be quite large (Papanicolaou-stained cytospin, × 50).

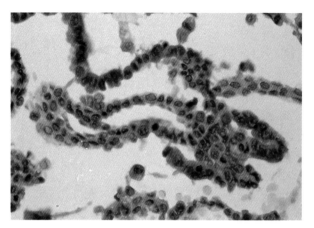

FIGURE 4–28C. Benign Mesothelial Cells, peritoneal washing specimen. In cell block sections, the flat sheets appear instead as thin ribbons of cells that sometimes have a pseudoglandular appearance as they fold over themselves (hematoxylin- and eosin-stained cell block, × 150).

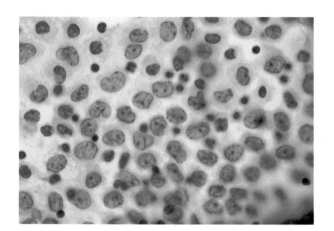

FIGURE 4–28B. Benign Mesothelial Cells, peritoneal washing specimen, same specimen as Figure 4–28A. In peritoneal washings there is often more variation in the nuclear contour and size of mesothelial cells than in effusions. The chromatin texture of these cells, however, is fine and regular (Papanicolaou-stained cytospin, × 250).

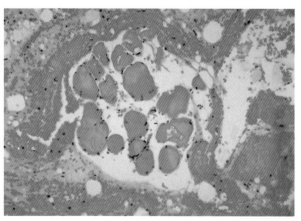

FIGURE 4–29. Skeletal Muscle, peritoneal washings. Skeletal muscle is commonly encountered in these specimens (hematoxylin- and eosin-stained cell block, × 50).

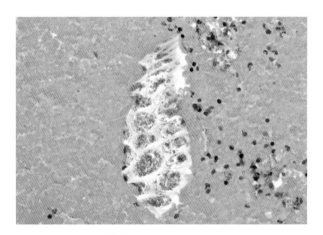

FIGURE 4–30. Vegetable Matter, peritoneal washings. The refractile cellulose membranes of this partially digested vegetable matter are still visible. This patient's washings were preceded by an endometrial curettage complicated by uterine and sigmoid colon perforation (hematoxylin- and eosin-stained cell block, × 100).

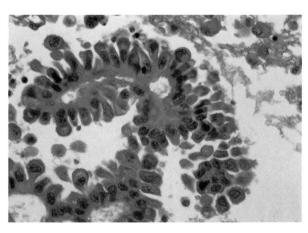

FIGURE 4–31B. Papillary Serous Borderline Tumor of the Ovary, peritoneal washings. The papillary arrangement, cellular tufting, and nuclear atypia are especially well demonstrated in this cell block preparation (hematoxylin- and eosin-stained cell block, × 150).

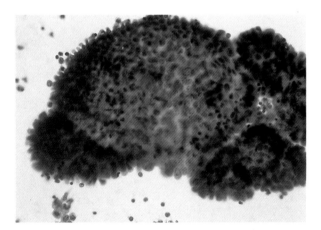

FIGURE 4–31A. Papillary Serous Borderline Tumor of the Ovary, peritoneal washings. The distinction between a carcinoma and a borderline tumor (tumor of low malignant potential) is based on the histologic features of the primary tumor and cannot be made reliably on the cytologic characteristics of cells in a fluid specimen. Both tumors are marked by nuclear atypia and cellular piling and are distinguished on this basis from normal mesothelium. Illustrated here is a large, three-dimensional cluster of malignant cells with variation in nuclear size and shape as well as abnormalities in chromatin texture. Around the edge of the cluster, the tumor cells have a columnar configuration not normally seen with sheets of benign mesothelium (Papanicolaou-stained cytospin, × 100).

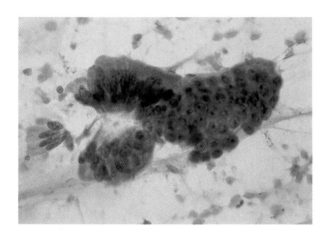

FIGURE 4–32A. Mucinous Borderline Tumor of the Ovary, peritoneal washings. The specimen is composed of well-differentiated columnar tumor cells that show a honeycomb pattern similar to that seen with endocervical cells on a Papanicolaou smear. The hyperchromatic, elongated nuclei may sometimes resemble intestinal carcinomas. This patient presented with ascites (Figs. 4–16A and 4–16B), but malignant cells were not identified in the original peritoneal fluid. Examination of the resected ovary revealed a borderline mucinous tumor (Papanicolaou-stained smear, × 150).

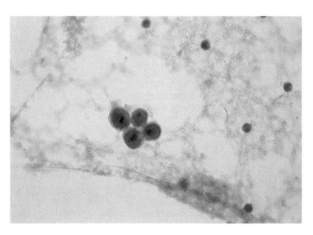

FIGURE 4–33A. Dysgerminoma of the Ovary, peritoneal washings. The tumor cells are typically present as single cells or as loose clusters and have prominent nucleoli. Lymphocytes, which are often a prominent component of the tumor, are present in the background (Papanicolaou-stained smear, × 150).

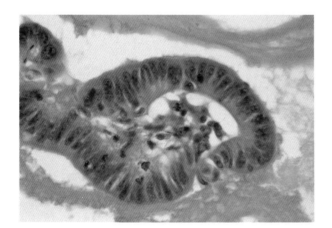

FIGURE 4–32B. Mucinous Borderline Tumor of the Ovary, peritoneal washings, same specimen as Figure 4–32A. The papillary architecture as well as the nuclear hyperchromasia and crowding are well appreciated on the cell block preparation (hematoxylin- and eosin-stained cell block, × 150).

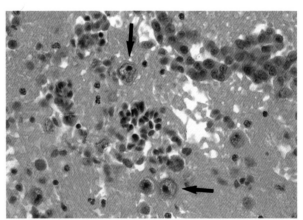

FIGURE 4–33B. Dysgerminoma of the Ovary, peritoneal washings. The cell block shows occasional single tumor cells with large, irregular nuclei and prominent nucleoli (arrows). Lymphocytes and benign mesothelial cells are present in the background (hematoxylin- and eosin-stained cell block, × 150).

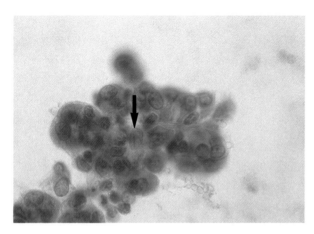

FIGURE 4–34A. Granulosa Cell Tumor, peritoneal washings. These cells are arranged in large, cohesive sheets. The cells are somewhat crowded but not especially pleomorphic, and they may be difficult to distinguish from mesothelial cells. Many have nuclear grooves, however, that are characteristic of this neoplasm (arrow) and not usually seen in mesothelial cells (Papanicolaou-stained smear, × 250).

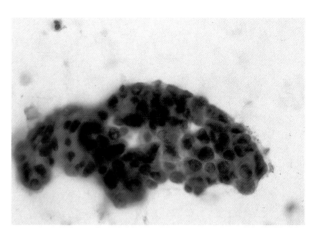

FIGURE 4–35A. Adenocarcinoma of the Endometrium, peritoneal washings. The tumor cells of this well-differentiated carcinoma have subtle cytologic changes allowing their distinction from mesothelial cells, i.e., the tumor cells are larger, somewhat more hyperchromatic, and more haphazardly arranged than mesothelial cells. A honeycomb pattern is not apparent (Papanicolaou-stained smear, × 150).

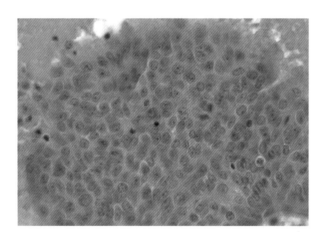

FIGURE 4–34B. Granulosa Cell Tumor, peritoneal washings. Nuclear grooves can also be identified in the cell block preparation. Comparison of these cells with the resected ovarian tumor was helpful in establishing the diagnosis (hematoxylin- and eosin-stained cell block, × 150).

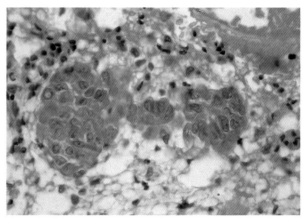

FIGURE 4–35B. Adenocarcinoma of the Endometrium, peritoneal washings, same specimen seen in Figure 4–35A. Comparison of the cells in the cell block sections with sections of the resected uterus (see Fig. 4–35C) were helpful in arriving at a diagnosis (hematoxylin- and eosin-stained cell block, × 150).

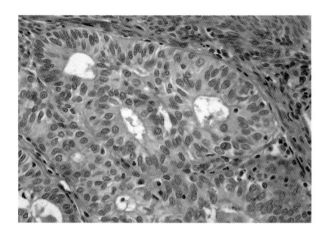

FIGURE 4–35C. Adenocarcinoma of the Endometrium, invading myometrium, same patient as in Figures 4–35A and 4–35B. Although well differentiated, the tumor penetrated through more than two thirds of the thickness of the myometrium, and implants were identified in the endocervix and fallopian tube (hematoxylin- and eosin-stained tissue section, × 150).

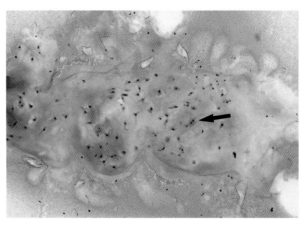

FIGURE 4–36. Chondrosarcoma of the Pelvis, pelvic peritoneal washings. The specimen was composed of large masses of cartilage, identified as well-circumscribed masses of pale purple extracellular matrix containing atypical chondrocytes. Note the binucleate chondrocyte (arrow), a characteristic of malignancy (Papanicolaou-stained smear, × 25).

DIFFERENTIAL GROUPING

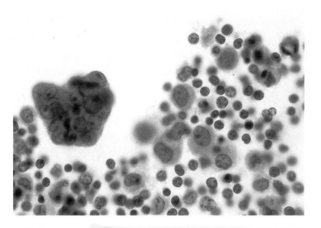

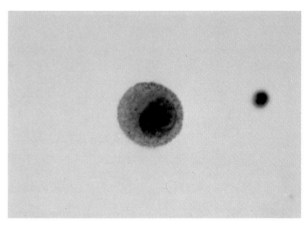

FIGURE 4–37. Metastatic Breast Cancer, Pleural Fluid. The best way to recognize malignant cells is to identify a population of benign mesothelial cells and then contrast them with any cells that may be suspect. The individual cells in the cell cluster are not especially large or pleomorphic. However, the nuclei are consistently different from those of the surrounding mesothelial cells; they all have very prominent nucleoli, and the nuclear to cytoplasmic ratio is much increased. The size of the cell cluster by itself raises the suspicion of malignancy (Papanicolaou-stained cytospin, × 250).

FIGURE 4–38B. Malignant Melanoma, Pleural Fluid. If there is a history of melanoma and the cells look suspicious, the slides should be carefully screened for pigmented cells, which may be few in number. As seen here, melanin pigment within malignant cells has a fine, even granularity (Papanicolaou-stained cytospin, × 375).

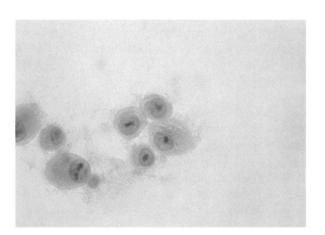

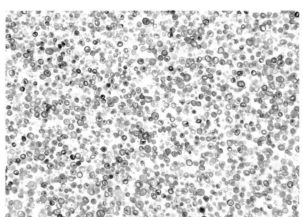

FIGURE 4–38A. Malignant Melanoma, Peritoneal Fluid. Like some adenocarcinomas, melanomas may show little in the way of cell clustering. When not pigmented (amelanotic), they may mimic reactive mesothelial cells. However, as seen here, they often have especially prominent and irregular nucleoli. Nucleoli in highly reactive mesothelial cells can be quite prominent and may be multiple, but not as large as some of these (Papanicolaou-stained smear, × 250).

FIGURE 4–38C. Malignant Melanoma, Pleural Fluid. If the findings are equivocal and no pigment is identified, the cells of a malignant melanoma may be identified by their positive reactivity for HMB-45, the so-called "melanoma-specific antigen" (immunoperoxidase method for HMB-45, cell block, × 50).

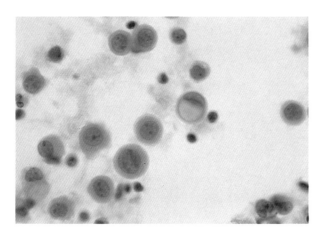

FIGURE 4–39A. Vacuolated Mesothelial Cell, Pleural Fluid. The cell in the center is similar in size to adjacent recognizable benign mesothelial cells. Although compressed to one side, the nucleus appears regular in outline with a normal chromatin pattern (Papanicolaou-stained cytospin, × 250).

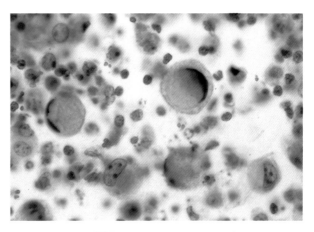

FIGURE 4–39C. Adenocarcinoma of the Stomach (Signet Ring Cell Type), Pleural Fluid. These cells are very enlarged and have hyperchromatic nuclei. Although not necessary for a diagnosis of malignancy, special stains for mucin and carcinoembryonic antigen were positive and confirmed the impression of an adenocarcinoma (Papanicolaou-stained cytospin, × 250). *attenuated nucleus*

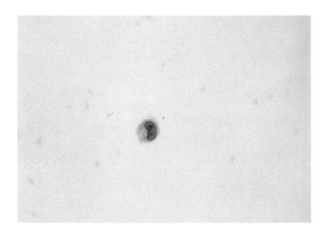

FIGURE 4–39B. Vacuolated Histiocyte, Pleural Fluid. Histiocytes may be indistinguishable from mesothelial cells. The two together are the most common vacuolated cells in effusions. It is less important to identify the exact cell type than it is to determine that a cell is benign. This cell is most likely a histiocyte by virtue of its bean-shaped nucleus and finely vacuolated cytoplasm (Papanicolaou-stained cytospin, × 250).

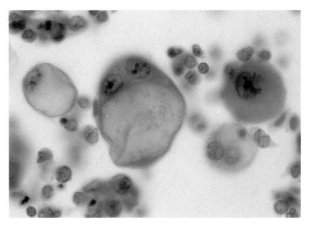

FIGURE 4–39D. Malignant Mesothelioma, Peritoneal Fluid. Some mesotheliomas are composed of a population of vacuolated cells. These cells are obviously malignant but their marked vacuolization made adenocarcinoma a diagnostic possibility. The cells showed a staining pattern (see Table 4–1) characteristic of mesothelial cells, and electron microscopy confirmed the diagnosis of malignant mesothelioma (Papanicolaou-stained cytospin, × 250).

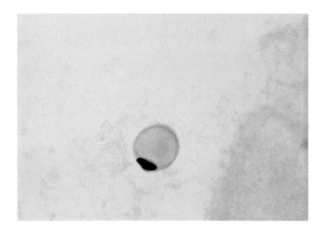

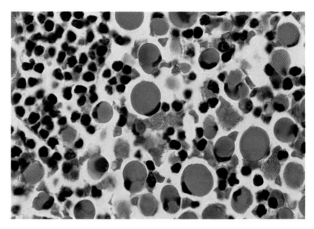

FIGURE 4–39E. Signet Ring Cell Lymphoma, Peritoneal Fluid. The cells of this tumor may easily be confused with benign mesothelial cells or histiocytes. The nucleus is difficult to evaluate because of its compression to one side (Papanicolaou-stained smear, × 250).

FIGURE 4–39G. Signet Ring Cell Lymphoma, retroperitoneal lymph node biopsy, same patient as in Figures 4–39E and 4–39F. The cells of the resected tumor bear a striking resemblance to those seen in the previous fluid specimen. This unusual form of lymphoma is characterized by malignant cells, which accumulate large amounts of cytoplasmic immunoglobulin (hematoxylin- and eosin-stained tissue section, × 250).

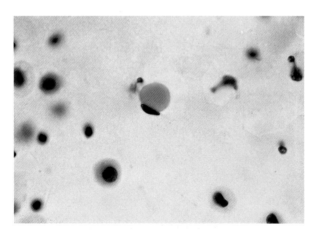

FIGURE 4–39F. Signet Ring Cell Lymphoma, Peritoneal Fluid, same specimen as Figure 4–39E. Some cells contain a large eosinophilic cytoplasmic globule. There is often a prominent population of lymphoid cells. A diagnosis of malignant lymphoma was made when immunoperoxidase studies showed staining of the malignant cells for one but not the other immunoglobulin light chain (Papanicolaou-stained smear, × 250).

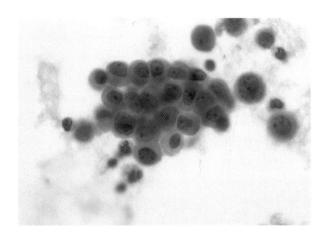

FIGURE 4–40A. Reactive Mesothelial Cells, Pleural Fluid.
Although most mesothelial cells in effusions are dyshesive
and randomly dispersed on the slide, occasional clusters
such as this one are encountered. It is uncommon, however, for a benign condition to produce clusters containing
much more than 20 cells (Papanicolaou-stained cytospin,
× 250).

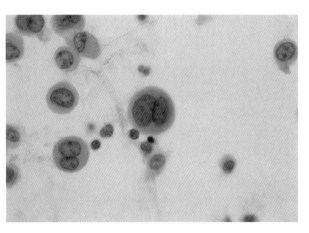

**FIGURE 4–41A. Reactive Mesothelial Cells, Peritoneal
Fluid.** Benign reactive mesothelial cells are often binucleated and may have a coarsely clumped chromatin
texture as well as irregular nuclear contours, as seen here.
Prominent nucleoli may also be present (Papanicolaou-
stained cytospin, × 250). *nucleoli much more prominent in RS cell*

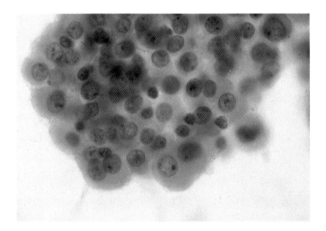

FIGURE 4–40B. Malignant Mesothelioma, Pleural Fluid,
same specimen as Figures 4–26A and 4–26B. Although
these malignant mesothelial cells are larger than the benign
cells in the previous illustration (Fig. 4–40A), there is little
in the way of nuclear pleomorphism, hyperchromasia, or
increase in nuclear to cytoplasmic ratio. A diagnosis of
malignancy was made primarily on the basis of the aggregation of these cells into large clusters; a part of one of
these is apparent in this field (Papanicolaou-stained smear,
× 250).

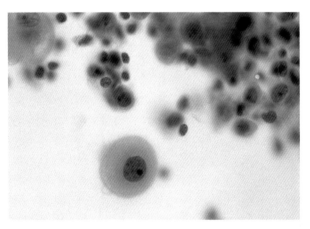

FIGURE 4–41B. Malignant Mesothelioma, Pleural Fluid,
same specimen seen in Figure 4–27. Some cases of mesothelioma cannot be diagnosed with certainty by cytologic
methods alone, especially cases in which the malignant
cells are dispersed as single cells and obscured by abundant
inflammation. The single, enlarged cell seen here is representative of this specimen. Cases like this are impossible
to distinguish from reactive fluids because there is no
unusual cell clustering, no increase in nuclear to cytoplasmic ratio, and only minimal nuclear atypia (Papanicolaou-stained cytospin, × 250).

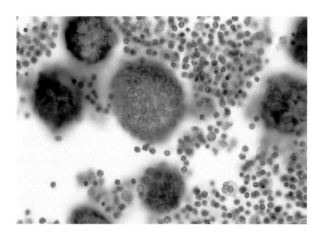

FIGURE 4–42A. Breast Cancer, Pleural Fluid. The tumor cells are arranged in ball-like clusters with smooth outer contours. By focusing with the microscope, the hollowness of many of these spheres can be appreciated (Papanicolaou-stained cytospin, × 150).

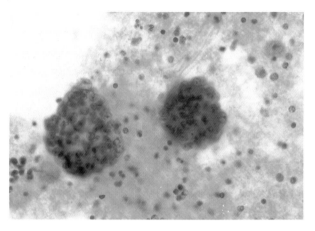

FIGURE 4–43A. Malignant Mesothelioma, Pleural Fluid. The cells are arranged in clusters and at first glance appear similar to those in Figure 4–42A but with slightly more scalloped edges, which is characteristic of mesotheliomas. By focusing with the microscope, the spheres do not appear hollow (Papanicolaou-stained cytospin, × 150).

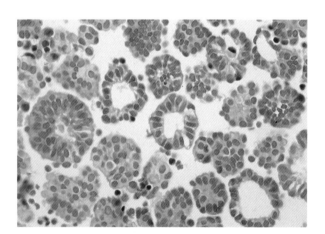

FIGURE 4–42B. Breast Cancer, Pleural Fluid. The fact that many of these spheres are hollow is best appreciated in cell block sections. Such gland-like (or acinar) structures are common in adenocarcinomas but rare in mesotheliomas and may provide a clue to the correct identification of the tumor (hematoxylin- and eosin-stained cell block, × 150).

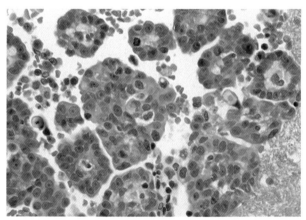

FIGURE 4–43B. Malignant Mesothelioma, Pleural Fluid. Acinar arrangements are uncommon in mesotheliomas. Instead, these tumors often exfoliate as papillary fragments, with cells arranged around a solid, cellular core, as seen here. Such papillary fragments, however, occasionally can be seen in some adenocarcinomas (hematoxylin- and eosin-stained cell block, × 150).

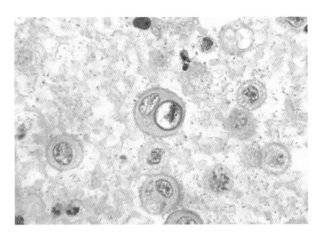

FIGURE 4–44. Adenocarcinoma of the Lung, Pleural Fluid.
A definitive distinction between mesothelioma and adenocarcinoma often depends on histochemical and immunocytochemical studies. This tumor was identified as an adenocarcinoma on the basis of the positive staining with periodic acid–Schiff. The mucin vacuole has a bright red center surrounded by a halo and then a bright red ring (PAS-D–stained cell block, × 250).

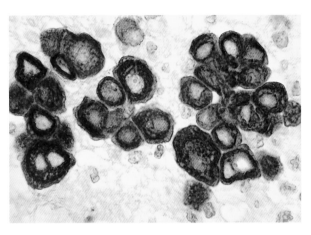

FIGURE 4–46. Malignant Mesothelioma, Peritoneal Fluid.
Tumor cells are strongly positive for keratin with a perinuclear accentuation of staining intensity, a pattern highly characteristic of mesothelial cells (immunoperoxidase method, cell block, × 250).

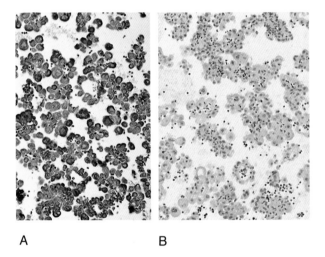

A   B

FIGURE 4–45. Malignant Mesothelioma, Pleural Fluid, same case as in Figures 4–26A and 4–26B and 4–40B. Tumor cells are strongly positive for keratin (A) and negative for carcinoembryonic antigen (B) (immunoperoxidase method, cell block, both × 50).

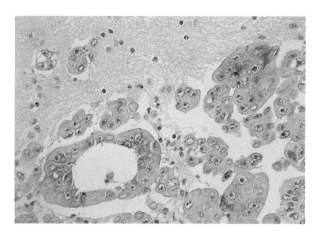

FIGURE 4–47. Breast Cancer, Pleural Fluid. These tumor cells show immunoreactivity for carcinoembryonic antigen, virtually never encountered in mesotheliomas (immunoperoxidase method for carcinoembryonic antigen, cell block, × 100).

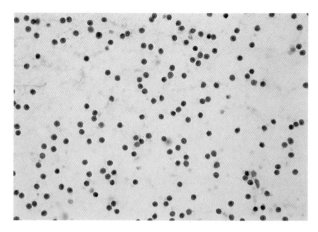

FIGURE 4–49A. Tuberculous Effusion, Pleural Fluid. The cells are all small, mature lymphocytes. A pleural biopsy specimen revealed caseating granulomas and acid-fast organisms (Papanicolaou-stained smear, × 100).

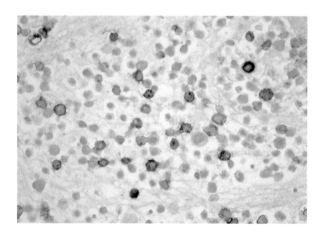

FIGURE 4–48. Adenocarcinoma of the Stomach, Peritoneal Fluid. Tumor cells show strong staining for Ca 19–9, a cellular antigen commonly expressed in adenocarcinomas, especially those of the stomach, colon, and pancreas, and not seen in mesotheliomas (immunoperoxidase method for Ca 19–9, cell block, × 100).

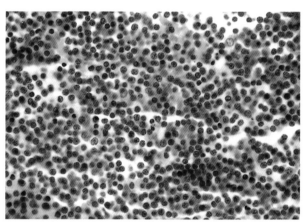

FIGURE 4–49B. Tuberculous Effusion, Pleural Fluid, same specimen seen in Figure 4–49A (hematoxylin- and eosin-stained cell block, × 150).

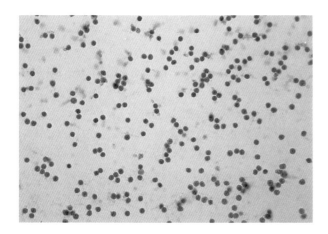

FIGURE 4–50A. Chronic Lymphocytic Leukemia, Pleural Fluid. These cells are indistinguishable from those in Figure 4–49A. A distinction would depend on demonstrating a clonal population of B cells on air-dried cytospins or performing kappa/lambda analysis on fresh fluid by flow cytometry (Papanicolaou-stained smear, × 100).

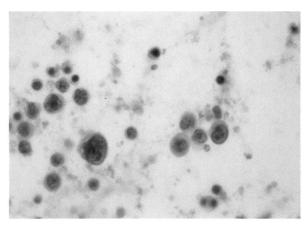

FIGURE 4–51A. Malignant Lymphoma, Pleural Fluid. The lymphoid cells have enlarged, hyperchromatic nuclei with irregular nuclear contours and prominent nucleoli (Papanicolaou-stained cytospin, × 250).

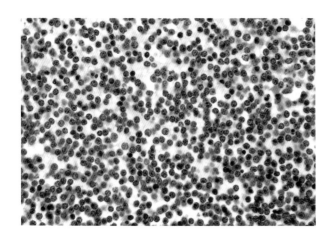

FIGURE 4–50B. Chronic Lymphocytic Leukemia, Pleural Fluid, same specimen seen in Figure 4–50A (hematoxylin- and eosin-stained cell block, × 150).

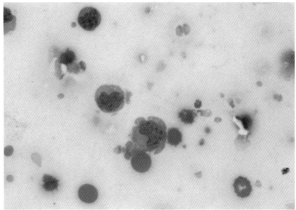

FIGURE 4–51B. Malignant Lymphoma, Pleural Fluid, same specimen as in Figure 4–51A. The irregular contours are best appreciated on the air-dried Wright-stained preparations. Although a diagnosis of malignancy is possible in cases like this, establishing the precise subtype of lymphoma often necessitates examination of solid tissue (Wright-stained cytospin, × 250).

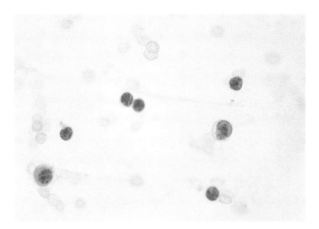

FIGURE 4–52A. Reactive Lymphocytes, Pleural Fluid. This patient had a history of a high-grade B-cell lymphoma treated with bone marrow transplantation. This pleural effusion contained a population of small, benign-appearing lymphocytes but also occasional larger cells, some with irregular nuclei or plasmacytoid shapes, which raised the possibility of recurrent lymphoma (Papanicolaou-stained smear, × 250).

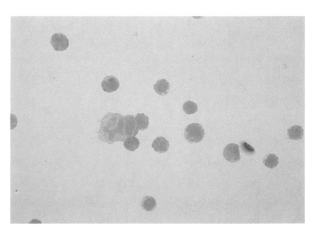

FIGURE 4–52C. Reactive Lymphocytes, Pleural Fluid, same specimen as in Figures 4–52A and 4–52B. Immunoperoxidase studies showed that all the lymphocytes, including the larger cells, stained as T cells (T11 immunoperoxidase, × 250).

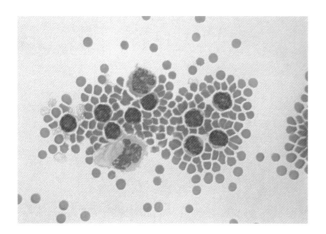

FIGURE 4–52B. Reactive Lymphocytes, Pleural Fluid, same specimen as in Figure 4–52A (Wright-stained cytospin, × 250).

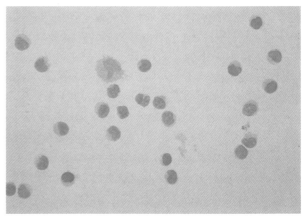

FIGURE 4–52D. Reactive Lymphocytes, Pleural Fluid, same specimen as in Figures 4–52A through 4–52C. None of the cells stained as B cells. These findings supported a benign diagnosis (Dako pan-B [DB-10] immunoperoxidase, × 250).

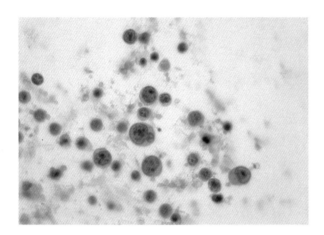

FIGURE 4–53. Malignant Lymphoma, Pleural Fluid. The malignant cells with their irregular nuclear contours and prominent nuclear blebs typically show no tendency for cluster formation. The lymphoid nature of these cells can be confirmed with immunoperoxidase studies for leukocyte common antigen (Papanicolaou-stained cytospin, × 250).

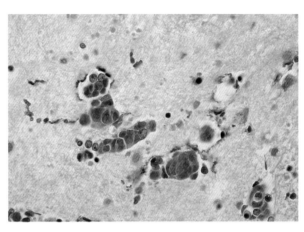

FIGURE 4–54B. Small-Cell Carcinoma of the Lung, Pleural Fluid, same specimen as Figure 4–54A (hematoxylin- and eosin-stained cell block, × 150).

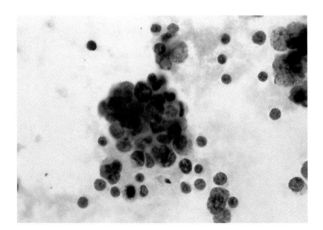

FIGURE 4–54A. Small-Cell Carcinoma of the Lung, Pleural Fluid. The cells of small-cell carcinoma have scant cytoplasm, dark nuclei with granular chromatin, and small nucleoli. Although similar in size to those of many lymphomas, the cells are cohesive and mold to each other's contours. This is very rarely seen in lymphomas (Papanicolaou-stained cytospin, × 250).

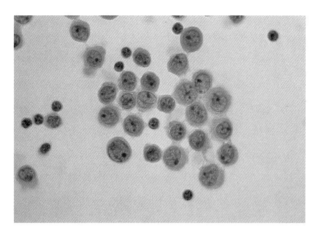

FIGURE 4–55A. Lobular Carcinoma of the Breast, Pleural Fluid. Unlike the cells of infiltrating ductal carcinoma of the breast, the cells of this tumor are small and typically exfoliate as single cells. They are often inconspicuous and may not be recognized as malignant, being confused with mesothelial cells. Even when recognized as atypical, they may be misinterpreted as malignant lymphoma, especially in cases where nuclear contour irregularity is pronounced. As seen here, the cells are small, the nuclei are folded, cleaved, and irregular, and cytoplasm is scant (Papanicolaou-stained cytospin, × 250).

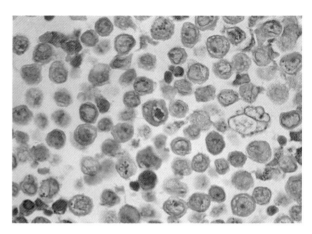

FIGURE 4–55C. Lobular Carcinoma of the Breast, Pleural Fluid, same case as seen in Figures 4–55A and 4–55B. Most of these tumors are positive for mucin, which helps distinguish them from reactive mesothelial cells and lymphoma. Fortunately, it is rare for breast cancer to manifest itself initially as a positive fluid; in most cases there already is a documented malignancy. Knowledge of the histologic subtype and comparison of the biopsy material to the fluid specimens are very important for correct identification (periodic acid–Schiff stain with diastase, cell block, × 250).

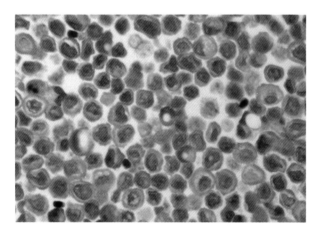

FIGURE 4–55B. Lobular Carcinoma of the Breast, Pleural Fluid, same case as seen in Figure 4–55A. The nuclear irregularity of these cells can be appreciated on cell block preparations. Occasional cytoplasmic vacuoles are present (hematoxylin- and eosin-stained cell block, × 250).

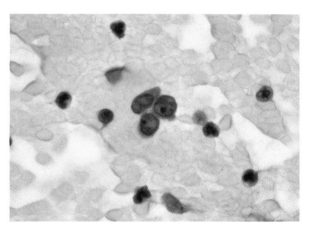

FIGURE 4–56. Ewing Sarcoma-Neuroepithelioma-Askin Tumor, Pleural Fluid. These small, malignant cells were identified in a 14-year-old girl who had a pleural effusion and a mass involving the ribs and chest wall. The cells had round or irregular nuclei, moderately prominent nucleoli, and scant cytoplasm. Small-cell aggregates like this one suggested a nonlymphoid tumor, but precise classification was not possible on cytologic examination alone. Fluid submitted for cytogenetic analysis revealed a translocation of the long arms of chromosomes 11 and 22, which is characteristic of tumors classified as Ewing sarcoma, neuroepithelioma, and Askin tumor. This finding has suggested a common histogenesis for these childhood neoplasms (hematoxylin- and eosin-stained smear, × 250).

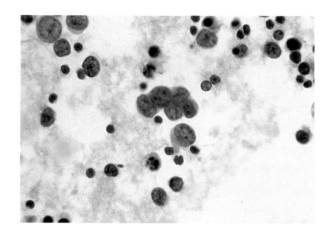

FIGURE 4–57A. Alveolar Rhabdomyosarcoma, Peritoneal Fluid. These tumors, composed of small to medium-sized cells, can resemble lymphomas and other small-cell tumors. The nuclei are hyperchromatic, have a granular chromatin texture, and very scant cytoplasm (Papanicolaou-stained cytospin, × 250).

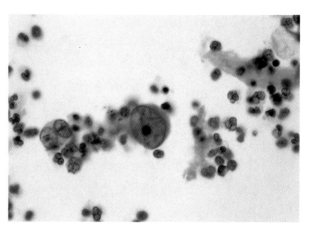

FIGURE 4–58. Large-Cell Undifferentiated Carcinoma of the Lung, Pericardial Fluid. Large malignant cells may be seen in poorly differentiated carcinomas of many sites. Note the very large nucleus, prominent nucleolus, and scant cytoplasm (Papanicolaou-stained cytospin, × 250).

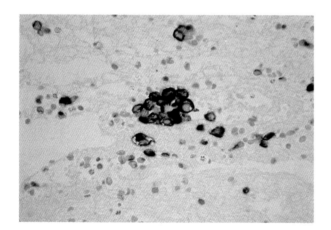

FIGURE 4–57B. Alveolar Rhabdomyosarcoma, Peritoneal Fluid, same specimen as in Figure 4–57A. These tumors are strongly positive for desmin, a marker of muscle differentiation, which allows distinction from other small-cell neoplasms (immunoperoxidase method for desmin, × 150).

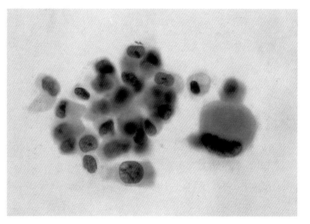

FIGURE 4–59. Malignant Schwannoma, Pleural Fluid (malignant peripheral nerve sheath tumor), same case as seen in Figures 4–19A and 4–19B. The cells of some sarcomas may be very pleomorphic and may resemble poorly differentiated carcinomas. This sarcoma is negative for keratin proteins and positive for S-100 protein. Some sarcomas, however, can be keratin positive. An exact identification was aided by comparison of these cells with the previously resected neoplasm (Papanicolaou-stained cytospin, × 250).

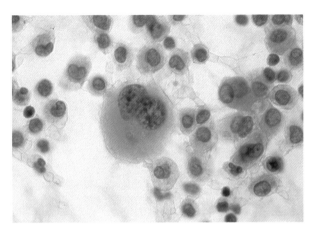

FIGURE 4–60A. Malignant Mesothelioma, Peritoneal Fluid. The cells of some mesotheliomas can be quite large. The large malignant cell seen here has a peripheral halo (brush border) and dense cytoplasm that suggests mesothelial derivation (Papanicolaou-stained smear, × 250).

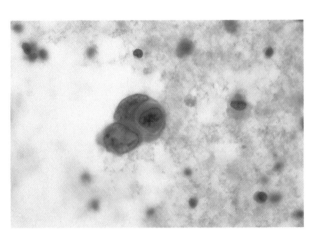

FIGURE 4–61. Nonseminomatous Germ Cell Tumor, Pleural Fluid. These tumors shed large, highly atypical cells that may be single or arranged in clusters. Note the large areas of chromatin clearing in the nucleus, which is seen in many of these tumors. This patient had a history of a testicular tumor. A good knowledge of the patient's history and comparison of the fluid with previous specimens are crucial for a correct diagnosis (Papanicolaou-stained cytospin, × 250).

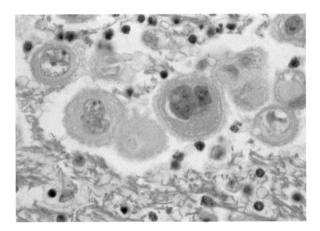

FIGURE 4–60B. Malignant Mesothelioma, Peritoneal Fluid. The brush border of some malignant mesothelial cells can be appreciated on cell block preparations also (hematoxylin- and eosin-stained cell block, × 250).

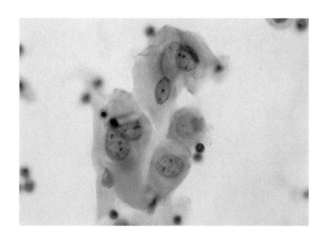

FIGURE 4–62A. Mesothelial Cell Atypia Due to Treatment, peritoneal washing. There is marked nuclear and cytoplasmic enlargement, but the normal nuclear to cytoplasmic ratio appears to be preserved (Papanicolaou-stained cytospin, × 250).

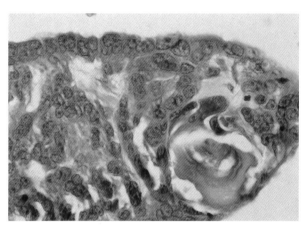

FIGURE 4–63. Papillary Serous Adenocarcinoma of the Ovary, peritoneal washing. This is the patient's initial peritoneal washing, before treatment; it provides a frame of reference for interpreting subsequent washings. The malignant cells seen here and photographed at the same magnification as Figure 4–62B are quite different from the atypical cells, due to treatment effect seen in Figures 4–62A and 4–62B, i.e., the nuclei are large and more variable in size, the chromatin texture is more coarse, nucleoli are prominent, and the nuclear to cytoplasmic ratio is significantly increased. Multiple peritoneal biopsies taken concurrently with the specimen in Figures 4–62A and 4–62B were negative for the diagnosis of tumor (hematoxylin- and eosin-stained cell block, × 150).

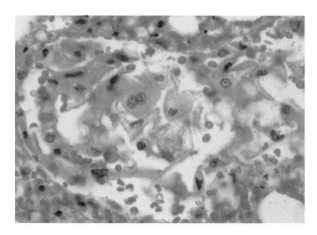

FIGURE 4–62B. Mesothelial Cell Atypia Due to Treatment, peritoneal washing, same specimen as Figure 4–63. In the cell block, there are occasional cells with hyperchromatic, angular nuclei (hematoxylin- and eosin-stained cell block, × 150).

C·H·A·P·T·E·R

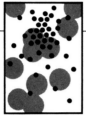

5

CEREBROSPINAL FLUID CYTOLOGY

Edmund S. Cibas

Compared with other fluid specimens, the amount of cerebrospinal fluid (CSF) available for cytologic examination is limited. The total volume of CSF in the adult is about 150 ml. Under normal circumstances, fluid is produced by the choroid plexus, predominantly in the lateral ventricles, circulates through the third and fourth ventricles, and then exits the ventricular system at the base of the brain through the foramina of Luschka and Magendie to bathe the subarachnoid spaces of the brain and spinal cord. Fluid is then reabsorbed by the arachnoid granulations into the venous system.

Normal CSF contains less than five cells/mm³, mostly lymphocytes and monocytes (Figs. 5–1 to 5–3). Choroidal, ependymal, and arachnoid lining cells are rarely seen; when a few benign, cuboidal cells are encountered, they are often presumed to be of choroidal or ependymal origin (Figs. 5–4 and 5–5). The occasional benign spindle cell encountered in CSF is often presumed to be of arachnoidal origin. Frequent contaminants include squamous cells (presumably from the skin) and starch particles (from gloves, see Fig. 5–11A).

Cerebrospinal fluid is most commonly obtained by passing a needle through the intervertebral space of the lumbar portion of the spinal column with the patient on his or her side (lumbar puncture). Less frequently, the cisternum magnum at the base of the skull is used. Ventricular fluid can also be aspirated through an operative hole in the skull; such specimens often contain fragments of normal brain tissue (Figs. 5–5 and 5–6). Patients with documented tumors are often treated with intrathecal chemotherapy instilled through an Ommaya reservoir, a small pouch under the scalp with a cannula leading into a lateral ventricle; fluid can be withdrawn from the ventricle via this reservoir for cytologic examination.

Tumor cells in CSF are not necessarily very numerous. Therefore, although volumes as small as 1 ml are often submitted for evaluation, a volume of at least 3 ml is preferred. The more fluid submitted, the greater the likelihood of detection of abnormal cells. Ideally, CSF should be collected fresh, without fixative, and submitted for preparation as quickly as possible because cells in CSF deteriorate rapidly. If any delay in preparation is anticipated, specimens may be collected in Saccomano carbowax fixative. This guarantees excellent specimen preservation but precludes the preparation of air-dried slides, which are useful in the evaluation of lymphomas and leukemias (discussed later). A variety of preparatory techniques are used, most commonly cytocentrifugation and membrane filtration. Depending on the volume and cellularity of the specimen, the author routinely prepares two to four slides, some of which are alcohol-fixed and Papanicolaou-stained and some of which are air-dried and Wright-stained.

One pitfall of CSF cytology is the bloody (traumatic) tap. Contamination of CSF by peripheral blood can be a source of diagnostic error if the elements of circulating blood are interpreted as intrinsic to the CSF. Thus, the neutrophils normally found in blood may be misinterpreted as acute meningitis, or leukemic blasts may be interpreted as involvement of the central nervous system by leukemia. It has been shown that very little blood is needed to significantly alter the cellular composition of CSF. Because alcohol fixation often lyses red cells, contamination by blood is best recognized on air-dried Wright-stained preparations, which preserve red cell morphology. If numerous red cells are present, the possibility of a traumatic tap should be considered and discretion is advised in diagnosis. Similarly, it is advisable to stain CSF samples separately to avoid "floaters," since a diagnosis of malignancy in CSF is often made on the basis of relatively few cells.

NON-NEOPLASTIC CONDITIONS

Most central nervous system (CNS) infections result in nonspecific alterations in the cellular composition of CSF. Acute bacterial infections lead to an increase in polymorphonuclear leukocytes (Fig. 5–7); viral infections typically result in an increase in mononuclear cells, predominantly lymphocytes (Figs. 5–12A to 5–12C); and parasitic infections may lead to an increase in eosinophils. The only organism identified with any frequency in CSF is the fungus *Cryptococcus neoformans* (Fig. 5–11B). Bacteria may be seen with Papanicolaou or Wright stain, but exact identification requires culture. Most viral meningoencephalitis is produced by the enterovirus group of viruses (e.g., coxsackievirus and echovirus), which do not produce identifiable viral changes such as inclusions. Herpes simplex and herpes zoster, however, can occasionally be recognized in CSF by virtue of their characteristic cytopathic changes. These enlarged, altered cells can be misinterpreted as malignant, and therefore viral infection should be considered in the differential diagnosis of large atypical cells in CSF (see Table 5–5). The protozoan *Toxoplasma gondii*, the causative agent in cerebral toxoplasmosis, is occasionally identified in CSF as a small, 3 to 6 μ, bow-shaped organism (Fig. 5–10). Amebic organisms have been identified in CSF, as has

Angiostrongylus cantonensis, but the organisms in most parasitic CNS infections, including cerebral cysticercosis, are generally not seen in CSF.

Cytology laboratories are occasionally asked to evaluate CSF from patients suspected of having a benign recurrent aseptic meningitis (Mollaret disease). This is a very rare disorder characterized by periodic attacks of fever, nausea, vomiting, headache, and neck stiffness, which can last for up to seven days. Signs and symptoms disappear rapidly but recur days to years later. The cause is unknown, and the disease is usually self-limited. Diagnosis depends on the typical clinical presentation and the exclusion of other causes. The cytologic changes are nonspecific. There may be a pleocytosis of lymphocytes and neutrophils, but the hallmark of this disorder is the presence of large mononuclear cells called Mollaret cells, which have a fragile-appearing cytoplasm and a large, irregular nucleus (Figs. 5–9A and 5–9B). These cells are thought to be monocytes; they are neither specific nor essential for the diagnosis.

Cerebrospinal fluid is rarely examined in patients with cerebral infarction, but the cells encountered are similar to those seen in the underlying damaged parenchyma (neutrophils and foamy macrophages). Subarachnoid hemorrhage may be distinguished from a traumatic tap if erythrophagocytosis and hemosiderin-laden macrophages are present. Demyelinating diseases, such as multiple sclerosis, and idiopathic inflammatory disorders, such as Guillain-Barré syndrome, may result in a nonspecific CSF pleocytosis. Cerebrospinal fluid is paradoxically unremarkable in such devastating illnesses as Alzheimer disease, Jacob-Creutzfeldt disease, Parkinson disease, and Huntington chorea. Foamy macrophages, presumably containing abnormal accumulations of cellular metabolites, have been described in CSF from patients with storage diseases such as Tay-Sachs disease, Hunter-Hurler syndrome, and Sanfilippo syndrome.

NEOPLASTIC CONDITIONS

Malignant cells, in most instances, are identified without difficulty in CSF because they are unlike any of the normal cells of CSF. Metastatic tumors are more commonly encountered than are primary CNS tumors. Although not all tumors involving the leptomeninges shed recognizable malignant cells, studies suggest that the sensitivity of CSF cytology is approximately 60%. The most difficult malignancies to identify reliably in CSF are lymphomas and leukemias. In general, it is advisable to give every case a primary diagnosis or general categorization such as "negative," "suspicious," or "positive," followed by a descriptive diagnosis that further characterizes the cells identified. Most CSF samples can be easily categorized as negative or positive, but in some cases the findings may be inconclusive because of scant evidence or poor cellular preservation.

DIFFERENTIAL DIAGNOSES

Small (Lymphocyte-Like) Cells

By common consensus, one of the most difficult challenges in CSF cytology is the specimen composed of lymphoid cells with varying degrees of atypia

(Table 5–1). Unfortunately, the cellularity of the specimen is not always helpful in distinguishing benign from malignant fluids. Meningitis and noninfectious CNS disorders such as multiple sclerosis are characterized by an increased number of reactive lymphoid cells that, on occasion, may be difficult to distinguish from leukemia or lymphoma. These specimens typically show a mixed population of mature lymphocytes with scant cytoplasm, condensed chromatin, and regular nuclear outlines, together with larger cells with more abundant cytoplasm, larger nuclei with prominent nucleoli, and irregular nuclear contours (Figs. 5–12A and 5–12B). These larger cells represent stimulated lymphocytes, including immunoblasts and plasmacytoid cells. In general, benign fluids show a somewhat heterogeneous mixture of lymphoid cells with predominantly small mature lymphocytes; neoplasms are typically more monomorphous and immature in their appearance, but exceptions to this rule occur.

Cerebrospinal fluid examination in patients with acute lymphoblastic leukemia (ALL) is especially important, because prophylactic CNS treatment has reduced the incidence of recurrence in the CNS from about 60% to 10% and has significantly increased survival. The disease is predominantly seen in children, and as in all the leukemias and lymphomas, air-dried Wright-stained samples are helpful in the evaluation of cellular morphology. The leukemic blasts in alcohol-fixed, Papanicolaou-stained slides have hyperchromatic nuclei with granular chromatin, prominent nucleoli, occasionally irregular nuclear contours, and scant cytoplasm (Fig. 5–13A). This is in contrast to their appearance in Wright-stained preparations, where the chromatin has an evenly distributed, pale (so-called blastic) appearance (Fig. 5–13B). A marker that is helpful in confirming a diagnosis of ALL is terminal deoxytransferase (TDT), a DNA polymerase that is not present in normal lymphocytes or in nonlymphoblastic leukemias (Fig. 5–13C).

Although prophylactic CNS treatment has not improved survival in acute nonlymphocytic leukemia, CSF examination is valuable in guiding therapy (Figs. 5–14A and 5–14B). The nonlymphocytic blasts (e.g., myelocytes and myelomonocytes) may be indistinguishable from ALL blasts on Papanicolaou-stained material, but Wright stain may show cytoplasmic granules not usually seen in lymphoblasts, or it may show Auer rods (red, rod-like structures in the cytoplasm), which are diagnostic of acute myelogenous leukemia. In CSF, it is usually sufficient simply to identify the presence of blasts because the definitive diagnosis regarding cell type rests with the bone marrow biopsy.

Chronic lymphocytic leukemia (CLL) very rarely involves the CNS, and the cells are morphologically indistinguishable from mature lymphocytes. This diagnosis should be made with extreme caution in CSF after excluding the possibility of specimen contamination with blood, and preferably other evidence, such as immunocytochemistry or flow cytometry (discussed later) should support the diagnosis.

Approximately 4% of patients with systemic malignant lymphoma develop meningeal involvement. A lymphoma with diffuse histology or of the large-cell "histiocytic" type more commonly involves the CNS than one with nodular histology or of the small-cell "lymphocytic" type. Lymphoblastic and undifferentiated lymphomas have a high incidence of CNS involvement. Evidence of Hodgkin disease and well-differentiated lymphocytic lymphoma is rarely seen in CSF. As with the leukemias, it is important to differentiate lymphoma from a reactive condition. A hypercellular specimen composed of large atypical lymphoid cells with irregular nuclear contours, prominent nucleoli, and abundant cytoplasm in a patient with a history of a large-cell lymphoma is usually straightforward. A less cellular sample or a sample composed predominantly of small lymphoid cells is often difficult. Features that favor a diagnosis of lymphoma include a monomorphous population, prominent nucleoli, and marked nuclear contour irregularity (Figs. 5–12D, 5–12E, and 5–15A). In some cases, however, definitive diagnosis may not be possible without lymphoid marker studies. Unstained air-dried cytospins are reacted with antibodies against a pan–B-cell marker, a pan–T-cell marker, and kappa and lambda immunoglobulin light chains. Reactive and inflammatory fluids are composed primarily of T cells, whereas most lymphomas that involve the CNS are B-cell neoplasms (Fig. 5–12F). The T-cell lymphomas, including mycosis fungoides, typically have very prominent nuclear irregularity that facilitates diagnosis even without markers. Conversely, a predominantly B-cell infiltrate is highly suspicious for lymphoma in CSF, and the diagnosis can be established by demonstrating light chain clonality (a marked preponderance of either kappa or lambda expression). These lymphocyte markers can also be measured by flow cytometry, but more fluid (8 to 12 ml of a moderately cellular specimen) is required for this technique.

A variety of other small-cell neoplasms may on occasion be confused with lymphoma or leukemia. Medulloblastoma, a tumor of the cerebellum seen in children, is composed of small cells with scant cytoplasm that may resemble leukemic blasts or lymphoma (Fig. 5–15B). It is morphologically identical to other small-cell neoplasms such as neuroblastoma, retinoblastoma, and small-cell carcinoma of the lung (Figs. 5–15C and 5–15D). What distinguishes all these nonlymphoid tumor cells from lymphoid cells is their tendency to cluster and exhibit nuclear molding. A word of caution is advised: on occasion, lymphocytes (and the cells of lymphoma or leukemia) cluster together on cytospin preparations and may mimic small-cell neoplasms, such as medulloblastoma and small-cell carcinoma (Figs. 5–15F to 5–15H). Caution should be exercised if the nuclear features are poorly preserved (Fig. 5–15F). The differential diagnosis of small cells in CSF is summarized in Table 5–1.

Plasma Cells

Plasma cells are occasionally seen in CSF (Table 5–2). If present in large numbers, they raise the possibility of a plasma cell neoplasm, such as multiple myeloma or plasmacytoma, which on rare occasions may involve the meninges. Plasma cells may be seen in a variety of benign conditions, such as multiple sclerosis, viral and tuberculous meningitis (Fig. 5–8), Lyme disease, neurosyphilis, and cerebral cysticercosis. The diagnosis of multiple myeloma or plasmacytoma may be confirmed by demonstrating a preponderance of immunoreactivity for either kappa or lambda light chains.

Eosinophils

Eosinophils are also rarely seen in CSF (Table 5–3), the most frequent cause of their presence being parasitic infection. The two parasites most likely to provoke a CSF eosinophilia both invade the CNS. Some (but not all) patients with cerebral cysticercosis caused by *Taenia solium* have a pleocytosis with increased eosinophils. Cerebral angiostrongyliasis, also known as eosinophilic meningitis (caused by *Angiostrongylus cantonensis*), is characterized by a high percentage (sometimes more than 90%) of eosinophils. A rare fungal meningitis caused by *Coccidioides immitis* has been reported to be associated with increased eosinophils, as have certain bacterial infections, such as tuberculosis and syphilis. Malignancies involving the CNS may show an eosinophilic pleocytosis, the best documented being lymphoma. Foreign material introduced via shunts and hypersensitivity reactions has also been implicated. In some patients, a cause for the presence of the eosinophils is never established.

Histiocytes

Histiocytes are encountered in CSF in a variety of conditions (Table 5–4). These are large cells derived from monocytes with round to oval, sometimes folded, nuclei and abundant cytoplasm that may be foamy or granular (Fig. 5–16A). Histiocytes may be seen in meningitis of any cause, in subarachnoid hemorrhage (showing erythrophagocytosis or filled with hemosiderin), in cerebral infarction, and postoperatively or after diagnostic procedures such as myelography. Macrophages with foamy cytoplasm have been reported in CSF from patients with storage diseases such as Tay-Sachs disease and Hunter-Hurler and Sanfilippo syndromes. Large neoplastic lymphoid cells in lymphomas are usually easily distinguished from benign histiocytes by virtue of their marked nuclear atypia. Large atypical histiocytes can be seen in the rare group of disorders termed histiocytosis X as well as in the malignant histiocytoses.

Large Atypical Cells

Cells from both metastatic and primary CNS tumors, if present in CSF, are usually easily identified as malignant, either by virtue of their large size (Fig. 5–16B) or by their tendency to cluster. Identifying the exact origin of these cells depends on a good clinical history (age of patient, radiographic findings, or previously diagnosed malignancy); immunohistochemical studies may be helpful (discussed later).

Metastatic tumor cells may be abundant or very few in number, and there may be either a very marked or very mild inflammatory reaction. Once a positive diagnosis is established and therapy has been instituted, patients are frequently followed by periodic CSF examination to monitor the effect of treatment. The disease may wax and wane; subsequent fluids may show no residual tumor cells, but often a small number of malignant cells are still recognizable. Comparison with the initial diagnostic specimen is often helpful because in this circumstance even one cell similar to the original tumor is significant and may be sufficient for a positive diagnosis.

Virtually any tumor may metastasize to the leptomeninges and result in a positive CSF. The most common, however, are carcinomas of the lung and breast, melanoma, and lymphoma. Adenocarcinomas are encountered more commonly than squamous or transitional cell carcinomas; metastatic sarcomas and germ cell tumors in CSF are rare. Small-cell carcinomas (in particular those of the lung) are commonly identified in the CSF.

Determining the origin of malignant cells usually depends on a good clinical history. In most instances, a primary tumor has already been diagnosed, in which case the cells in a malignant CSF may be described as "consistent with origin from known breast cancer." It is extremely uncommon, in fact, for breast cancer to metastasize to CSF before the primary tumor has been detected. But some tumors, notably carcinomas of the lung (adenocarcinoma and large-cell and small-cell undifferentiated carcinomas), melanoma, and gastric adenocarcinoma may initially present as a positive CSF. If a primary CNS tumor is suspected, careful review of the history and radiologic findings is essential because many primary CNS tumors have very characteristic clinical and radiographic presentations.

The differential diagnosis of large atypical cells in CSF is listed in Table 5–5. Adenocarcinomas can appear as single cells or clusters and usually have large, variably sized nuclei with prominent nucleoli. Cytoplasm may be scant or abundant, and vacuoles may be present. In particular, adenocarcinomas of the breast often have scant cytoplasm (Fig. 5–17), and those of the lung may have abundant, finely vacuolated cytoplasm (Fig. 5–21). In addition, breast cancer cells have more of a tendency to form cellular rows and even occasional gland structures than does lung cancer (Figs. 5–18 and 5–19), but these features cannot always be relied upon to identify the cell type. Note that the less common lobular type of breast cancer is composed of small cells and is in the differential diagnosis of small-cell tumors. The cells of malignant melanoma, if not pigmented, may resemble those of adenocarcinoma. There is less of a tendency to cluster formation in the former, and the nuclei usually contain a more prominent macronucleolus. A definite diagnosis depends on identifying cytoplasmic melanin.

Rare melanomas may arise in the meninges (Fig. 5–22). Melanin by itself, however, is not pathognomomic of melanoma because the meninges may be pigmented in a condition called melanosis cerebri, and this pigment may be phagocytized by macrophages. Large-cell "histiocytic" lymphomas exfoliate as single cells and should be considered if there is no convincing cell clustering. On rare occasions, cells with herpetic inclusions have been mistaken for adenocarcinoma.

In patients with no known malignancy and a solitary CNS mass, the possibility of a glial tumor should be considered. The most common large-cell CNS tumors to shed in CSF are the astrocytic neoplasms (astrocytomas or glioblastoma multiforme). The amount of hyperchromasia and pleomorphism of the cells depends on the grade of the neoplasm, but these tumors may shed very large, hyperchromatic cells that are either single or grouped. Fine cytoplasmic extensions (the glial fibrils) may be seen and are helpful in pointing to a glial origin (Fig. 5–23). Medulloblastomas and astrocytomas or glioblastomas multiforme account for about 65% of all primary CNS tumors identified in CSF; other CNS tumors exfoliate less commonly.

Oligodendroglioma, a glial neoplasm, can shed either as single cells or in clusters. The cells typically have round nuclei and, when clustered, have a syncytial quality. Tumors that are mixtures of oligodendroglioma and astrocytoma commonly occur, and even pure oligodendrogliomas have a tendency to become more anaplastic with each recurrence, so that distinction of these tumors from astrocytoma or glioblastoma and from metastatic adenocarcinomas is often impossible in CSF. Germ cell tumors of the pineal gland (e.g., germinoma, embryonal carcinoma, endodermal sinus tumor, choriocarcinoma, and teratoma) are included in this differential diagnosis (Fig. 5–24), as is chordoma (Fig. 5–25). Chordoma is a slow-growing tumor that tends to invade locally but that can metastasize. The tumor is composed of large cells, some of which develop abundant bubbly cytoplasm (physaliferous cells); the cells are positive on periodic acid–Schiff (PAS) and mucin stains, and they express keratin, epithelial membrane antigen, and S-100 protein. They can be easily confused with adenocarcinoma.

Immunohistochemical stains are useful in characterizing malignant cells of unknown origin in CSF (Table 5–6). Antibodies raised against keratin proteins, epithelial membrane antigen, and carcinoembryonic antigen identify metastatic carcinomas. If no known primary tumor exists, carcinoma of the lung or stomach should be strongly considered. Leukocyte common antigen can identify the lymphomas, and HMB-45 (the so-called melanoma-specific antigen) can identify melanomas. Glial tumors mark for glial fibrillary acidic protein. Histiocytic neoplasms can be identified with the KP1 antibody and with antibodies to lysozyme. Because none of these antibodies is always reliable if used alone, it is recommended that a panel be chosen to help with this differential.

Clusters of Medium-Sized Cuboidal Cells

Some CNS tumors exfoliate as clusters of cuboidal cells with round to oval nuclei (Table 5–7). Most ependymomas, for example, are well-differentiated tumors composed of bland, oval nuclei. In CSF they may look like clusters of benign columnar or cuboidal cells indistinguishable from normal ependymal or choroidal cells, or they may suggest adenocarcinoma. Some ependymomas are anaplastic and may mimic either small-cell tumors, such as medulloblastoma (see Table 5–1) or metastatic adenocarcinoma (see Table 5–5).

The choroid plexus, which is specialized ependyma, may give rise to choroid plexus papillomas (Fig. 5–26A), identified in CSF as cohesive clusters of medium-sized cells. Carcinoma of the choroid plexus, on the other hand, may be morphologically indistinguishable from an adenocarcinoma. The pineal gland, a small midline structure posterior to the third ventricle, may give rise either to germ cell tumors (above) or primary pineal cell tumors. There are two varieties of primary pineal tumors: a well-differentiated pineocytoma, which may resemble an ependymoma, and the more primitive-looking pineoblastoma, which is indistinguishable from medulloblastoma (see Table 5–1). Pituitary adenomas rarely exfoliate in CSF, where they have a bland cuboidal or columnar appearance. Last, a metastatic, well-differentiated papillary adenocarcinoma may mimic any of these well-differentiated CNS neoplasms, and a correct identification may depend on having a thorough clinical history.

Bibliography

Bigner SH, Johnston WW: Cytopathology of the Central Nervous System. New York: Masson, 1983.
Burger PC, Scheithauer BW, Vogel FS: Surgical Pathology of the Nervous System and Its Coverings. New York: Churchill Livingstone, 1991.
Rosenthal DL: Cytology of the Central Nervous System. Basel: Karger, 1984.

ACKNOWLEDGMENTS

The author would like to thank Geraldine S. Pinkus, M.D., of the Brigham and Women's Hospital for performing the immunoperoxidase studies and Ms. Robin Lee for her expert editorial assistance.

Table 5–1. DIFFERENTIAL DIAGNOSIS OF SMALL CELLS IN CSF

Lymphocytes	Metastatic small-cell tumors
Meningitis (especially viral)	Small-cell carcinoma of the lung
Multiple sclerosis, inflammatory CNS disorders	Retinoblastoma
Leukemia	Neuroblastoma (e.g., adrenal)
Lymphoma	Rhabdomyosarcoma
Medulloblastoma	Lobular carcinoma of the breast
Other CNS tumors	
Anaplastic ependymoma	
Pineoblastoma	
Neuroblastoma	

Table 5–2. DIFFERENTIAL DIAGNOSIS OF PLASMA CELLS IN CSF

Meningitis (viral, tuberculosis)	Neurosyphilis
Multiple sclerosis	Cerebral cysticercosis
Lyme disease	Multiple myeloma or plasmacytoma

Table 5–3. DIFFERENTIAL DIAGNOSIS OF EOSINOPHILS IN CSF

Peripheral blood contamination	Malignancy (lymphoma)
Parasitic infection	Foreign material
Fungal infection (*Coccidiodes immitis*)	Hypersensitivity (vaccination, drugs)
Bacterial infection (tuberculosis, syphilis)	Idiopathic

Table 5–4. DIFFERENTIAL DIAGNOSIS OF HISTIOCYTES AND HISTIOCYTE-LIKE CELLS IN CSF

Meningitis	Storage diseases	Histiocytosis X
Hemorrhage or infarction	Lymphoma	Malignant histiocytoses
Postmyelography		

Table 5–5. DIFFERENTIAL DIAGNOSIS OF LARGE ATYPICAL CELLS IN CSF

Carcinoma	CNS tumors	Histiocytes
Lung	Astrocytoma or glioblastoma	Viral infection (especially herpetic)
Breast (ductal)	Oligodendroglioma	
Other	Ependymoma	
Melanoma	Choroid plexus carcinoma	
Lymphoma	Pineocytoma	
Other metastatic tumors	Pineal germ cell tumors	
	Chordoma	

Table 5–6. IMMUNOHISTOCHEMICAL STUDIES IN THE EVALUATION OF MALIGNANT CELLS
OF UNKNOWN ORIGIN IN CSF

Reagents	Tumor
Keratin	Carcinoma
Epithelial membrane antigen	Carcinoma
Carcinoembryonic antigen	Carcinoma
Leukocyte common antigen	Lymphoma
Glial fibrillary acidic protein	Glial tumors
HMB-45	Melanoma
Lysozyme, KP1	Histiocytes and true histiocytic neoplasms

Table 5–7. DIFFERENTIAL DIAGNOSIS OF GROUPS OF MEDIUM-SIZED CUBOIDAL CELLS

Benign choroid or ependymal cells	Pineocytoma
Choroid plexus papilloma	Pituitary adenoma
Ependymoma	Well-differentiated (papillary) adenocarcinoma

 •

NORMAL CELLS

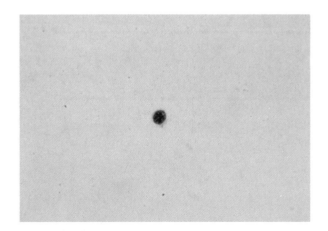

FIGURE 5–1. **Benign Lymphocyte.** Note the round nucleus, peripherally clumped chromatin, and scant cytoplasm (Papanicolaou stain, × 250).

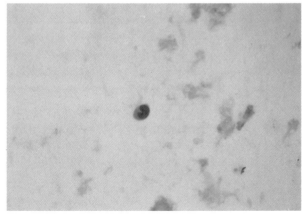

FIGURE 5–2. **Monocyte.** These cells are larger than lymphocytes and typically have a folded or kidney bean shaped nucleus, a more dispersed chromatin pattern, and more abundant cytoplasm (Papanicolaou stain, × 250).

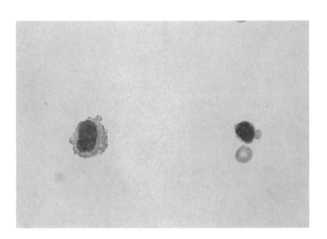

FIGURE 5–3. Lymphocyte and Monocyte (Wright stain, × 250).

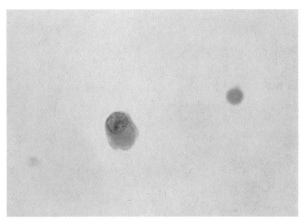

FIGURE 5–4B. Choroidal Cell, same specimen as that seen in Fig. 5–4A. This cell is similar to that seen in Figure 5–4A except that the cytoplasm has a lucent peripheral rim suggesting a brush border. This benign cell most likely exfoliated from the choroid plexus, the cells of which have long microvilli (Papanicolaou stain, × 250).

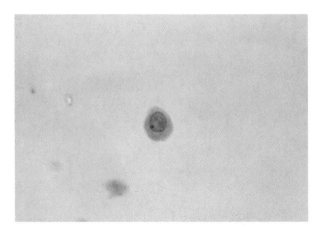

FIGURE 5–4A. Ependymal-Choroidal Cell. This cuboidal cell is benign because of its bland chromatin pattern, small nucleolus, and ample cytoplasm. Occasional benign cuboidal cells, present as single cells or in groups (see Fig. 5–26B), are usually interpreted as ependymal or choroidal cells (Papanicolaou stain, × 250).

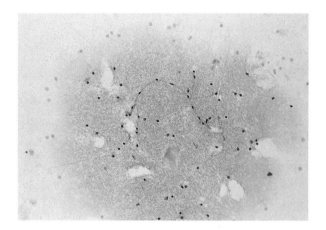

FIGURE 5–5. Brain Tissue. Ventricular specimens often contain fragments of brain tissue (either gray or white matter). Note the fuzzy contour and fine capillaries (Papanicolaou stain, × 50).

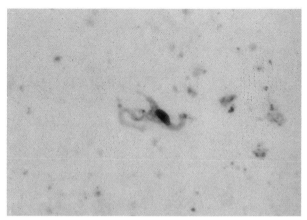

FIGURE 5–6. Neuron. These cells are rare in CSF but may be occasionally seen in ventricular specimens. They are identified by their triangular shape and long cytoplasmic processes (Papanicolaou stain, × 250). (Courtesy of Barbara Atkinson, M.D.)

INFLAMMATORY CONDITIONS

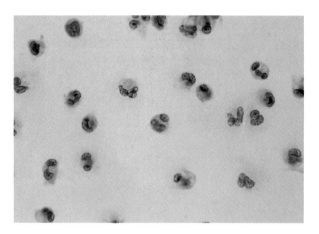

FIGURE 5–7. Polymorphonuclear Leukocytes. These inflammatory cells are most commonly seen in **acute bacterial meningitis** (Papanicolaou stain, × 250).

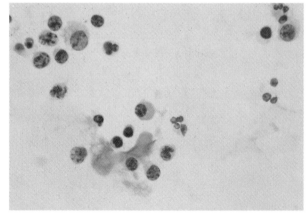

FIGURE 5–8. Plasma Cells, Tuberculous Meningitis. The plasma cell in the center has an eccentrically placed nucleus and abundant cytoplasm. The patient had multiple pulmonary nodules. Acid-fast organisms were cultured from CSF, urine, and gastric and synovial fluids. Plasma cells and plasmacytoid lymphocytes may also be seen in viral and fungal meningitis as well as in multiple sclerosis (Papanicolaou stain, × 250).

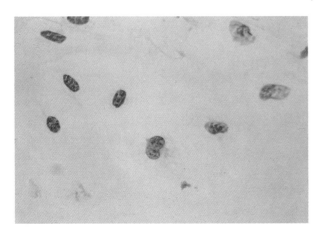

FIGURE 5–9A. Mollaret Meningitis. Sample of CSF from a 27-year-old woman who over several years was admitted to the hospital four times for the acute onset of severe headache, neck stiffness, and low-grade fever. Cultures and titers for organisms (including tuberculosis, syphilis, and Lyme disease) were negative, and these episodes subsided spontaneously. The cells in her sample of CSF were large monocytoid cells with faint, wispy cytoplasm, characteristic of this disorder (Papanicolaou stain, × 250).

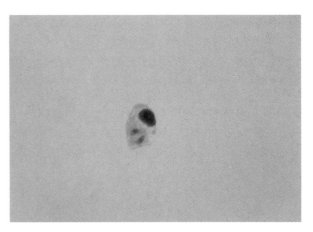

FIGURE 5–10. *Toxoplasma gondii*. This histiocyte contains two intracytoplasmic organisms diagnostic of toxoplasma. The organisms are crescentic or bow shaped and have tiny nuclei. The patient was being treated for malignant lymphoma (Papanicolaou stain, × 375).

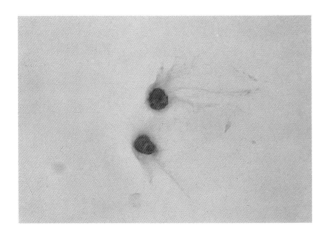

FIGURE 5–9B. Mollaret Meningitis, same specimen as that seen in Figure 5–9A (Wright stain, × 250).

DIFFERENTIAL GROUPING

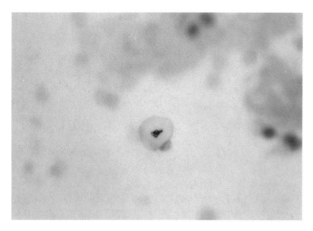

FIGURE 5–11A. Starch Particle. This is a common contaminant of CSF and is identified by its refractile center, which is shaped like a Maltese cross under polarized light (Papanicolaou stain, × 250).

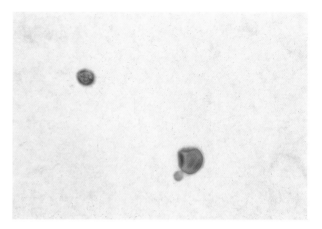

FIGURE 5–11B. Cryptococcus. These fungal organisms are somewhat variable in size (5- to 15-μ diameter) and stain deep purple or pink with the Papanicolaou stain. In CSF they appear as rounded yeast forms, some of which show a characteristic thin-necked budding (lower right). The wall of these organisms is often indented, trapping air under the cover slipping medium, which results in a crystal-like, refractile artifact. This artifact, however, does not form a Maltese cross under polarized light. Some of the organisms have a thick capsule, which stains positive on mucin stains. There may or may not be an inflammatory background (Papanicolaou stain, × 250).

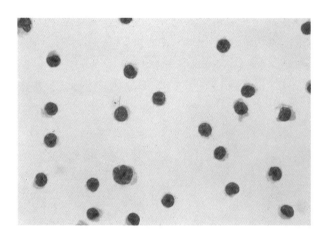

FIGURE 5–12A. Viral Meningitis. This hypercellular sample is composed predominantly of small lymphocytes with only occasional larger, irregular lymphoid cells (lower left) (Papanicolaou stain, × 250).

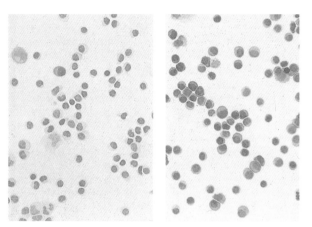

FIGURE 5–12C. Viral Meningitis, same specimen as in Figures 5–12A and 5–12B. Most of the cells were immunoreactive for a T-cell marker (right), and only rare cells stained as B cells (left). This finding supports a benign diagnosis (× 50).

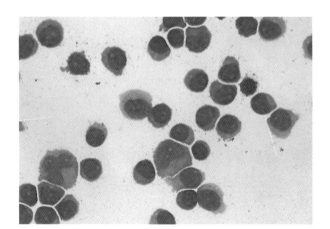

FIGURE 5–12B. Viral Meningitis. This air-dried Wright-stained slide is from the same sample as that of Figure 5–12A and photographed at the same magnification. Many of the small lymphocytes have plasmacytoid features. As in Figure 5–12A, there are occasional larger, irregular forms. Such specimens raise the possibility of a lymphoma. Most lymphomas, however, are composed of a more homogeneous population of atypical cells.

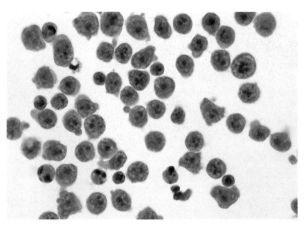

FIGURE 5–12D. Malignant Lymphoma. This hypercellular specimen is composed mostly of large, atypical lymphoid cells with prominent nucleoli. Notice the highly irregular pattern of chromatin clumping, the variation in nuclear shape, and the presence of karyorrhexis, all of which are commonly seen in lymphomas. Occasionally, small, benign lymphocytes (arrow) are admixed (Papanicolaou stain, × 250).

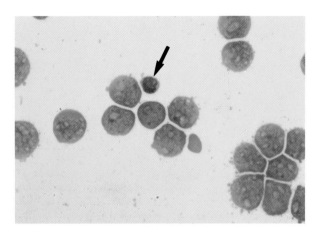

FIGURE 5–12E. Malignant Lymphoma. Large, atypical lymphoid cells with prominent nucleoli are present, as is a small, benign lymphocyte (arrow) (Wright stain, × 250).

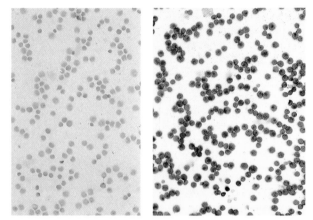

FIGURE 5–12G. Malignant Lymphoma. The majority of the cells stain for lambda light chains (right); there is no detectable staining for kappa light chains (left). Demonstrating monoclonality helps confirm the diagnosis of malignant lymphoma (× 50).

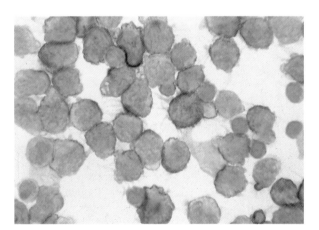

FIGURE 5–12F. Malignant Lymphoma. All the large, atypical cells stain as B cells. The small, benign-appearing cells are nonreactive and therefore are probably T cells (L26 immunoperoxidase, × 250).

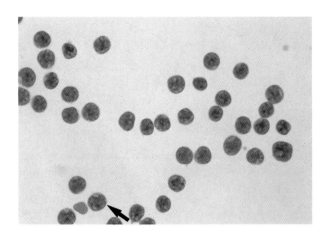

FIGURE 5–13A. Acute Lymphoblastic Leukemia. These dispersed, single cells are quite uniform in appearance. They are larger than normal, mature lymphocytes, and their nuclear chromatin appears somewhat lighter (contrast with Fig. 5–1). Nucleoli can be identified (see arrow) (Papanicolaou stain, × 250).

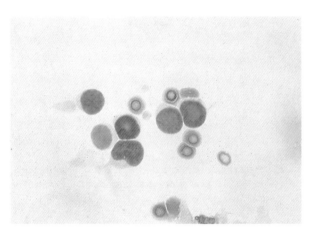

FIGURE 5–13C. Acute Lymphoblastic Leukemia, same specimen as that seen in Figures 5–13A and 5–13B. Most of the cells are immunoreactive for the nuclear enzyme terminal deoxytransferase, which is specific for lymphoblasts. Note the brown staining within the nuclei of leukemic cells. (Surrounding red cells appear refractile as a result of cover-slipping artifact.)

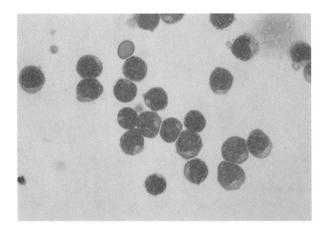

FIGURE 5–13B. Acute Lymphoblastic Leukemia, same specimen as that shown in Figure 5–13A. The paler, more dispersed chromatin of the leukemic cells is better appreciated on this air-dried Wright stain (× 250).

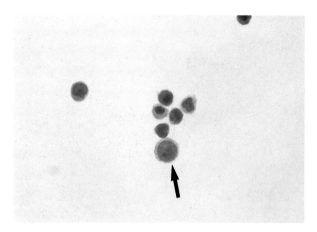

FIGURE 5–14A. Acute Myelogenous Leukemia. Two large blasts are seen among some degenerate and inflammatory cells. One myeloblast (arrow) has an especially prominent nucleolus (Papanicolaou stain, × 250).

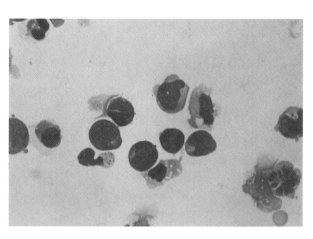

FIGURE 5–14B. Acute Myelogenous Leukemia, same specimen as that seen in Figure 5–14A. Some of the blasts in this case have irregular nuclear contours. Other cells, representing more mature cells, or myelocytes, contain cytoplasmic granules (Wright stain, × 250).

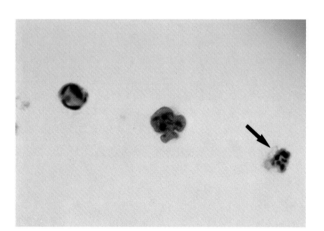

FIGURE 5–15A. Malignant Lymphoma. Lymphoma cells often may have extremely irregular nuclear contours. Single-cell necrosis (arrow) is characteristic of these cells, even prior to therapy. Both of these features, however, can be seen in other tumors. The cells of a lymphoma, however, tend not to cluster (Papanicolaou stain, × 375).

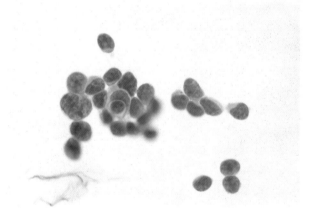

FIGURE 5–15B. Medulloblastoma. This tumor of the cerebellum is characterized by small cells that have scant cytoplasm. They tend to form clusters, and cell molding is common. The differential diagnosis includes small-cell carcinoma of the lung. Because medulloblastoma is a tumor principally of childhood, the age of the patient is of great help in distinguishing between these two possibilities. Other small-cell tumors, however, such as neuroblastoma and retinoblastoma, may be seen in childhood; additional clinical and radiographic findings are therefore crucial for a correct diagnosis (Papanicolaou stain, × 250). (Courtesy of William Kupsky, M.D., Children's Hospital Medical Center, Boston, Mass.)

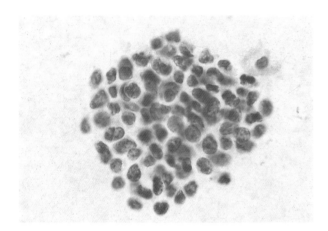

FIGURE 5–15C. Small-Cell Carcinoma of the Lung. These cells are indistinguishable morphologically from the cells of medulloblastoma (Papanicolaou stain, × 250).

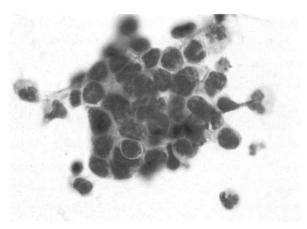

FIGURE 5–15E. Pineoblastoma. This uncommon tumor of the central nervous system is composed of undifferentiated cells that form clusters and show cell molding. It is morphologically indistinguishable from medulloblastoma, small-cell carcinoma, and any of the other nonhematopoietic small-cell tumors (see Table 5–1) (Papanicolaou stain, × 250). (Courtesy of William Kupsky, M.D., Children's Hospital Medical Center, Boston, Mass.)

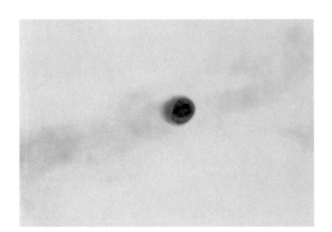

FIGURE 5–15D. Small-Cell Carcinoma of the Lung. When present as single cells, these tumor cells look like lymphocytes, and it may be impossible to identify them as malignant. A careful search should be made for diagnostic cell clusters; these are sometimes identified only on subsequent samples of CSF (Papanicolaou stain, × 375).

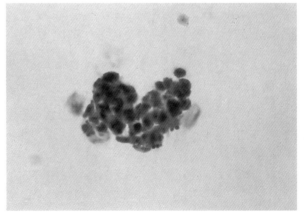

FIGURE 5–15F. Clusters of Poorly Preserved Lymphocytes. This 21-year-old woman presented with classic symptoms of viral meningitis: headache, stiff neck, fever, chills, and myalgia. Her CSF contained occasional tight clusters of poorly preserved cells. The clustering raised the possibility of a small-cell tumor such as medulloblastoma, but the results of computed tomographic and magnetic resonance imaging scans were negative, as were repeat CSF samples. Her symptoms resolved spontaneously. As if to prove that nothing is sacred, this case illustrates the fact that lymphocytes do on occasion form clusters, especially in cytospin preparations, and may be a source of diagnostic confusion when the cells are poorly preserved (Papanicolaou stain, × 250).

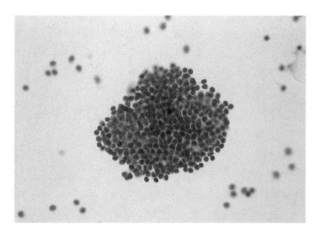

FIGURE 5–15G. Lymphocytes in a Cluster. When well preserved, as in this case, identifying the cells as lymphocytes is not difficult even when they cluster (Papanicolaou stain, × 100).

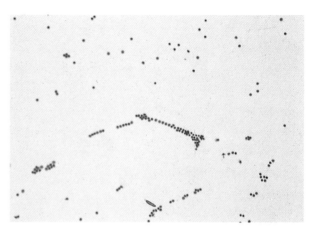

FIGURE 5–15H. Lymphocytes in Rows. As in Figure 5–15G, identifying these cells as lymphocytes is not difficult, even when they are arranged in rows (Papanicolaou stain, × 50).

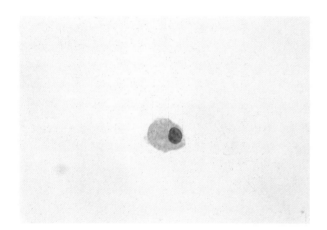

FIGURE 5–16A. Histiocyte. Malignant cells are usually identified without difficulty, given an understanding of the normal elements of CSF. Histiocytes may be worrisome, however, because of their larger size. This cell is identified as benign because of its abundant cytoplasm and its round nucleus, even nuclear membrane, and bland chromatin pattern. It contains occasional pigment granules, representing hemosiderin. If abundant hemosiderin-laden macrophages are present, intracerebral, subdural, or subarachnoid hemorrhage should be considered (Papanicolaou stain, × 250).

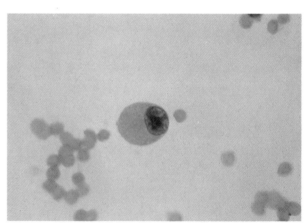

FIGURE 5–16B. Malignant Cell, Unknown Origin. This cell, photographed at the same magnification as Figure 5–16A, is identified as malignant because its nucleus is much larger and more atypical. Note the prominent nucleolus and coarsely clumped chromatin pattern. Some malignant cells, like this one, may have abundant cytoplasm. This 52-year-old patient had no history of malignancy and presented with headaches and hydrocephalus. The results of yearly mammograms and a chest radiograph were negative (Papanicolaou stain, × 250).

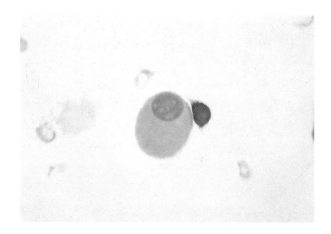

FIGURE 5–16C. Specimen from same patient shown in Figure 5–16B. Additional fluid was received, and six air-dried cytospins were examined by the immunoperoxidase technique. The malignant cells were negative for leukocyte common antigen. An adjacent benign lymphocyte is positive (Leukocyte common antigen immunoperoxidase, × 250).

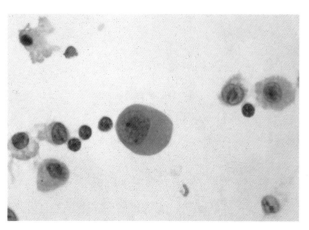

FIGURE 5–16E. Pleural Fluid, same patient as in Figures 5–16B through 5–16D. Nine months after initial presentation, the patient's test results showed pleural fluid that contained malignant cells similar to those in her CSF. A few months later, the patient died and an autopsy revealed a carcinoma of the lung. This case illustrates the fact that some tumors, especially lung cancer, may metastasize very early to the leptomeninges (Papanicolaou stain, × 250).

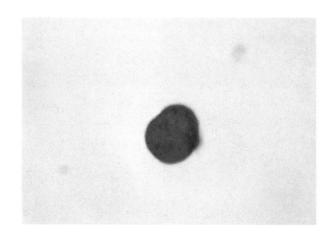

FIGURE 5–16D. Specimen from same patient shown in Figures 5–16B and 5–16C. The tumor cells were strongly positive for carcinoembryonic antigen. The cells also showed strong staining for keratin proteins (AE1/AE3) and epithelial membrane antigen (not shown). Stains for glial fibrillary acidic protein (GFAP) and HMB-45 were negative. These findings excluded lymphoma-plasmacytoma, melanoma, sarcoma, and primary glial tumor; a diagnosis of metastatic carcinoma was made, most likely of lung or stomach origin. A decision was made not to pursue any further clinical evaluation, and the patient was treated with intrathecal methotrexate.

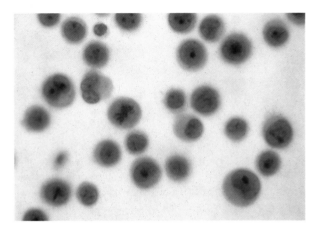

FIGURE 5–17. Metastatic Breast Cancer. Cerebrospinal fluid from this patient with known breast cancer contained numerous large malignant cells with coarse chromatin and prominent nucleoli. Mitoses were numerous (Papanicolaou stain, × 250).

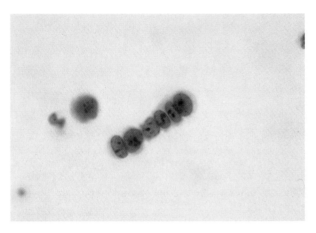

FIGURE 5–19. Metastatic Breast Cancer. Cell rows are not diagnostic of lobular carcinoma; this patient's breast cancer was ductal (Papanicolaou stain, × 250).

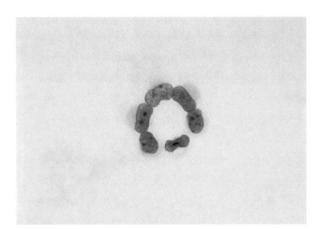

FIGURE 5–18. Metastatic Breast Cancer. Although not common in CSF, adenocarcinomas may occasionally form gland-like structures (Papanicolaou stain, × 250).

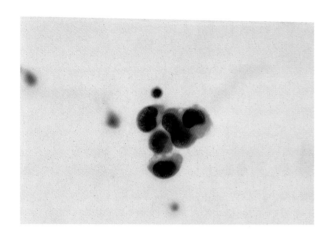

FIGURE 5–20. Metastatic Transitional Cell Carcinoma of the Bladder. Without a history of known malignancy it is usually impossible to determine the primary site from the morphologic features of the metastatic cells alone in CSF. This patient had a known history of bladder cancer, and the malignant cells were similar to those seen on a previous biopsy (Papanicolaou stain, × 250).

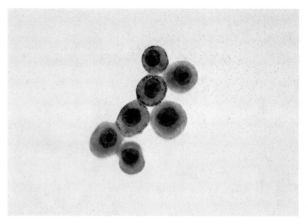

FIGURE 5–22. Malignant Melanoma. A diagnosis of melanoma was established in this patient based on the malignant features of the cells (large cells, huge nucleoli, irregular nuclear contours) and the presence of melanin pigment. Melanoma may rarely arise from the leptomeninges. After an extensive search, no primary site was found elsewhere; thus, a presumptive diagnosis of primary leptomeningeal melanoma was made. Without intracytoplasmic melanin, these cells may be mistaken for adenocarcinoma (Papanicolaou stain, × 250).

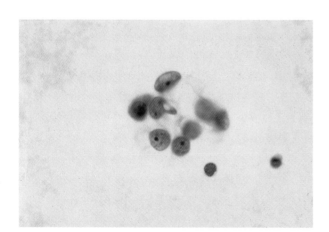

FIGURE 5–21. Metastatic Adenocarcinoma of the Lung. The large cells in this cluster have a finely clumped chromatin pattern, irregular nuclear shapes, prominent nucleoli, and vacuolated cytoplasm. The findings are diagnostic of malignancy (Papanicolaou stain, × 250).

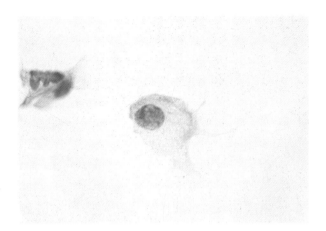

FIGURE 5–23. Astrocytoma. High-grade astrocytoma and glioblastoma multiforme have many patterns of exfoliation in CSF, from small, anaplastic cells to huge, multinucleated cells, either of which can be arranged as single cells or clusters. The cells occasionally preserve their characteristic cytoplasmic processes in CSF, which can offer a clue to their glial origin (Papanicolaou stain, × 250). (Courtesy of William Kupsky, M.D., Children's Hospital Medical Center, Boston, Mass.)

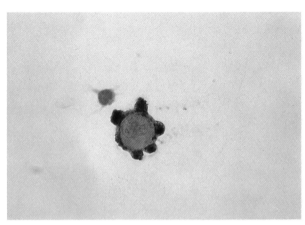

FIGURE 5–25. Chordoma. This 19-year-old woman had a biopsy-confirmed chordoma of the base of the skull. This subsequent cytologic specimen of CSF showed large cells with round nuclei, prominent nucleoli, and abundant cytoplasm. The cytoplasm of this cell has a strong positive reaction to the periodic acid–Schiff stain, and the positivity is accentuated within peripheral cytoplasmic blebs. These cells may be easily confused with adenocarcinoma. A subsequent autopsy confirmed extensive leptomeningeal spread of chordoma (Periodic acid–Schiff stain, × 250). (Courtesy of William Kupsky, M.D., Children's Hospital Medical Center, Boston, Mass.)

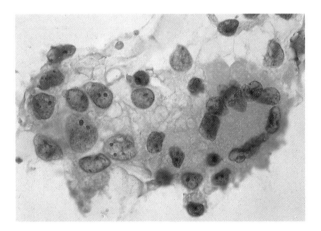

FIGURE 5–24. Choriocarcinoma of the Pineal Gland. This 4-year-old boy with a third ventricular tumor had elevated levels of human chorionic gonadotropin in the serum and CSF. Cytologic specimens of CSF showed numerous large malignant cells with features of cytotrophoblast and syncytiotrophoblast (Papanicolaou stain, × 250). (Courtesy of William Kupsky, M.D., Children's Hospital Medical Center, Boston, Mass.)

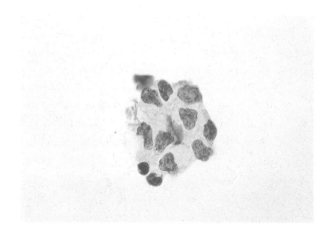

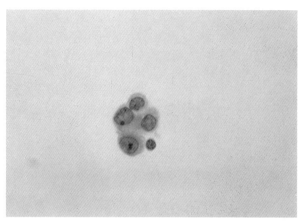

FIGURE 5–26A. Choroid Plexus Papilloma. This CSF was obtained from a ventriculoperitoneal shunt catheter immediately prior to resection of a choroid plexus papilloma of the lateral ventricle in a 7-year-old boy. The specimen contained occasional tight groups of medium-sized cells with irregular nuclear contours and abundant cytoplasm. This pattern may also be seen with ependymoma, pineocytoma, pituitary adenoma, and some well-differentiated papillary adenocarcinomas (Papanicolaou stain, × 250). (Courtesy of William Kupsky, M.D., Children's Hospital Medical Center, Boston, Mass.)

FIGURE 5–26B. Ependymal-Choroidal Cells, same specimen as in Figs. 5–4A and 5–4B). Compare this small cluster of benign-appearing cuboidal cells of presumed choroidal-ependymal origin with those in Figure 5–26A. Although the cells are smaller and the nuclei less irregular than those of the papilloma, the possibility of a neoplasm cannot be entirely excluded on morphologic grounds alone, since these tumors may deviate very little in their appearance from benign choroid plexus cells. Clinical and radiographic correlation are important. This specimen was obtained from a young patient with acquired immune deficiency syndrome who had no evidence of a central nervous system tumor (Papanicolaou stain, × 250).

C·H·A·P·T·E·R

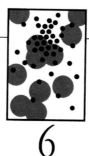

6

STEREOTACTIC BIOPSY OF THE CENTRAL NERVOUS SYSTEM

Sandra H. Bigner

Allan H. Friedman

Peter C. Burger

The advent of sophisticated radiologic imaging techniques, such as computed tomography (CT) and magnetic resonance imaging, has stimulated a renewed interest in percutaneous brain biopsies. Using image-guided stereotaxis, the surgeon can deliver the tip of a biopsy probe to a precise destination within the cranium. Since this biopsy procedure is performed through a small opening in the skull made under local anesthesia, the patient's hospital stay and recovery time are short.

Over the past 15 years, specific indications for stereotactic-guided brain biopsies have emerged. Stereotactic biopsies have proved to be invaluable in establishing the diagnosis of deep brain or irresectable lesions that are entangled in eloquent areas of the brain. Reports of large series of brain biopsies have shown that even the best radiologic techniques are not a substitute for morphologic diagnosis. Brain biopsies have been used to monitor ongoing processes and the effects of therapy. For instance, standard radiologic tests are poor in differentiating recurrent tumor from radiation necrosis. Stereotactic-guided biopsies can be used to establish a diagnosis and to direct therapy in patients who are too medically ill to undergo a standard craniotomy. This technique can also have a therapeutic role in draining cysts and abscesses.

Optimal use of this technique requires intimate cooperation between the pathologist and the surgeon, since the pathologist is confronted with the task of making a diagnosis from small bits of tissue. The most critical step in correctly interpreting samples obtained stereotactically is generating a differential diagnosis based on clinical history, age of the patient, location of the lesion, radiographic appearance, and previous therapeutic intervention. In addition, one must be familiar with the morphologic presentation of these lesions in samples prepared by different methods and aware of the limitations of each preparatory technique. Finally, a close interaction between the surgeon and pathologist provides the opportunity for repeat sampling to ensure that adequate tissue is obtained to permit a definite diagnosis prior to terminating the biopsy procedure.

The preparative method for stereotactic biopsies depends on the size and consistency of the sample obtained. Solid tissue fragments obtained through a large needle are usually evaluated by frozen section for immediate diagnosis and by formalin fixation and paraffin embedding for final diagnosis. This procedure can be supplemented by imprints of the fragments and by filter and cytospin preparation of needle washings to display detailed cellular morphology and to provide material for additional studies such as immunohistochemistry. Smaller fragments obtained through a fine needle are usually smeared or squashed on a slide, whereas cystic contents are evaluated by cytospin or filter methods.

HYPOCELLULAR SAMPLES

One of the most commonly encountered situations in interpreting stereotactic biopsies from any intracranial site is the hypocellular sample in which one must distinguish a reactive process from a low-grade astrocytoma. In this situation, it is crucial to know whether there is a distinct mass on CT scan or whether the lesion consists only of a diffuse enlargement. In the former situation, a hypocellular specimen containing only normal cells, edema, or gliosis indicates that the lesion has not been sampled and that the specimen is from the surrounding region. If, on the other hand, the lesion is poorly defined on the CT scan, one would expect to see a hypocellular lesion, and the distinction between edema, gliosis, cerebritis, and low-grade astrocytoma becomes critical. These conditions all result in cohesive tissue from which cells exfoliate poorly; thus, one usually obtains solid cores of tissue that do not smear easily and are best processed histologically. Although some observers advocate a squash technique, the lesions considered are extremely difficult to differentiate from one another in these preparations.

Parameters that distinguish low-grade astrocytomas from non-neoplastic processes include increased cellularity, nuclear pleomorphism, and hyperchromasia (Figs. 6–1 and 6–2). An important characteristic is that the cells make up a distinct population rather than representing a mixture of oligodendroglia and astrocytes that are present in normal and reactive white matter. This feature is particularly apparent in pilocytic astrocytomas composed of a uniform population of bipolar astrocytes of a morphologic cell type that is infrequently seen in non-neoplastic conditions. This lesion often contains waxy bodies known as Rosanthal fibers. Microcystic changes and calcification are often seen in low-grade astrocytomas, although these features alone are insufficient to distinguish a neoplastic process from reactive conditions. Finally, it is important to be aware that low-grade astrocytomas are among the most difficult intracranial lesions to diagnose, even when large fragments are obtained by open craniotomy. Unless clear-cut features of neoplasia are present, one should avoid making a definitive diagnosis or request additional tissue.

HYPERCELLULAR LESIONS

A common group of entities that are often sampled stereotactically includes cellular lesions in which the cells are relatively bland, lacking frank malignant criteria. In this setting, the differential diagnosis includes infarct, oligodendroglioma, ependymoma, and anaplastic astrocytoma. Although these lesions occur most frequently in the cerebral hemipheres of adults, they are occasionally seen in children and sometimes occur in the posterior fossa. These conditions all exfoliate readily, and the individual cells have distinctive features. Macrophages that comprise subacute infarcts are identified by their bean-shaped nuclei, indistinct cytoplasic borders, and phagocytized material within the cytoplasm (Figs. 6–3A and 6–3B). If these cells present a diagnostic problem, staining with pan-leukocytic antibodies usually distinguishes macrophages from cells of gliomas. Oligodendrocytes have round regular nuclei with finely granular chromatin, visible but not prominent nucleoli, and wispy cytoplasm (Figs. 6–3C and 6–3D). Cells of ependymomas are smaller than those of oligodendroglia; the nuclei are more ovoid, and the cell shape is slightly elongated (Figs. 6–4A and 6–4B). Anaplastic astrocytomas have irregular hyperchromatic nuclei, nucleoli that may be visible although not prominent, and moderate amounts of cytoplasm that may display processes (Figs. 6–4C and 6–4D). All of these glial neoplasms express glial fibrillary acidic protein (GFAP), which may be used to distinguish them from nonglial neoplasms but not from one another. In addition to the cytologic features shown here, tissue fragments processed histologically demonstrate distinct architectural characteristics for each of these lesions (Figs. 6–3A, 6–3C, 6–4A, and 6–4C). Infarcts show regions of gliosis surrounding a center of macrophages. Oligodendrogliomas are composed of nests of cells within a reticulovascular network. Ependymomas typically form pseudorosettes and sometimes contain true rosettes as well. Anaplastic astrocytomas form sheets of cells and, although they may be highly vascularized, lack the endothelial proliferation and necrosis characteristic of glioblastomas. Anaplastic astrocytomas are highly infiltrative, whereas oligodendrogliomas and ependymomas usually have discrete borders.

MALIGNANT NEOPLASMS

When a stereotactic biopsy of a cerebral mass in an adult reveals a hypercellular lesion in which the cells display malignant criteria, malignant gliomas, lymphoma (either primary or metastatic), metastatic carcinoma, and malignant melanoma should all be considered (Figs. 6–5 and 6–6). Useful features in separating gliomas from these other tumor types include the presence of cytoplasmic processes, infiltrative pattern, and the characteristic necrosis with a periphery of pseudopalisading cells (Figs. 6–7 and 6–8). The glial nature of the cells is best confirmed by the immunohistochemical demonstration of GFAP. Individual cells of large-cell lymphoma can be quite similar to these other tumors, but the perivascular pattern in tissue sections and the lack of processes and cohesion are helpful features. Demonstration of reactivity with pan-leukocyte antibodies as well as lack of reactivity with GFAP, S-100, HMB-45, and cytokeratin is useful in establishing this diagnosis.

Occasionally, a lesion is clearly lymphoid, but it may be difficult to distinguish between lymphoma and a non-neoplastic lymphocytic infiltrate. Here, antibodies against lymphocytic subsets are helpful in identifying monoclonal populations. Metastatic tumors are generally well circumscribed. The cells are cohesive and frequently have prominent macronucleoli and a high mitotic rate. Expression of cytokeratins and carcinoma-associated antigens, such as Tag-72, EMA, and CEA, may be useful in distinguishing carcinoma. Melanoma, in contrast, is negative for these reagents but expresses HMB-45 and ME1-14. S-100 is of limited use in this differential diagnosis since it is expressed by most primary central nervous system (CNS) tumors as well as melanoma and approximately one third of metastatic carcinomas also express S-100.

In cytologic preparations one must be cautious concerning cell shape. In smear preparations, all tumors have a tendency to appear sheet-like, and tumors other than gliomas may have cytoplasmic extensions that mimic processes. The single-cell presentation of melanoma and lymphoma may be difficult to ascertain in smears. However, in needle washings and cyst fluids prepared on filters or by cytocentrifugation, all cells tend to round up and ball up, minimizing the appearance of process formation in gliomas.

GRADING OF HIGH-GRADE GLIOMAS

Astrocytic neoplasms are divided into three grades: astrocytoma, anaplastic astrocytoma (AA), and glioblastoma multiforme (GBM). The distinction between the first two is based on greater cellularity, nuclear hyperchromasia, and pleomorphism in AA than in astrocytomas—features that can be identified on smears as well as in histologic sections. Both AA and GBM show hypercellularity, and pleomorphism may be present or absent (Figs. 6–7 and 6–8). Although endothelial proliferation in glomeruloid tufts is often seen in GBM, these structures are usually at the periphery of the lesion and may not be sampled by a stereotactic biopsy. The most definitive characteristic of GBM that is not seen in AA is the presence of necrosis, which may occur in confluent areas or may consist of a serpentine pattern surrounded by pseudopalisading cells (Figs. 6–7B and 6–7D). This feature is often demonstrable in tissue fragments but is usually impossible to identify with certainty in smears or squash preparations. The inability to determine the presence or absence of necrosis is a limitation of small stereotactic biopsies obtained through a fine needle, since the distinction between AA and GBM is critical for clinical staging. For this reason, many neurosurgeons use a large needle for solid intracranial lesions, obtaining large tissue fragments that can be processed histologically.

CYSTIC LESIONS

When a lesion with a lucent center is encountered in any intracranial location, a common practice is to aspirate the liquid contents stereotactically. In this setting the differential diagnosis includes cysts, abscesses, granulomata, and tumors with necrotic centers. These samples are processed similarly to any other fluid, using membrane filters, smears, cytocentrifugation, or cell block preparation. Frequently, clear fluid is obtained containing only macrophages (see Fig. 6–10A). Here, it is usually impossible to determine whether the lesion is a non-neoplastic cyst or represents a cystic astrocytoma or cystic hemangioblastoma. If the fluid is turbid and contains polymorphonuclear leukocytes or amorphous necrotic debris, abscesses of bacterial or fungal etiology should be considered, and specific organisms should be sought by culture and by morphologic identification on both routine and fungal stains (Fig. 6–9). In the immunosuppressed patient, including those with AIDS, *Nocardia, Mucor, Candida,* and *Aspergillis* should be considered. Particularly in AIDS patients, if a granulomatous infiltrate is recovered, tubercular bacilli and *Toxoplasma gondii* should be sought.

When abundant mature squamous epithelial cells are obtained, epidermoid and dermoid cysts should be considered (Fig. 6–10B). If the lesion is in the suprasellar region, fragments of benign cuboidal epithelium representing adamantinomatous elements should be sought since their presence indicates that the lesion is a craniopharyngioma rather than a dermoid or epidermoid cyst. Central necrosis is a feature of both GBM and metastases. When this material is aspirated, a common problem is difficulty in identifying well-preserved diagnostic cells (Figs. 6–10C and 6–10D). Sometimes they simply are not present, and a repeat sample from the periphery of the mass rather than from the necrotic center should be requested.

STEREOTACTIC BIOPSIES IN CHILDREN

The differential diagnosis for supratentorial lesions in children is similar to the lesions seen in adults except that low-grade astrocytomas occur considerably more frequently than high-grade tumors and that metastases and primary lymphomas are less common than in adults. A significant difference in childhood brain tumors is that the majority of them are located in the posterior fossa either as gliomas or ependymomas involving the brainstem or as cerebellar astrocytomas or medulloblastomas. An additional site for tumors in children and adolescents is the pineal region where germ cell tumors, pineoblastomas, and pineocytomas as well as gliomas may all occur. The morphologic presentation of childhood gliomas has been described in previous sections.

Tumor types that are frequent in childhood but occur uncommonly as primary CNS tumors in adults are small-cell tumors (Fig. 6–11). These lesions, referred to by some observers as primitive neuroectodermal tumors (PNETs), are composed of small cells with round hyperchromatic nuclei and scant cytoplasm. They may occur in sheets, with or without regions of necrosis, and may form rosettes. This same morphologic cell type may arise in the cerebellum as a medulloblastoma, in the pineal gland as a pineoblastoma, in the retina as a retinoblastoma, or in the cerebral hemispheres or adrenal medulla as a neuroblastoma. Since many of these tumors show some degree of neuronal differentiation, as demonstrated by synaptophysin or neural-cell adhesion molecule (N-CAM), they are most appropriately distinguished from one another by the site of origin rather than immunophenotype. However, expression of synaptophysin and neurofilament protein is useful in distinguishing these lesions from gliomas and from non-neurogenic small-cell tumors, such as sarcomas and lymphomas.

SPECIMENS OBTAINED WITH THE CAVITRON ULTRASONIC SURGICAL ASPIRATOR

The cavitron ultrasonic surgical aspirator (CUSA), which allows tissue dissection by fragmentation, is used to remove central or peripheral nervous system tumors adjacent to or within vital structures. Such tumors include meningiomas (Fig. 6–12), acoustic neuromas, and schwannomas, particularly when they are near the venous sinuses, cranial or spinal nerves, or major arteries. Pineal tumors and some childhood tumors in the posterior fossa are also removed by this means. The aspirated fragments must be retrieved from the suction line and are usually adequate for cytologic and histologic examination. The fragments may be evaluated by filter, smear, or cytospin methods or may be processed histologically as cell blocks or small biopsies.

Bibliography

Bigner SH, Johnston WW: Cytopathology of the Central Nervous System. New York: Masson, 1983, pp 75–116, 125–143.
Burger PC, Scheithauer BW, Vogel FS: Surgical Pathology of the Nervous System and Its Coverings, 3rd Edition. New York: Churchill Livingstone, 1991.
Chandrasoma PT, Apuzzo MLJ: Stereotactic Brain Biopsy. Tokyo: Igaku-Shoin, 1989.
Silverman JF, Jones FD, Unverferth M, Berns L: Cytopathology of neoplasms of the central nervous systems in specimens obtained by the cavitron ultrasonic surgical aspirator. Acta Cytol 33:576–582, 1989.

DIFFERENTIAL GROUPINGS

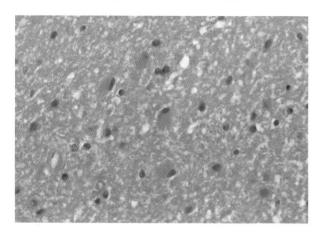

FIGURE 6–1. Comparison of gliosis and low-grade astrocytoma (hematoxylin- and eosin-stained needle biopsies, × 40).
A. Gliosis. These cells are taken from the region surrounding a metastasis and are easy to diagnose as benign, based on the reactive astrocytes with abundant pink cytoplasm. These cells are scattered within a background of neuropil containing astrocytes and oligodendroglia with inconspicuous cytoplasm.

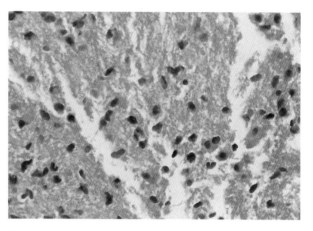

C. Low-grade Astrocytoma. Tumor is more obvious here than the lesion shown in Figure 6–1B, since it is moderately hypercellular and the cells are pleomorphic. The cells have hyperchromatic nuclei and form a distinct population.

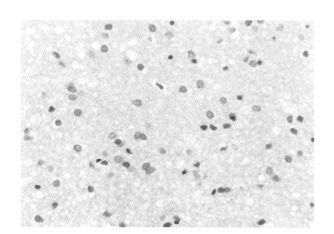

B. Low-grade Astrocytoma. This is a subtle lesion, since the only appreciable finding is an increase in the number of bland astrocytic nuclei within a background of brain tissue. Important features are that the astrocytic nuclei are the dominant cell type seen and that these cells constitute a monomorphic population.

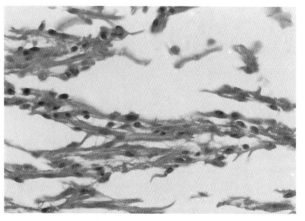

D. Pilocytic Astrocytoma. This example shows a uniform population of spindle-shaped cells, which would be unusual in a reactive condition.

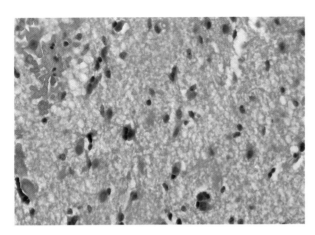

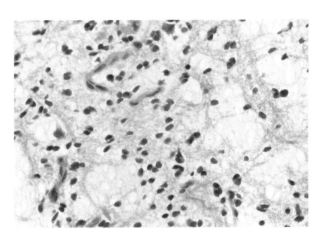

FIGURE 6–2. Comparison of gliosis and low-grade astrocytoma (Figs. 6–2A and 6–2C—hematoxylin- and eosin-stained needle biopsies; 6–2B and 6–2D, Papanicolaou-stained needle washings, × 40).

A. Gliosis. This smear contains an increased number of reactive astrocytes. This biopsy was taken from the deep cerebral gray matter and thus contains neurons, which should not be mistaken for neoplastic cells.

C. Microcystic Astrocytoma. Tumor is readily apparent, since the lesion is hypercellular and is composed of a distinct population of cells surrounding microcystic cavities.

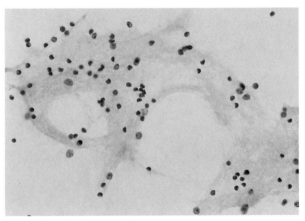

B. Reactive Astrocytosis. This needle washing from the specimen shown in A shows the same features, which are reactive astrocytes scattered within a mixture of normal brain elements. In cases such as this, it may be impossible to exclude the possibility that the edge of a low-grade glioma has been sampled, but the important point is that A and B contain insufficient evidence to diagnose an astrocytic neoplasm.

D. Microcystic Astrocytoma. The same features, with microcyst formation, are apparent in the needle washing specimen of this case.

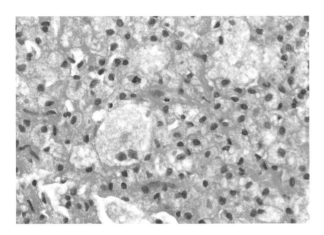

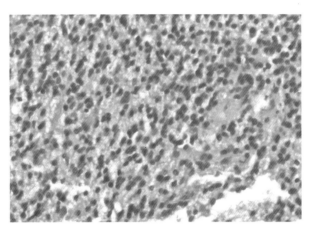

FIGURE 6–3. Differential diagnosis of hypercellular lesions—infarct versus oligodendroglioma (Figs. 6–3A and 6–3C, hematoxylin- and eosin-stained needle biopsies; 6–3B and 6–3D, Papanicolaou-stained needle washings, × 40).

A. Cerebral Infarct. This smear is composed of a dense population of macrophages with round to bean-shaped nuclei and phagocytized material within abundant cytoplasm.

C. Oligodendroglioma. A hypercellular lesion composed of cells with round to oval nuclei and indistinct cytoplasm is present. Nuclear regularity distinguishes this tumor from the anaplastic astrocytoma, and the degree of cellularity is too great for a low-grade astrocytoma.

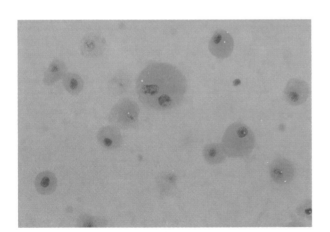

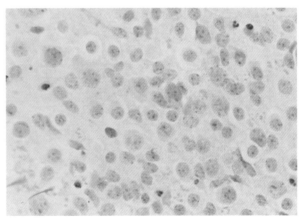

B. Cerebral Infarct. Almost all cells in the cytologic preparation of this infarct are macrophages. The largest ones are easy to recognize but many smaller ones are also present.

D. Oligodendroglioma. Regular cuboidal cells with round nuclei, finely granular chromatin, and moderate amounts of wispy cytoplasm are readily apparent.

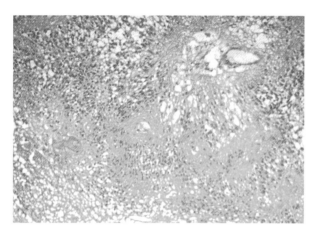

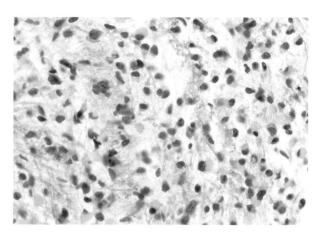

FIGURE 6–4. Differential diagnosis of hypercellular lesions—ependymoma versus anaplastic astrocytoma (Figs. 6–4A and 6–4C, hematoxylin- and eosin-stained needle biopsies, Figs. 6–4B and 6–4D, Papanicolaou-stained needle washings, Fig. 6–4A, × 25; Figs. 6–4B to 6–4D, × 40).

A. Ependymomas. In histologic preparations, these tumors are cellular, and eosinophilic regions surrounding blood vessels, termed pseudorosettes, are apparent.

C. Anaplastic Astrocytoma. This tumor is composed of cells that retain an astrocytic morphology as manifested by process formation. In contrast to low-grade astrocytomas, infarcts, ependymomas, and oligodendrogliomas, these nuclei are hyperchromatic and pleomorphic.

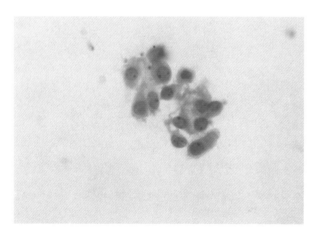

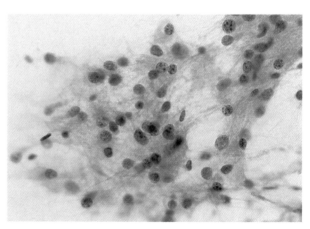

B. Ependymomas. These cells are small and cuboidal or columnar in shape, with round to oval, regular nuclei.

D. Anaplastic Astrocytoma. This tumor shows the same features described in Figure 6–4D, although the nuclear hyperchromasia and pleomorphism are more obvious.

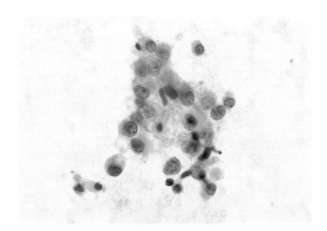

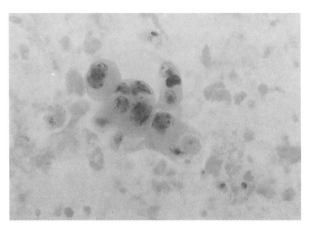

FIGURE 6–5. Cytologically malignant lesions: glioblastoma and metastatic carcinoma (Fig. 6–5A—needle washing, Papanicolaou stain; Fig. 6–5B, needle washing, immunocytochemistry for glial fibrillary acidic protein; Fig. 6–5C, cyst fluid, Papanicolaou stain; Fig. 6–5D, hematoxylin- and eosin-stained needle biopsy specimen, × 40).

A. Glioblastoma. Cells have hyperchromatic, pleomorphic nuclei and wispy cytoplasm. The cytologic features of glioblastomas are indistinguishable from those of anaplastic astrocytomas.

C. Metastatic Adenocarcinoma. These cells have more coarsely clumped, irregular chromatin and more prominent nucleoli than are generally seen in gliomas. As is illustrated here, cells of metastases are usually larger than those of glioblastomas.

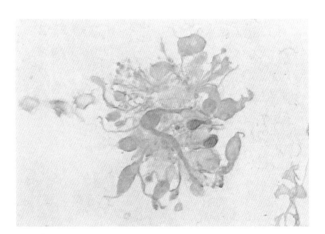

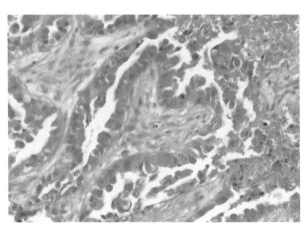

B. Glioblastoma. This preparation, using an antibody against glial fibrillary acidic protein, nicely demonstrates the cytoplasmic processes of cells and also stains the cytoplasm of their cell bodies.

D. Metastatic Adenocarcinoma. This tumor from a lung primary shows a distinct papillary pattern.

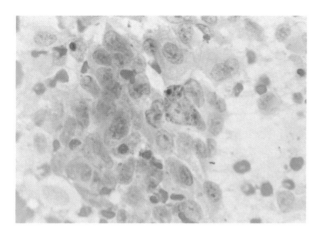

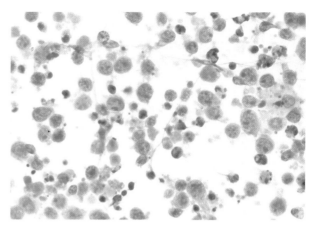

FIGURE 6–6. Cytologically malignant lesions: melanoma and lymphoma (Fig. 6–6A, needle washing, Fig. 6–6C, imprint, Papanicolaou stain; Figs. 6–6B and 6–6D, hematoxylin- and eosin-stained needle biopsies, × 40).

A. Melanoma. Cells are similar to those of large-cell undifferentiated carcinoma. In this field, pigment is not apparent.

C. Large-cell Lymphomas. Cells show pronounced malignant nuclear features and scant cytoplasm. The single-cell presentation helps in distinguishing these tumors from other malignancies.

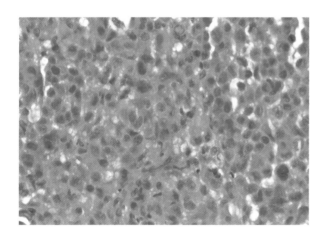

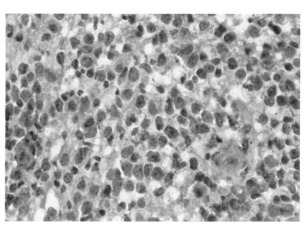

B. Melanoma. The same tumor as shown in Figure 6–6A demonstrates intracytoplasmic melanin pigment, which allows a specific diagnosis.

D. Lymphoma. In histologic preparations, lymphomas must be distinguished from oligodendrogliomas. Cells from lymphoma display more nuclear atypicality and contain higher nuclear to cytoplasmic ratios than do cells of oligodendrogliomas.

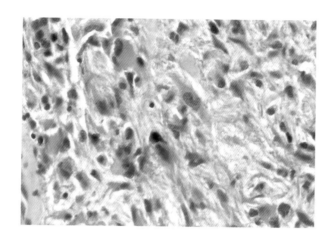

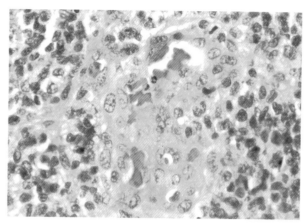

FIGURE 6–7. Histologic features of Glioblastoma Multiforme (Figs. 6–7A to 6–7C, hematoxylin and eosin stain, × 40; Fig. 6–7D, × 25).

A. Glioblastoma. Tumors are composed of pleomorphic cells with hyperchromatic, irregular nuclei, variable amounts of cytoplasm, and astrocytic morphology.

C. Glioblastoma. Glomeruloid tufts formed by plump, proliferating capillary endothelial cells are a typical, although not necessary, feature of these tumors.

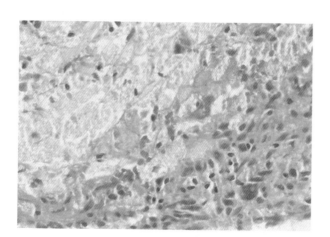

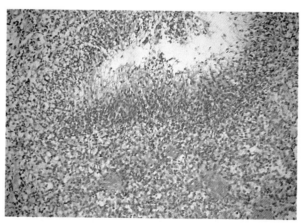

B. Glioblastoma. Necrosis is a required feature of these tumors. It often occurs in confluent areas, as is shown here.

D. Glioblastoma. This pattern of serpentine regions of necrosis surrounded by pseudopalisading cells is a characteristic feature of glioblastomas. Prominent endothelial proliferation is also present in this field.

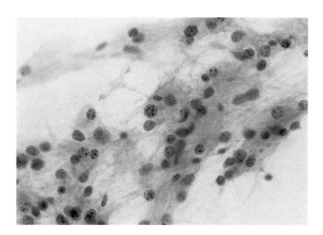
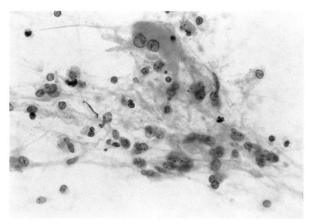

FIGURE 6–8. Comparison of anaplastic astrocytoma and glioblastoma multiforme.
FIGURES 6–8A and 6–8C, Anaplastic Astrocytoma. Smear preparations, Papanicolaou stain, × 40.

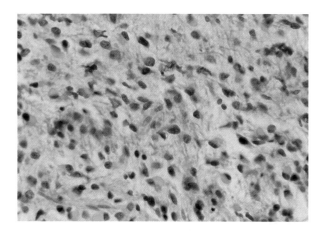
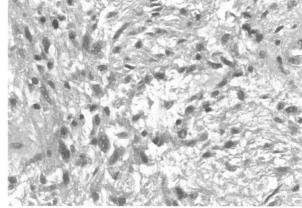

FIGURES 6–8B and 6–8D, Glioblastoma. Hematoxylin- and eosin-stained biopsies, × 40.

It is virtually impossible to distinguish anaplastic astrocytoma (Figs. 6–8A and 6–8B) from glioblastoma (Figs. 6–8C and 6–8D) using cytologic features alone. Although glioblastomas are classically considered to be highly pleomorphic with large multinucleate giant cells, as shown in Fig. 6–8C, many of these tumors actually show considerable cellular uniformity (as shown in Fig. 6–5A). This particular example of anaplastic astrocytoma (Figs. 6–8A and 6–8B) shows cellular regularity, but these tumors can also be pleomorphic. Because the presence of necrosis is the most reliable way to distinguish glioblastoma from anaplastic astrocytoma, histologically processed biopsy specimens are generally required to make this distinction.

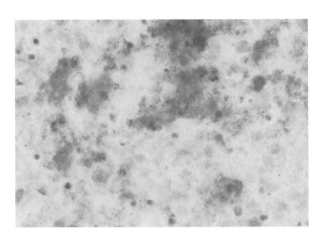

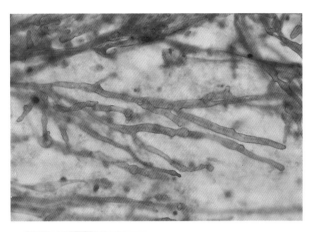

FIGURE 6–9. Differential diagnosis of Cystic Lesions— Infectious Conditions. Cyst fluids, Papanicolaou stain (Fig. 6–9A); Gram stain (Fig. 6–9B); period acid–Schiff stain (Fig. 6–9C) methenamine silver stain of cell block (Fig. 6–9D), × 40.

A. Bacterial Abscess. This smear shows necrotic contents of the abscess cavity in which the tiny organisms can barely be seen.

C. Mucor. Thick, ribbon-like, nonseptate *mucor hyphae* in a brain abscess from a patient on steroids.

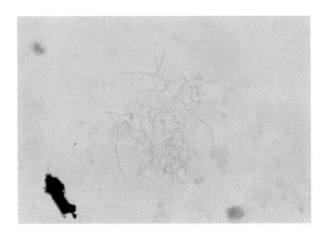

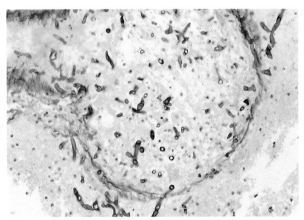

B. Nocardia. Fine, filamentous, gram-positive forms of *Nocardia* from an abscess from a patient with acquired immune deficiency syndrome.

D. Mucor. In this cell block preparation, *Mucor hyphae* can be seen growing through a vessel wall, producing thrombosis and infarction.

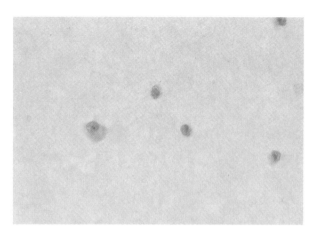

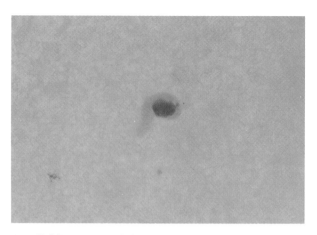

FIGURE 6–10. Differential diagnosis of cystic lesions and cyst fluids. (Papanicolaou stain, × 40).

A. Cystic Astrocytoma. This fluid contains macrophages that are indistinguishable from those seen in non-neoplastic cysts. The diagnosis of cystic astrocytoma usually necessitates surgical resection with examination of solid tumor areas surrounding the cystic cavity or evaluation of mural nodules of tumor tissue that may be present.

C. Glioblastoma Multiforme. Rare malignant astrocytes can be identified in cyst contents.

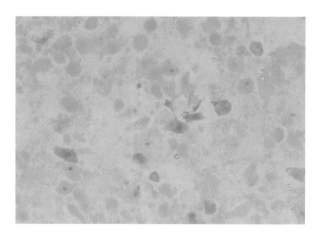

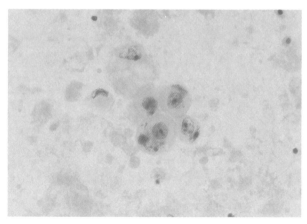

B. Craniopharyngioma. These keratinized squamous cells are similar to the contents of dermoid and epidermoid cysts. The presence of cohesive columnar adamantinomatous components is necessary to diagnose craniopharyngiomas with certainty.

D. Metastatic Adenocarcinoma. Within the cystic, necrotic debris, occasional well-preserved tumor fragments are found.

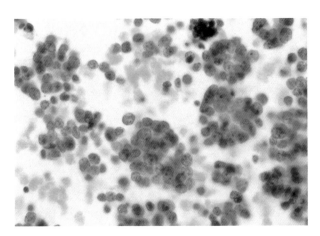

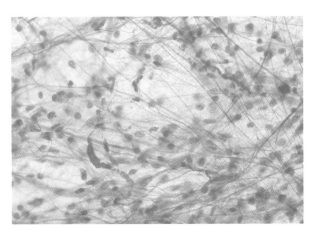

FIGURE 6–11. Childhood brain tumors—pineoblastoma and pilocytic astrocytoma. Figures 6–11A and 6–11B, needle washing; Figure 6–11A, Papanicolaou stain; Figure 6–11B, immunocytochemistry using an antibody against neural-cell adhesion molecule (N-CAM); Figure 6–11C, imprint, Papanicolaou stain; Figure 6–11D, hematoxylin- and eosin-stained biopsy × 40.

A. Pineoblastoma. This tumor is similar to the other types of small-cell central nervous system tumors, such as medulloblastoma, retinoblastoma, and cerebral neuroblastoma, in that the cells have round, hyperchromatic nuclei, scant cytoplasm, and frequently form rosettes.

C. Childhood Glioma. This tumor shows the spindle-shaped piloid astrocytes that frequently characterize childhood gliomas.

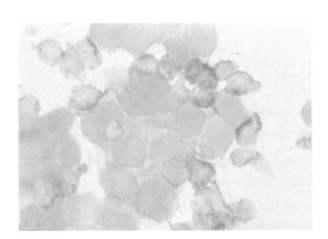

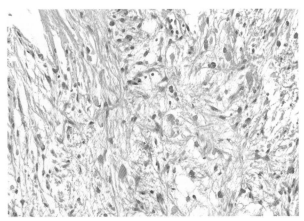

B. Pineoblastoma. Small-cell neurogenetic tumors usually express neural and neuroectodermal markers. This figure demonstrates reactivity with anti-N-CAM antibody UJ13-A.

D. Pilocytic Astrocytoma. The waxy, eosinophilic structures, which are particularly evident in this imprint are Rosenthal fibers.

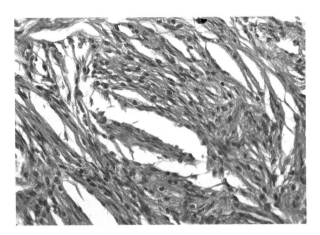

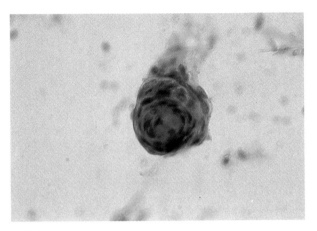

FIGURE 6–12. Meningioma sample obtained by a Cavitron ultrasonic aspirator. Figure 6–12A, hematoxylin- and eosin-stained cell block; Figures 6–12B to 6–12D, cyto-centrifuged preparation (Fig. 6–12A, × 25, Fig. 6–12B, × 40, Figs. 6–12C and 6–12D, × 60).

A. Meningioma. This histologic preparation shows the typical oval nuclei and indistinct cell borders of meningiomas. Although meningioma cells are often spindle shaped, here, cellular degeneration artifactually accentuates this feature.

C. Meningioma. Whorl formation is characteristic of meningiomas.

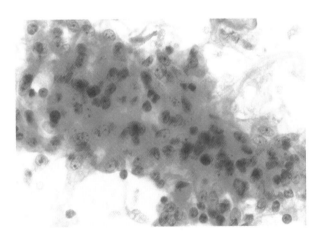

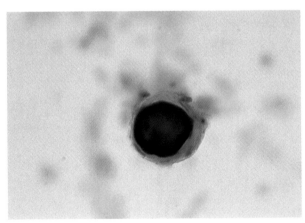

B. Meningioma. This cytologic preparation more accurately represents the features of this particular meningioma, which is composed of sheets of oval cells with bland nuclei arranged in syncytia.

D. Meningioma. Psammoma bodies are also a typical feature of meningioma.

C·H·A·P·T·E·R

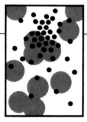

7

GASTROINTESTINAL CYTOLOGY

Linda Green

Cytology of the alimentary tract is used primarily as an adjunctive test in association with direct endoscopic visualization and biopsy for the diagnosis of neoplastic conditions. It is occasionally also helpful in diagnosis of non-neoplastic conditions such as inflammatory lesions or infections. This chapter discusses such sites as the oral cavity, esophagus, stomach, and intestine. There are many similarities in appearance of a tumor type from one site to the next, but some specific diagnoses should be considered for each site.

The oral mucosa is examined most commonly by scraping superficial cells from a suspicious lesion with a spatula or gauze-wrapped finger. The material is smeared onto a slide and then fixed immediately in alcohol for routine Papanicolaou stain or air-dried for the Romanowsky type of stains (e.g., May-Grunwald-Giemsa, Wright, or Diff-Quick).

A technique used exclusively in the esophagus is the inflatable balloon abrasion method, which consists of passing a noninflated balloon into the stomach, expanding the balloon and withdrawing it. This technique results in a cytologic specimen that has sampled the entire length of the esophagus. A new technique, the suction abrasive cytology tube, has been developed to obtain cellular samples from the esophagus in order to screen asymptomatic populations at higher risk of developing esophageal carcinoma. There are three standard techniques used to obtain specimens from the esophagus, stomach, intestine, or colon: lavage, washings, and brushings and salvage cytology. To obtain a lavage sample, a plastic tube is placed near the lesion and the patient swallows a normal saline solution either with or without a mucolytic enzyme such as papain to break down the mucin; then this is reaspirated through the tube. The fluid removed from three washes is collected and centrifuged, and the cellular material is then spread onto glass slides, and a cell block may be prepared. The main advantage of this cumbersome, blind sampling technique is that it may detect neoplastic cells derived from a small flat carcinoma that might be missed endoscopically.

Endoscopic visualization with brushing of lesions and salvage cytology are the most commonly used techniques. Their cumulative diagnostic accuracy is reported to be from 88 to 99%. Cellular material is obtained by vigorously brushing any lesion identified during endoscopy. The brush is used to spread the sample on glass slides that are then fixed immediately for staining. The brush may then be washed in a fixative and the fluid centrifuged, or it may be washed in saline from which membrane filter preparations are made. Brushings should be obtained prior to endoscopic biopsies because postbiopsy bleeding may obscure the area and result in false-negative results.

Salvage cytology specimens are collected by aspirating the biopsy channel of the endoscope into a mucus trap between each biopsy to recover the material that is clinging to the outside of the biopsy forceps and has been dislodged within the endoscope. The material in the mucus trap is rapidly fixed and centrifuged; then smears are prepared, and a cell block made from any particulate material. Other methods used to obtain gastrointestinal specimens include endoscopic fine needle aspiration, endoscopic jet washing, and the endoscopic suction technique.

All techniques can demonstrate carcinoma; however, compared with other techniques, brushing material may show cells that have a relatively bland appearance and less nuclear hyperchromasia, more delicate nuclear borders, and less prominent nucleoli. To avoid false-positive diagnosis, strict cytologic criteria for malignancy must be met for brush specimens.

NORMAL CYTOLOGIC FINDINGS

The oral cavity sheds squamous epithelial cells that are similar to the superficial and intermediate cells of the cervix and vagina (Fig. 7–1). Abundant superficial keratinized anucleated cells may be present normally, especially from scrape smears of the palate. Nuclear pyknosis is not observed. Central nuclear chromatin bars similar to those seen in Anitschkow cells of rheumatic heart disease are common.

The cytologic material obtained from the esophagus is composed of either sheets or single superficial or intermediate squamous cells. Parabasal cells and numerous anucleated squamous cells are not normally seen. Large numbers of basal cells in the specimen suggest trauma, inflammation, or erosion. Rarely, squamous "pearls" may be noted. Brushing and abrading usually remove only a few cells from a normal esophageal mucosa. These may occasionally be accompanied by macrophages and ciliated columnar cells of respiratory origin. Lavage, wash, and salvage cytology specimens often contain foreign material, especially food and plant cells.

Specimens from the gastroesophageal junction may contain a mixture of squamous epithelium and columnar cells of gastric origin. The normal gastric mucosa only sheds a few superficial epithelial cells, which are present as either cohesive clusters or less commonly as single cells (Fig. 7–2). The cell clusters and sheets display a honeycomb appearance and rosette-like formations. The cells have round or oval nuclei with dispersed, lace-like chromatin. They focally display a columnar shape and may have a mucin vacuole at the luminal portion of the cell. Rarely, cells of the gastric fundic glands (parietal and chief cells) may be found. The parietal cells are round to triangular with a foamy or granular cytoplasm, whereas the chief cells are much smaller with a cuboidal shape and a granular, eosinophilic cytoplasm and indistinct borders.

The most commonly sampled sites in the small bowel are the duodenum and the ampulla of Vater. The specimen obtained is composed of rare honeycomb-like sheets of cells, with occasional goblet cells forming clear windows (Fig. 7–3). Single cells and small cell clusters are seen. Cells have columnar shapes with brush borders and basilar ovoid nuclei. Paneth cells are recognized by coarse eosinophilic granular cytoplasm. Argentaffin cells from the base of the crypts of Lieberkühn are not found on cytologic specimens.

Cytologic material obtained from the colon consists of a few to moderate number of groups or sheets of cells that have a loose honeycomb-like pattern (Fig. 7–4). There is a predominance of goblet cells that have intracytoplasmic mucin and basilar nuclei. Relatively few absorptive type cells are interspersed. The clusters are often three dimensional, with the absorptive type cells and goblet cells on different planes of focus.

INFLAMMATORY CONDITIONS

Inflammatory conditions of the alimentary tract can be separated into infectious and noninfectious causes. Infections include bacterial, fungal, viral, or parasitic etiologies. Noninfectious lesions include, in the oral cavity, pemphigus vulgaris, vitamin deficiencies, and Darier's disease and, in the esophagus, reflux esophagitis, trauma, Plummer-Vinson syndrome, vitamin deficiencies, and Barrett syndrome.

Inflammation of the mucosa of the oral cavity and esophagus results in the shedding of more cells than normal, often with numerous basal or parabasal cells. There may be a background of necrotic cellular debris, fibrinoid material, and acute or chronic cells. These may be single, clustered, and/or intermixed with necrotic cellular debris. The inflammatory infiltrate may contain a mixture of neutrophils, eosinophils, lymphocytes, plasma cells, histiocytes, and erythrocytes. The inflammatory mixture depends on the condition producing it and on the presence of ulceration. The epithelial cells usually show degenerative changes such as diffuse hyperchromasia, pyknosis, and cytoplasmic disruption. Regenerating squamous epithelial cells may be seen in cohesive groups or sheets. The nuclei are enlarged and have washed-out or pale granular chromatin, a thin nuclear rim, and prominent round and regular macronucleoli. The cytoplasm of the cells may be thick and granular with eosinophilic or cyanophilic staining.

The most commonly encountered infections of the oral cavity and esophagus are herpetic or fungal, often *Candida*. The cytologic findings in herpetic infections of the oral cavity and esophagus are similar. There may be a few or numerous multinucleated cells with molded ground-glass nuclei showing margination of the chromatin against the nuclear membranes with intranuclear eosinophilic inclusions (Fig. 7–5). The same cytopathic effects may be observed in the glandular cells of the rest of the alimentary tract, but their occurrence in these sites is rare. Candidal infections reveal few or many hyphae, yeast forms often intermixed with exudate, and anucleated, necrotic squamous cells (Fig. 7–6). The organism can usually be identified on routine Papanicolaou stain but can be more readily detected by special stains for the organisms, including Gomori's methenamine silver, periodic acid–Schiff, and nonspecific fluorescent whiteners.

In the stomach the most common cytologically encountered inflammatory lesion is gastric ulceration, which must be distinguished from an ulcerating carcinoma. In ulcers, abundant to rare necrotic and inflammatory cells are found in the smear background. In most cases, the epithelial cells are present in cohesive clusters of various sizes with very few single cells, making this the best criterion (Fig. 7–7). Intestinal metaplasia may produce cells with brush borders and goblet cells. The most significant cytologic manifestation is the presence of regenerative changes of glandular epithelium occurring at the edge of the ulceration. These cells may show enlarged nuclei, increased nuclear to cytoplasmic ratio, prominent nucleoli, and mitotic figures. These nuclear changes may range from slight to conspicuous. Features used to distinguish changes of repair from carcinoma include preservation of polarity, uniformity of cell size with minimal pleomorphism, cohesiveness of cells, and the lack of numerous single cells.

Gastric and peptic ulcer disease is associated with *Helicobacter pylori* infection. *H. pylori* is a curved, S-shaped, gram-negative, flagellated bacillus that may be seen cytologically in the exudate on Papanicolaou stain (Fig. 7–8). It is best demonstrated by special stains such as Warthin-Starry, Dieterle, or Giemsa.

In the intestine and colon, the cytologic diagnosis of duodenitis and colitis remains nonspecific unless specific causative agents are found, such as giardiasis (Fig. 7–9), strongyloidiasis (Fig. 7–10), *Entamoeba histolytica* infection (Fig. 7–11), or cryptosporidiosis (Fig. 7–12). Inflammatory bowel disease may prove a diagnostic dilemma with focal cells with larger irregularly shaped nucleoli.

NEOPLASIA

The most common malignant neoplasm of the oral cavity and esophagus is squamous cell carcinoma. Carcinoma in situ (CIS) is more easily detected in the oral cavity than in the esophagus. Single cells and small clusters of abnormal squamous cells are seen that have predominately eosinophilic cytoplasm, moderate nuclear hyperchromasia, nuclear irregularity, and a decreased nuclear to cytoplasmic ratio (Fig. 7–13). These cells and groups resemble CIS of the cervix. Invasive squamous cell carcinoma can be detected cytologically with a high sensitivity (over 90%), but it is possible to determine the degree of differentiation. Cells from well-differentiated tumors (Figs. 7–14 and 7–15) have prominent keratinizing cytoplasm, bizarre shapes, anisocytosis, and scattered pyknotic and hyperchromatic nuclei. Pearl formations may be seen. Moderately differentiated tumors (Figs. 7–16 and 7–17) have less abundant cytoplasm with less differentiation toward keratinizing squamous cells. Nuclear chromatin is more variable with some hyperchromatic and pyknotic nuclei, but some have a more vesicular pattern. Poorly differentiated tumors (Figs. 7–18 and 7–19) have enlarged cells with a high nuclear to cytoplasmic ratio, nuclear hyperchromasia, irregular nuclear rims, and irregular nuclear chromatin centers and/or nucleoli.

Adenocarcinoma is the most common malignancy of the alimentary tract. Regardless of the alimentary origin, adenocarcinomas have distinctive cytopathologic features (Figs. 7–20 to 7–25). They exfoliate in sheets, in small clusters, and as single cells. The cells are enlarged, and anisocytosis is prominent, as is anisokaryosis and increased nuclear to cytoplasmic ratios. Nuclear atypia is prominent, as demonstrated by irregular, indented nuclear outlines, hyperchromasia, irregularly distributed chromatin, enlarged irregular nucleoli, and abnormal mitotic figures. Nuclear molding is also prominent, and cell within cell or "cannibalism" may be noted. There is usually an associated tumor diathesis composed of inflammatory cells, cellular debris, and red blood cells. The cytoplasm may be scant to abundant with a finely vacuolated, cyanophilic appearance. Occasionally, cytoplasmic vacuoles may be large and may fill the entire cytoplasm, forming signet ring cells (Fig. 7–26). Stains for mucin, i.e., Mayer mucicarmine and Alcian blue, may be used to demonstrate this feature (Fig. 7–27) but are not necessary.

Carcinoids generally originate in the deep layers of the epithelium and are seldom identified in cytologic material unless superficial ulceration occurs. The use of endoscopic fine needle aspiration of submucosal lesions may improve diagnostic yield in the future. Cells from carcinoids occur in small clusters or as scattered single cells (Figs. 7–28 and 7–29). The nuclei are relatively uniform in size and round or ovoid in shape, with a fine uniformly distributed chromatin and small distinct nucleoli. These cells have scant granular cytoplasm and may form small rosette-like or acinar forms. Lack of pleomorphism together with the characteristic nuclear chromatin is the best cytologic criterion.

Lymphomas arise in the submucosa and are only detectable by exfoliative cytology when they have ulcerated. Large-cell lymphoma (histiocytic lymphoma) sheds single cells or loosely cohesive aggregates of cells with scant cytoplasm (Fig. 7–30). The cells have round or irregular nuclei with clumped chromatin and large nucleoli either centrally or eccentrically located. The background may contain proteinaceous granular debris, and there may be impressive lymphocyte karyorrhexis. Small-cell lymphoma may be exceedingly difficult to distinguish morphologically from chronic gastritis or pseudolymphoma (Fig. 7–31). If adequate material is obtained, immunohistochemistry can be used to determine if the lymphocytic population is monoclonal.

Melanoma may shed single cells or small clusters of cells or may appear as large cellular groups (Fig. 7–32). These cells have many different and varied cytologic features but are similar to melanoma cells elsewhere. They are often composed of large pleomorphic cells with large irregular nuclei, or they may have moderate-sized cells with uniform nuclei. They usually have large macronucleoli. Melanin granules are often found in the cytoplasm and are brown-black, granular, and nonrefractile. Amelanotic melanomas may present as a malignant neoplasm mimicking similar adenocarcinoma or sarcoma.

Sarcomas very rarely are detected by brushing or salvage techniques and then only when the tumor has ulcerated. Elongated, spindle-shaped pleomorphic cells may be seen singly or in a few small groups. The nuclei are often oblong in shape with "squared-off" ends and have hyperchromatic chromatin and irregular nuclear chromatin centers (Fig. 7–33).

Bibliography

Drake M: Gastroesophageal Cytology. Basel: S. Karger, 1985.

Fenoglio-Preiser CM, Lantz PE, Listrom MB, et al.: Gastrointestinal Pathology: An Atlas and Text. New York: Raven Press, 1989, pp. 943–958.

Gupta JP, Jain AK, Agrawal BK, Gupta S: Gastroscopic cytology and biopsies in the diagnosis of gastric malignancies. J Surg Oncol 22:62–64, 1983.

Takeda M: Atlas of Diagnostic Gastrointestinal Cytology. New York: Igaku-Shoin Medical Publishers Inc, 1983.

Winawer SJ, Leidner SD, Hajdu SI, Sherlock P: Colonoscopic biopsy and cytology in the diagnosis of colon cancer. Cancer 42:2849–2853, 1978.

● ●

NORMAL CELLS AND INFECTIONS

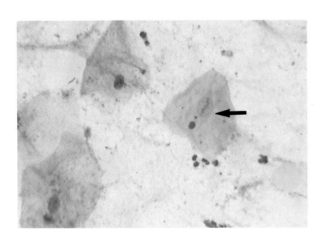

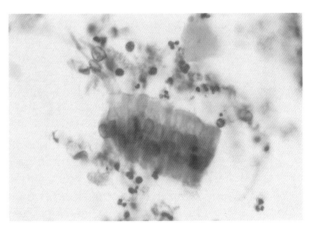

FIGURE 7–1. Normal Squamous Cells (Esophagus). Desquamated uniform superficial and intermediate cells are seen with abundant cytoplasm demonstrating varying degrees of keratinization. These cells have uniform, small, delicate nuclei with evenly distributed chromatin and occasional chromatin bars (arrow) (esophageal brush, Papanicolaou stain, × 400).

FIGURE 7–2. Normal Glandular Epithelium (Stomach). A strip of mucus-producing columnar cells is demonstrated. The cells have a more centrally placed and uniform nucleus than do cells in the lower gastrointestinal tract. The chromatin pattern is delicate and dispersed, with occasional round, small nucleoli. Only rarely are single cells found (salvage cytology, Papanicolaou stain, × 400).

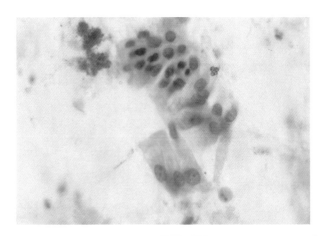

FIGURE 7–3. Normal Glandular Epithelium (Duodenum). An irregular three-dimensional strip or sheet of columnar cells is demonstrated. This sheet focally demonstrates a flat, striated, luminal surface that focally may have cilia. Nuclei are basal in location and round or oval in shape, with focal small nucleoli. The cytoplasm is cyanophilic, but other normal cells may have acidophilic cytoplasm (salvage cytology, Papanicolaou stain, × 400).

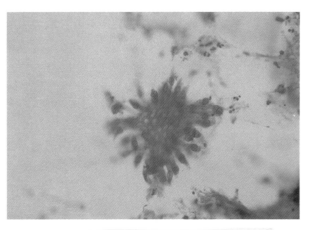

FIGURE 7–4. Normal Glandular Epithelium (Colon). The columnar cells are shed as a sheet (arrow). They have uniform oval nuclei with small, round nucleoli or chromatin centers or both. Interspersed goblet cells contain a large intracytoplasmic mucin droplet. The cell clusters are not numerous and may have accompanying macrophages, leukocytes, and superficial squamous cells of anal origin (brushing cytology, Papanicolaou stain, × 400).

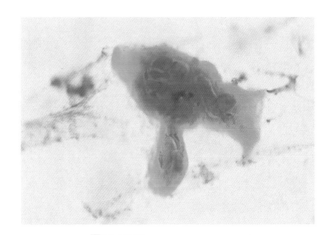

FIGURE 7–5. Epithelial Cell Infected with Herpes Virus (Esophagus). Two infected epithelial cells demonstrate the cytopathic effects of the herpes virus. The cells are enlarged and contain multiple nuclei that show nuclear molding and "smudged" or "ground glass" intranuclear inclusions surrounded by a clear halo (salvage cytology, Papanicolaou stain, × 630).

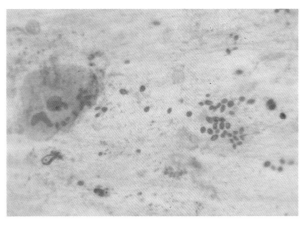

FIGURE 7–6. Candida Organisms (Esophagus). On a Papanicolaou stain, small, red, oval budding yeast are seen with a background of necrotic debris and superficial squamous cells. The associated inflammation is composed of both acute and chronic inflammatory cells. Often, both yeast and pseudohyphae may be seen in *Candida albicans*. In the present example only yeast are seen because this esophagitis resulted from a different *Candida* species (salvage cytology, Papanicolaou stain, × 400).

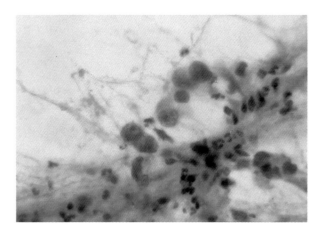

FIGURE 7–7A. Epithelial Repair Associated with Acute Ulceration (Stomach). A small strip of glandular epithelium is surrounded by necrotic debris and acute inflammatory cells. The nuclear to cytoplasmic ratio is increased, and a few cells are degenerated. In the preserved reactive cells, the nuclei are enlarged, with dispersed, "washed-out" chromatin. The nuclear rims remain thin and regular, and cellular adhesion is maintained, unlike carcinomas that demonstrate numerous single cells with coarse chromatin and irregular nuclear rims (salvage cytology, Papanicolaou stain, × 400).

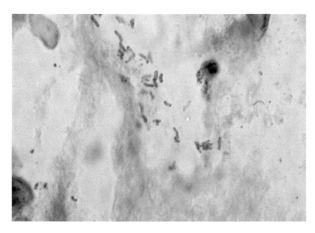

FIGURE 7–8. *Helicobacter pylori* (Stomach). These S-shaped bacilli are embedded in the surface gastric mucus and have been associated with both acute and chronic inflammation and ulcerations (salvage cytology, Warthin-Starry stain, × 1000).

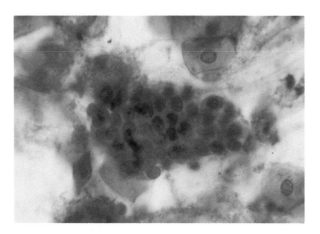

FIGURE 7–7B. Epithelial Repair Associated with Ulceration (Esophagus). A large, cohesive group of epithelial cells is seen in the center surrounded by superficial squamous cells and debris. The central cluster is composed of cells of repair with uniform nuclei, each containing a small, distinct nucleolus. There is no pleomorphism, and no single cells are present, as in carcinoma or dysplasia (salvage cytology, Papanicolaou stain, × 400).

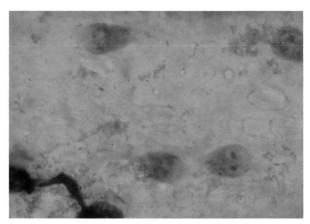

FIGURE 7–9. *Giardia lamblia* (Duodenum). Four trophozoites of *Giardia lamblia* are demonstrated. They are flat, pear-shaped, binucleated organisms with four pairs of flagella. They may be mistaken for histiocytes but the binucleation and the central line created by their sucker plate should aid in their recognition (brushing cytology, Papanicolaou stain, × 1000).

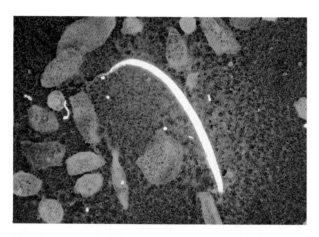

FIGURE 7–10. Rhabditiform Larvae of *Strongyloides stercoralis* (Stomach). This rhabditiform larvae can be identified by its short buccal structure, capsule esophagus, pointed tail, and length of about 200 to 300 μ. With preparation of a wet mount, motility may be demonstrated. The larva can be seen on routine staining or by the use of fluorescent whitening stains examined under a fluorescent microscope (gastric washing, Tinopal CBS-X [Whitener Fluorescent Stain], × 225).

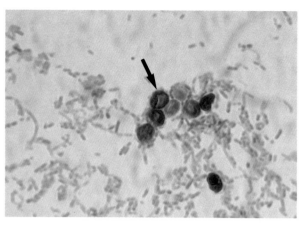

FIGURE 7–12. Cryptosporidium (Rectum/Sigmoid Colon). This parasitic organism, which may be seen in immunocompromised patients and children, consists of cysts (arrow), which are round or oval structures (2 to 4 μ) commonly associated with an acute inflammatory infiltrate. The red- or pink-stained cysts are surrounded by bacilli representing normal colonic flora. These cysts are best demonstrated by a Giemsa stain or a modified acid-fast staining technique, as seen here (washing cytology, modified acid-fast stain, × 1000).

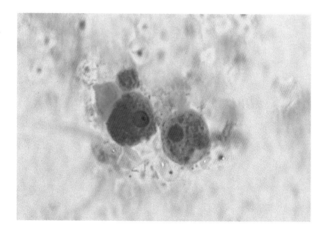

FIGURE 7–11. Amoeba *(Entamoeba histolytica)* (Colon). Trophozoites as seen here may be mistaken for histiocytes on colonic cytologic specimens. They are about 15 to 25 μ in diameter, with a single, round nucleus with clumped chromatin at the nuclear membrane and a central, nuclear, dark-staining round structure, the karyosome. Their cytoplasm contains abundant glycogen, which can be demonstrated with special stains such as periodic acid-Schiff. Rarely, intracytoplasmic, ingested red blood cells may be seen (washing cytology, Papanicolaou stain, × 1000).

MALIGNANT TUMORS

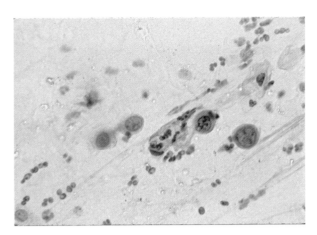

FIGURE 7–13. Squamous Cell Carcinoma in Situ (Esophagus). Single, small cells comparable with the size of parabasal cells are scattered amid acute inflammatory cells. As in the cervix, there is an increased nuclear to cytoplasmic ratio and the nuclei have a clumped, dense, irregular chromatin pattern. Unlike cervical carcinoma in situ, the cells from the esophagus and oral cavity may have occasional prominent nucleoli. As seen here, the cytoplasm can show varying degrees of keratinization (brushing cytology, Papanicolaou stain, × 400).

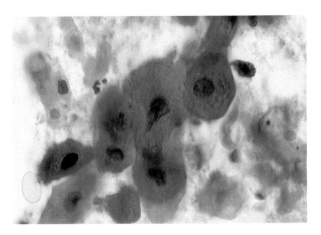

FIGURE 7–14B. Invasive, Well-Differentiated Squamous Cell Carcinoma (Esophagus). Both single cells and loose or tightly packed cell clusters or sheets are visible, all of which show cytoplasmic keratinization. The nuclei are hyperchromatic, with irregular shapes and thick nuclear rims. Occasionally, nucleoli may be seen. The cell clusters contain both nonviable degenerate cells with pyknotic nuclei, as well as large vesicular nuclei of viable cells (lavage cytology, Papanicolaou stain, × 630).

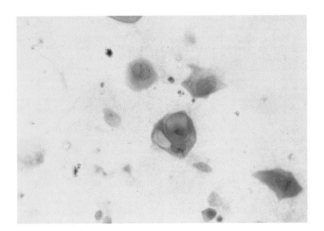

FIGURE 7–14A. Invasive, Well-Differentiated Squamous Cell Carcinoma (Esophagus). A cell grouping, or "pearl," is seen in the center as a wrapping formation, with one cell surrounding another to form a three-dimensional structure (salvage cytology, Papanicolaou stain, × 630).

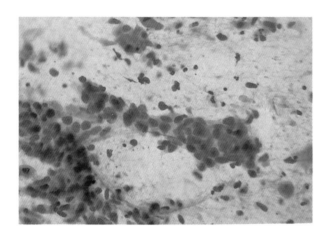

FIGURE 7–15A. Moderately Differentiated Squamous Cell Carcinoma (Esophagus). There are fewer recognizably keratinized cells, and the nuclear to cytoplasmic ratio is increased compared with that of well-differentiated tumors. The nuclei are enlarged, with irregular nuclear shapes and clumped, irregular chromatin. Nucleoli are prominent and may be irregular in shape (salvage cytology, Papanicolaou stain, × 400).

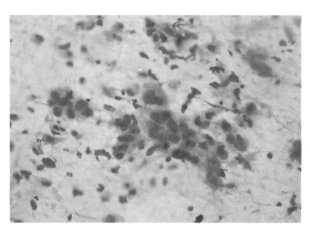

FIGURE 7–16A. Poorly Differentiated Squamous Cell Carcinoma (Esophagus). A central, loosely cohesive group of cells is seen amid a necrotic background. The nuclei are large and irregular, with a prominent nucleolus. No keratinization is identified. The cells resemble those of adenocarcinoma and in some instances cannot be identified with certainty as squamous cell carcinoma (salvage cytology, Papanicolaou stain, × 160).

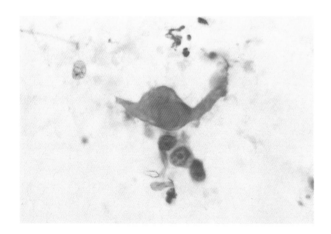

FIGURE 7–15B. Moderately Differentiated Squamous Cell Carcinoma (Esophagus). The tumor cells have an increased nuclear ratio, clumped chromatin, and prominent nucleoli. An anucleated "ghost" keratinizing cell with "tadpole" features is also present, suggesting that a well-differentiated component is also present (salvage cytology, Papanicolaou stain, × 400).

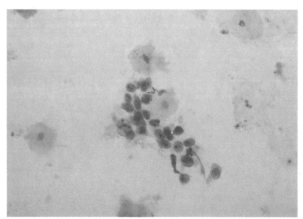

FIGURE 7–16B. Poorly Differentiated Squamous Cell Carcinoma (Esophagus). A loose aggregate of cells with a high nuclear to cytoplasmic ratio is seen in the center. The chromatin is clumped, and multiple nucleoli and/or chromatin centers are present. Single cells are also present, with a suggestion of polygonal cytoplasm. This suggests that the cells are squamous in origin even though no keratinization is seen (salvage cytology, Papanicolaou stain, × 160).

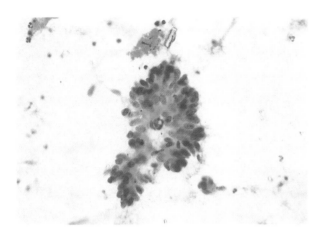

FIGURE 7–17A. Well-Differentiated Adenocarcinoma (Stomach). Large clusters with pseudoglandular formations, as well as small clusters, are seen. Only a few single cells may be found. In this case of intestinal-type adenocarcinoma, the cellular organization shows minimal disruption, but there is focal crowding, overlapping, and loss of polarity (brushing cytology, Papanicolaou stain, × 160).

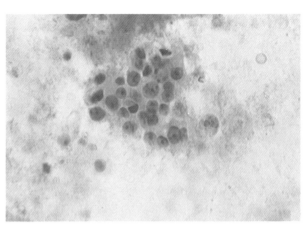

FIGURE 7–18A. Moderately Differentiated Adenocarcinoma (Stomach). The degree of nuclear abnormality seen in the sheet of loosely cohesive cells falls in between those of a well-differentiated and a poorly differentiated adenocarcinoma. Both single cells and cellular clusters are seen with gland-like arrangements and focal intracytoplasmic mucin production. Pleomorphism of nuclear size and shape is more evident, and nuclear molding may be prominent. Large nucleoli and irregular chromatin centers are prominent (salvage cytology, Papanicolaou stain, × 400).

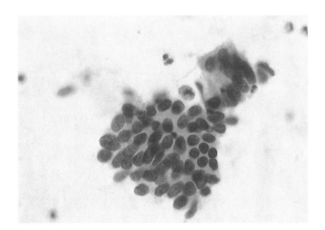

FIGURE 7–17B. Well-Differentiated Adenocarcinoma (Stomach). The cells from the case illustrated in Figure 7–17A show focal mild pleomorphism, nuclear membrane irregularity, and occasional prominent nucleoli (brushing cytology, Papanicolaou stain, × 400).

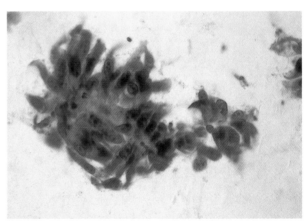

FIGURE 7–18B. Moderately Differentiated Adenocarcinoma (Colon). A cluster of loosely cohesive enlarged cells is seen with nuclear crowding, hyperchromasia, and multiple irregular chromatin centers. The cytoplasm is granular, as described in Figure 7–18A, and a gland-like structure is formed (brushing cytology, Papanicolaou stain, × 400).

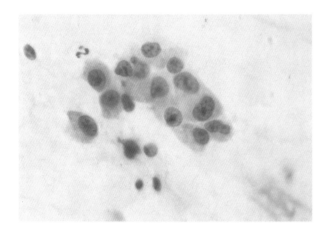

FIGURE 7–19A. Poorly Differentiated Adenocarcinoma (Stomach). The cells are in small clusters, with scattered, single cells. The cells are enlarged, with nuclear enlargement, nuclear irregularity, and loss of polarity. Nucleoli are prominent, multiple, and irregular. The cytoplasm is abundant to scant in amount, with an increased nuclear to cytoplasmic ratio, and cytoplasmic vacuoles may be rare. They are absent in this example (salvage cytology, Papanicolaou stain, × 400).

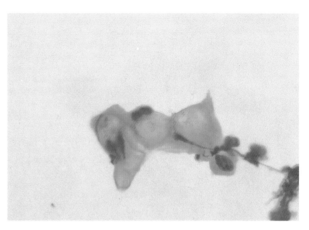

FIGURE 7–20A. Signet Ring Adenocarcinoma (Stomach). The cells are seen as small, loosely cohesive groups, as shown here, or often as single cells. The cells have an eccentrically placed, hyperchromatic, irregular nucleus that is pushed to the edge of the cytoplasm by a large intracytoplasmic mucin droplet, which may be single or multivacuolated (salvage cytology, Papanicolaou stain, × 630).

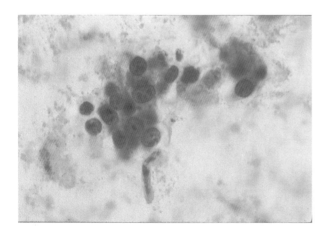

FIGURE 7–19B. Poorly Differentiated Adenocarcinoma (Colon). There is an irregular cluster of cells that was accompanied by numerous scattered single cells. There is anaplasia and nuclear irregularity. Cytoplasmic and intranuclear vacuoles, not demonstrated here, may be seen and are representative of mucin production (salvage cytology, Papanicolaou stain, × 630).

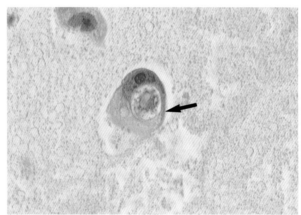

FIGURE 7–20B. Signet Ring Adenocarcinoma (Stomach). A single signet ring cell is present, with an eccentric, enlarged nucleus containing a large nucleolus. Nucleoli are often not found in these cells, which are often degenerating, but when the cells are well-preserved, they can demonstrate prominent nucleoli, as seen here. The cytoplasm has both large and small vacuoles, which contain pink-staining mucin (arrow) (cell block from salvage cytology, mucicarmine stain, × 630).

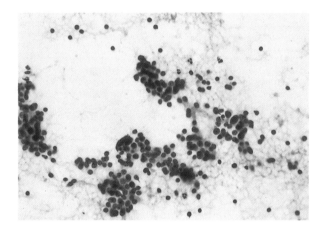

FIGURE 7–21A. Carcinoid (Small Intestine). This carcinoid tumor consists of small groups, cords, large clusters, and scattered, single, uniform cells with regular, round nuclei that vary little in size or shape. The cells are cuboidal and may form small pseudoacinar structures. The cells differ from normal epithelium, which is columnar and sheds as few large sheets and groups of cells, with more cytoplasm (endoscopic fine needle aspiration, Papanicolaou stain, × 225).

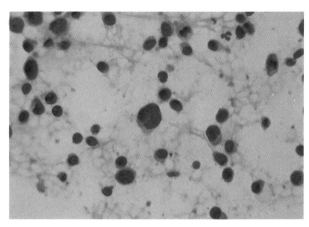

FIGURE 7–22. Large-Cell Lymphoma (Stomach). The cells shed are single and loosely clustered and are three to five times the size of mature lymphocytes. The cells have scant, cyanophilic, delicate cytoplasm, and the nuclei have coarse granular and vesicular chromatin. Irregular nucleoli or chromatin centers are generally prominent. The background may be necrotic, with inflammation and single dead or "ghost" cells because these lesions are submucosal and must be ulcerated in order to shed cells on washings or brushings (salvage cytology, Papanicolaou stain, × 400).

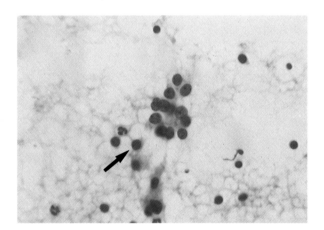

FIGURE 7–21B. Carcinoid (Small Intestine). A small group of cells forming a "rosette-like" pseudoglandular structure is present in the center, surrounded by single tumor cells (arrow). The nuclei are uniform in size and shape. The chromatin is more granular than normal epithelium, and small, eccentric nucleoli are present (endoscopic fine needle aspiration, Papanicolaou stain, × 400).

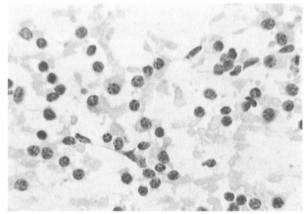

FIGURE 7–23. Small-Cell Lymphomas (Stomach). The cells are seen as small, loosely cohesive sheets and single cells. They have an open and coarsely clumped chromatin pattern, focal nuclear irregularity, and occasional nucleoli or multiple chromatin centers. There is then some rim of cyanophilic delicate cytoplasm that often is disrupted, as is seen here by the brushing procedure or slide preparation. In this example, the nuclei are eccentric, with "clock-face" chromatin resulting in a plasmacytoid appearance. Unlike reactive chronic inflammatory processes, which are polymorphic, these lymphocytes are uniform in size. The cells differ from carcinoid and small-cell carcinoma by the lack of cohesion or "molding" (salvage cytology, Papanicolaou stain, × 400).

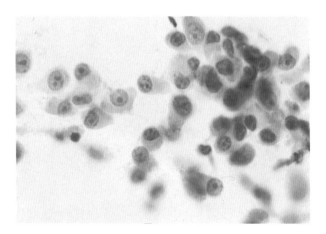

FIGURE 7–24. Melanoma (Small Intestine). In this example of metastatic melanoma, the cells are seen in small clusters and as single cells that have large, eccentric nuclei with striking macronucleoli. This case is that of an amelanotic melanoma; it may be difficult to differentiate from an adenocarcinoma. In such a case, special stains may be necessary. A trichrome stain may demonstrate intracytoplasmic melanin as black granules. S-100 or HMB-45 immunoperoxidase stains may stain melanomas but would be negative in carcinomas (salvage cytology, Papanicolaou stain, × 400).

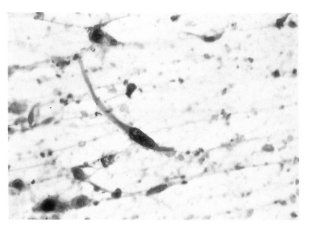

FIGURE 7–25. Leiomyosarcoma (Cecum). This leiomyosarcoma sheds as large single, spindled cells with stretched out cytoplasm and elongated oval to "cigar-shaped" nuclei with blunt ends. The chromatin is hyperchromatic and coarse (salvage cytology, Papanicolaou stain, × 225).

DIFFERENTIAL GROUPS

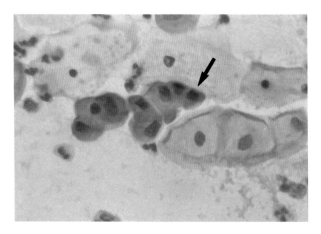

FIGURE 7–26. Human Papilloma Virus (Esophagus). The cells present occur as a sheet and cluster of cells with irregular, "raisin-like" nuclei. Some cells have perinuclear zones. When the cells are clustered and lack the characteristic perinuclear halos (arrow), they must be distinguished from squamous cell carcinoma. Squamous cell carcinomas have an increased nuclear to cytoplasmic ratio and abnormal cell shapes are common, whereas this is not true of papillomas (brushing cytology, Papanicolaou stain, × 400).

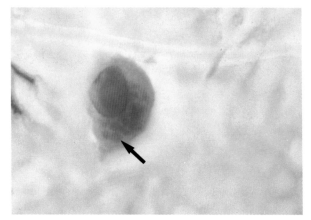

FIGURE 7–27. Cytomegalovirus Infection (Stomach). The epithelial cell is infected with CMV. It is enlarged and has a large nucleus with "glassy" or "smudged" chromatin. It differs from carcinoma because of its 1) smooth, regular nuclear rim; 2) lack of coarse, hyperchromic nucleus; 3) lack of nucleolus; 4) presence of a perinuclear "halo" around the inclusion, which may stain either red or purple; and 5) abundant cyanophilic cytoplasm. In this cell, there are also blue, dense granules (arrow), which probably represent viral coat protein or complete viral units (salvage cytology, Papanicolaou stain, × 1000).

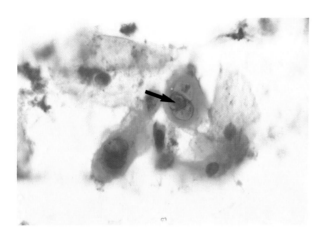

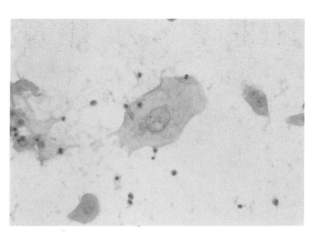

FIGURE 7–28. Herpes Infection (Esophagus). The epithelial cells are enlarged and contain two or more enlarged, molded nuclei with "washed-out" chromatin as a result of the presence of an intranuclear inclusion (arrow), which represents live and dead virions. The inclusion is separated from the nuclear rim by an artifactual cleft, resulting in the perinuclear "halo." Although multinucleated carcinoma cells occur, their nuclei are irregular, hyperchromatic, and usually contain nucleoli (salvage cytology, Papanicolaou stain, × 630).

FIGURE 7–30. Folic Acid Deficiency (Esophagus). As in radiation atypia, the epithelial cell shows cellular enlargement with concomitant enlargement of the nucleus. There can also be multinucleation and cytoplasmic vacuolization. Nuclear folding may be seen but the nuclear rim remains smooth. These changes are reversible after appropriate therapy (salvage cytology, Papanicolaou stain, × 400).

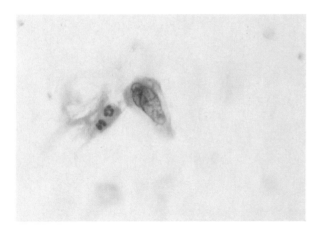

FIGURE 7–29. Epithelial Atypia Secondary to Radiation (Esophagus). The epithelial cell is greatly enlarged, with both cytoplasmic and nuclear enlargements. The nucleus has pale, "washed-out" chromatin with "cleared-out" areas. The cytoplasm is delicate and vacuolated, with membrane disruption secondary to fragility. In contrast, a carcinoma usually will have an enlarged, irregular, dense nucleus and an increased nuclear to cytoplasmic ratio, as seen in Figures 7–16A and 7–16B (salvage cytology, Papanicolaou stain, × 400).

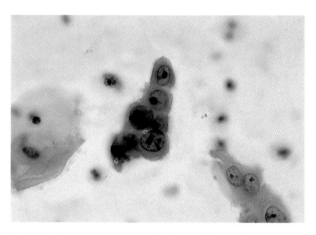

FIGURE 7–31. Pemphigus Vulgaris (Oral). A cluster of parabasal cells is seen with enlarged nuclei and irregular, "bar-shaped" nucleoli. Unlike carcinoma, the nuclei have "open" chromatin and are uniform in size and shape (oral scrape, Papanicolaou stain, × 400). (Courtesy of Ibrahim Ramzy, M.D.)

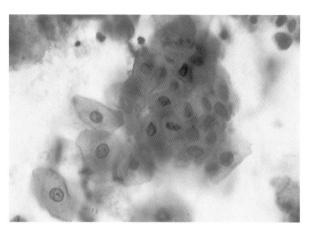

FIGURE 7–32B. Atypia in Reflux Esophagitis (Esophagus). A group of superficial squamous cells is seen that were shed among numerous numbers of both cell groups and single cells. The nuclei are not uniformly oval or round. There are irregular nuclei with increased nuclear to cytoplasmic (N/C) ratios suggesting atypia. The nuclei seen are not hyperchromatic, as in squamous cell carcinoma (salvage cytology, Papanicolaou stain, × 400).

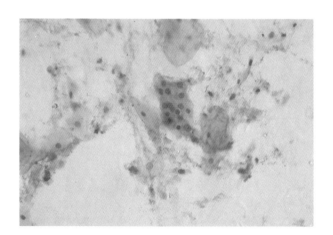

FIGURE 7–32A. Reflux Esophagitis (Esophagus). A central cluster of basal epithelial cell is seen amidst necrotic, inflammatory material and superficial squamous cells. These cells are not normally seen unless inflammation or ulceration or both are occurring. The nuclei are uniform and bland, with vesicular chromatin pattern (salvage cytology, Papanicolaou stain, × 225).

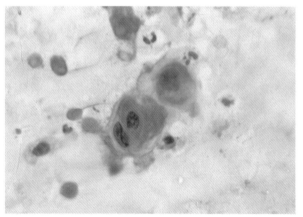

FIGURE 7–32C. Dysplasia in Esophagitis (Esophagus). A loosely cohesive atypical cell group is seen with the keratinizing cytoplasm. There is abundant cytoplasm, and the nuclei are granular or "washed out." The nuclear rim is indistinct as a result of degeneration. Unlike in carcinoma, the chromatin is not irregular, and thickened nuclear rims are not evident. The cells were scarce and embedded in acute inflammatory, necrotic debris (salvage cytology, Papanicolaou stain, × 400).

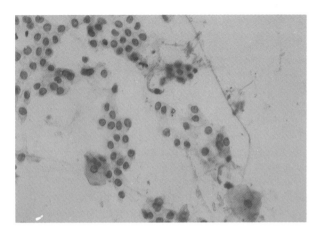

FIGURE 7–33. Barrett Esophagus (Esophagus). Numerous benign columnar cells are seen intermixed with superficial squamous cells. A cytologic specimen from a Barrett esophagus may look exactly like specimens obtained from the gastroesophageal function. It is therefore important to know the exact location in the esophagus from which the specimen was taken (salvage cytology, Papanicolaou stain, × 225).

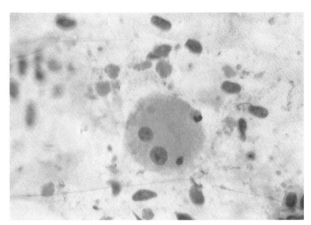

FIGURE 7–35. Mucinophages (Stomach). A lipid-laden and mucin-laden histocyte, as seen here, has uniform nuclear rims and bland chromatin. The nucleolus is smaller than those seen in signet ring carcinoma and lacks irregularity. If the histiocytic nucleus is degenerated or pyknotic, it may be difficult to distinguish from an isolated carcinoma cell. Unlike signet ring carcinoma cells, in which the nucleus is completely pushed to the cytoplasmic membrane by the cytoplasmic vacuole, the histiocyte nucleus is eccentric but still maintains a rim of cytoplasm around itself. It maintains a round shape and is not deformed by the vacuoles. Special stains for mucin are not helpful because both will stain positively for intracellular mucin (salvage cytology, Papanicolaou stain, × 400).

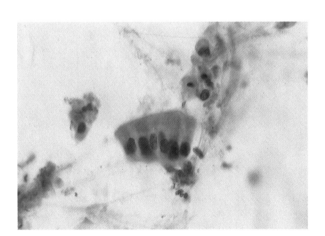

FIGURE 7–34. Intestinal Metaplasia (Stomach). The central row of detached cells is shed from intestinal metaplastic epithelium; these cells are larger than normal gastric cells. They are columnar in shape and have enlarged, uniform, round nuclei and abundant, opaque cytoplasm. The cytoplasm may contain a single cytoplasmic vacuole. Cells such as these may be seen in the esophagus in Barrett esophagitis or in the stomach in chronic gastritis or pernicious anemia. Unlike those in carcinoma, they demonstrate uniformity and organization (salvage cytology, Papanicolaou stain, × 400).

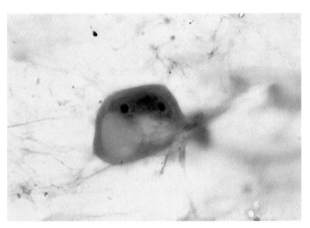

FIGURE 7–36. Signet Ring Adenocarcinoma (Stomach). In this well-preserved, binucleated cell, the enlarged nucleus has granular chromatin, an irregular nuclear rim, and prominent nucleoli. The nuclei are displaced eccentrically by the large mucin vacuoles. Histiocytes may contain a single cytoplasmic vacuole also, but multivacuolated cytoplasm is more common in carcinoma cells. The malignant characteristics of the nucleus are the only reliable features that identify signet ring carcinoma (salvage cytology, Papanicolaou stain, × 630).

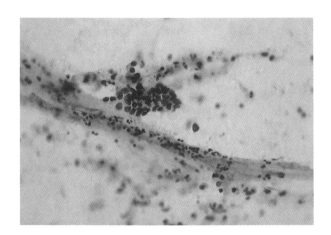

FIGURE 7–37A. Regenerative Atypia in Acute Ulceration (Stomach). An aggregate of cohesive epithelial cells is seen amid acute inflammatory cells and mucin. There is an increase in the nuclear to cytoplasmic ratio but the nuclei remain fairly uniform. No single cells are seen. The lack of single cells helps differentiate atypia from the well-differentiated type of adenocarcinoma (salvage cytology, Papanicolaou stain, × 225).

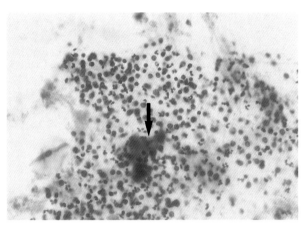

FIGURE 7–38. Acute Gastritis (Stomach). In this case of acute gastritis secondary to the use of nonsteroidal anti-inflammatory drugs, there is prominent acute inflammation, necrotic debris, and both a group (arrow) and scattered single degenerating epithelial cells. The cytoplasm is "stripped" and there are bare, pyknotic nuclei (salvage cytology, Papanicolaou stain, × 225).

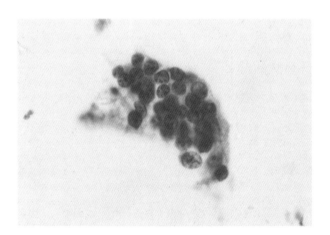

FIGURE 7–37B. Regenerative Epithelial (in Ulcers) Atypia (Stomach). A sheet of relatively uniform cells is seen with an increase in nuclear to cytoplasmic ratio. The chromatin is granular and evenly distributed. A prominent nucleolus is present but is uniform in size and shape. The cells remain cohesive and do not shed as scattered single cells, as seen in adenocarcinoma. Although the nuclei are atypical, the cells are still uniform and polarity is maintained (salvage cytology, Papanicolaou stain, × 400).

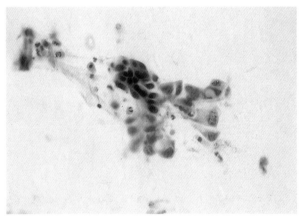

FIGURE 7–39. Chronic Gastritis with Atypia (Stomach). The background is free of necrosis and the cells are loosely aggregated, but single cells are conspicuously absent. The nuclei are enlarged, with occasional nucleoli, and the nuclear to cytoplasmic ratio is increased. Unlike those in carcinoma, the nuclear membranes remain thin and regular and polarity is maintained. Some pleomorphism is evident, with benign epithelial cells transforming into atypical cells (salvage cytology, Papanicolaou stain, × 400).

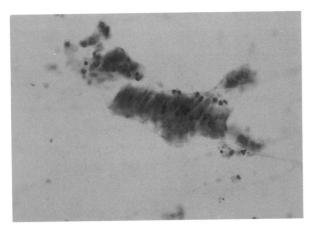

FIGURE 7–40. Hyperplastic Polyp (Colon). Small clusters and groups of columnar cells are present. The cells have the features of normal colonic mucosa. Goblet cell clusters may predominate. The brushing smears are more cellular than those taken from a normal colon. Unlike adenomatous polyps, mucin production and goblet cells are still evident (brushing cytology, Papanicolaou stain, × 225).

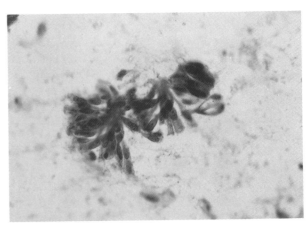

FIGURE 7–42A. Villous Adenoma/Polyp (Rectum). A large cluster of columnar cells with elongated to oval nuclei is seen. The tapered, granular cytoplasm has a flat edge with a brush border. The nuclei are crowded and appear to be "jumbled." Mitotic figures may be observed, but they are "normal" in appearance. The nuclei are uniform in size, with thin, regular nuclear rims and small nucleoli (brushing cytology, Papanicolaou stain, × 400).

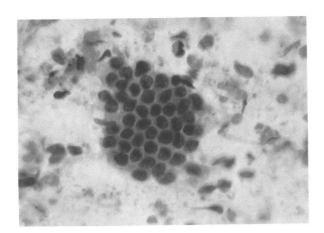

FIGURE 7–41. Adenomatous Polyp (Colon). An adenomatous polyp produces a cellular sample of cell clusters and groups. The group seen here has a slight increase in nuclear to cytoplasmic ratio, as compared with that of normal colonic epithelium. Cellular polarity is maintained, as is uniformity of cell shape and size. Unlike normal colonic epithelium or hyperplastic polyps, mucin vacuoles or goblet cells are absent (brushing cytology, Papanicolaou stain, × 400).

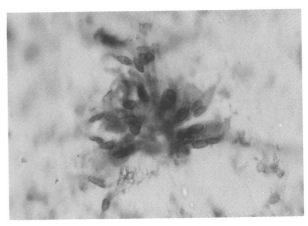

FIGURE 7–42B. Villous Adenoma/Polyp (Rectum). The small cluster of columnar cells is "jumbled" and three dimensional. The nuclei have "washed-out," finely granular chromatin, and the nuclear rims are thin. They lack the pleomorphism, hyperchromasia, and increased nuclear to cytoplasmic ratios seen in carcinoma (brushing cytology, Papanicolaou stain, × 630).

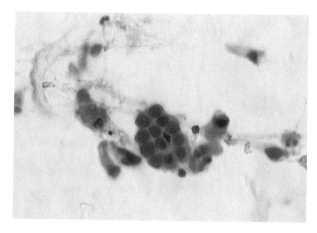

FIGURE 7–43. Adenomatous Polyps with Dysplasia (Colon). In this cellular cluster of columnar cells, there are changes of dysplasia, including increase in the nuclear to cytoplasmic ratio; nuclear crowding; prominent round, regular nucleoli; and more granular chromatin. Unlike malignant neoplasms, the cells still remain fairly uniform in size and shape and lack the hyperchromasia and dense, irregular nuclear rims of adenocarcinoma. The cells still show glandular architectural groups. As in adenomatous polyps without dysplasia, mucin production is not evident (brushing cytology, Papanicolaou stain, × 225).

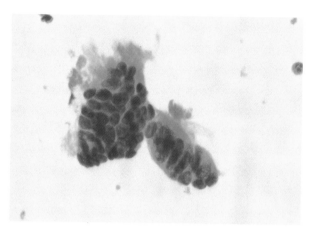

FIGURE 7–45. Adenocarcinoma Arising in an Adenomatous Polyp (Colon). The two cellular aggregates were shed from an adenomatous polyp containing adenocarcinoma. There is marked nuclear crowding, with overlapping, irregularly shaped, hyperchromatic nuclei. There is an attempt to polarity, but because of an increase in the nuclear to cytoplasmic ratio, "molding" is present. Benign adenomatous cell clusters (not pictured) were intermixed with both aggregates and single cells, as shown (brushing cytology, Papanicolaou stain, × 400).

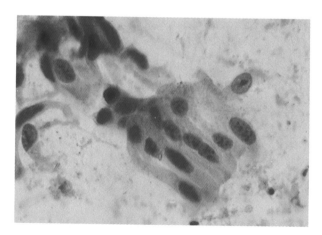

FIGURE 7–44. Villous Adenoma with Dysplasia (Colon). The cellular group consists of a sheet of columnar cells with elliptical nuclei. There is slight nuclear crowding and nuclei varying in size and shape. Prominent nucleoli are seen. Carcinomas, in contrast to dysplasia, often lose the "cigar-shaped" nuclei, have less cytoplasm with an increased nuclear to cytoplasmic ratio, and have irregular nuclear contours (brushing cytology, Papanicolaou stain, × 630).

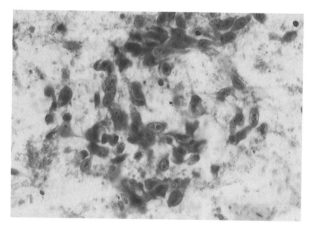

FIGURE 7–46. Adenocarcinoma Arising in a Villous Adenoma (Rectum). These cells have lost their cohesion and are seen as a loose aggregate of pleomorphic cells with scant cytoplasm resulting from an increased nuclear to cytoplasmic ratio. No polarity remains, and the cells possess both macronucleoli and irregular chromatin centers. These cells were seen interspersed with classic epithelial clusters of villous adenoma (see Figs. 7–42A and 7–42B) (brushing cytology, Papanicolaou stain, × 225).

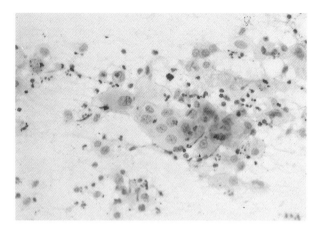

FIGURE 7–47. Mucoepidermoid Carcinoma (Oral Cavity). There are two cell types present: a well-differentiated keratinizing squamous cell carcinoma that may show "pearl" formations and an adenocarcinoma component. The cells of the adenocarcinoma component have granular or vesicular chromatin and moderate to abundant vacuolated or clear cytoplasm. The smear is cellular, with both single cells and clustered cells. Mucoepidermoid carcinoma always has a well-differentiated squamous cell component. In contrast, adenosquamous cell carcinoma always has a poorly differentiated squamous cell component (brushing cytology, Papanicolaou stain, × 225).

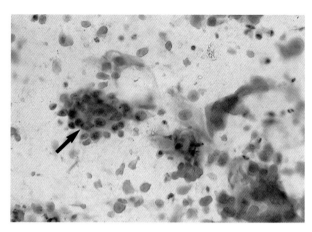

FIGURE 7–49. Adenosquamous Cell Carcinoma (Stomach). The two components seen here are both poorly differentiated, with prominent pleomorphism, hyperchromasia, and anaplasia. The squamous differentiation can be seen as polygonal cells with orangeophilic keratinizing cytoplasm and scattered, degenerating individual cells. The glandular components (arrow) consist of a cell cluster or "ball" with a high nuclear to cytoplasmic ratio and dense, granular chromatin. A mucicarmine stain demonstrated focal mucin production in cell clusters (touch preparation, Papanicolaou stain, × 225).

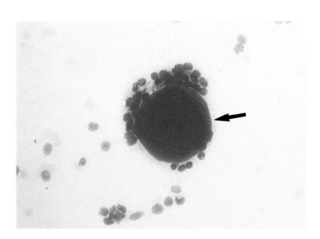

FIGURE 7–48. Adenoid Cystic Carcinoma (Salivary Gland). As seen in this Diff-Quik stain, the amorphous hyaline material is bright purple (arrow) and is within an acinar formation. The associated epithelial cells are seen as sheets or spherules, with bland and regular nuclei (fine needle aspiration, Diff-Quik stain, × 225).

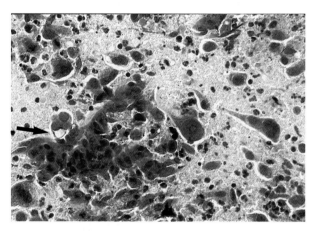

FIGURE 7–50. Squamous Cell Carcinoma (Stomach). In this air-dried Giemsa smear there are numerous clustered and single cells with "dirty," necrotic backgrounds. The cells are pleomorphic in size and shape, with some multinucleated and polygonal cells that have pulled out cytoplasm. Degenerative vacuoles are seen (arrow) and should not lead to the erroneous diagnosis of adenocarcinoma. Macronucleoli may be seen, which is a feature more typical of adenocarcinomas. Occasionally, in such cases, a mucin stain may help to distinguish an adenocarcinoma, and cell block material may be helpful in visualizing intercellular bridging or polygonal shapes of squamous cell differentiation. Occasionally, only a diagnosis of carcinoma can be made with certainty (salvage cytology, Giemsa stain, × 225).

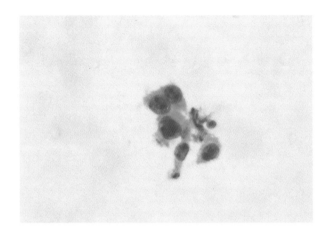

FIGURE 7–51. Adenocarcinoma in Situ (Stomach). There is a small group of epithelial cells with high nuclear to cytoplasmic ratios, irregular chromatin, and prominent, irregular nucleoli. In contrast to invasive adenocarcinoma, the background is clean and lacks the necrotic and inflammatory background. This finding is suggestive but not diagnostic of adenocarcinoma in situ. The cells differ from atypia of repair by the irregularity of the nuclear rim and irregularity of the prominent nucleoli (salvage cytologic specimen, Papanicolaou stain, × 400).

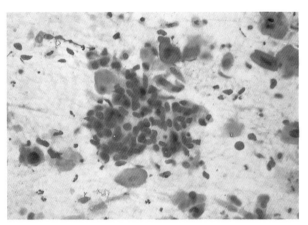

FIGURE 7–53A. Adenocarcinoma Arising in Barrett Esophagus (Esophagus). A central aggregate of columnar cells with high nuclear to cytoplasmic ratios, nuclear irregularity, and disorganization is present amid a necrotic background containing superficial squamous cells. This specimen was taken from the midesophagus and represents an adenocarcinoma arising in a Barrett esophagus. The patient had a microinvasive, well-differentiated adenocarcinoma (salvage cytology, Papanicolaou stain, × 225).

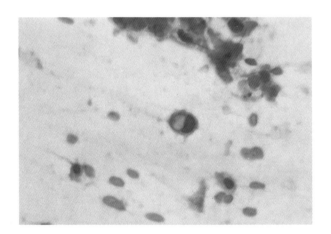

FIGURE 7–52. Signet Ring Adenocarcinoma in Situ (Stomach). Single cells and naked nuclei are seen. The cells have an eccentric, enlarged nucleus with intracytoplasmic mucin vacuoles. The nuclear morphology is the same as that of an invasive signet ring carcinoma. In situ signet ring carcinoma lacks the necrotic and inflammatory background of its invasive counterpart. No aggregates are noted, and the cells may be missed when few in number (salvage cytology, Papanicolaou stain, × 400).

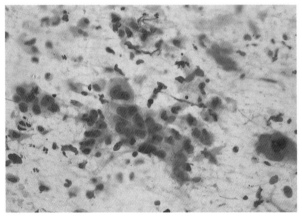

FIGURE 7–53B. Adenocarcinoma Arising in Barrett Esophagus (Esophagus). A loosely cohesive sheet of cells that have large pleomorphic nuclei with prominent nucleoli is seen amid necrotic debris. Single cells were numerous, whereas superficial squamous cells were scarce. This patient had an invasive, poorly differentiated adenocarcinoma arising in a Barrett esophagus. The specimen was taken in the midesophagus of a known Barrett esophagus patient (salvage cytology, Papanicolaou stain, × 225).

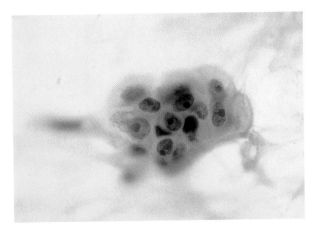

FIGURE 7–54A. Mucinous Adenocarcinoma (Colon). The background of the smear is hazy, with strands of blue representing mucin. The cell cluster is composed of pleomorphic cells with large, irregular nuclei and prominent nucleoli. Abundant foamy, vacuolated cytoplasm is present. This variant of adenocarcinoma may also have smaller cuboidal cells in small pseudoglandular aggregates (salvage cytology, Papanicolaou stain, × 400).

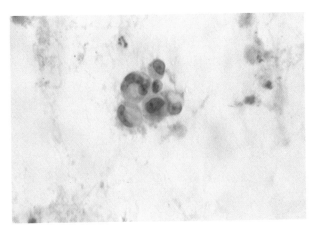

FIGURE 7–55A. Adenocarcinoma, Gastric Type (Stomach). A cell cluster of large cells with an increased nuclear to cytoplasmic ratio is seen. Single cells in such cases are more frequent than cell clusters or groups. The nuclei are eccentric, with cytoplasmic mucin vacuoles. Signet ring carcinoma is a poorly differentiated adenocarcinoma, gastric type, when found in the stomach (salvage cytology, Papanicolaou stain, × 400).

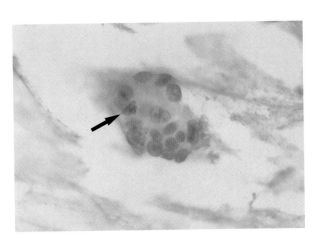

FIGURE 7–54B. Mucinous Adenocarcinoma (Colon). The cell cluster shows nuclear pleomorphism and crowding, with irregular nuclear rims and multiple chromatin centers. Focally, intracytoplasmic mucin (arrow) is identified on this mucicarmine stain as a bright pink-red. The background shows wispy, thin strands of pink material and represents the mucinous background seen in Figure 7–54A (salvage cytology, mucicarmine stain, × 400).

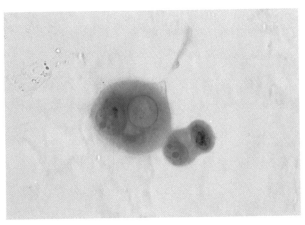

FIGURE 7–55B. Adenocarcinoma, Gastric Type (Stomach). The cell cluster demonstrates pleomorphism of size and shape and dense chromatin with multiple nucleoli. The small cells have scant granular cytoplasm. The large central cell has granular cyanophilic cytoplasm and a cytoplasmic vacuole (arrow) representing mucin production (salvage cytology, Papanicolaou stain, × 1000).

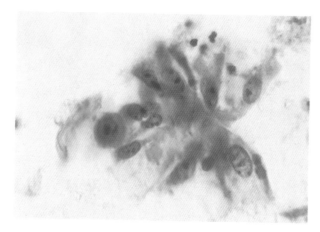

FIGURE 7–56A. Adenocarcinoma, Intestinal Type (Stomach). A cluster of columnar cells with elongated cytoplasm and ovoid basally oriented nuclei is seen. There is nuclear crowding, and prominent, irregular nucleoli are present. Single cells are present but the majority of the cells are shed as clusters. The gastric type of adenocarcinoma is more pleomorphic, with many single cells (salvage cytology, Papanicolaou stain, × 630).

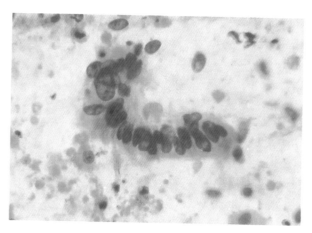

FIGURE 7–57. Adenocarcinoma Arising in Inflammatory Bowel Disease (Colon). A large strip of epithelium is seen, with a background of necrotic and inflammatory debris. Nuclear pleomorphism, irregular, dense chromatin, and nuclear crowding are present. Reactive atypia would be more uniform in size and would retain thin, regular nuclear shapes (salvage cytology, Papanicolaou stain, × 400).

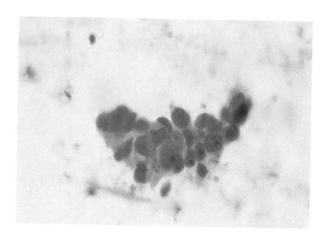

FIGURE 7–56B. Adenocarcinoma, Intestinal Type (Stomach). A large cellular group is seen, with enlarged, crowded hyperchromatic nuclei with molding. In this poorly differentiated adenocarcinoma of the intestinal type, the columnar nature of the cells is less evident, but suggested. Clustered cells predominate in this case, with only scattered single cells (brushing cytology, Papanicolaou stain, × 400).

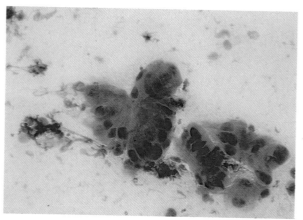

FIGURE 7–58. Adenocarcinoma Arising in an Adenomatous Polyp (Colon). In this air-dried Diff-Quik–stained smear, several clusters of glandular epithelial cells are present amid a "dirty" or inflamed background. Unlike benign epithelial cells, the cells are pleomorphic, with disorderly, large, irregular nuclei. An attempt at glandular formation is evident. The cells present cannot be distinguished from adenocarcinomas, in which remaining adenomatous polyp is not evident. If numerous benign clusters with the features described in Figure 7–41 are intermixed with the carcinoma, then adenocarcinoma arising in an adenomatous polyp can be suggested (brushing cytology, Giemsa stain, × 225).

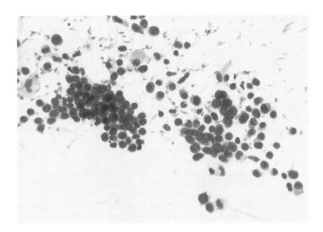

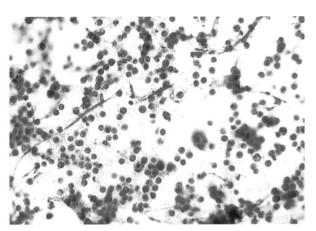

FIGURE 7–59A. Carcinoid (Rectum). Aggregates of cohesive and noncohesive cells are present that are fairly uniform in size and shape with round nuclei, some of which contain distinct, small nucleoli. The cells lack the pleomorphism of size and shape of adenocarcinomas. In cases in which an adenocarcinoma is mixed with carcinoid, a two-cell population is seen (salvage cytology, Papanicolaou stain, × 225).

FIGURE 7–60A. Lymphoma (Stomach). In this air-dried Diff-Quik stain, a diffuse, monomorphic population of cells is observed. The cells are predominantly single or in loose clusters. At this power, it is evident that the cells are three to four times larger than mature lymphocytes. The differential in such a case may include pseudolymphoma or carcinoid tumor. Carcinoid tumor occurs in nests and clusters, with few single cells. It has more cytoplasm, and the nuclear chromatin is diffuse and finely granular, not coarse as in lymphoma or clumped as in carcinoma. Pseudolymphoma has a polymorphic population of lymphocytes with numerous intermixed, small, mature lymphocytes and plasma cells (salvage cytology, Diff-Quik, × 225).

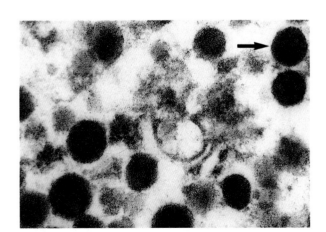

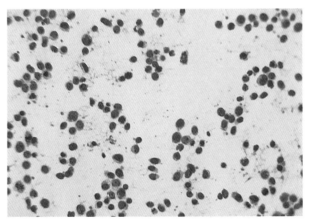

FIGURE 7–59B. Electron Microscopy of Carcinoid (Rectum). The tumor seen in 7–59A, ultrastructurally, is found to contain round, membrane-bound, electron-densed structures (arrow) in the cytoplasm. These structures represent the neurosecretory granules of carcinoid tumors (glutaraldehyde-fixed salvage cytology material, uranyl acetate/lead citrate, transmission electron micrograph, × 7100).

FIGURE 7–60B. Lymphoma (Stomach). A Papanicolaou-stained smear of a large-cell lymphoma, B-cell type, demonstrates the characteristic large cells with scant cytoplasm that are predominantly shed as single cells. In the better-preserved cells, the chromatin is granular and a prominent nucleolus can be seen. Some melanomas may shed large single cells with scant cytoplasm. They usually differ from lymphomas in that their nuclei have clumped chromatin and distinct macronucleoli (salvage cytology, Papanicolaou stain, × 225).

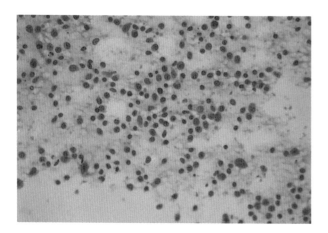 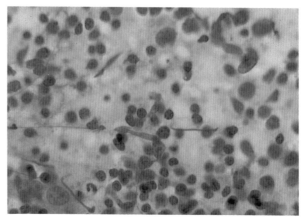

FIGURES 7–61A and 7–61B. Pseudolymphoma (Stomach). A large collection of lymphoid cells and debris is present. The population is a mixture of cells of different sizes with scant cytoplasm. There is no uniformity of cell type, as seen in lymphoma (salvage cytology, Papanicolaou stain, × 225 and × 400).

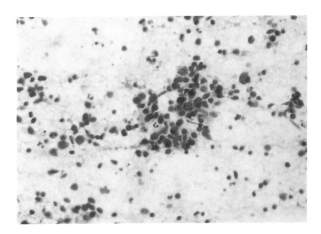

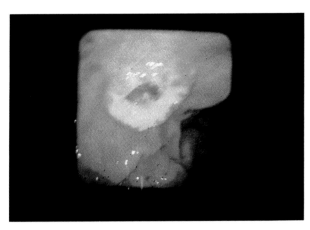

FIGURE 7–62A. Metastatic Small-Cell Carcinoma (Stomach). The smear demonstrates clusters and loosely cohesive sheets of cells with irregular nuclei and scant cytoplasm. The cells are "molding" in relation to one another, and the background is inflammatory, with scattered necrotic debris. Unlike in lymphoma, the majority of cells are clusters, although single cells are also seen. The cells differ from those of carcinoid tumor in that carcinoid tumor lacks the characteristic "molding" of nuclei seen here, cells from carcinoid tumors have more cytoplasm, and may have gland-like patterns (salvage cytology, Papanicolaou stain, × 400).

FIGURE 7–63. Endoscopic Appearance of a "Volcano-like" Lesion of Metastatic Neoplasm to the Gastrointestinal Tract (Stomach). On the lesser curvature, a "volcano-like" lesion is evident. The nodular mass has raised edges, and a central "ulcerated" depression is observed. This appearance is characteristic of metastatic lesions, which arise in the submucosa secondary to vascular access. The mucosa is preserved at the edges overlying the tumor, but because of lack of vascularity, ulceration occurs in the center. Often these lesions are multiple and produce "bull's eye" lesions on radiography with contrast. Although lymphomas also arise submucosally, they are irregular, usually larger, and lack the "volcano-like" appearance (view on upper gastrointestinal endoscopy).

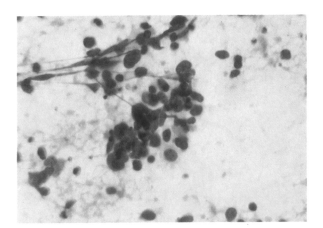

FIGURE 7–62B. Metastatic Small-Cell Carcinoma (Stomach). The nuclei present are three to five times the size of those of a mature lymphocyte. The cytoplasm is scant, and molding is evident. The fragility of the nuclei results in focal "blue" streaks or "crushed" aggregates. In the well-preserved cells, distinct irregular nucleoli can be seen. Distinguishing a primary small-cell carcinoma from a metastatic carcinoma is impossible on cytologic or histologic specimens alone. The endoscopic appearance of the lesion and the clinical history are necessary in order to distinguish a primary from a secondary lesion (salvage cytology, Papanicolaou stain, × 630).

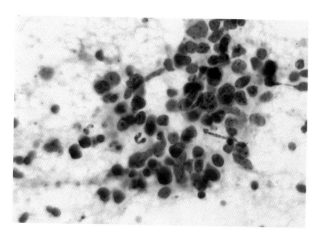

FIGURE 7–64A. Primary Small-Cell Carcinoma (Undifferentiated Carcinoma of the Stomach). The small, anaplastic cells are seen as a large, irregular cluster amid an inflammatory background. The chromatin is coarse, and nuclear molding and scant cytoplasm are present. As in the metastatic small-cell carcinoma, the differential diagnosis would include large-cell lymphoma and carcinoid tumor. Some authors suggest that the presence of nucleoli implies that the malignancy is primary in the gastrointestinal tract. In reality, the presence of nucleoli usually only signals that the cells are better preserved and that nucleoli may be seen in either primary or metastatic small-cell carcinoma. Pleomorphism may be present. The size of cells in extrapulmonary small-cell carcinoma is 10 to 60 μ although the majority range from 10 to 20 μ (brushing cytology, Papanicolaou stain, × 630).

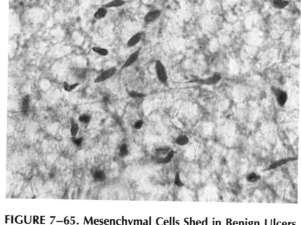

FIGURE 7–65. Mesenchymal Cells Shed in Benign Ulcers (Stomach). Bland, uniform, elliptical cells with elongated, scant cytoplasm are seen against a necrotic background. These cells are seldom shed from the base of gastric ulcers but when seen may be misinterpreted as cells from a spindle cell neoplasm. The cells are few in number and have evenly dispersed nuclear chromatin. In contrast, sarcomas would be more cellular and would demonstrate pleomorphism with irregular nuclear shapes and sizes (salvage cytology, Papanicolaou stain, × 400).

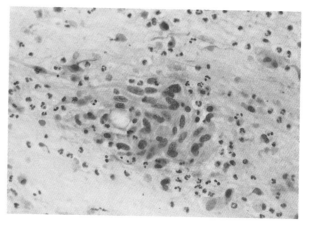

FIGURE 7–66. Leiomyoma (Small Intestine). A cluster of spindle cells with elliptical, "blunt-ended" nuclei is seen forming a "whorled" pattern. The background is inflammatory secondary to ulceration of the mucosa overlying this leiomyoma. The cells have characteristic cigar-shaped nuclei, which are uniform in shape and size with evenly dispersed chromatin. The cells are similar to normal smooth muscle cells. The presence of large numbers of such cells in the clinical setting of a submucosal mass suggests the diagnosis of leiomyoma. The presence of numerous nucleoli or mitotic figures suggests the possibility of leiomyosarcoma because leiomyomas should not have mitotic activity (salvage cytology, Papanicolaou stain, × 225).

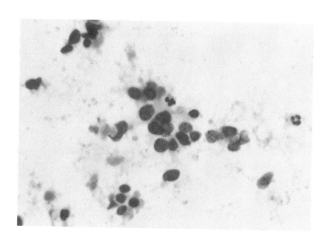

FIGURE 7–64B. Primary Small-Cell Carcinoma (Esophagus). A cluster of irregularly shaped nuclei surrounded by scant to absent cytoplasm is present in the center and is surrounded by single cells and bare nuclei. Primary small-cell carcinoma, like its metastatic counterpart, is fragile. Cytoplasm may be stripped, and nuclei may be "pulled out" or crushed. "Molding" of the nuclei is the most consistent feature (brushing cytology, Papanicolaou stain, × 630).

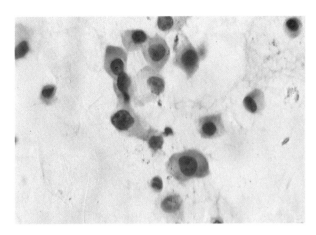

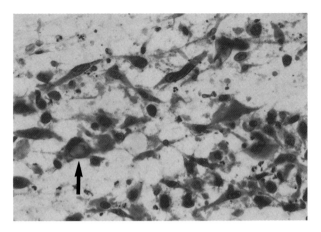

FIGURE 7–67. Leiomyoblastoma (Stomach). The cells seen are round to polygonal, with a moderate amount of cyanophilic cytoplasm. The irregular, coarse nuclei are centrally located. Single cells predominate, as seen here, but small clusters may occur. Neither multinucleated forms nor mitotic figures are as prominent as in leiomyosarcomas. Carcinomas are more cohesive, with more abundant vacuolated cytoplasm, and have prominent nucleoli. Melanomas may be difficult to distinguish from leiomyoblastomas but melanomas show more pleomorphism and may demonstrate macronucleoli (brushing cytology, Papanicolaou stain, × 400).

FIGURE 7–68B. Pleomorphic Leiomyosarcoma (Cecum). The smear is very cellular, with large or "gigantic" pleomorphic cells with "pulled-out" cytoplasm and triangular shapes. The nuclei are bizarre, with abnormal shapes, hyperchromasia, and irregular nucleoli. One cell (arrow) has a clearing in the cytoplasm, mimicking an adenocarcinoma cell. This vacuolization represents only degenerative change. The differential includes those entities described in 7–68A. In sarcomas, transition from benign epithelium to tumor cells is not observed, but instead, there is a two-cell population of benign mucosal epithelium and pleomorphic malignant cells. The vacuolization observed in pleomorphic leiomyosarcoma results in a vacuole with granular material, not the empty space with the central dense material that is sometimes observed in mucin vacuoles of adenocarcinoma (fine needle aspiration, Papanicolaou stain, × 220).

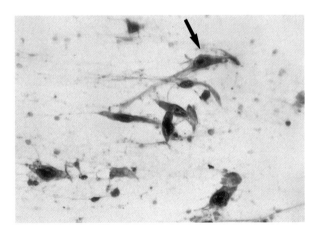

FIGURE 7–68A. Leiomyosarcoma (Small Intestine). Single, elongated spindle cells with a high nuclear to cytoplasmic ratio and clumped chromatin. Prominent nucleoli are evident (arrow). Sarcomatoid carcinomas may mimic mesenchymal lesions but may still show areas of aggregation focally. Differential diagnoses include synovial sarcoma, liposarcoma, fibrosarcoma, and malignant fibrous histiocytoma. In many instances, cell block material, immunoperoxidase stains, and electron microscopy would be necessary to arrive at a diagnosis other than that of sarcoma (fine needle aspiration, Papanicolaou stain, × 400).

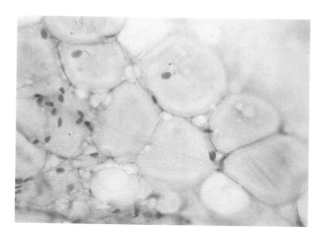

FIGURE 7–69. Lipoma (Large Bowel). The fat cells are seen as a small cluster of cells with small, delicate, oval nuclei eccentrically placed as a result of a large intracytoplasmic fat vacuole. The presence of such cell groups suggests the diagnosis of lipoma, since fat should not otherwise be seen on endoscopic cytology specimens (salvage cytology, Papanicolaou stain, × 225).

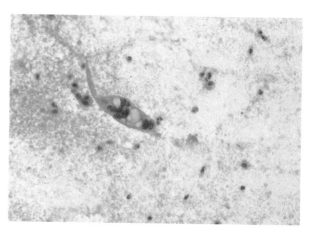

FIGURE 7–71. Sarcomatoid Carcinoma (Stomach). The cell in the center is greatly enlarged and multinucleated, with abundant "pulled-out" cytoplasm containing intracytoplasmic vacuoles. These vacuoles represent mucin production. Most carcinomas contain classic cellular groups as well as single bizarre cells. If only large, spindled bizarre cells are present, a sarcoma must be considered in the differential. In some difficult cases, immunoperoxidase stains for epithelial and mesenchymal antigens or electron microscopy or both are necessary to arrive at a correct diagnosis (salvage cytology, Papanicolaou stain, × 225).

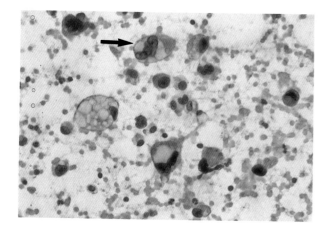

FIGURE 7–70. Liposarcoma (Colon). Single, bizarre, pleomorphic cells are seen amid a bloody background. Characteristic lipoblasts are present (arrows) and contain single and multiple lipid vacuoles. The nucleus is distorted or scalloped by the expanding lipid droplets and may or may not have convolutions (touch preparation, hematoxylin and eosin stain, × 225).

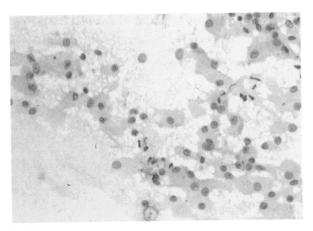

FIGURE 7–72A. Granular Cell Tumor (Esophagus). A uniform population of loosely adhesive cells with abundant granular cytoplasm is seen. The nuclei are round and bland in appearance, and the nuclear to cytoplasmic ratio is increased in comparison with that of epithelial cells. The differential might include leiomyoblastoma, which has less cytoplasm. If the cells are few in number, they may be mistakenly dismissed as histiocytes (fine needle aspiration, Papanicolaou stain, × 225).

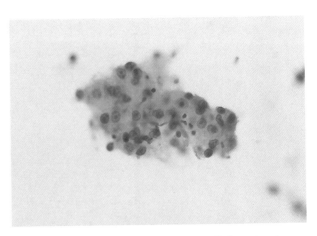

FIGURE 7–73. Metastatic Hepatocellular Carcinoma (Stomach). A central, cohesive cluster of large cells with abundant granular cytoplasm and prominent nuclei with macronuclei are seen. The hepatic origin of the cells can be confirmed by the identification of intracytoplasmic bile or alphafetoprotein by special stains or immunoperoxidase stains. Adenocarcinomas do not usually have such abundant cytoplasm or macronucleoli. The differential diagnosis would include hepatoid adenocarcinoma, which contains both hepatocellular carcinoma and adenocarcinoma. In such a case, two-cell populations (hepatoma and adenocarcinoma) would be observed. This metastatic hepatoma would endoscopically have the appearance of that seen in Figure 7–63 (salvage cytology, Papanicolaou stain, × 225).

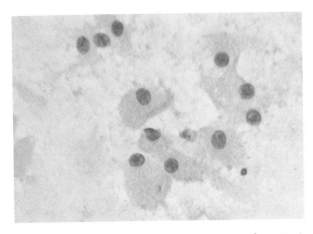

FIGURE 7–72B. Granular Cell Tumor (Esophagus). A higher power view of the case in Figure 7–72A demonstrates the uniform sheet of cells with abundant granular cytoplasm and slightly eccentric nuclei. Ultrastructurally, the granularity is a result of abundant lysozymes in the cytoplasm (fine needle aspiration, Papanicolaou stain, × 400).

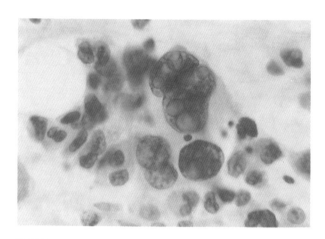

FIGURE 7–74. Metastatic Adenocarcinoma of the Lung (Stomach). A sheet of loosely cohesive bizarre cells demonstrating nuclear pleomorphism is seen. The case shown here is an adenocarcinoma; it is impossible on solely cytologic grounds to make this distinction. Clinical history and endoscopic appearance (Fig. 7–63) are the most important factors in arriving at an accurate diagnosis of metastatic carcinoma (salvage cytology, Papanicolaou stain, × 400).

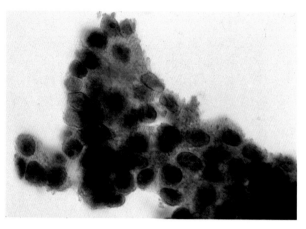

FIGURE 7–75B. Metastatic Adenocarcinoma of the Prostate (Duodenum). A prostate-specific antigen immunoperoxidase stain (PSA) of a smear from the case seen in Figure 7–75A demonstrates prominent positive staining of the cytoplasm, seen as the red-brown areas. This confirms the diagnosis of metastatic prostate carcinoma; PSA positive material would not be seen in a primary adenocarcinoma of the gastrointestinal tract (salvage cytology, PSA stain, × 400).

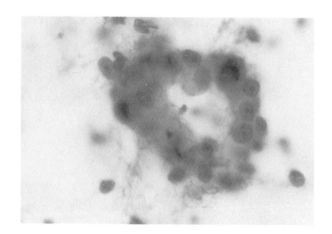

FIGURE 7–75A. Metastatic Adenocarcinoma of the Prostate (Duodenum). A glandular arrangement of cells with prominent, round nuclei and distinct, prominent macronucleoli is seen. Mucin production is absent. In the same smear, large acinar or cribriform cell clusters are evident. The large macronuclei in cells with fairly uniformly sized nuclei should alert the cytologist to the possibility of metastatic prostate carcinoma. The endoscopic appearance of the lesion or lesions would be that seen on Figure 7–63 (salvage cytology, Papanicolaou stain, × 400).

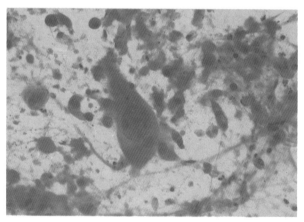

FIGURE 7–76. Squamous Cell Carcinoma with Radiation Cytopathic Effect (Esophagus). Numerous single and loosely clustered cells are seen amid a necrotic background. The central cell's nucleus and cytoplasm are greatly increased in size as compared with those of the adjacent cells. The chromatin is granular but open, and an irregular nucleolus is evident. The malignant features remain. The effects of the radiotherapy include focal size increase of both the nucleus and cytoplasm and more open, granular chromatin (salvage cytology, Papanicolaou stain, × 225).

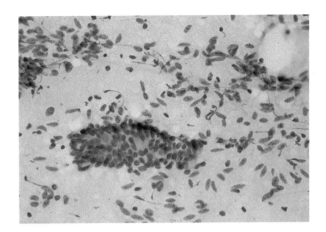

FIGURE 7–77A. Gangliocytic Paraganglioma (Duodenum). The cellular specimen consists of a mixture of single or loosely aggregated uniform spindle cells and large sheets of uniform cells resembling carcinoid tumor. The aggregates have pink fibrillary material in the gland-like spaces (touch preparation, Papanicolaou stain, × 225).

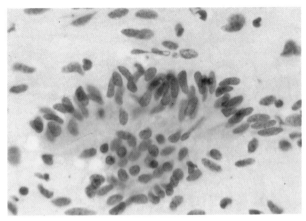

FIGURE 7–77B. Gangliocytic Paraganglioma (Duodenum). A cluster of cells with elliptical, bland nuclei is seen amid a background of single cells with scant cytoplasm. The nuclei are palisading, with a pattern similar to that of Verocay bodies of neurilemomas. These cells stain for neurosecretory granules, and neural and carcinoid-like features are seen ultrastructurally. Differential diagnosis would include carcinoid tumor and neurilemoma. This lesion is submucosal but may ulcerate and shed cells (touch preparation, Papanicolaou stain, × 400).

C·H·A·P·T·E·R

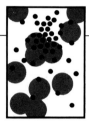

8

FINE NEEDLE ASPIRATION OF THE LIVER AND PANCREAS

Barbara S. Ducatman

LIVER

Aspiration of the liver and pancreas is usually guided by imaging techniques. At present, computed tomography (CT) is probably the most widely used modality to guide needle placement; ultrasound may also be utilized. Magnetic resonance imaging (MRI) has also been adapted for aspiration with special plastic needles. On rare occasions, large hepatic lesions may be aspirated by palpation alone.

The presence of a pathologist in the radiology suite is helpful. Although most experienced radiologists are skilled at needle placement, the percentage of successful aspirations increases when a judgment as to specimen adequacy can be rendered immediately. Other important information can also be obtained and synthesized. Aspirates should start with a smaller gauge needle; if few cells are aspirated, a larger needle is employed. Larger gauge needles (18 and 20 gauge) should not be used for the first pass because they may cause continued bleeding, dilution of the cellular sample, and interference with subsequent attempts. When present, the pathologist can also comment on the radiologist's techniques. Such feedback is especially helpful with inexperienced personnel. A final advantage is the ability of the pathologist to effectively triage cellular material, a precious resource. On many occasions, a previously unsuspected disease is diagnosed. In these cases, the sample is split to give material for adjunct procedures such as electron microscopy, flow cytometry, estrogen receptors, cell surface markers, and cultures. This may spare the patient a second invasive (and expensive) procedure to collect diagnostic material for studies not performed on the first aspiration.

A variety of stains may be used for immediate cytologic diagnosis. At Beth Israel Hospital, a portable cart with two staining setups (an interchangeable toluidine blue–eosin and hematoxylin-eosin tray and a Diff-Quik setup) is taken to radiology. Material is expressed onto glass slides, and the needle is rinsed in 50% ethanol, Sacomanno fixative, or a balanced electrolyte solution for cytospin slides. One or two air-dried smears are stained with Diff-Quik, and one or two alcohol-fixed smears are stained with either toluidine blue–eosin or hematoxylin-eosin. Immunocytochemical markers can be performed reliably on the cytospin material. A second or third pass can be made to collect additional material for adjunct technologies. In general, a single smear is made to check adequacy before preparing the sample for adjunct techniques.

The major drawback is the time required for this approach. An immediate interpretation takes from 10 minutes for an uncomplicated positive case (which does not need special studies) to 90 minutes when multiple passes are inadequate and/or special studies are deemed necessary. However, the referring clinician, radiologist, and cytopathologist render optimal patient care when they work together as a team.

Aspiration cytology of the liver is used to diagnose specific benign and malignant diseases. Since a partial hepatectomy is undertaken in only select cases, a cytology diagnosis is rarely confirmed by subsequent histology. Follow-up information may be available only after a postmortem examination. Therefore, special studies to confirm the diagnosis or to determine the site of primary tumor are more commonly done on cytologic material obtained from the liver in contrast with those sites easier to biopsy surgically. In addition, a pathologist often feels more pressure to render a definite diagnosis when this is the only sample that is obtained.

Major Disease of the Liver

Benign Conditions

Normal hepatocytes may be seen in an unsuccessful aspirate, as background for another pathologic process, and in the absence of disease. They are polygonal cells with abundant granular cytoplasm and central nuclei (Fig. 8–1). Benign liver cells are seen as small or large clusters and single cells. Pigment is often plentiful—this may represent bile, hemosiderin, or lipofuscin (Fig. 8–2). Nuclei are round or oval with granular chromatin and small but prominent nucleoli. Intracytoplasmic nuclear inclusions are sometimes noted.

Occasionally, aspirates from the liver contain bile ducts, which present as tight clusters or sheets of cells having either a mosaic or palisade arrangement. Cell borders are distinct; nuclei are round to oval with finely granular chromatin and inconspicuous nucleoli. Small blood vessels and spindle-shaped endothelial cells may also be observed either singly or in small clusters. Kupffer cells may be noted as single cells, often with kidney-bean shaped nuclei, and phagocytized material. Vacuolated cells may be aspirated from a liver with fatty changes, which might be confused with the mucin vacuoles of an adenocarcinoma (Fig. 8–3).

Infectious Conditions

The differential diagnosis of all multiple and single lesions of the liver includes infectious conditions. A hepatic abscess yields a cellular aspirate with many single cells, predominantly polymorphonuclear leukocytes. Rare degenerating or benign hepatocytes may also be observed. A hepatic abscess must be differentiated from carcinoma with cystic or necrotic degeneration. The presence of benign hepatocytes is a useful feature.

Granulomatous disease is also an increasing problem that usually presents with a characteristic picture. Granulomas are three-dimensional aggregates of histiocytes (both mono- and multinucleated), lymphocytes, and plasma cells (Fig. 8–4). Although special stains for organisms may be necessary, fungi can often be seen on standard cytologic preparations. *Mycobacterium avium-intracellulare* often gives histiocytes a finely vacuolated cytoplasm with ''negative images'' highly suggestive of the organism (Fig. 8–5). Acid-fast stains confirm the diagnosis (Fig. 8–6). Sarcoidosis is an entity to consider when no organisms are identified.

Hydatid cysts are usually not aspirated, since any leakage of contents may give rise to anaphylactic shock. Aspiration yields characteristic hooklets (Fig. 8–5); occasionally, entire scolices are also found. Other parasitic diseases that may present as a liver mass are amebiasis *(Entamoeba histolytica)* and schistosomiasis *(Schistosoma mansoni).*

Cirrhosis and Reactive Conditions

Unfortunately for cytopathologists, the liver responds to a variety of insults with hepatocellular unrest. The diagnosis of cirrhosis rests on the histologic picture of regenerative nodules. Reactive changes present the same cytologic picture, whether from cirrhosis, adjacent metastatic disease, viral hepatitis, chemotherapy, or other metabolic injuries (Fig. 8–7). Reactive hepatocytes often exist in a continuum ranging from unequivocally benign to very atypical cells (Fig. 8–8) and may be easily confused with low-grade hepatocellular carcinoma (Table 8–1). The cells are single and in dyshesive sheets and clusters. The polygonal cells contain central nuclei. Nuclear pleomorphism may be striking, and binucleated cells may be seen. The chromatin pattern may be coarsely granular and irregular with intranuclear inclusions and prominent nucleoli (Fig. 8–9). Bile pigment may be present within the hepatocytes; cells of bile ductal epithelium are also more commonly noted in aspirates of cirrhosis than from a normal liver (Fig. 8–10).

Malignant Neoplasms of the Liver

Hepatocellular carcinoma is often a diagnostic problem. Well-differentiated hepatocellular carcinoma is often quite difficult to distinguish from cirrhosis and other reactive conditions. The cells have abundant polygonal granular cytoplasm, which may contain bile. The trabeculae, clusters, and sheets of hepatocytes are characteristically surrounded by endothelial cells and separated by sinusoidal capillaries (Figs. 8–11 and 8–12). Nuclear spacing is irregular; nuclei are central with an increased nuclear to cytoplasmic ratio. Prominent macronucleoli are seen (Fig. 8–13). Multinucleated tumor cells are also a useful feature (Fig. 8–14).

In contrast, poorly differentiated hepatocellular carcinoma is difficult to distinguish from metastatic carcinoma (Table 8–2). In such instances, sinusoidal capillaries, bile within tumor cells, and the endothelial cells surrounding tumor cells are helpful since they indicate hepatocellular carcinoma. Many naked nuclei and intranuclear cytoplasmic inclusions are also seen. Nuclei are central and round with macronucleoli. Immunocytochemical stains for alphafetoprotein (AFP) can also be of use in confirming the diagnosis, as can serum AFP.

Cholangiocarcinoma

Well-differentiated cholangiocarcinoma may closely resemble normal bile duct epithelium. There are loosely cohesive sheets of cells and some single cells (Fig. 8–15). However, the cellularity of the specimen is increased, principally the bile duct type component with only rare hepatocytes. Although nuclear enlargement and pleomorphism are not prominent findings, there is nuclear crowding (Fig. 8–16). Poorly differentiated cholangiocarcinoma cannot be reliably distinguished from tumors arising in extrahepatic bile ducts or from metastatic carcinoma (Fig. 8–17 and Table 8–2). As with hepatocellular carcinoma, positive staining for AFP may be a useful feature in reaching the diagnosis. Mixed hepatocellular and cholangiocarcinoma can be seen, in which both elements are present.

Metastatic Carcinoma

The liver often contains metastases that may arise from many primary sites, including adenocarcinoma of gastrointestinal (colon, stomach, or pancreas), breast, or pulmonary origin. The cytologic picture is classic for adenocarcinoma with clusters and balls of cells with nuclear pleomorphism and irregularity. Cytoplasmic vacuoles may be seen. Nuclei are commonly eccentric in position.

The pathologist is often asked to make a judgment as to the site of origin. The current cytologic material should, whenever possible, be compared to previous histologic or cytologic material and correlated with the clinical findings (Fig. 8–18). When the primary site is not known, there are a few criteria that may suggest the site of origin (Table 8–3). Colorectal carcinomas typically are "tall, dark, and necrotic." These cells have abundant cytoplasm arranged in a palisaded fashion with elongated nuclei and dense, hyperchromatic chromatin (Fig. 8–19). Nucleoli are not prominent. Breast carcinoma presents a variable picture (Fig. 8–20). One pattern that is fairly characteristic is an Indian-file arrangement of cells with signet ring features, suggesting lobular carcinoma. Estrogen-receptor (ER) positivity on immunostaining is an indirect marker that may be helpful if the primary tumor was ER-positive but is not specific for breast cancer.

A patient with a neuroendocrine tumor may present with liver metastases. Such neoplasms have eccentric nuclei with the typical "salt and pepper" chromatin pattern. The cells are present singly or in loosely cohesive clusters or rosettes (Fig. 8–21). Positive immunocytochemical staining for chromogranin may help confirm this diagnosis. Small-cell carcinoma has a typical appearance similar to that seen in the lung. There are single and tightly molded cells that have scant cytoplasm. The nuclei are hyperchromatic with coarsely granular chromatin (Fig. 8–22).

Squamous carcinoma, particularly the keratinizing variant, is easy to identify. It is not possible, however, to identify the specific site of origin. Poorly differentiated, nonkeratinizing squamous cancer may be more difficult to distinguish from a poorly differentiated adenocarcinoma or other large cell tumors.

Nonepithelial Malignancies

Lymphoma demonstrates the same typical cytologic picture that it has in other sites—a monomorphic population of atypical lymphoid cells. Spindle-cell neoplasms include sarcomatoid carcinoma and sarcoma. Immunocytochemical studies for leukocyte common antigen (LCA), keratin, epithelial membrane antigen (EMA), and vimentin may be applied (Table 8–4). If vimentin is positive, then other more specific antigens may be tried, including desmin (muscle origin) and myoglobin (skeletal muscle).

Melanoma shares three cytologic characteristics with hepatocellular carcinoma: (1) abundant granular cytoplasm with pigment, (2) macronucleoli, and (3) intranuclear cytoplasmic inclusions. In general, melanin pigment is finer than bile or hemosiderin. In addition, the cells of melanoma are often predominantly single. A battery of immunoperoxidase stains, including S-100 (positive) and HMB-45 (positive) as well as AFP (negative) and keratin (negative) may be applied, which would suggest melanoma (Table 8–4).

Other unusual tumors may also metastasize to liver, such as germ cell tumors (Fig. 8–23). Unfortunately, germ cell neoplasms may also exhibit positive staining for AFP. As with other types of metastatic disease, any previous material must be reviewed.

Use of Immunocytochemistry and Electron Microscopy

In undifferentiated malignancies, immunocytochemistry and/or electron microscopy may be used for classification of tumor, particularly in metastatic and inoperable tumors. In these instances, a surgical procedure would not be therapeutic, but a definite diagnosis is necessary for chemotherapy selection and prognosis. Therefore, when undifferentiated malignant cells are identified on immediate interpretation, material should be set aside for immunocytochemistry and electron microscopy. If adjunct techniques are not available, material should be collected for submission to a referral institution.

PANCREAS

Intraoperative Cytology

Few cytologic consultations are as stressful for the pathologist as the intraoperative aspiration of a pancreatic mass. A positive (or suspicious) diagnosis may result in an extensive resection. When malignancy is suspected, multiple needle passes should be performed until a definitive malignant diagnosis is reached or the area has been adequately sampled. As with needle aspiration of other sites, a positive diagnosis is reserved for those cases with unequivocal cytologic features of malignancy; any doubt should lead, at most, to a suspicious diagnosis. Slides for immediate diagnosis may be either air-dried for Diff-Quik staining or alcohol-fixed and stained with toluidine blue–eosin, hematoxylin–eosin, or a fast Papanicolaou stain. Only appropriately smeared, well-fixed material with adequate cellularity should be evaluated. In general, any direct smear with five to six or more groups of cells is adequate for diagnosis, provided that the cytologic detail can be evaluated.

Radiologic-Guided Procedures

As radiologic imaging of the abdomen improves, more pancreatic aspirates will be seen in the radiology suite and fewer in the operating room. Positive results lead to definitive treatment or a decision not to treat. Since patients with pancreatic carcinoma often present with advanced or inoperable disease, they may be spared an operative procedure. The techniques for aspiration of the pancreas localized by radiologic procedures are identical to those previously described for the liver.

Alternative methods for sampling biliary tract and pancreatic lesions include biliary drainage specimens and intrabiliary brush lesions obtained under fluoroscopic guidance (Fig. 8–24). The endoscopist may also sample via retrograde pancreatico-duodenoscopy brushes. The cytologic interpretation is the same as for needle aspirations, but the cellularity is much higher. In contrast to a needle aspiration, many benign sheets, clusters, and single cells are seen, which might erroneously lead to a diagnosis of well-differentiated carcinoma. Therefore, it is important to know both the type and site of the specimen.

Major Diseases of the Pancreas and Biliary Tract

Benign Conditions

Aspiration of normal pancreas tissue usually yields both acinar and ductal epithelium. Exocrine epithelial cells are present in acinar and cohesive clusters with abundant granular cytoplasm (Fig. 8–25). Nuclei are uniform, small, round, and regular with even granular chromatin and inconspicuous nucleoli. Naked nuclei are common. Ductal epithelium usually demonstrates monolayers of cells that have distinct cell borders (Fig. 8–26). Biliary tract epithelium, including the gallbladder, is also seen as monolayers of cells with round, regular nuclei (Figs. 8–27 and 8–28); occasional stones in the biliary tract may be seen on drainage or brush specimens with distinctive cholesterol crystals (Fig. 8–29).

Pancreatitis. Pancreatitis may show a variable number of inflammatory cells, both acute and chronic, interspersed with pancreatic epithelial cells. These often exhibit regenerative atypia that can be quite pronounced and may be confused with pancreatic adenocarcinoma (Fig. 8–30) (Table 8–5). Benign mesenchymal tissue from resultant fibrosis may also be a prominent component (Fig. 8–31). Foamy macrophages from the accompanying fat necrosis are noted in the background, as are mucus and debris (Figs. 8–32 and 8–33).

The cytologic appearance of an aspirate of a pancreatic pseudocyst is nonspecific and often depends on the cause. Commonly, pseudocysts developing after pancreatitis demonstrate mucinous debris, inflammatory cells, and degenerating epithelial cells (Fig. 8–34). The smear may also be acellular or have only inflammatory cells.

Malignant Diseases

Adenocarcinomas. The cytologic diagnosis of well-differentiated pancreatic adenocarcinoma is a problem. The cells are usually present in sheets similar to reactive atypia; however, nuclear crowding, nuclear pleomorphism, and cellular dyshesion are more pronounced (Figs. 8–35 and 8–36). Nuclear membranes are irregular. Single malignant cells are also noted. Although the nuclei and nucleoli of carcinoma are larger than those seen in reactive epithelium, this distinction may be difficult to appreciate. Mitotic figures may also be seen.

Poorly differentiated adenocarcinomas are usually easily diagnosed as malignant. Atypical cells are numerous and are found both singly and in dyshesive clusters. Cells have nuclear molding and crowding and may have vacuolated cytoplasm (Fig. 8–37). Nuclei are large and irregular with coarsely granular chromatin and large prominent nucleoli (Fig. 8–38). Naked nuclei may be seen. Undifferentiated pancreatic carcinoma may be quite variable in appearance and often has spindle-shaped and multinucleated cells (Figs. 8–39 and 8–40). When a tumor presents as a large, poorly defined mass on CT scan and has bizarre cytology, then sarcomatoid pancreatic carcinoma and retroperitoneal sarcoma are diagnostic considerations (Table 8–6). Careful examination of the smears of pancreatic carcinoma often show more typical cells of adenocarcinoma with mucus vacuoles (Fig. 8–41).

Neuroendocrine (Islet Cell) Tumors. An islet cell tumor is a neuroendocrine tumor and has a classic appearance as described previously. It usually has eccentric nuclei, regular and coarsely granular ("salt-and-pepper") chromatin, inconspicuous nucleoli, and abundant granular cytoplasm. Cells are usually single but may be seen in dyshesive clusters and rosettes (Figs. 8–42 and 8–43). As with other neuroendocrine tumors, immunocytochemical studies, particularly chromogranin, are useful.

Unusual Tumors of the Pancreas

Cystic mucinous neoplasms often occur in the distal portion of the pancreas and must be differentiated from pseudocysts and retention cysts. Mucinous cystadenomas show small clusters with a honeycomb appearance and single cells with abundant cytoplasm distended by mucus. Nuclei are small and regular, with a low nuclear to cytoplasmic ratio and inconspicuous nucleoli. Mucinous cystadenocarcinomas are more cellular and display clusters of cells with malignant nuclear features (Figs. 8–44A to 8–44C). Since mucinous cystadenomas have the potential to transform focally to cystadenocarcinomas, such lesions should be completely excised.

The solid and papillary epithelial neoplasm is an unusual low-grade tumor of young women. The aspirates contain papillary fronds lined by uniform cells with a fibrovascular core (Fig. 8–45A). The cytoplasm may either be dense or vacuolated, and nuclei are small and regular (Fig. 8–45B). Myxoid globules may also be interspersed among the cells.

Bibliography

Bottles K, Cohen MB, Holly EA, et al: A step-wise logistic regression analysis of hepatocellular carcinoma. An aspiration biopsy study. Cancer 62:558–563, 1988.

Koss LG, Woyke S, Olszewski W: Aspiration Biopsy. Cytologic Interpretation and Histologic Basis. New York: Igaku-Shoin, 1984, pp 350–394.

Noguchi S, Yamamoto R, Tatsuta M, et al: Cell features and patterns in fine-needle aspiration of hepatocellular carcinoma. Cancer 58:321–328, 1986.

Orell SR, Sterrett GF, Walters MN-I, Whitaker D: Manual and Atlas of Fine Needle Aspiration Cytology. New York: Churchill Livingstone, 1986, pp 146–155 and 170–181.

Table 8–1. DIFFERENTIAL DIAGNOSIS OF ATYPICAL HEPATOCYTES

	Reactive Processes Including Cirrhosis, Hepatitis, and Toxic-Metabolic and Metastatic Disease (Figs. 8–46A, 8–46C, and 8–46E)	Hepatocellular Carcinoma (Figs. 8–46B, 8–46D, and 8–46F)
CT picture	Diffuse lesion or multiple nodules	Single large lesion; occasionally multiple nodules
Cellularity	Low to high; generally moderate	High
Cellular arrangements	Dyshesive sheets and clusters, single cells, fibrous tissue	Dyshesive sheets and clusters, single cells, trabeculae, irregular nuclear spacing
Nuclear pleomorphism	Mild to moderate; occasional binucleated cells	Marked; multinucleated tumor giant cells; increased N/C ratio
Chromatin pattern	Finely to coarsely granular chromatin; micronucleoli	Coarsely granular chromatin; macronucleoli
Serum alphafetoprotein	Low	Low to high

Table 8–2. DIFFERENTIAL DIAGNOSIS OF POORLY DIFFERENTIATED CARCINOMA IN LIVER

	Hepatocellular Carcinoma (Fig. 8–47A)	Intrahepatic (Figs. 8–47B, 8–47C) and Extrahepatic (Fig. 8–47D) Cholangiocarcinoma	Metastatic Adenocarcinoma Colonic (Fig. 8–47E) and Pancreatic (Fig. 8–47F)
Cellularity	High	Moderate to high	High
Two cellular populations	No	Reactive hepatocytes are sometimes seen in addition to tumor cells	Reactive hepatocytes are sometimes seen in addition to tumor cells
Cellular arrangements	Sinusoidal capillaries; endothelial cells around dyshesive clusters and sheets of tumor cells; many single cells and naked nuclei	Dyshesive sheets, clusters, and palisades; rare single cells	Dyshesive clusters, sheets, and single cells
Bile	May be present between and within tumor cells	May be present between tumor cells	Not present in tumor cells
Nuclei	Pronounced pleomorphism; central nuclei; coarsely granular chromatin; macronucleoli; multinucleated tumor giant cells; intranuclear cytoplasmic inclusions	Eccentric; finely to coarsely granular chromatin; minimal pleomorphism	Variable; finely to coarsely granular chromatin; mild to marked pleomorphism
Special stains			
AFP	+	+/−	−
Naphthylamidase	+	+	−
Keratin—low molecular weight (CAM 5.2)	+	+	+
Keratin—high molecular weight (AE1/AE3)	− or +/− (focal, weak)	+	+

Table 8–3. DIFFERENTIAL DIAGNOSIS OF METASTATIC ADENOCARCINOMA
WITHOUT KNOWN PRIMARY TUMOR IN LIVER

	Colon (Figs. 8–48A and 8–48B)	Breast (Fig. 8–48C) and Pancreas (Fig. 8–48D)
Background	Necrotic	Usually bloody or clean
Cellular arrangements	Clusters; palisades	Variable; usually dyshesive clusters and sheets; "Indian files" suggest breast cancer
Nuclei	Elongate; dense chromatin hyperchromatic	Variable
Cytoplasm	Elongate; abundant	Variable
Other	—	Estrogen receptors suggest breast or ovary cancer; prostatic acid phosphatase or prostate specific antigen suggests prostate cancer

Table 8–4. DIFFERENTIAL DIAGNOSIS OF PREDOMINANTLY SINGLE MALIGNANT CELLS
IN LIVER AND/OR PANCREAS

	Hepatocellular Carcinoma (Fig. 8–49A)	Metastatic Melanoma (Fig. 8–49B)	Neuroendocrine Tumor (Fig. 8–49C)	Lymphoma (Fig. 8–49D)	Poorly Differentiated Adenocarcinoma or Pancreatic Adenocarcinoma (Figs. 8–49E and 8–49F)
Cellular Arrangement	Endothelial cells around dyshesive clusters; sheets; naked nuclei	Predominantly single cells; rare loose aggregates	Predominantly single cells; rare loose clusters; rosettes	Single cells; no aggregation	Single cells; dyshesive clusters and sheets with nuclear molding
Nuclei	Central; may be multinucleated; macronucleoli; pronounced pleomorphism; intranuclear cytoplasmic inclusions	Mild to marked pleomorphism; may be multinucleated; intranuclear cytoplasmic inclusions; macronucleoli	Minimal pleomorphism; eccentric nuclei; granular salt-and-pepper chromatin; inconspicuous nucleoli	Monomorphic; central nuclei; coarsely granular chromatin; nucleoli variable	Eccentric; irregular; pleomorphic; nucleoli present—often multiple
Cytoplasm	Abundant granular, polygonal; bile present	Melanin pigment; scant to abundant cytoplasm	Granular cytoplasm	Scant cytoplasm	Abundant; coarsely or finely vacuolated; granular
Immunocytochemistry					
Alphafetoprotein	+	−	−	−	−
Keratin	+	−	+	−	+
Chromogranin	−	−	+	−	−
S-100	−	+	−	−	−
HMB 45	−	+	−	−	−
Leukocyte common antigen	−	−	−	+	−

Table 8–5. DIFFERENTIAL DIAGNOSIS OF SHEETS OF ATYPICAL PANCREATIC DUCTAL CELLS

	Chronic Pancreatitis (Figs. 8–50A and 8–50C)	Well-Differentiated Pancreatic Adenocarcinoma (Figs. 8–50B and 8–50D)
Cellularity of ductal epithelial cells	Few	Numerous
Background	Inflammatory cells; debris; fat necrosis; fibrous tissue	Inflammatory cells; necrotic cells; fat necrosis
Cellular arrangements	Cohesive sheets with distinct cell boundaries	Cohesive and dyshesive sheets with nuclear crowding and overlapping; rare single epithelial cells and mitotic figures
Nuclei	Normal size; round and regular; even chromatin distribution	Larger than normal; irregular contour; pleomorphic; hyperchromatic; molded
Nucleoli	Inconspicuous	Small but prominent; sometimes multiple

Table 8–6. DIFFERENTIAL DIAGNOSIS OF SPINDLE-SHAPED CELLS FROM THE REGION OF THE PANCREAS

	Pleomorphic Carcinoma (Figs. 8–51A and 8–51C)	Retroperitoneal Sarcoma (Figs. 8–51B and 8–51D)
Cellular arrangements	Loose sheets and syncytia; clusters; single cells; nuclear molding may be visible	Loose sheets and syncytia; single cells
Cytoplasm	Spindled and round; granular; vacuolated	Spindle-shaped; granular
Nuclei	Prominent nucleoli; finely to coarsely granular chromatin; vesicular nuclei	Inconspicuous nucleoli; finely to coarsely granular chromatin
Giant cells	Common	Rare, except in malignant fibrous histiocytoma
Immunocytochemistry		
Keratin	+	−
Vimentin	+/−	+

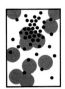

NORMAL CELLS AND BENIGN CONDITIONS, LIVER

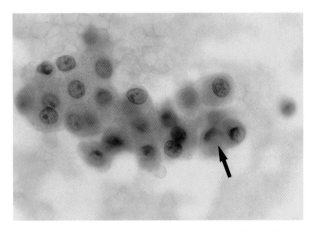

FIGURE 8–1. Benign Hepatocytes. These polygonal cells are arranged in a cohesive cluster with regular nuclear spacing. The cytoplasm is abundant and granular. Nuclei are central and round, with some variability in size and shape. Chromatin clumping is often apparent. A single cell (arrow) is pigmented (Papanicolaou stain, × 250).

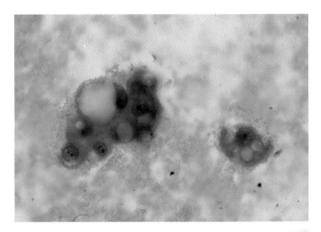

FIGURE 8–3. Benign Hepatocytes with Fatty Changes. The cells contain coarse cytoplasmic vacuoles; however, the nuclei are small, round, and regular, without any malignant features. Elsewhere in the smear, benign hepatocytes resembling those with the fat vacuoles should be seen (Papanicolaou stain, × 250). (Courtesy of Barbara F. Atkinson, M.D., Philadelphia, Pa.)

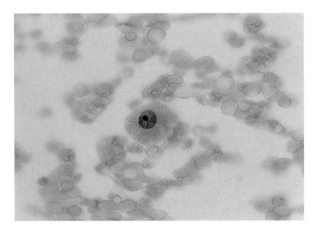

FIGURE 8–2. Benign Hepatocyte. This cell has a small, slightly eccentric nucleus and granular cytoplasm. As seen here, the nucleoli of benign hepatocytes are often quite prominent (Papanicolaou stain, × 250).

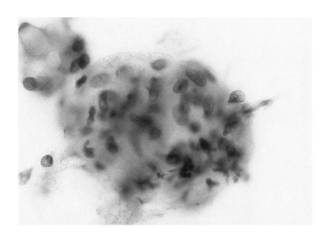

FIGURE 8–4. Hepatic Granuloma in an AIDS Patient. Note the tight cluster of epithelial-like histiocytes, which are quite spindled. There is considerable depth of focus. Such lesions may have to be differentiated from both stromal and epithelial neoplasms of the liver. The abundant cytoplasm and kidney-bean nuclei are typical of histiocytes (Papanicolaou stain, × 250).

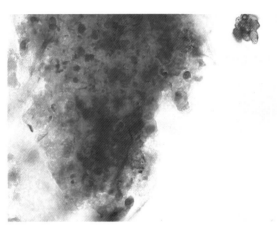

FIGURE 8–6. *Mycobacterium avium-intracellulare* **in an AIDS patient.** Acid-fast stain from the preceding case with numerous acid-fast bacilli noted (Papanicolaou stain, × 250).

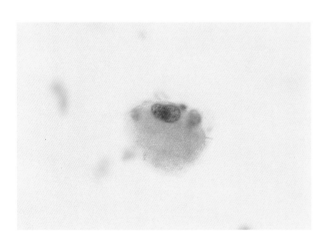

FIGURE 8–5. Single Histiocyte from Liver Aspiration of AIDS Patient Infected with *Mycobacterium avium-intracellulare.* The granular cytoplasm is filled with acid-fast bacilli which appear as negative images in the cytoplasm (Papanicolaou stain, × 250).

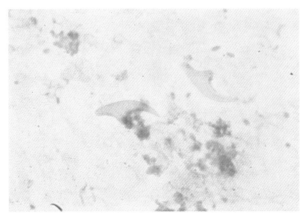

FIGURE 8–7. Echinococcal Cyst. Note the refractile hooklets in the background of cystic debris (Papanicolaou stain, × 100). (Courtesy of Edmund S. Cibas, M.D., Boston, Mass.)

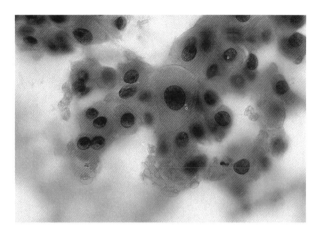

FIGURE 8–8. Atypical, Reactive Hepatocytes. These cells demonstrate marked nuclear pleomorphism. However, there is a spectrum of changes ranging from benign to atypical in contrast to those in well-differentiated hepatocellular carcinoma (Papanicolaou stain, × 250).

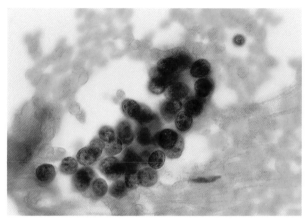

FIGURE 8–10. Bile Duct Aspirated from a Patient with Cirrhosis. Elsewhere in the smear, reactive hepatocytes were noted. Note the tight cellular cohesion of the three-dimensional duct structure with regularly spaced nuclei and lack of nuclear pleomorphism (Papanicolaou stain, × 250).

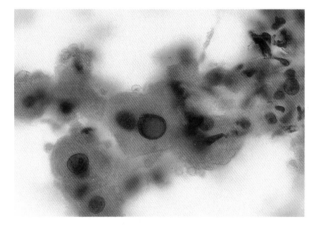

FIGURE 8–9. Reactive Hepatocytes from a Case of Cirrhosis. Note the enlarged nucleus and prominent intranuclear inclusion of the cell in the center of the field (Papanicolaou stain, × 250).

MALIGNANT TUMORS, LIVER

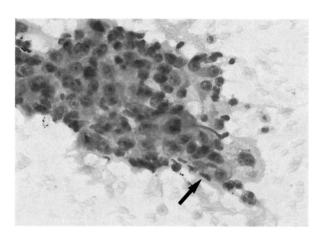

FIGURE 8–11. Hepatocellular Carcinoma. Note the irregular nuclear spacing and overlapping. There is more pronounced nuclear pleomorphism than with cirrhosis. In contrast to those in cirrhosis, all of these cells are very atypical. Endothelial cells surround the cluster (arrow) (Papanicolaou stain, × 100).

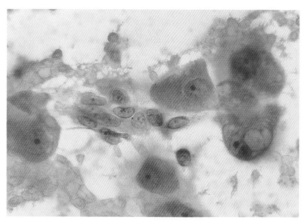

FIGURE 8–13. Fibrolamellar Hepatocellular Carcinoma. This aspiration is from a young woman with a history of a previous fibrolamellar hepatocellular carcinoma, which had been resected. The hepatocytes are atypical, with abundant oncocytic cytoplasm and enlarged vesicular pleomorphic nuclei. Benign stromal cells are also seen in the middle of the field (toluidine blue and eosin stain, × 250).

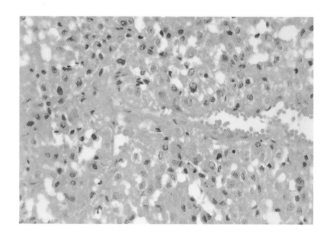

FIGURE 8–12. Hepatocellular Carcinoma (Cell Block). Note the thick trabeculae with too many layers of cells and lack of biliary tract structures (hematoxylin and eosin stain, × 25).

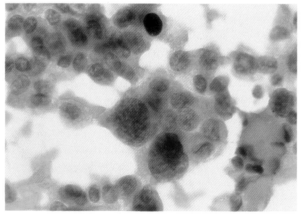

FIGURE 8–14. Poorly Differentiated Hepatocellular Carcinoma. Multinucleated tumor cells are seen. In such cases, it is difficult to recognize the hepatic origin of the tumor cells, but the scant cytoplasm is granular and reminiscent of hepatocytes. In such instances, either positive staining of tumor cells for alphafetoprotein or elevated levels of serum alphafetoprotein are very useful (Papanicolaou stain, × 250).

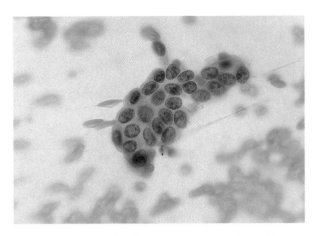

FIGURE 8–15. Well-Differentiated Cholangiocarcinoma. This case was called suspicious on aspiration, based on the cellularity of the sample, along with a mild degree of nuclear pleomorphism, atypicality, and crowding. Note the similarity of this case to benign bile ducts (see Fig. 8–10) (Papanicolaou stain, × 250).

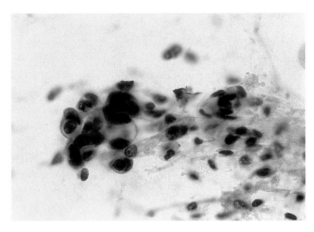

FIGURE 8–17. Cholangiocarcinoma. This specimen was obtained via a brush. It is less differentiated than the previous case. Note the irregular nuclei and the yellowish bile present within the sample (Papanicolaou stain, × 250).

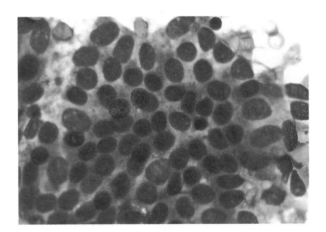

FIGURE 8–16. Well-Differentiated Cholangiocarcinoma. Sheets of bile duct-type epithelium with nuclear crowding and overlapping and a mild degree of nuclear enlargement are seen. This photograph corresponds to Figure 8–15 (Diff-Quik stain, × 250).

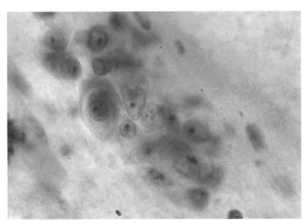

FIGURE 8–18. Metastatic Pancreatic Adenocarcinoma to the Liver. There are molded, vesicular nuclei and nucleoli. This could also be metastatic from other sites, such as the stomach or breast in a female patient. Pancreatic origin was presumed on the basis of a large mass in the pancreas (toluidine blue and eosin stain, × 250).

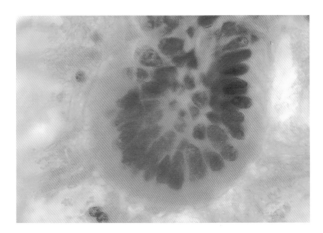

FIGURE 8–19. Metastatic Colonic Adenocarcinoma to the Liver. The specimen was very cellular, with many such groups of cells. Note the tall and columnar cells with elongated, hyperchromatic nuclei (Papanicolaou stain, × 250).

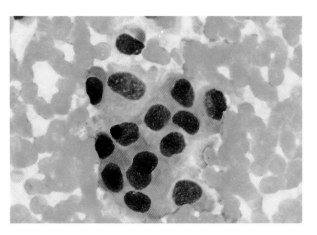

FIGURE 8–21. Metastatic Carcinoid to the Liver. Note the abundant granular cytoplasm, eccentric nuclei with coarsely granular chromatin, and lack of nucleoli (Diff-Quik stain, × 250).

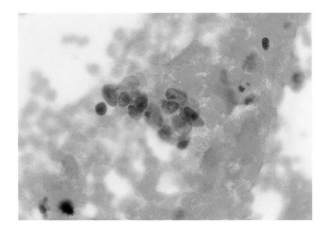

FIGURE 8–20. Metastatic Breast Carcinoma to the Liver. The cells are present in dyshesive sheets and clusters, with hyperchromatic, irregular nuclei. Although this picture is consistent with a breast primary, it cannot be differentiated from other forms of metastatic or primary adenocarcinoma with certainty unless the original slides are available for comparison.

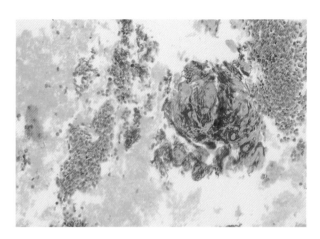

FIGURE 8–22. Cell Block of Metastatic Small-Cell Carcinoma to the Liver. There is much necrosis and crush artifact similar to that which would be seen in a bronchial biopsy. The cells are quite uniform (hematoxylin and eosin stain, × 250).

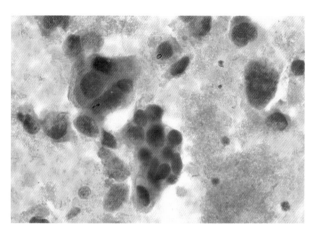

FIGURE 8–23. Metastatic Germ Cell Tumor to the Liver. This aspirate is from a 22-year-old woman with an ovarian tumor and a metastasis to the liver. These cells do resemble hepatocellular carcinoma, and they stained positively for alphafetoprotein. The tumor was determined to be metastasis from an ovarian primary based on the patient's history (Papanicolaou stain, × 250). (Courtesy of Barbara F. Atkinson, M.D., Philadelphia, Pa.)

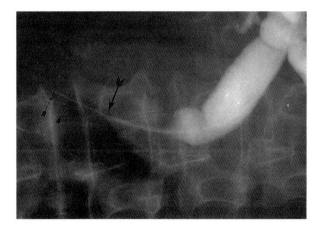

FIGURE 8–24. Radiograph Demonstrating Brush Technique. The patient has a pancreatic carcinoma with obstruction of the common duct. There is a sheath positioned in the middle of the lesion with a large arrow marking the sheath's tip. The two smaller arrows show a small ureteral biopsy brush that was used. (Courtesy of Barbara F. Atkinson, M.D., Philadelphia, Pa.)

NORMAL CELLS AND BENIGN CONDITIONS, PANCREAS

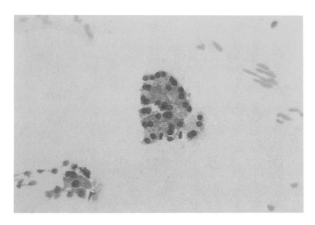

FIGURE 8–25. Benign Acinar Cells of the Pancreas. Note the abundant granular cytoplasm and small, round, regular nuclei (Papanicolaou stain, × 100). (Courtesy of Rosario Granados, M.D., Boston, Mass.)

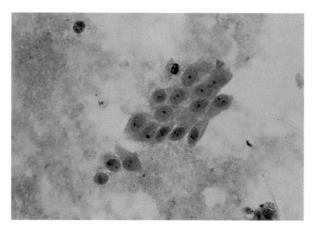

FIGURE 8–27. Brush Specimen of a Normal Biliary Duct. Note the regular cells with granular cytoplasm and nuclei with finely granular chromatin and inconspicuous nucleoli (Papanicolaou stain, × 250). (Courtesy of Barbara F. Atkinson, M.D., Philadelphia, Pa.)

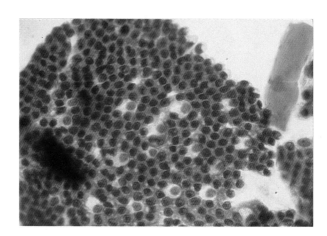

FIGURE 8–26. Benign Pancreas. Note the cohesive sheet of cells with a honeycomb appearance and bland nuclei (Papanicolaou stain, × 100). (Courtesy of Barbara F. Atkinson, M.D., Philadelphia, Pa.)

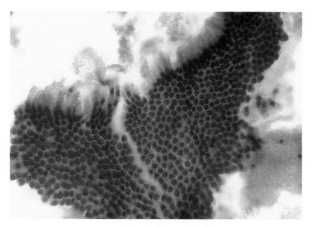

FIGURE 8–28. Brush Specimen of Normal Gallbladder Epithelium. The cells are arranged in a sheet with palisade arrangement at the border and honeycomb within. The nuclei are round and regular (Papanicolaou stain, × 100). (Courtesy of Barbara F. Atkinson, M.D., Philadelphia, Pa.)

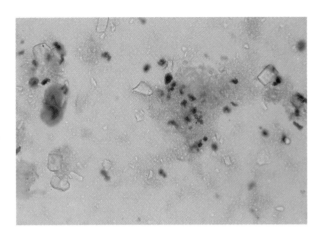

FIGURE 8–29. Gallstone. Refractile cholesterol crystals are visible (Papanicolaou stain, × 250). (Courtesy of Barbara F. Atkinson, M.D., Philadelphia,Pa.)

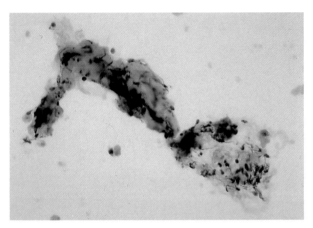

FIGURE 8–31. Fibrous Tissue from Chronic Pancreatitis. Generally in chronic pancreatitis, only scant cells are aspirated. If there are tissue fragments, these are generally collagen or benign connective tissue components (Papanicolaou stain, × 200).

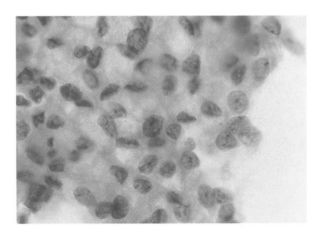

FIGURE 8–30. Reactive Atypia of Pancreatic Ductal Cells. The cells are arranged in a sheet with somewhat distinct cytoplasmic boundaries and no overlapping of nuclei. Nuclear pleomorphism is minimal (Papanicolaou stain, × 250).

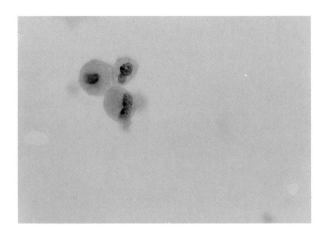

FIGURE 8–32. Fat Necrosis in Chronic Pancreatitis. The vacuolated histiocytes have typical kidney-bean nuclei and should not be confused with signet ring cells (Papanicolaou stain, × 250).

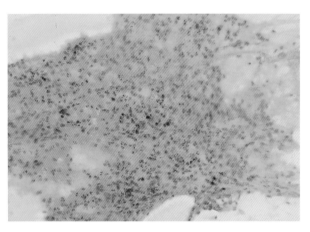

FIGURE 8–34. Pancreatic Pseudocyst. This aspirate shows debris that contains acute inflammatory cells and degenerating pancreatic ductal epithelial cells (Papanicolaou stain, × 100).

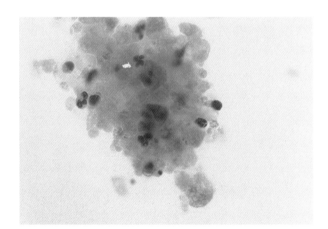

FIGURE 8–33. Chronic Pancreatitis. Amorphous debris and inflammatory cells (Papanicolaou stain, × 250).

MALIGNANT TUMORS, PANCREAS

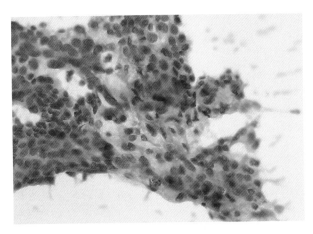

FIGURE 8–35. Well-Differentiated Pancreatic Adenocarcinoma. The specimen is highly cellular. The sheets of cells show some structure but are disordered, with pronounced nuclear crowding and overlapping (Papanicolaou stain, × 250).

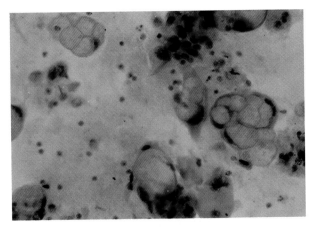

FIGURE 8–37. Mucinous Pancreatic Adenocarcinoma. The mucin actually stains pink on the periodic acid-Schiff stain. Note the many single cells filled with large vacuoles of mucin. These should be contrasted with histiocytes such as those in fat necrosis (see Fig. 8–32) (Papanicolaou stain, × 100). (Courtesy of Barbara F. Atkinson, M.D., Philadelphia, Pa.)

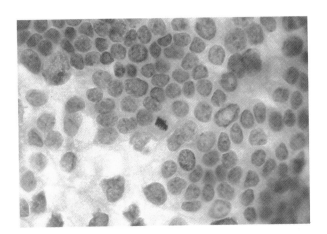

FIGURE 8–36. Well-Differentiated Pancreatic Adenocarcinoma. The cells are dyshesive, with nuclear crowding and a mitotic figure in the center of the field. This would be unusual in benign or reactive pancreatic cells (Papanicolaou stain, × 250).

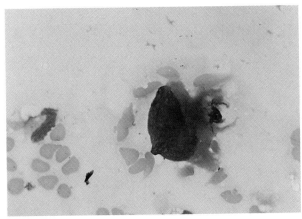

FIGURE 8–38. Pancreatic Adenocarcinoma. There is a single, huge malignant cell with marked nuclear atypia (Diff-Quik stain, × 250).

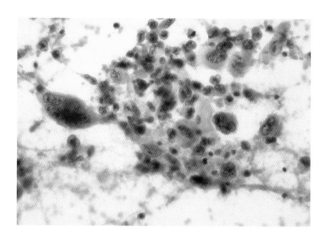

FIGURE 8–39. Pleomorphic Giant Cell Carcinoma of the Pancreas. This was aspirated from a 38-year-old female. Note the lack of cohesion, cellular pleomorphism, and the multinucleated tumor giant cell (Papanicolaou stain, × 100).

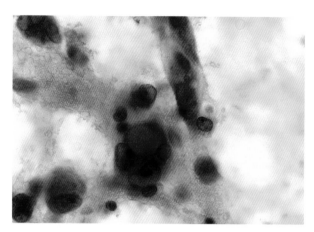

FIGURE 8–41. Pleomorphic Giant Cell Carcinoma of the Pancreas. Note the vacuolated single epithelial cell demonstrating the epithelial nature of the malignancy (contrast with Figs. 8–39 and 8–40) (toluidine blue and eosin stain, × 250).

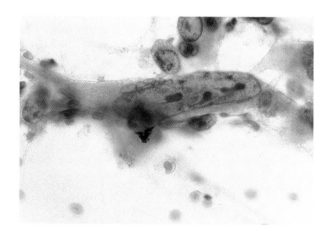

FIGURE 8–40. Pleomorphic Giant Cell Carcinoma of the Pancreas. This is a malignant spindle cell (Papanicolaou stain, × 250).

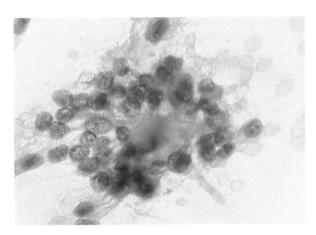

FIGURE 8–42. Islet Cell Tumor of the Pancreas. A rosette of cells surrounds amorphous material that did not stain for amyloid. The nuclei are relatively uniform in size, with a finely granular, "salt-and-pepper" chromatin pattern. There is scant and delicate cytoplasm (Papanicolaou stain, × 250).

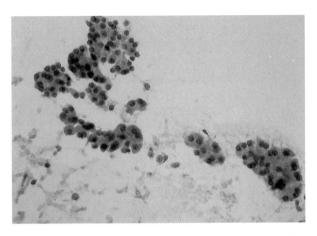

FIGURE 8–44A. Mucinous Cystadenocarcinoma of the Pancreas. The specimen is cellular, with many clusters of tightly and loosely cohesive cells (Papanicolaou stain, × 100). (Case courtesy of Rosario Granados, M.D., Boston, Mass.)

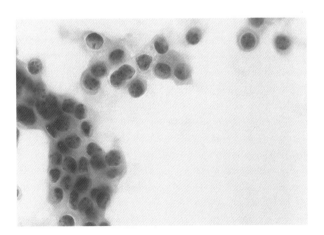

FIGURE 8–43. Pancreatic Islet Cell Tumor. The cells are loosely cohesive and single, with very eccentric nuclei and granular chromatin. The distinctive "salt-and-pepper" chromatin, with eccentric granular cytoplasm, should help differentiate this from the ordinary pancreatic adenocarcinoma. However, such cases may resemble lobular carcinoma, and in such instances, immunocytochemical stains, such as chromogranin, may be very useful (Papanicolaou stain, × 250).

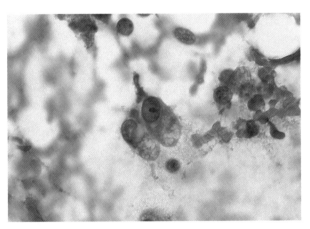

FIGURE 8–44B. Mucinous Cystadenocarcinoma of the Pancreas. This higher power view shows the vacuolated cytoplasm (Papanicolaou stain, × 250).

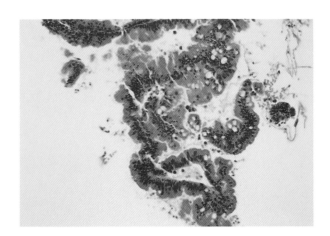

FIGURE 8–44C. Cell Block of Mucinous Cystadenocarcinoma of the Pancreas. Note the nuclear stratification and hyperchromasia (hematoxylin and eosin stain, × 25).

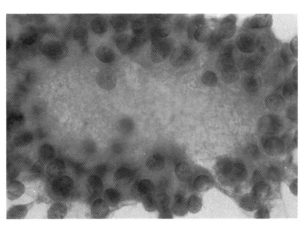

FIGURE 8–45B. Papillary and Solid Epithelial Neoplasm. The papillary fronds are lined by uniform cells with dense cytoplasm and small and regular nuclei (Papanicolaou stain, × 250).

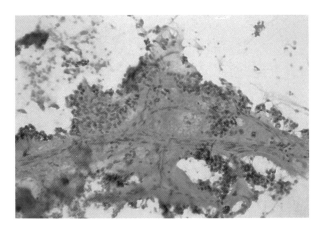

FIGURE 8–45A. Papillary and Solid Epithelial Neoplasm. This specimen was aspirated from a young woman. Note the papillary structures surrounding delicate fibrovascular cores (Papanicolaou stain, × 50). (Case courtesy of Rosario Granados, M.D., Boston, Mass.)

DIFFERENTIAL GROUPING

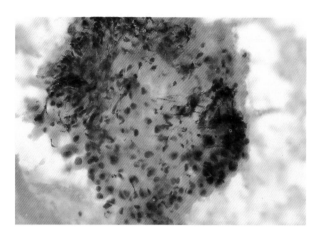

FIGURE 8–46A. Hepatic Cirrhosis. Note the fibrous tissue and atypical hepatocytes. However, benign-appearing hepatocytes are also seen, with a spectrum ranging from benign to atypical (Papanicolaou stain, × 100).

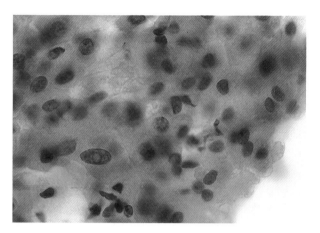

FIGURE 8–46C. Hepatic Cirrhosis. Nuclei are slightly enlarged, with an occasional intranuclear cytoplasmic inclusion and mild pleomorphism. In contrast to that of hepatocellular carcinoma, the degree of atypia and pleomorphism is not as pronounced, and benign cells are seen as well (Papanicolaou stain, × 250).

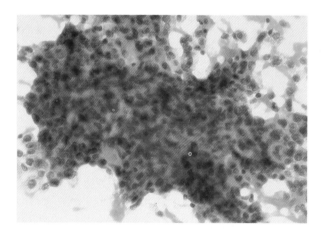

FIGURE 8–46B. Well-Differentiated Hepatocellular Carcinoma. Note the increased cellularity and irregular nuclear spacing as compared with that in Fig. 8–40 (Papanicolaou stain, × 100).

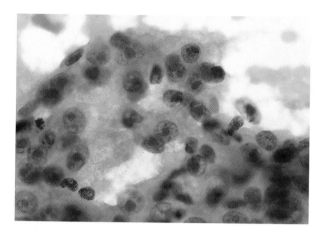

FIGURE 8–46D. Well-Differentiated Hepatocellular Carcinoma. Note the prominent macronucleoli. The cytoplasm resembles that of benign hepatocytes and is granular and polygonal, and an endothelial cell surrounds the cluster of hepatocytes (Papanicolaou stain, × 250).

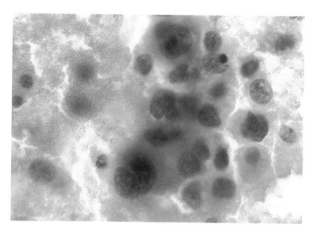

FIGURE 8–46F. Hepatocellular Carcinoma. In contrast to those in the previous figure, the nuclear contours are irregular, and multinucleated tumor giant cells are seen. Pronounced crowding of nuclei has occurred (Papanicolaou stain, × 250).

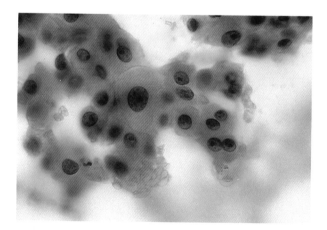

FIGURE 8–46E. Hepatic Cirrhosis. The reactive hepatocytes have round and regular nuclei. The nuclear size is variable, but the nuclear contour is smooth; more benign-appearing cells are also noted (Papanicolaou stain, × 250).

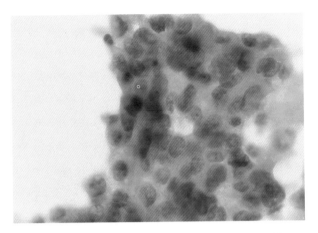

FIGURE 8–47A. Hepatocellular Carcinoma. The cells appear in a trabecular arrangement and have granular cytoplasm and nuclear overlapping. Useful features to make a diagnosis of hepatocellular carcinoma are endothelial cells surrounding such trabeculae, granular and polygonal cytoplasm, macronucleoli, and intracytoplasmic nuclear inclusions. When bile is seen, it is also a useful feature (Papanicolaou stain, × 250).

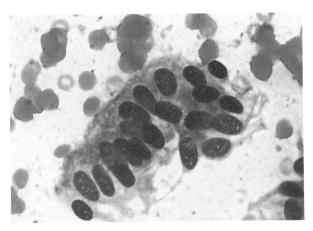

FIGURE 8–47C. Well-Differentiated Cholangiocarcinoma. The cells are in a palisade arrangement. The nuclei are elongated and eccentric compared with those in Fig. 8–47A (hepatocellular carcinoma) (Diff-Quik stain, × 250).

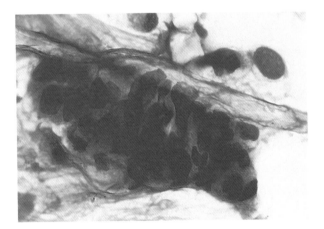

FIGURE 8–47B. Well-Differentiated Cholangiocarcinoma. The aspirate was cellular, with tightly cohesive clusters of cells. The diagnosis is based on cellularity, slight nuclear pleomorphism, atypia, and the presence of single cells (Diff-Quik stain, × 250).

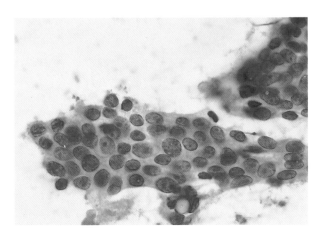

FIGURE 8–47D. Carcinoma of the Gallbladder. These cells could not be differentiated from cholangiocarcinoma or other metastatic adenocarcinomas. Note the cluster of cells in ductal-type arrangement, with enlarged, somewhat pleomorphic nuclei and small but prominent nucleoli. The nuclei are crowded and slightly irregular (hematoxylin and eosin stain, × 250).

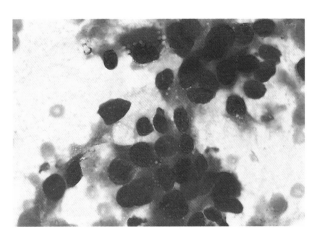

FIGURE 8–47F. Metastatic Pancreatic Carcinoma to the Liver. The origin of this tumor could not be determined on cytologic grounds alone, although the arrangement of cells in clusters and acini, lack of endothelial cells, and lack of macronucleoli differentiate it from a hepatocellular carcinoma. It would be useful to compare the cytologic features of this tumor with any previous material, either cytologic or histologic (Diff-Quik stain, × 250).

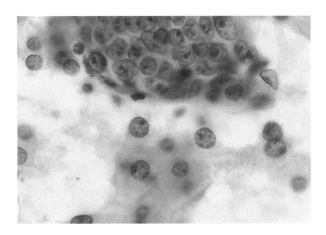

FIGURE 8–47E. Metastatic Adenocarcinoma of the Colon. Note that there are two cellular populations with reactive hepatocytes and a cluster of malignant cells with hyperchromatic nuclei and nucleoli (Papanicolaou stain, × 250).

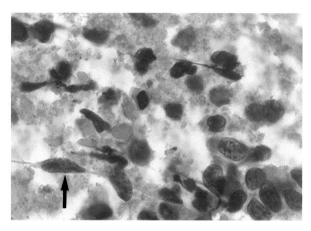

FIGURE 8–48A. Metastatic Adenocarcinoma of the Colon. This picture demonstrates the classic features of colonic carcinoma (tall, dark, and necrotic). Occasional spindle cell nuclei are seen (arrow). The necrotic cells may bear a resemblance to keratinized cells, and colonic carcinoma may be confused with squamous cell carcinoma. It is useful to find tall and columnar cells to differentiate these lesions (Papanicolaou stain, × 250).

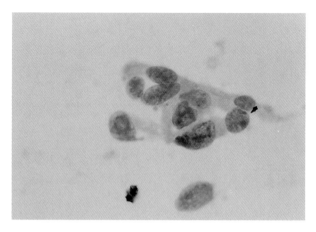

FIGURE 8–48C. Metastatic Breast Carcinoma. The cells are dyshesive, with delicate cytoplasm and irregular nuclei. Although this picture is consistent with a breast primary, comparison with previous material is necessary to confirm the diagnosis. If this is unavailable, estrogen receptors are sometimes useful (Papanicolaou stain, × 250).

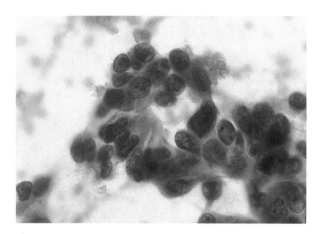

FIGURE 8–48B. Metastatic Adenocarcinoma of the Colon. These cells are tall and columnar, with oval, hyperchromatic nuclei (Papanicolaou stain, × 250).

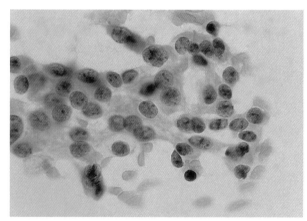

FIGURE 8–48D. Metastatic Pancreatic Adenocarcinoma. These cells are arranged in loose sheets, with nuclear overlapping and nuclear pleomorphism. There is some irregularity of the nuclear membrane. This patient had a large mass in the pancreas and multiple nodules in the liver. On this basis, a presumptive diagnosis of pancreatic adenocarcinoma was made (Papanicolaou stain, × 250).

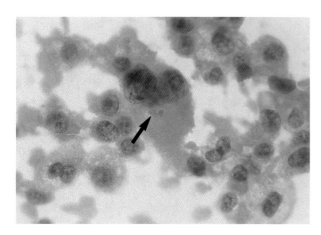

FIGURE 8–49A. Hepatocellular Carcinoma. Many single cells are present, with a binucleated tumor cell in the center of the field. This tumor cell has malignant nuclear characteristics, and bile pigment is present in the cytoplasm (arrow) (Papanicolaou stain, × 250).

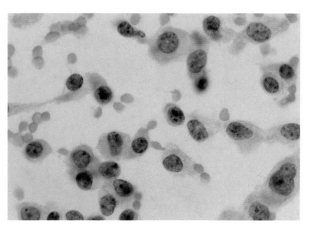

FIGURE 8–49C. Metastatic Islet Cell Tumor to the Liver. Note the eccentric nuclei and "salt-and-pepper" chromatin pattern. These cells stained positively for chromogranin (Papanicolaou stain, × 250).

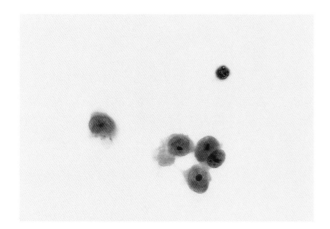

FIGURE 8–49B. Metastatic Melanoma to the Liver. Note the granular and dusty appearance of the cytoplasm, which is suggestive of pigment. Nucleoli are prominent. These cells stained positively with HMB-45, confirming the diagnosis of metastatic melanoma (Papanicolaou stain, × 250).

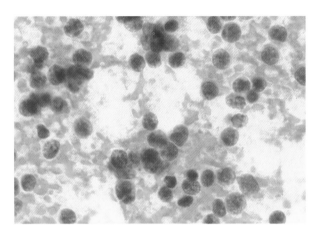

FIGURE 8–49D. Non-Hodgkin's Lymphoma in an Aspiration of a Liver. These cells are monomorphic and single, with scant cytoplasm. In contrast to those of Figure 8–49C, there is less cytoplasm, and the nuclei are central. These cells stained positively for LCA (Papanicolaou stain, × 250).

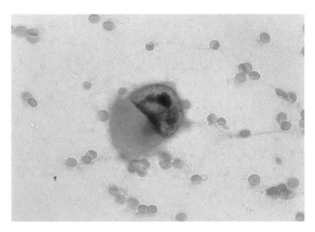

FIGURE 8–49F. Undifferentiated Pancreatic Carcinoma Metastatic to the Liver. This cell is huge, with a vesicular chromatin pattern of the nucleus and a prominent nucleolus. The eccentric location of the nucleus and granular cytoplasm is suggestive of an adenocarcinoma. The cells stained positively for EMA and keratin and negatively for HMB-45, S-100, and LCA (Papanicolaou stain, × 250).

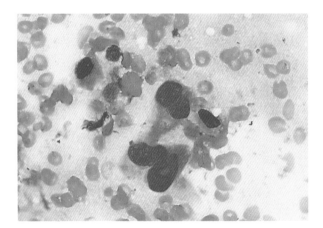

FIGURE 8–49E. Poorly Differentiated Pancreatic Adenocarcinoma Metastatic to the Liver. These single cells have eccentric nuclei and are very pleomorphic (Diff-Quik stain, × 250).

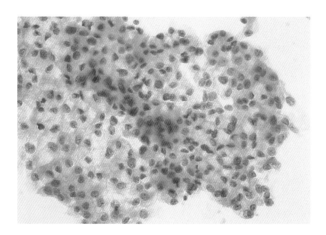

FIGURE 8–50A. Reactive, Atypical Ductal Cells in Chronic Pancreatitis. Cells are present in sheets, with distinct cell boundaries and lack of nuclear crowding or pleomorphism (Papanicolaou stain, × 100).

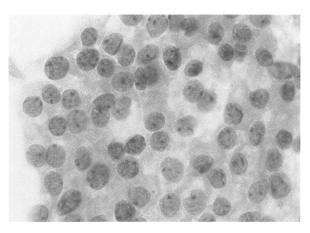

FIGURE 8–50C. Chronic Pancreatitis. This high-power view demonstrates the round and regular nuclei of chronic pancreatitis (Papanicolaou stain, × 250).

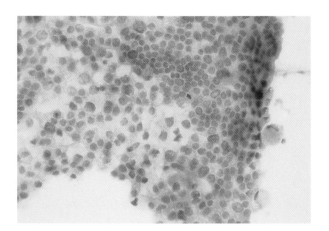

FIGURE 8–50B. Well-Differentiated Adenocarcinoma. The changes are extremely subtle, as contrasted with those in the previous figure. Although the nuclei are still round, slight irregularities of the nuclear membrane exist. Pronounced nuclear crowding and overlapping are present. The edges of the sheet were dyshesive. A mitotic figure is evident in the center of the field (Papanicolaou stain, × 100).

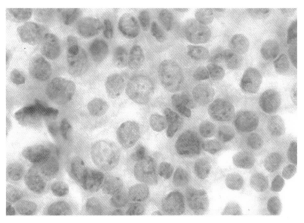

FIGURE 8–50D. Well-Differentiated Pancreatic Carcinoma. In contrast to the previous figure, more nuclear crowding is present, and the nuclear contours are irregular (Papanicolaou stain, × 250).

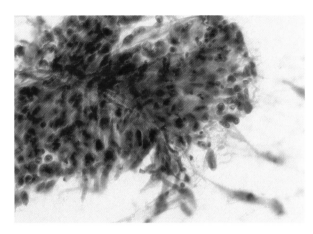

FIGURE 8–51A. Pleomorphic Carcinoma of the Pancreas. Note the prominent spindle cell pattern. This figure should be contrasted with the granuloma in Figure 8–4; it is more cellular, and the nuclei are irregular and lack the distinctive kidney-bean appearance of histiocytes (Papanicolaou stain, × 100).

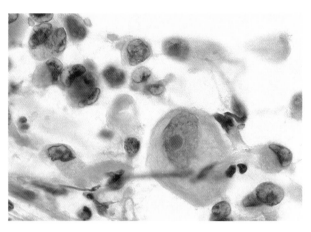

FIGURE 8–51C. Pleomorphic Carcinoma of the Pancreas. Careful examination of this smear may also disclose cells more reminiscent of adenocarcinoma, with prominent nucleoli and eccentric nuclei with cytoplasmic vacuolization (Papanicolaou stain, × 250).

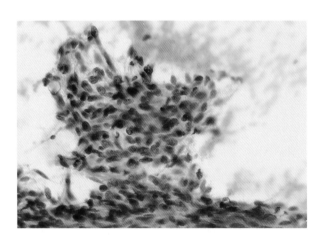

FIGURE 8–51B. Primary Sarcoma of the retroperitoneum. This is indistinguishable from the pleomorphic carcinoma in the previous photograph. Immunocytochemical stains are necessary to make a distinction when only the spindle component of a pleomorphic carcinoma is present on an aspirate (Papanicolaou stain, × 100).

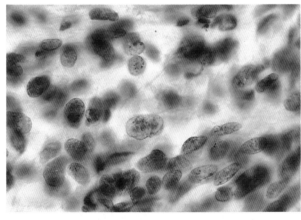

FIGURE 8–51D. Primary Sarcoma of the Retroperitoneum. This high-power view demonstrates monotonous spindle cells with a coarsely granular chromatin pattern (Papanicolaou stain, × 250).

C·H·A·P·T·E·R

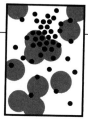

9

URINARY CYTOLOGY

Lori J. Elwood
Christine King
Jean M. Colandrea

ROLE OF URINARY CYTOLOGY

Cytologic evaluation of the urine is useful in a variety of clinical situations. It is a valuable screening test for patients at high risk for developing urothelial malignancy. It provides a noninvasive method to follow patients treated conservatively for superficial bladder neoplasms and to monitor residual urothelium after surgical treatment for malignant bladder tumors. Urine cytology is also a useful diagnostic tool in the initial evaluation of patients presenting with signs or symptoms of urologic disease.

The sensitivity of urine cytology as a screening test ranges from less than 50% to greater than 90%, depending on the grade of the underlying neoplasm. Urine cytology is very sensitive in detecting high-grade, cytologically malignant urothelial tumors in high-risk patients. In contrast, it is relatively insensitive for screening for low-grade papillary neoplasms. This is due, in part, to the tendency of these lesions not to exfoliate. Furthermore, since the cells of many low-grade tumors lack cytologic criteria of malignancy, a definite cytologic diagnosis of neoplasia may not be possible. Fortunately, experts agree that low-grade urologic tumors are indicative of nonaggressive clinical behavior characterized by multiple recurrences with little effect on overall survival. Thus, the clinical consequences of a negative urine cytology in the presence of a low-grade papillary tumor may be minor.

Urine cytology is used in combination with cystoscopy to follow patients previously treated for urologic tumors. In this capacity, cytology is superior to cystoscopy for detecting the flat lesions of carcinoma in situ, which may not be visible to the cystoscopist, and in monitoring areas not accessible to the cystoscope, such as ureters, Brunn's nests, and prostatic ducts.

Urine cytology is also a useful tool for the evaluation of patients presenting with hematuria or symptoms of urinary tract disease such as dysuria or frequency. The cytologic features of local inflammatory processes, renal parenchymal disease, and urothelial neoplasia are distinct and can provide direction for further evaluation in many cases.

SPECIMEN COLLECTION

A random voided urine obtained by midstream clean-catch technique usually provides adequate material for cytologic evaluation. First-morning voided urine may be more cellular, but degeneration caused by prolonged exposure of the cells to the hypertonic milieu of urine can preclude optimal cytologic evaluation. Similarly, urine from 24-hour urine collections and external collection bags is unacceptable for cytologic evaluation. Use of midstream clean-catch technique avoids the obscuring and possibly confusing effects of genital contamination in voided specimens.

Instrumented specimens, including cystoscopy urine, catheterized urine, and bladder washings, are more cellular than voided specimens and often show better preservation. These benefits have not been shown to be of sufficient diagnostic utility, however, to justify the risk associated with an invasive procedure for routine specimen procurement.

Specimens obtained by washing or brushing the ureters and pelves are useful for the evaluation of radiologically demonstrated lesions of the upper collecting system and for localizing the source of malignant urothelial cells not appearing to originate in the bladder. In both situations, obtaining bilateral specimens for comparison is extremely useful.

Surveillance of ureters following cystectomy for urothelial malignancy can be accomplished by cytologic evaluation of urine obtained through an ileal conduit. For optimal evaluation, the specimen must be freshly obtained and not collected from stagnant urine in an external collection bag.

SPECIMEN PREPARATION

Use of preservatives to reduce degeneration and to inhibit bacterial growth is usually unnecessary since optimal cytologic evaluation can be obtained from specimens refrigerated without fixatives for up to 48 hours. Preservatives can be used, however, when longer delays in processing cannot be avoided.

The three basic methods commonly used to prepare urine specimens for cytology include direct smearing, membrane filtration, and cytocentrifugation. All three methods can provide excellent preparations; however, each has associated advantages and disadvantages, and use of a given method is a matter of personal preference. Cell block preparations are unsatisfactory for routine cytologic evaluation of urine.

Specimens are routinely stained by the Papanicolaou method, which optimally demonstrates nuclear detail and cytoplasmic keratin. Air-dried, modified Wright-stained preparations can be useful for intraoperative evaluation of material obtained by ureteral or pelvic brushing.

CELLULAR COMPONENTS OF NORMAL VOIDED URINE

Normal voided urine specimens are characterized by low cellularity and contain urothelial cells of predominantly superficial (umbrella) and intermediate types. Umbrella cells are large, often larger than superficial squamous cells, and have a rigid shape with at least one flat or concave side (Fig. 9–1). The cytoplasm is more dense than that of a squamous cell and is sometimes vacuolated. These cells may be multinucleated with round or oval nuclei containing finely granular and evenly dispersed chromatin and often eosinophilic micronucleoli. They can show marked reactive features, including nuclear enlargement, hyperchromasia, coarse chromatin, and macronucleoli. Even when they are reactive, the nuclear to cytoplasmic ratio remains low, and as long as they can be recognized as superficial cells, they can be considered benign. The intermediate cells are oval in shape in voided specimens and are smaller than the superficial cells, approximating the size of parabasal squamous cells (Figs. 9–2 and 9–3). They are often present in small loose groups on the slide. They have small nuclei similar in character to resting superficial cells and dense cytoplasm, which may contain abundant glycogen.

Squamous cells are often present in preparations of voided urine and may represent contaminants from the vulva, vagina, or urethra of a female or the distal urethra or prepuce of a male (Fig. 9–2). Squamous cells can also exfoliate from an area of physiologic or pathologic metaplasia in the urinary bladder. Squamous metaplasia of the trigone is a normal variant in females and is rarely seen in males. Widespread squamous metaplasia can be associated with chronic inflammatory states such as schistosomiasis. Squamous cells are usually distinguishable from urothelial cells by their extreme cytoplasmic thinning and often pyknotic nuclei.

Rare renal epithelial cells can be found in normal voided urine. Two types are readily discernible. The first type is of convoluted tubule origin (Fig. 9–4 and 9–5). The convoluted cells are usually smaller than the transitional cells but occur in a broad range of sizes from 10 to 60 μ in greatest dimension. The largest cells arise from the proximal tubules and the smallest from the distal tubules. They are oval in shape and have extremely granular cytoplasm and eccentric, small round nuclei showing varying degrees of degeneration. Because of the extreme cytoplasmic granularity, anucleate convoluted cells resemble small granular casts, and multinucleate convoluted cells resemble degenerated renal tubular cell casts.

The second type of renal cell seen in urine specimens is the small (12 to 14 μ in diameter) polygonal cell of collecting duct origin (Fig. 9–6). Collecting duct renal cells occur singly or in small fragments. They have centrally placed, small round nuclei with dense chromatin and relatively scant, soft cytoplasm with angulated cytoplasmic borders. They can be mistaken for histiocytes or lymphocytes in Papanicolaou-stained material, particularly when they are degenerated. The presence of numerous renal cells of either type is pathologic.

Normal voided urine can contain rare red blood cells and inflammatory cells including lymphocytes, monocyte/macrophages, and polymorphonuclear leukocytes. If origin from the genital tract is excluded, the presence of large numbers of either red cells or inflammatory cells is pathologic.

Frequently, the epithelial cells in urine specimens contain distinct, dense, usually eosinophilic, and rarely turquoise-staining inclusions in their cytoplasm (Fig. 9–7). The cells containing these inclusions usually show marked degeneration of both cytoplasm and nuclei, and their presence is felt to be a manifestation of degeneration. These cytoplasmic inclusions can be particularly numerous in the epithelial cells in ileal conduit specimens (Fig. 9–14). Although they are a nonspecific finding, they are usually found in the urine of patients with some form of urinary tract disease or history of nephrotoxic drug exposure.

CELLULAR COMPONENTS OF NORMAL INSTRUMENTED SPECIMENS

Catheterized specimens are similar to voided specimens with two exceptions. First, they lack contamination from the external genitalia and vagina. Second, they are more cellular and often contain pseudopapillary fragments of urothelial cells due to the traumatic effects of the catheter. These fragments show maintained polarity and are often surfaced by umbrella cells (Fig. 9–8). Component cells have well-defined cell borders and uniform nuclei with a powdery chromatin pattern. Nuclear borders can show slight irregularity or marked degenerative wrinkling; however, markedly abnormal nuclear contours are not present. The presence of benign urothelial tissue fragments in catheterized specimens makes it difficult to diagnose low-grade papillary urothelial neoplasia, which often appears similar.

Bladder washings are usually richly cellular and show superior preservation of urothelial cells that occur singly, in monolayered sheets, and in pseudopapillary fragments similar to those present in catheterized specimens. Cells from the deep layers of the urothelium, characterized by their small size, are often present (Figs. 9–9 and 9–10). In these specimens, the intermediate and deep urothelial cells can assume a columnar configuration and umbrella cells can show extreme multinucleation (Figs. 9–11 and 9–12). Nuclei can appear hypochromatic with relatively prominent nucleoli, particularly if hypotonic solutions have been used to wash the bladder. Since the area sampled is limited to the area of urothelium that is washed, and since pseudopapillary fragments obscure the diagnosis of low-grade urothelial neoplasia, these specimens are less suitable for routine screening than voided specimens.

Specimens obtained through an ileal conduit are distinguished by high cellularity and a dirty background due to the presence of mucus and bacteria (Figs. 9–13 and 9–14). Although rare urothelial cells can be seen, the epithelial cells are predominantly columnar cells of ileal epithelial origin. The columnar cells are present singly and in three-dimensional groups. Degeneration is often so advanced that columnar configuration is not recognizable, and these cells can be mistaken for neoplastic urothelial cells. In the evaluation of these specimens, nuclear criteria of malignancy must be found in preserved cells before a malignant diagnosis is made.

NONCELLULAR COMPONENTS OF URINE

Mucus can be seen in normal urine and appears as faint purple, blue, or red amorphous streaks. When associated with inflammation, mucus can be abundant or present in the configuration of Curschmann spirals (Figs. 9–15 and 9–16). Fibrin, appearing as faint fibrillar red or blue streaks, can be seen in urine from patients with glomerular disease or from those with hematuria (Fig. 9–17).

Crystals are commonly found in urine specimens. Their presence is dependent on solute concentrations, pH, and specimen temperature. Since solvents used in fixation and staining of cytologic material can dissolve some crystals and since urinalysis results, including pH, are not always available to the cytopathologist, cytologic material is not ideal for evaluating crystals. When present, however, the morphology of many crystals is characteristic enough to allow identification in cytologic preparations (Fig. 9–18 to 9–24). Crystals frequently seen in Papanicolaou-stained material include amorphous phosphates, amorphous urates, triple phosphate, uric acid, calcium oxalate, and ammonium biurate (Table 9–1). Although these crystals are usually clinically insignificant, familiarity with their appearance facilitates the identification of pathologic crystals when they occur. Those that can be seen in Papanicolaou-stained material include tyrosine, leucine, cystine, and bilirubin.

Casts are often found in urine specimens and can be either physiologic or pathologic. Physiologic casts are of either hyaline or granular types and are composed predominately of Tamm-Horsfall (tubular type) protein that has precipitated in the tubular lumen. Hyaline casts appear in Papanicolaou-stained material as transparent, homogeneous, purple or green cylinders (Figs. 9–25 and 9–34). They can be particularly numerous in specimens obtained from patients after vigorous exercise or after diuretic therapy. Granular casts can also be found in the urine of individuals with normal renal function and can be increased in number following strenuous exercise or prolonged fever. These are characterized by the presence of fine or coarse cyanophilic granular debris within the protein matrix of the cast representing precipitated plasma protein or degenerated cells (Figs. 9–26 and 9–31).

Most pathologic casts contain cells or cellular debris within the protein matrix of the cast. Erythrocyte casts are composed of erythrocytes or ghosts of erythrocytes in a cast configuration (Fig. 9–27). They can be bound together by fibrin and, therefore, may not have a recognizable protein matrix. Red blood cell casts are almost pathognomonic of renal glomerular disease. Leukocyte casts contain lymphocytes, histiocytes, or polymorphonuclear leukocytes in a protein matrix (Fig. 9–28). When degeneration is marked, the various types of leukocytes may be indistinguishable in these casts. They are associated with the presence of leukocytes in the renal interstitium and are thus seen in pyelonephritis and other inflammatory tubulointerstitial diseases, such as lupus nephritis and vasculitis, including renal allograft rejection. Renal tubular epithelial casts contain renal tubular cells in the protein matrix (Figs. 9–29 and 9–30). They can be found in the urine of patients with almost any renal parenchymal disease. Cellular constituents of renal tubular epithelial casts are sometimes identifiable as typical convoluted or collecting duct cells but often appear markedly reactive with cellular and nuclear enlargement, hyperchromasia, prominent nucleoli, and vacuolated cytoplasm.

As the components of cellular casts degenerate, granular casts are formed. The granular material within the cast matrix usually appears green or blue in Papanicolaou-stained material, although hemoglobin pigment can be recognized as red coloration in granular casts derived from erythrocyte casts (Figs. 9–31 and 9–32). Pathologic granular casts are usually found in urines showing other features characteristic of renal parenchymal disease. Waxy casts are acellular and appear as very dense cyanophilic cylinders (Fig. 9–33). They have very well defined borders, blunt ends, and often "cracks" in the matrix. They are formed after long-term retention of cellular casts within the tubular lumen, and represent an end stage of degeneration. Their presence is characteristic of urinary stasis as occurs in chronic renal failure, especially with oliguria. Casts with large caliber casts (so-called broad casts) are a particularly ominous finding in the urine sediment since they reflect tubular dilation as seen in end-stage renal disease (Fig. 9–34). Fatty casts can be found in the urine samples of patients with nephrotic syndrome (Figs. 9–35 and 9–36). They have the rigid configuration of other casts but are composed of variably sized fat vacuoles.

Urine may be contaminated with exogenous material. Lubricant, as is commonly used by the cystoscopist, appears as homogeneous, basophilic, translucent or opaque globules of varying sizes (Fig. 9–37). Pollen grains, more abundant in the air during certain seasons, can appear differently depending on the plant of origin and how well they take up stain (Figs. 9–38 and 9–39). All varieties of pollen are, however, characterized by the absence of a nucleus and the presence of a refractile cell wall that is more or less well demonstrated. *Alternaria* is a pigmented mold that appears yellow-brown. The macroconidia, commonly encountered laboratory contaminants, appear dark brown and are characterized by the presence of both longitudinal and transverse septae (Fig. 9–40). Rarely, the hair of the carpet beetle larva is seen in urine cytology specimens. It has a distinctive fish-head and skeleton appearance and is brown in color (Fig. 9–41).

CONTAMINANTS FROM THE GENITAL SYSTEM

Squamous cells of female reproductive tract origin can often be distinguished from squamous metaplasia of the bladder in a voided urine specimen by their association with vaginal bacterial flora (Fig. 9–42). These contaminating squamous cells can appear normal or reflect pathologic processes occurring in the tissue of origin, such as squamous intraepithelial lesions (dysplasias) (Fig. 9–43). Endometrial cells shed during menses may also contaminate urine specimens of female patients (Fig. 9–44). Their presence can be misleading because they often appear as three-dimensional groups of small degenerated cells that are difficult to identify and may raise a suspicion of malignancy. Close examination reveals the nuclear wrinkling and hypochromasia characteristic of endometrial cells. Furthermore, the background usually shows marked vaginal contamination and red blood cells.

Rarely, specimens from male patients contain prostate or seminal vesical epithelial elements. This is most likely to occur in a specimen obtained following prostatic massage. Benign prostatic epithelium usually appears as loose sheets of cells with low nuclear to cytoplasmic ratios; eccentric, round, often pyknotic nuclei; and soft, vacuolated cytoplasm (Fig. 9–45). Seminal vesical epithelial cells appear in small groups with a more haphazard arrangement (Fig. 9–46). They characteristically show anisonucleosis, a powdery chromatin pattern, and abundant vacuolated cytoplasm containing lipofuscin pigment. Such specimens may also contain prostatic concretions or spermatozoa (Fig. 9–47). Spermatozoa can also be seen in first morning specimens from male patients, and they can be found in urine from either gender following coitus.

INFECTIONS

Bacterial infection of the urinary tract is common and usually due to coliform bacteria or staphylococci (Fig. 9–48). Acute inflammatory cells, red blood cells, and a monomorphic population of bacteria are seen unless the infection is in the early stages or partially treated. Urothelial cells are often found in greater numbers than in noninfected urine and frequently show reactive features, including nuclear enlargement, hyperchromasia, prominent nucleoli, and cytoplasmic vacuolization (Fig. 9–62).

Fungal infection occurs in the bladder and is most often due to invasive candidiasis (Figs. 9–49 and 9–50). Depending on the species of *Candida* present, the organism is identifiable as budding yeast with or without a pseudohyphal component (Fig. 9–51). The background generally shows blood and inflammatory cells unless immunosuppression with neutropenia precludes an inflammatory response. The transitional cells can show reactive features.

The most frequent viral infection of the urinary bladder is polyoma. The cytopathic effects of polyoma virus are often seen in urine specimens of immunosuppressed patients and, rarely, in urine specimens of individuals with normal immune status. Affected cells are enlarged and have markedly increased nuclear to cytoplasmic ratios. The nucleus is usually in an extremely eccentric position, and the cytoplasm is often degenerated, trailing behind the nucleus. This overall appearance has prompted their description as "comet-like" (Fig. 9–52). Diagnostic cells can be few and contain gelatinous, grey-blue intranuclear inclusions either filling the nucleus and displacing the chromatin to a peripheral ring or associated with a thin peri-inclusion clear zone (Figs. 9–53 and 9–54). Chromatin in infected cells, even when they do not contain a diagnostic inclusion, is usually peripherally displaced and shows a reticular pattern of degeneration. Since polyoma urinary tract infection is usually asymptomatic, its importance lies in the associated cytopathic changes that can simulate malignancy.

Cytomegalovirus-infected cells are rarely seen in the urine of immunosuppressed patients, particularly renal allograft recipients. Infected patients present with hematuria and features of transplant rejection. Diagnostic cells are enlarged renal tubular type cells that contain a single, dense, eosinophilic or basophilic intranuclear inclusion associated with peripherally clumped chromatin and a prominent peri-inclusion clear zone (Fig. 9–55). In addition, they contain multiple, small, often poorly visualized cytoplasmic inclusions. Specimens usually contain few diagnostic cells.

Herpes simplex virus can infect the urethra and urinary bladder, but infection of the genital tract is more common. Since infected cells from either site appear identical, it is not possible to distinguish the site of origin with certainty by voided urine cytology. Infected cells are enlarged, show squamous differentiation, and contain single or multiple inclusion–bearing nuclei. When multiple nuclei are present, pronounced molding is characteristic. The intranuclear inclusions are either of the ground-glass type or of the hard eosinophilic type with angular contours (Fig. 9–56 and 9–57).

Human papilloma virus–infected cells can originate in the urinary tract, but genital infection is more common. Associated cytopathic changes include koilocytosis, dyskeratosis, and often dyskaryosis indistinguishable from that seen in cervical and vaginal cytology specimens (Fig. 9–58).

Trichomonas vaginalis organisms can be seen in the urine, usually as contaminants from the genital tract. The organisms are pear-shaped, measure approximately 30 μ in the long axis, and generally stain poorly. A round nucleus, characteristic axostyle, and eosinophilic cytoplasmic granules can often be seen and aid in identification (Fig. 9–59).

Schistosoma haematobium ova can be seen in the urine as manifestations of bladder infection in patients from Africa and the Middle East. Ova are large (measuring from 112 to 180 μ in the long axis), oval, and transparent, superficially resembling uric acid crystals (Fig. 9–60). Identification is possible by recognition of the internal structure and characteristic terminal spine. Infection is associated with squamous metaplasia and in increased incidence of squamous cell carcinoma of the urinary bladder.

Rarely, eggs of the pinworm, *Enterobius vermicularis*, can be seen in urine specimens, usually from pediatric patients. They are oval with a characteristic flattened side and measure approximately 50 μ in greatest dimension. As with other helminth eggs, internal structure is characteristic and helps to distinguish the eggs from similar appearing noncellular objects in urine (Fig. 9–61).

NONINFECTIOUS INFLAMMATION

Various forms of noninfectious cystitis have been described. In interstitial cystitis (Hunner ulcer) there is infiltration of the bladder wall by mast cells, which can sometimes be found in the urine sediment. Eosinophilic cystitis is characterized by bladder wall infiltration by eosinophils, and affected patients can have eosinophiluria.

Malacoplakia is a rare disorder that may represent an aberrant host response to bacterial infection. In this disorder, the wall of the urinary bladder is infiltrated by closely packed macrophages with abundant granular cytoplasm. The cytoplasmic granularity is due to the presence of phagosomes containing bacterial debris. In addition, characteristic laminated calcified concretions (Michaelis-Gutmann bodies) are present both in the cytoplasm of some macrophages and extracellularly. Rarely, macrophages containing Michaelis-Gutmann bodies can be seen in the urine of affected patients.

Hemorrhagic cystitis may occur as a toxic drug reaction, particularly associated with cyclophosphamide therapy. The urine of affected patients contains gross or microscopic blood, inflammatory cells, and reactive urothelial cells. The reactive urothelial cells can show nuclear enlargement, hyperchromasia, undulation of the nuclear border, and prominent nucleoli, features that must be interpreted carefully with regard for the clinical setting (Fig. 9–62).

Inflammation due to nephrolithiasis and chronic outlet obstruction with bladder trabeculation is commonly associated with the presence of pseudopapillary fragments of urothelial cells in voided urine (Figs. 9–63 and 9–64). Although urothelial fragments occurring in these disorders can be virtually indistinguishable from those seen in low-grade transitional cell neoplasms, reactive nuclear features and cytoplasmic vacuolization favor one of these non-neoplastic conditions.

RENAL PARENCHYMAL DISEASE

Renal parenchymal diseases, such as glomerulonephritis, acute tubular necrosis, pyelonephritis, immune-mediated tubulointerstitial diseases, vasculitis, hypertension, and renal allograft rejection, are characterized by the presence of various combinations of renal tubular epithelial cells and pathologic casts as well as erythrocytes and inflammatory cells in urine specimens (Schumann, 1980). The various parenchymal lesions are not distinguishable by cytology alone, although some patterns are highly suggestive of specific lesions. Cellular specimens containing necrotic convoluted cells are characteristic of acute tubular necrosis or a drug reaction with similar pathogenesis (Figs. 9–65 and 9–66). Similarly, the finding of erythrocyte casts is fairly specific for glomerulonephritis (Fig. 9–27), and the finding of collecting duct cells in the urine of renal allograft recipients after Day 3 suggests rejection.

Either convoluted or collecting duct types of renal tubular epithelial cells can be seen in patients afflicted with almost any of the renal parenchymal diseases. In these conditions, tubular cells can display markedly reactive nuclear features and vacuolated cytoplasm, obscuring their classification as convoluted or collecting duct type (Fig. 9–67). In addition, they can exfoliate in fragments, sometimes making their distinction from neoplastic urothelial cells difficult (Fig. 9–68).

THERAPEUTIC EFFECT

Various agents used in treatment of benign and malignant diseases are associated with characteristic cellular features in urine specimens. Cyclophosphamide, via an active metabolite excreted in the urine, causes damage to submucosal vessels, smooth muscle, and urothelium. Characteristic urothelial abnormalities can occur, particularly after prolonged therapy, which are sometimes associated with hemorrhagic cystitis and include increased nuclear to cytoplasmic ratio, nuclear enlargement, eccentricity, hyperchromasia, and degeneration (Fig. 9–69). Nuclear contours may be irregular because of degeneration. The chromatin shows a reticular pattern of degeneration or peripheral clumping. In either case, the nucleus may be clear to the nuclear rim, creating an "empty" appearance. Cytoplasm is usually degenerated and granular or wispy. Since cyclophosphamide-affected cells exfoliate as single cells with enlarged, eccentric, hyperchromatic nuclei, they must be distinguished from cells of high-grade transitional cell carcinoma. Diagnostic errors can be avoided by requiring well-preserved cells, fulfilling criteria of malignancy to establish a malignant diagnosis. Cyclophosphamide-affected cells can also appear similar to cells infected with polyoma virus; however, diagnostic intranuclear inclusions are absent.

Mitomycin C and thio-TEPA denude the urothelium, and urine specimens reflect increased exfoliation. The most striking changes are seen in the superficial cells, which show reactive features with enlargement of both nucleus and cytoplasm and preservation of near-normal nuclear to cytoplasmic ratios (Fig. 9–70). Degenerative intranuclear and cytoplasmic vacuoles may be seen. Some cells show multinucleation and markedly reactive, sometimes bizarre, nuclei that may have nucleoli. Despite the significant nuclear changes, these cells can be recognized as superficial and benign by virtue of their low nuclear to cytoplasmic ratios. Any cells present in specimens from patients treated with these agents that show features resembling neoplasia are probably not due to therapeutic effect and warrant further investigation.

Changes caused by pelvic irradiation are similar to those described above for mitomycin C and thio-TEPA in that nuclear and cellular enlargement may be present with only mild alteration of nuclear to cytoplasmic ratios. Multinucleation, nuclear and cytoplasmic vacuolization, a smudged chromatin pattern, and cytoplasmic polychromasia are characteristic of irradiated cells (Figs. 9–71 and 9–72). Benign cells showing radiation effect lack the well-preserved nuclear changes and altered nuclear to cytoplasmic ratios required to make the diagnosis of neoplasia.

Intravesical bacille Calmette-Guérin (BCG) produces granulomatous inflammation with overlying mucosal ulceration similar to tuberculous cystitis. Urine cytology may show acute and chronic inflammation reflecting ulceration and multinucleated giant cells and lymphohistiocytic aggregates as manifestations of granulomatous inflammation (Fig. 9–73). Epithelial changes are reactive and nonspecific and do not simulate malignancy.

DYSPLASIA AND LOW-GRADE UROTHELIAL NEOPLASIA

Cells derived from urothelial dysplasia usually exfoliate in small groups, although rarely single dysplastic cells are seen (Figs. 9–74 to 9–76). Since dysplastic cells do not easily exfoliate, few diagnostic cells are present in any one specimen. Nuclei are slightly eccentrically located, enlarged, and hyperchromatic with evenly distributed chromatin that is more granular than that of normal urothelial cells. Nuclear borders can be slightly irregular and may show degenerative wrinkling, but markedly abnormal nuclear contours are not seen. Nucleoli are small or absent, in contrast to high-grade transitional cell carcinoma in which prominent nucleoli are seen in some cells. The cytoplasm lacks the glycogen often found in normal urothelial cells but is otherwise characteristic of transitional cells.

Epithelial fragments exfoliated from a low-grade papillary transitional neoplasm can be virtually indistinguishable from pseudopapillary urothelial fragments occuring in non-neoplastic conditions such as recent instrumentation, bladder trabeculation, and renal calculi (Fig. 9–77). At times, they are even surfaced by benign umbrella cells (Fig. 9–78). Cells derived from low-grade tumors may be slightly enlarged but can be smaller than normal urothelial cells. They are similar in character to dysplastic urothelial cells, containing hyperchromatic nuclei with granular, evenly dispersed chromatin, mildly irregular nuclear contours, and inapparent nucleoli; there is also homogeneous cytoplasm (Fig. 9–79). Since malignant nuclear features are often subtle in these tumors and degeneration is advanced, the presence of urothelial fragments in voided urine may be the only clue to the diagnosis. Although the absence of reactive nuclear features and lack of cytoplasmic vacuolization favor a diagnosis of neoplasia over other causes for papillary fragments in voided urine, clinical history is essential and follow-up cystoscopy is often required to arrive at a definitive diagnosis.

HIGH-GRADE UROTHELIAL NEOPLASIA

Carcinoma in situ and high-grade transitional cell carcinoma exfoliate readily, and urine specimens from affected patients usually contain numerous malignant cells. These high-grade lesions are cytologically indistinguishable (Figs. 9–80 to 9–84). They shed predominantly as single cells with scattered small clusters even when they arise from high-grade papillary tumors. Classic nuclear criteria of malignancy are seen, including nuclear pleomorphism, irregular nuclear borders, coarsely granular chromatin, irregular chromatin clearing, and sometimes abnormal nucleoli. Intermediate-grade tumors exfoliate in more papillary groups with fewer single cells and show more subtle malignant nuclear features (Figs. 9–85 and 9–86). The dense cytoplasm characteristic of transitional cells manifests in single cells as a sharp cytoplasmic edge and in cell groups as well-defined cell borders. Cytoplasmic vacuolization may be seen in cells from these higher-grade transitional cell carcinomas. Although mucin can be focally demonstrated, positive cells are rare, and other features of adenocarcinoma are not seen.

Although squamous cell carcinomas of the urinary bladder are rare, they occur with increased frequency in patients with chronic schistosomiasis and in those with exstrophy. They are most often well-differentiated keratinizing tumors exfoliating as single malignant cells. The cytologic features are identical to those seen in keratinizing squamous cell carcinomas occurring elsewhere (Figs. 9–87 and 9–88). Nuclei show classic malignant features or are opaque, without discernible chromatin structure. Dense orangeophilic or green-blue cytoplasm reveals the squamous nature of the malignant cells.

Primary adenocarcinomas of the bladder are rare, accounting for less than 2.5% of all primary neoplasms of the urinary bladder. They arise most frequently in the trigone, in an area of glandular metaplasia associated with chronic irritation. Other cases occur in patients with bladder exstrophy or in a urachal remnant in or near the dome of the bladder. Primary adenocarcinomas appear grossly as solitary masses without the multifocality of many transitional cell carcinomas. The majority are moderately to well differentiated mucinous adenocarcinomas with abundant extracellular mucin. They exfoliate predominantly as variably sized three-dimensional groups showing foci of nuclear palisading (Figs. 9–89 and 9–90). Intracellular and extracellular mucin is often abundant. Characteristically, cells of primary urothelial adenocarcinoma contain eccentric, vesicular nuclei with sometimes subtle nuclear criteria of malignancy, including parachromatin clearing and abnormal nuclear contours with or without prominent nucleoli. The cytoplasm is soft or vacuolated with often indistinct borders.

Although exceedingly rare, sarcomas may involve the urinary tract and also occur as single malignant cells. The most common primary sarcomas include rhabdomyosarcoma and leiomyosarcoma. Cells may be small and round or pleomorphic with nuclear features of malignancy and spindled cytoplasm. Sarcoma should be included in the differential diagnosis of any undifferentiated urinary tract malignancy.

MALIGNANCY SECONDARILY INVOLVING THE URINARY BLADDER

Malignant tumors not infrequently involve the urinary bladder by direct extension from an adjacent primary tumor, particularly of the rectum or prostate. Primary rectal adenocarcinomas are usually moderately to well differentiated mucinous adenocarcinomas both histologically and cytologically indistinguishable from most primary bladder adenocarcinomas (Figs. 9–91 and 9–92). Clinical correlation usually allows distinction.

Many prostatic adenocarcinomas have a characteristic appearance in urine cytology specimens. They exfoliate in variably sized syncytial groups with component cells showing large nuclei with powdery chromatin and prominent macronucleoli in almost every cell (Fig. 9–93). Cytoplasm is soft and usually contains no mucin. Immunocytochemically, most prostatic adenocarcinomas are distinct from adenocarcinomas arising in the urinary bladder and rectum as well as from transitional cell carcinomas. The prostatic tumors usually show reactivity with antibodies to prostatic alkaline phosphatase and/or prostate-specific antigen but not with antibody to carcinoembryonic antigen. The other three tumor types characteristically show the opposite staining pattern.

Difficult differential diagnoses are summarized in Table 9–2.

Bibliography

Droller MJ, Erozan YS: Thiotepa effects on urinary cytology in the interpretation of transitional cell cancer. J Urol 134:671–674, 1985.

Farrow GM: Pathologist's role in bladder cancer. Semin Oncol 6:198–206, 1979.

Farrow GM, Utz DC, Rife CC, Greene LF: Clinical observations on sixty-nine cases of in situ carcinoma of the urinary bladder. Cancer Res 37:2794–2798, 1977.

Graff L: Microscopic examination of the urinary sediment (crystals). In Graff L (ed.): A Handbook of Routine Urinalysis. Philadelphia: J.B. Lippincott, 1983, pp 83–107.

Highman WJ: Flat in situ carcinoma of the bladder: cytological examination of urine in diagnosis, follow-up, and assessment of response to chemotherapy. J Clin Pathol 41:540–546, 1988.

Koss LG: The urinary tract in the absence of cancer. In Koss LG (ed.): Diagnostic Cytology and its Histopathologic Basis. Philadelphia: J.B. Lippincott, 1979, pp 711–748.

Koss LG, Deitch D, Ramanathan R, Sherman AB: Diagnostic value of cytology of voided urine. Acta Cytol 29:810–816, 1985.

Murphy WM: Current status of urinary cytology in the evaluation of bladder neoplasms. Human Pathol 21:886–896, 1990.

Schumann GB: Urine sediment findings in various renal diseases. In Schumann GB (ed.): Urine Sediment Examination. Baltimore: Williams and Wilkins, 1980, pp 138–173.

Weiss MA: Urinary cytology of transitional cell neoplasms of the bladder. In Young RH (ed.): Pathology of the Urinary Bladder. New York: Churchill Livingstone, 1989, pp 245–284.

Table 9–1. CRYSTALS SEEN IN PAPANICOLAOU-STAINED PREPARATIONS

Morphology	Type	Urine pH	Clinical Significance
	Amorphous urates	≤7	none
	Amorphous phosphates	≥7	none
	Triple phosphate	≥7	usually none*
	Ammonium biurate	≥7	none
	Uric acid (brownish yellow)	≤7	usually none†
	Calcium oxalate	5 – 8	usually none‡
	Cystine	≤7	cystinuria due to inborn error of metabolism
	Bilirubin	≤7	bilirubinuria due to conjugated hyperbilirubinemia
	Leucine	≤7	aminoaciduria of severe liver disease
	Tyrosine	≤7	aminoaciduria of severe liver disease

*Can be seen in infected urine of alkaline pH.

†Can be seen in hyperuricemia with hyperuricosuria in conditions associated with increased nucleoprotein turnover (e.g., tumor lysis syndrome, high fever) or Lesch-Nyhan syndrome.

‡Can be seen in patients with oxalate calculi and in oxaluria due to fat malabsorption, ascorbic acid loading, hereditary oxaluria, or ethylene glycol poisoning.

Table 9–2. DIFFICULT DIFFERENTIAL DIAGNOSES

Low-grade transitional cell neoplasm versus urothelial fragments associated with renal calculi (Figs. 9–94A and 9–94B):
- Both present as benign-appearing urothelial fragments in voided urine.
- Reactive nuclear features (particularly prominent nucleoli) and vacuolated cytoplasm are cytologic features sometimes associated with renal calculi but not often with neoplasia.
- Since they are sometimes cytologically indistinguishable, clinical correlation is essential.
  Transitional cell fragments versus renal tubular epithelial fragments (Figs. 9–95A and 9–95B):
- Both can appear as three-dimensional clusters of cells with bland or reactive nuclear features.
- The cytoplasm of transitional cells is usually denser than that of renal tubular cells.
- Nuclei of transitional cells are usually centrally positioned, and those of renal cells are eccentric.
- Renal tubular cell fragments are usually found in urines showing other features of renal parenchymal disease.

High-grade transitional cell carcinoma versus cyclophosphamide therapeutic effect versus polyoma virus infection (Figs. 9–96A to 9–96D):
- All can be cellular specimens.
- All can be associated with single cells with large, degenerated, hyperchromatic nuclei in urine specimens of affected patients, and the presence of these cells in a urine specimen demands careful scrutiny of the specimen for preserved cells with diagnostic features.
- Cells diagnostic of high-grade transitional cell carcinoma contain nuclei with a well-preserved, granular chromatin, abnormal chromatin clearing, and abnormal nuclear contours.
- Cells characteristic of cyclophosphamide effect or polyoma virus infection are always degenerated with chromatin in a reticular pattern, often peripherally displaced or peripherally clumped.
- Cells diagnostic of polyoma virus infection contain gray-blue intranuclear inclusions usually filling the nucleus but sometimes associated with a narrow peri-inclusion clear zone.
  Necrotic transitional cell neoplasm versus ileal conduit specimen (Figs. 9–97A and 9–97B):
- Both contain numerous epithelial cells both singly and in three-dimensional fragments showing marked degeneration.
- Ileal conduit specimens often show a dirty background caused by mucus and bacteria.
- Specimens containing necrotic transitional cell carcinoma have a dirty background caused by cellular debris.
- Columnar configuration can sometimes be appreciated in some epithelial cells in ileal conduit specimens.
- Rare diagnostic malignant cells can usually be found in specimens containing necrotic neoplastic cells.
- Clinical history is helpful in making this distinction.
  Endometrial cells versus primary urothelial adenocarcinoma (Figs. 9–98A and 9–98B):
- Both can present with three-dimensional groups of cells containing hypochromatic nuclei with irregular nuclear borders in urine specimens.
- The irregular nuclear borders of endometrial cells are the result of degenerative wrinkling whereas those seen in adenocarcinoma are characteristic of malignancy.
- Prominent nucleoli are more characteristic of adenocarcinoma than endometrial cells.
- Most primary urothelial adenocarcinomas contain intracellular mucin, most endometrial cells do not.
- Endometrial cells are usually found in urine containing other evidence of contamination by the female genital tract.

Squamous dysplasia of genital tract origin versus squamous carcinoma (Figs. 9–99A and 9–99B):
- Both can present with abnormal keratinizing squamous cells in voided urine specimens.
- Urine containing squamous dysplasia of genital origin usually shows other evidence of genital contamination.
- In squamous dysplasia of genital origin abnormal cells are usually few in number, whereas in carcinoma numerous abnormal cells are present.
- In squamous dysplasia, nuclei are hyperchromatic with granular, evenly dispersed chromatin and rounded nuclear contours.
- In squamous carcinoma, some abnormal cells contain nuclei, fulfilling malignant criteria.

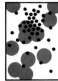

NORMAL CELLS

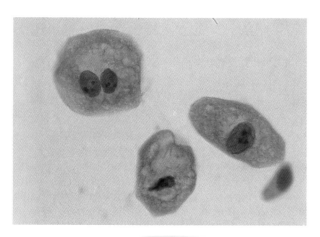

FIGURE 9–1. Superficial (Umbrella) Urothelial Cells (Papanicolaou-stained cytospin preparation, × 250).

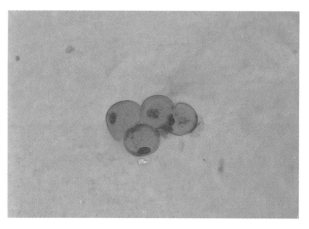

FIGURE 9–3. Intermediate Urothelial Cells containing cytoplasmic glycogen (Papanicolaou-stained filter preparation, × 250).

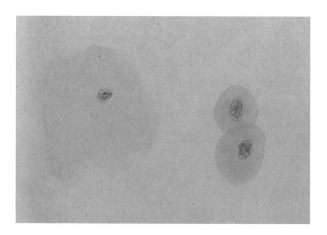

FIGURE 9–2. Normal Intermediate Urothelial Cells and a Squamous Cell. The thin, transparent cytoplasm of squamous cells is usually distinguishable from the denser cytoplasm of urothelial cells (Papanicolaou-stained filter preparation, × 250).

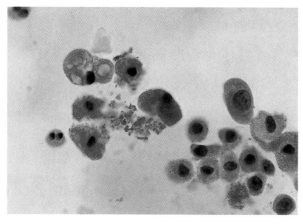

FIGURE 9–4. Renal Epithelial Cells of proximal (larger cells) and distal (smaller cells) convoluted tubular types. The granular cytoplasm and associated tubular debris distinguish these cells from urothelial cells. When convoluted tubular cells become degenerated or phagocytic, they can be difficult to distinguish from histiocytes. When anucleate, they resemble small granular casts, and when multinucleate, they resemble tubular epithelial casts. Familiarity with these variable appearances and attention to associated, more easily identified cells facilitate correct identification of tubular cells (Papanicolaou-stained cytospin preparation, × 250).

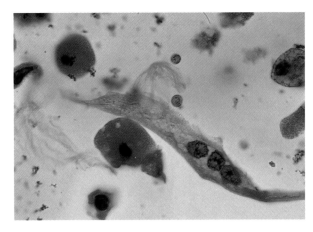

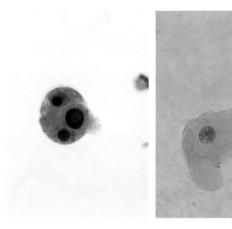

FIGURE 9–5. Umbrella Urothelial Cell with **Renal Epithelial Cells** of convoluted tubular type and a single polygonal collecting-duct–type renal cell (Papanicolaou-stained cytospin preparation, × 250).

FIGURE 9–7A,B. Degenerated Epithelial Cells containing eosinophilic and turquoise-staining **Cytoplasmic Inclusions.** These degenerated epithelial cells can be difficult to distinguish from histiocytes containing phagocytized debris. Familiarity with the characteristic appearance of the inclusions usually allows distinction. Also shown is a squamous cell (Papanicolaou-stained cytospin preparation, × 250).

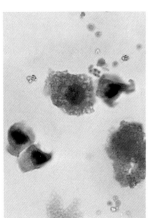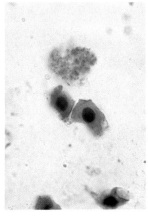

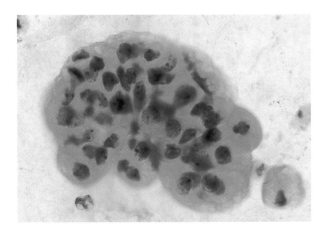

FIGURE 9–6A,B. Composite photograph showing polygonal-shaped, collecting-duct–type **Renal Epithelial Cells** associated with granular tubular debris and a single, granular, convoluted tubular cell (Fig. 9–6A). These cells are distinguishable from lymphocytes, which are of similar size, by their more abundant polygonal-shaped cytoplasm and characteristic round nuclei with finely granular, evenly distributed chromatin (Papanicolaou-stained cytospins, × 250).

FIGURE 9–8. Pseudopapillary Urothelial Fragment in instrumented urine. Note uniform oval nuclei with powdery chromatin, small nucleoli, and vacuolated cytoplasm. Although similar urothelial fragments can originate from a low-grade papillary urothelial neoplasm, the normochromasia, smooth nuclear borders, prominent nucleoli, and vacuolated cytoplasm seen in this fragment are characteristic of instrumented or reactive urothelium (Papanicolaou-stained filter preparation, × 250).

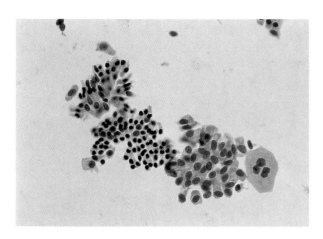

FIGURE 9–9. Urothelial Cells of Superficial, Intermediate, and Deep Types in an instrumented urine specimen (Papanicolaou-stained cytospin preparation, × 100).

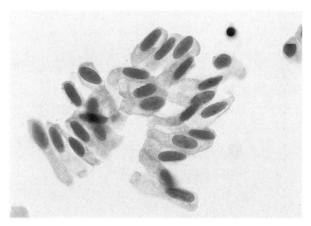

FIGURE 9–11. Intermediate Urothelial Cells assuming a columnar shape in instrumented urine (Papanicolaou-stained cytospin preparation, × 250).

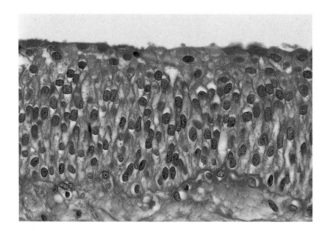

FIGURE 9–10. Normal Urothelium showing polarity, maturation, cytoplasmic clearing because of glycogen, and uniform, oval nuclei with powdery chromatin and small nucleoli (histologic section, × 160).

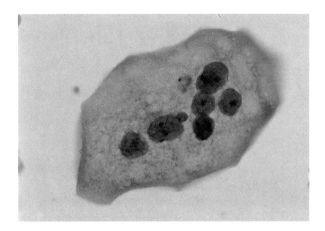

FIGURE 9–12. Multinucleated Umbrella Cell in instrumented urine (Papanicolaou-stained cytospin preparation, × 250).

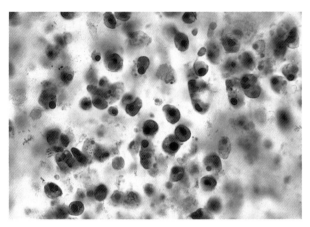

FIGURE 9–14. Ileal Conduit Urine containing numerous single degenerated epithelial cells with eosinophilic cytoplasmic inclusions and a background of mucus (Papanicolaou-stained filter preparation, × 250).

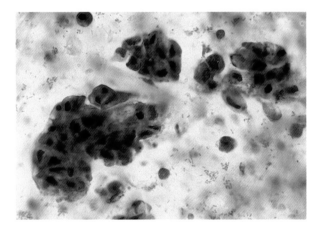

FIGURE 9–13. Ileal Conduit Specimen showing ileal epithelial cells singly and in fragments. Note cellular degeneration and a background of mucus and coliform bacteria (Papanicolaou-stained filter, × 250).

BENIGN CONDITIONS

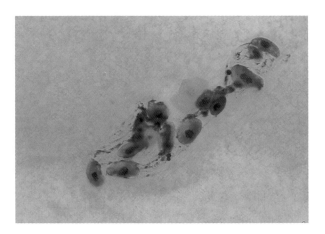

FIGURE 9–15. Blue-staining **mucus** strand with associated urothelial cells (Papanicolaou-stained filter preparation, × 250).

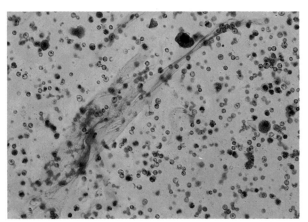

FIGURE 9–17. Fibrin associated with hematuria (Papanicolaou-stained filter preparation, × 100).

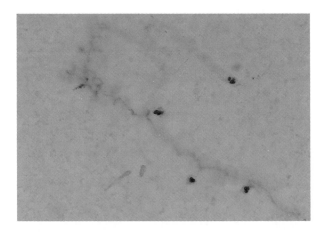

FIGURE 9–16. Mucus in the configuration of a Curschmann spiral (Papanicolaou-stained filter preparation, × 160).

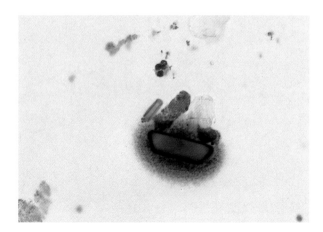

FIGURE 9–18. Triple Phosphate Crystals appearing as prisms, with oblique ends resembling "coffin lids." Note the granular halo reflecting partial dissolution of the crystal associated with processing (Papanicolaou-stained cytospin preparation, × 250).

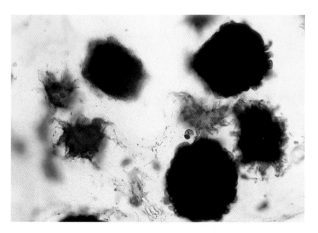

FIGURE 9–20. Ammonium Biurate Crystals showing spiculated "thorn apple" appearance and adjacent, blue-staining, partially dissolved crystals (Papanicolaou-stained cytospin preparation, × 250).

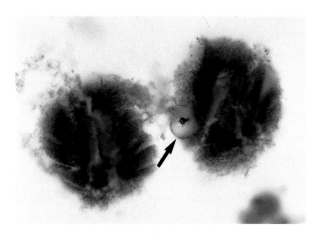

FIGURE 9–19. Amorphous Phosphates remaining in place of dissolved triple phosphate crystals. Note talc crystal (arrow) (Papanicolaou-stained cytospin preparation, × 250).

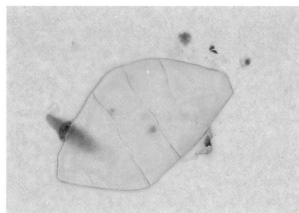

FIGURE 9–21. Uric Acid Crystal with "plate" shape. These crystals appear yellowish brown because they stain with urinary pigments (Papanicolaou-stained filter preparation, × 160).

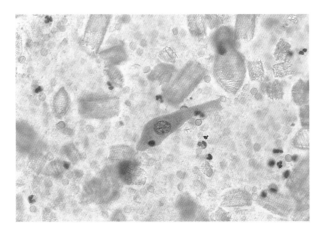

FIGURE 9–22. Reactive umbrella cell associated with numerous small **Uric Acid Crystals** and red blood cells (Papanicolaou-stained filter preparation, × 160).

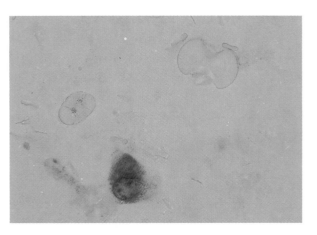

FIGURE 9–24. Calcium Oxalate Crystals in oval and dumbbell shapes. A reactive urothelial cell is partially in focus (Papanicolaou-stained filter preparation, × 250).

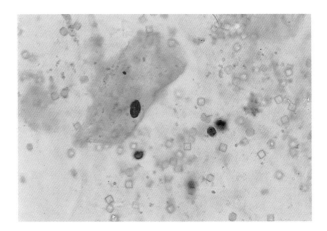

FIGURE 9–23. Tiny **Calcium Oxalate Crystals** appearing as colorless squares. Their six-sided architecture is not apparent in this photograph (Papanicolaou-stained smear preparation, × 250).

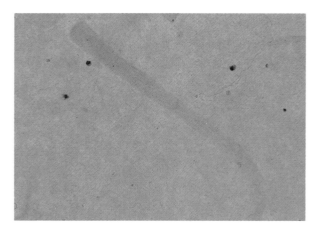

FIGURE 9–25. Hyaline Cast (Papanicolaou-stained filter preparation, × 100).

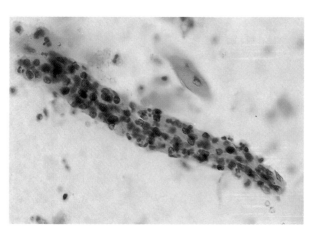

FIGURE 9–28. Leukocyte Cast containing lymphocytes and rare neutrophils (Papanicolaou-stained filter preparation, × 160).

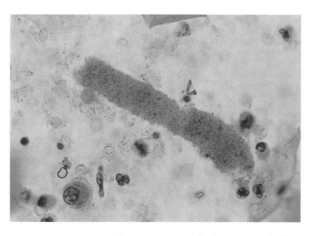

FIGURE 9–26. Granular Cast (Papanicolaou-stained filter preparation, × 250).

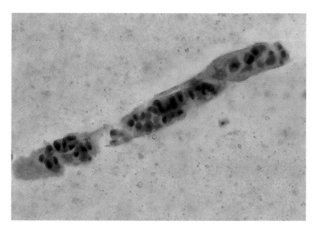

FIGURE 9–29. Renal Tubular Epithelial Cast with constituent cells of collecting-duct–type (Papanicolaou-stained filter preparation, × 160).

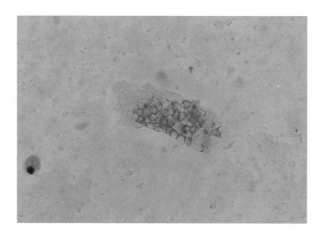

FIGURE 9–27. Erythrocyte Cast (Papanicolaou-stained filter preparation, × 250).

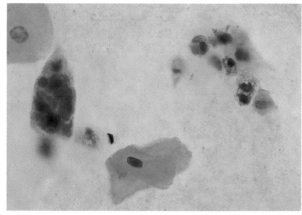

FIGURE 9–30. Renal Tubular Epithelial Cast and tubular cells showing reactive cytologic features. Squamous cells are also shown (Papanicolaou-stained filter preparation, × 250).

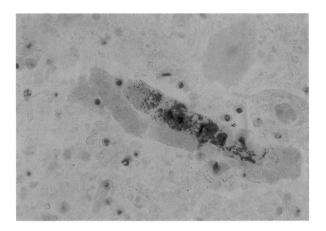

FIGURE 9–31. Coarse Granular Cast with adjacent erythrocyte cast (Papanicolaou-stained filter, × 160).

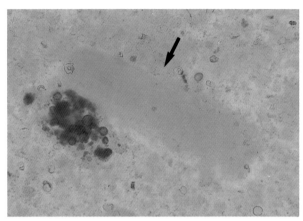

FIGURE 9–34. Broad Hyaline Cast (arrows) occurring in a pathologic sediment (Papanicolaou-stained filter preparation, × 250).

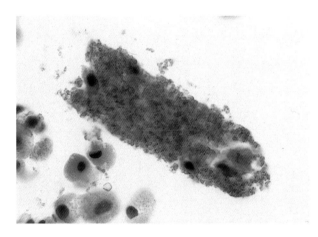

FIGURE 9–32. Hemoglobin Cast with associated renal tubular cells (Papanicolaou-stained cytospin preparation, × 250).

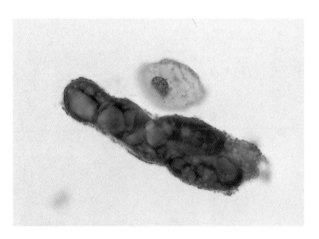

FIGURE 9–35. Fatty Cast. A urothelial cell is also shown (Papanicolaou-stained cytospin preparation, × 250).

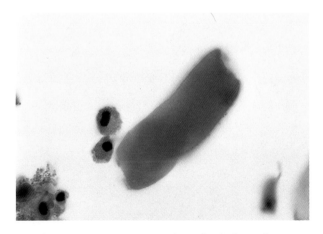

FIGURE 9–33. Waxy Cast and renal tubular cells (Papanicolaou-stained cytospin, × 250).

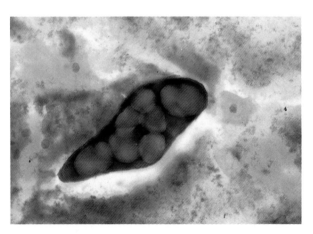

FIGURE 9–36. Fatty Cast with background of squamous cells and amorphous phosphates (Papanicolaou-stained filter, × 330).

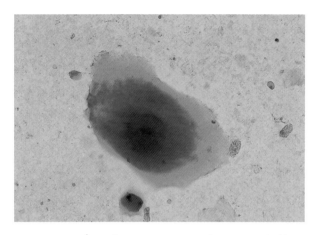

FIGURE 9–37. Lubricant (Papanicolaou-stained filter, × 100).

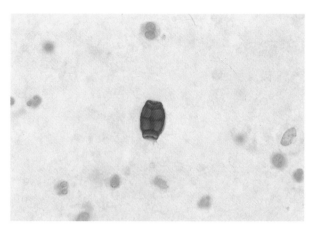

FIGURE 9–40. *Alternaria macroconidia* with characteristic longitudinal and horizontal striations (Papanicolaou-stained filter preparation, × 250).

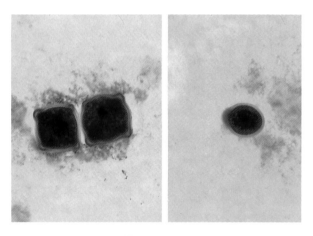

FIGURE 9–38A,B. Pollen in square and round shapes (Papanicolaou-stained filter preparations, × 250).

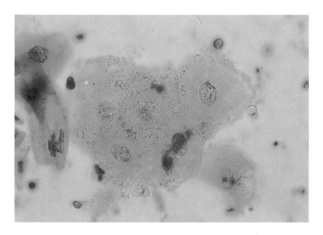

FIGURE 9–41. Carpet Beetle Larva Hair showing fish head and skeleton appearance (Papanicolaou-stained filter preparation, × 132).

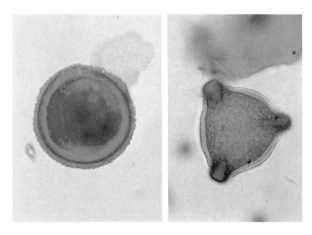

FIGURE 9–39A,B. Pollen showing round and triangular shapes and variable staining (Papanicolaou-stained filter preparations, × 330).

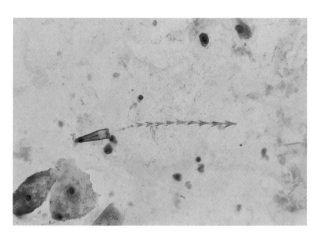

FIGURE 9–42. Squamous Cells of Vaginal Origin with associated vaginal flora bacteria (Papanicolaou-stained filter preparation, × 250).

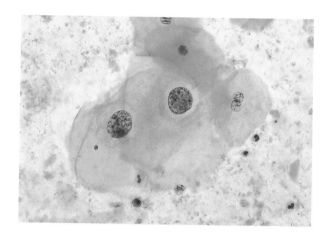

FIGURE 9–43. Urine containing cells exfoliated from a **Low-Grade Squamous Intraepithelial Lesion (mild dysplasia)** of the female reproductive tract. Note binucleate squamous cell with nuclei of normal size and chromasia. Although the nuclei of the dysplastic cells are similar in character to those seen in urothelial dysplasia, the squamous cytoplasm in these cells is clearly distinguishable from urothelial cytoplasm (Papanicolaou-stained filter preparation, × 160).

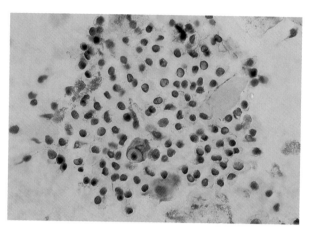

FIGURE 9–45. Prostatic Epithelial Cells in voided urine appearing as a loosely cohesive group of columnar cells with vacuolated cytoplasm. These cells could be mistaken for cells exfoliated from a focus of glandular metaplasia. A background showing spermatozoa, prostatic concretions, or seminal vesical epithelium facilitates their identification, as can clinical correlation (Papanicolaou-stained filter preparation, × 160).

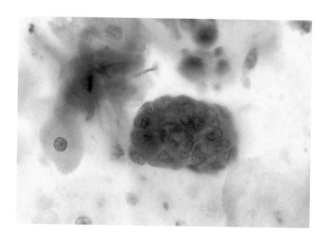

FIGURE 9–44. Endometrial Cells in a voided urine specimen present as three-dimensional groups of cells with wrinkled, hypochromatic nuclei. These cells resemble the cells of primary and secondary adenocarcinoma. The inapparent nucleoli and wrinkled nuclear membranes are more characteristic of benign endometrial cells. A background consistent with vaginal contamination and a corroborating clinical history allow correct identification of these cells. Note the fungal pseudohyphae in association with squamous cells of vaginal origin adjacent to the endometrial cells (Papanicolaou-stained filter preparation, × 250).

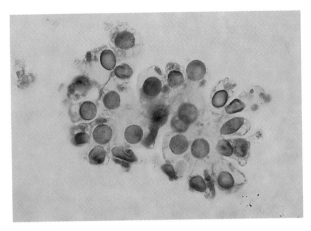

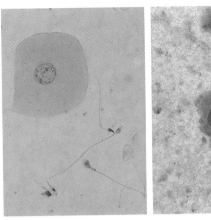

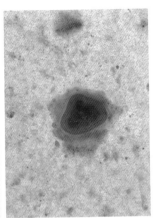

FIGURE 9–46. Seminal Vesicle Epithelial Cells in voided urine containing prominent cytoplasmic pigment. The powdery chromatin pattern characteristic of these cells is similar to that seen in prostatic adenocarcinoma. Lack of prominent nucleoli and the presence of cytoplasmic pigment allow correct identification (Papanicolaou-stained filter preparation, × 250).

FIGURE 9–47A. Spermatozoa with a urothelial cell in voided urine (Papanicolaou-stained filter preparation, × 250).

FIGURE 9–47B. Prostatic Concretion in voided urine (Papanicolaou-stained filter preparation, × 160).

INFECTIONS

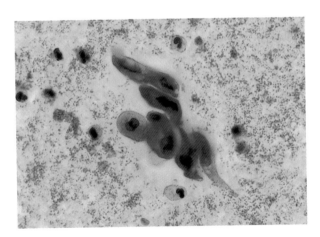

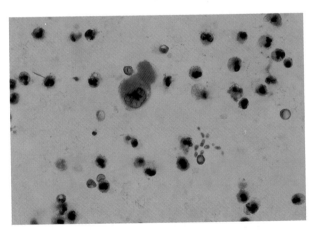

FIGURE 9–48. *Escherichia coli* Cystitis with reactive urothelial cells (Papanicolaou-stained filter preparation, × 250).

FIGURE 9–49. *Candida glabrata* Cystitis showing characteristic budding yeast together with red blood cells, neutrophils, and a reactive urothelial cell (Papanicolaou-stained filter preparation, × 250).

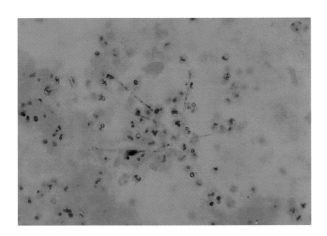

FIGURE 9–50. *Candida albicans* **Cystitis** showing pseudohyphae and associated inflammatory cells (Papanicolaou-stained filter preparation, × 160).

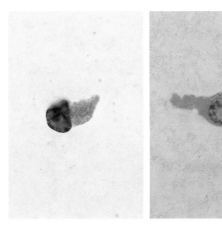

FIGURE 9–52A,B. "**Comet-shaped**" **Cells** in the urines of patients infected with polyoma virus. Indistinguishable degenerated cells can be seen in urines showing cyclophosphamide therapeutic effect and in high-grade transitional cell carcinoma. Diagnostic intranuclear inclusions should be found for definitive diagnosis of polyoma virus infection. Preserved cells with nuclei fulfilling criteria of malignancy must be found in order to diagnose malignancy. Cyclophosphamide therapeutic effect is a diagnosis of exclusion, since cyclophosphamide-treated patients are at greater risk for both polyoma virus infection and urothelial malignancy (Papanicolaou-stained filter preparation, × 250).

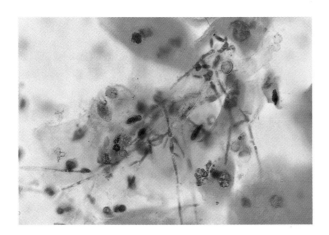

FIGURE 9–51. *Candida albicans* **Vaginitis** contaminating voided urine. Note typical shishkabob configuration of the squamous cells associated with the pseudohyphal form (Papanicolaou-stained filter, × 250).

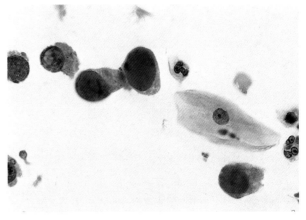

FIGURE 9–53. Polyoma Virus-infected cells with diagnostic grey-blue inclusions filling their nuclei. Also note the degenerated epithelial cells with large, markedly eccentric cytoplasm and the squamous cell (Papanicolaou-stained cytospin preparation, × 250).

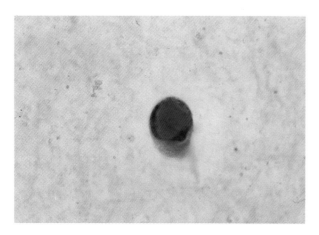

FIGURE 9–54. Epithelial cell containing diagnostic polyoma viral inclusion. The peripherally displaced chromatin is characteristic (Papanicolaou-stained filter preparation, × 250).

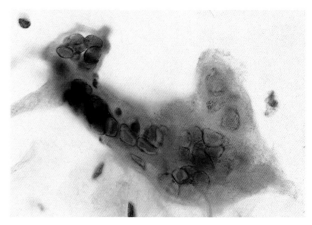

FIGURE 9–56. Herpes Simplex Virus. Infected cell with squamous cytoplasmic features and multiple molding nuclei containing eosinophilic intranuclear inclusions (Papanicolaou-stained filter preparation, × 250).

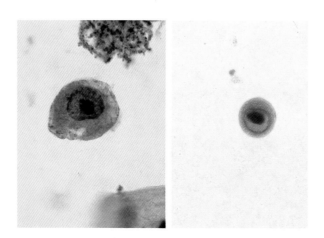

FIGURE 9–55A. Cytomegalic Inclusion Disease. This infected cell shows marked degeneration (Papanicolaou-stained cytospin preparation, × 330).
FIGURE 9–55B. Cytomegalic Inclusion Disease. This diagnostic cell contains a dense, intranuclear inclusion with a prominent peri-inclusion clear zone and peripherally displaced chromatin (Papanicolaou-stained filter preparation, × 250).

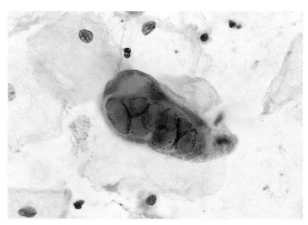

FIGURE 9–57. Herpes Simplex Virus. Infected cells showing glassy intranuclear inclusions (Papanicolaou-stained filter preparation, × 250).

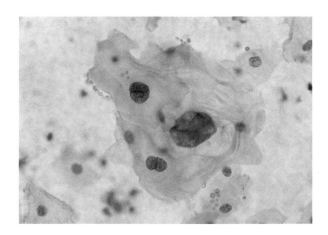

FIGURE 9–58. Human Papilloma Virus. Infected cells in voided urine showing koilocytosis and dyskaryosis (Papanicolaou-stained filter preparation, × 250).

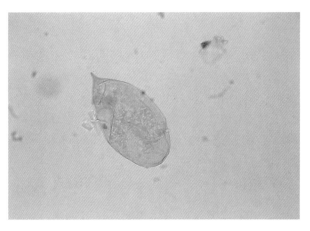

FIGURE 9–60. *Schistosoma haematobium* **Egg** showing a characteristic terminal spine (Papanicolaou-stained cytospin preparation, × 132).

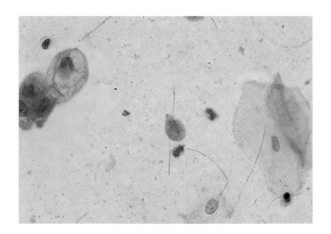

FIGURE 9–59. *Trichomonas vaginalis.* Organism has typical pear shape, poorly defined nucleus, and central axostyle. Note the associated filamentous bacteria that are frequently present in specimens containing trichomonads. Also shown are a squamous cell and urothelial cells (Papanicolaou-stained filter preparation, × 250).

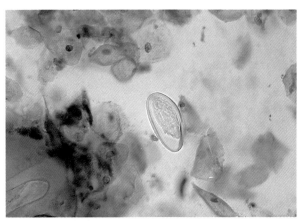

FIGURE 9–61. *Enterobius vermicularis* **(Pinworm) Egg** showing characteristic internal structure and flattened side. Numerous squamous cells and a triple phosphate crystal can also be seen (Papanicolaou-stained cytospin preparation, × 132).

REACTIVE, REPARATIVE, AND THERAPEUTIC EFFECTS

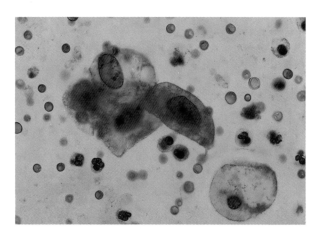

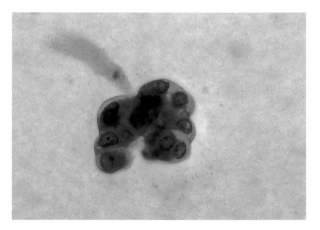

FIGURE 9–62. Reactive urothelial cells in **Hemorrhagic Cystitis**. These cells are characterized by cellular and nuclear enlargement, hyperchromasia, chromatin clearing, prominent nucleoli, and cytoplasmic vacuolization. They resemble cells that can be found in the presence of a high-grade urothelial malignancy. Attention to the reactive nuclear features, relatively low nuclear to cytoplasmic ratios, cytoplasmic vacuolization, lack of tumor cellularity, and background of blood and inflammation is helpful in the differential diagnosis. However, definitive diagnosis is not always possible, and follow-up cytology may be indicated (Papanicolaou-stained filter preparation, × 250).

FIGURE 9–64. Pseudopapillary urothelial fragment in the voided urine of a patient with **Renal Calculi** showing reactive nuclear features. The differential diagnosis includes a low-grade papillary neoplasm. The reactive nuclear features seen in these cells, particularly the prominent nucleoli, are more characteristic of a reactive process (Papanicolaou-stained filter preparation, × 160).

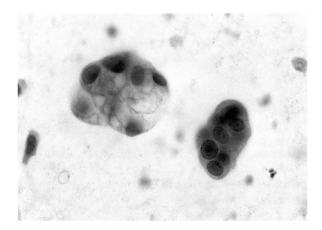

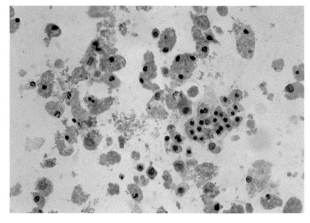

FIGURE 9–63. Pseudopapillary urothelial fragments in a patient with **Renal Calculi**. Note prominent cytoplasmic vacuolization. Although similar fragments can be seen in the voided urine specimens of patients with low-grade papillary neoplasms, the cytoplasmic vacuolization is more characteristic of a reactive process. Clinical and radiologic correlation should allow definitive diagnosis (Papanicolaou-stained filter preparation, × 250).

FIGURE 9–65. Acute Tubular Necrosis characterized by high cellularity with a predominance of necrotic renal epithelial cells of the proximal convoluted type (Papanicolaou-stained cytospin, × 66).

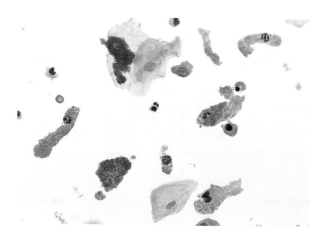

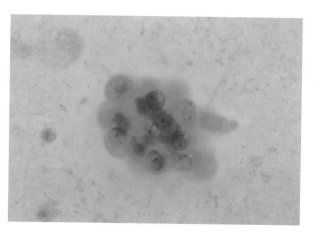

FIGURE 9–66. Acute Tubular Necrosis as a result of drug toxicity. The slide shows necrotic, convoluted-type renal tubular cells resembling small granular casts. The presence of nuclei, albeit degenerate, in some of the cells and the absence of a discernible cast matrix allows distinction (Papanicolaou-stained cytospin preparation, × 160).

FIGURE 9–68. Well-preserved **Reactive Renal Epithelial Cells** difficult to distinguish from urothelial cells because of their somewhat dense cytoplasm. The presence in the specimen of pathologic casts and other, more easily identified renal epithelial cells allows correct identification (Papanicolaou-stained filter preparation, × 250).

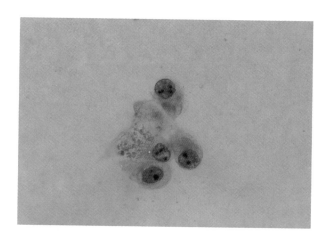

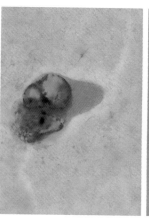

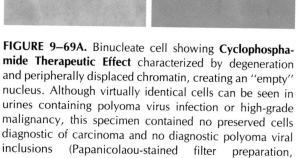

FIGURE 9–67. Renal Epithelial Cells showing reactive nuclear features. The soft cytoplasm and associated granular tubular debris allow differentiation from epithelium of urothelial origin (Papanicolaou-stained filter preparation, × 250).

FIGURE 9–69A. Binucleate cell showing **Cyclophosphamide Therapeutic Effect** characterized by degeneration and peripherally displaced chromatin, creating an "empty" nucleus. Although virtually identical cells can be seen in urines containing polyoma virus infection or high-grade malignancy, this specimen contained no preserved cells diagnostic of carcinoma and no diagnostic polyoma viral inclusions (Papanicolaou-stained filter preparation, × 250).
FIGURE 9–69B. Cell showing **Cyclophosphamide Therapeutic Effect** characterized by degeneration and an enlarged hyperchromatic nucleus with reticular chromatin pattern. The differential diagnosis includes a degenerated malignant cell and polyoma virus infection (Papanicolaou-stained filter, × 250).

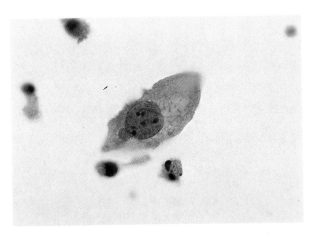

FIGURE 9–70. Benign umbrella cell showing **Effects of Topical Chemotherapy**, including abnormal nuclear contour, hyperchromasia, multiple prominent nucleoli, and cytoplasmic vacuolization (Papanicolaou-stained cytospin preparation, × 250).

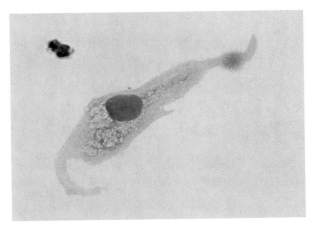

FIGURE 9–72. Radiated Umbrella Cell showing cellular enlargement, smudged chromatin, nuclear and cytoplasmic vacuolization, and cytoplasmic polychromasia (Papanicolaou-stained cytospin preparation, × 250).

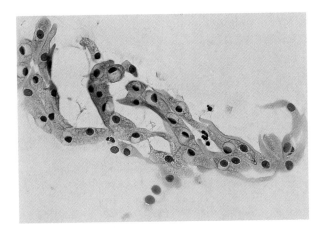

FIGURE 9–71. Sheet of benign urothelial cells demonstrating **Effects of Local Ionizing Radiation**, including cytoplasmic vacuolization (Papanicolaou-stained cytospin preparation, × 100).

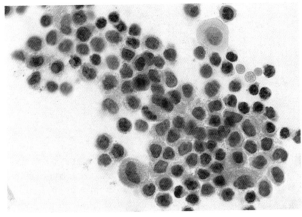

FIGURE 9–73. Lymphohistiocytic Aggregate exfoliated from patient treated with **BCG** (Papanicolaou-stained cytospin preparation, × 250).

DYSPLASIA AND LOW-GRADE MALIGNANCY

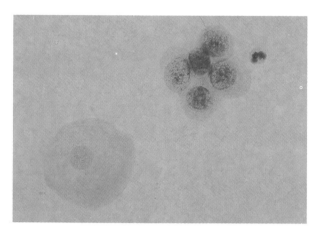

FIGURE 9–74. Dysplastic Urothelial Cells with adjacent normal urothelial cell. The small group of enlarged cells with hyperchromatic nuclei showing a granular, evenly distributed chromatin pattern, subtle irregularities of the nuclear contour, and inapparent nucleoli is characteristic of urothelial dysplasia. However, cells exfoliated from a low-grade papillary urothelial neoplasm can appear identical, and follow-up cystoscopy and biopsy are essential in the differential diagnosis (Papanicolaou-stained filter preparation, × 250).

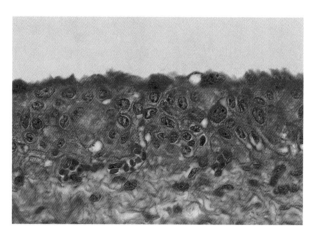

FIGURE 9–76. Urothelial Dysplasia characterized by nuclear enlargement, loss of cytoplasmic clearing because of glycogen, and altered polarity (histologic section, × 160).

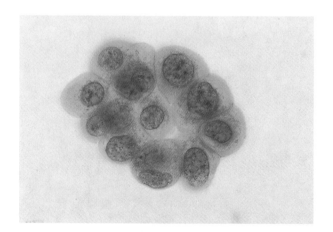

FIGURE 9–75. Urothelial Dysplasia. Small group of cells showing nuclear enlargement, slightly irregular nuclear contours, hyperchromasia, and a granular chromatin pattern. Nucleoli are not apparent. The differential diagnosis includes a low-grade papillary urothelial neoplasm (Papanicolaou-stained filter preparation, × 250).

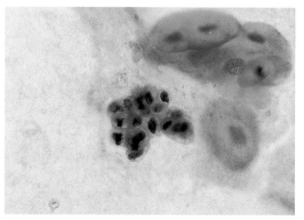

FIGURE 9–77. Degenerated epithelial fragment exfoliated from a **Low-Grade Papillary Transitional Cell Neoplasm.** Note the small size of the constituent cells. Similar degenerated papillary fragments can be seen in patients with renal calculi or bladder trabeculation related to chronic outlet obstruction. The subtle nuclear membrane abnormalities and absence of nucleoli favor a diagnosis of neoplasia. Cystoscopy is often necessary for definitive diagnosis (Papanicolaou-stained filter preparation, × 250).

MALIGNANT TUMORS

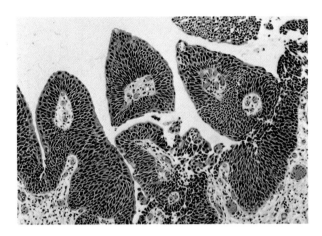

FIGURE 9–78. Low-Grade Papillary Transitional Cell Neoplasm. The uniform, hyperchromatic tumor cells show vertical polarity and are surfaced by umbrella cells (histologic section, × 66).

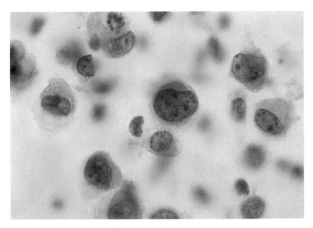

FIGURE 9–80. Numerous single malignant cells exfoliated from **Urothelial Carcinoma in Situ**. Note the high nuclear to cytoplasmic ratios and malignant nuclear features, including chromatin clearing, prominent nuclear membrane abnormalities, and prominent nucleoli in some cells. The high tumor cellularity of the specimen and the unequivocal malignant nuclear features exclude reactive processes from the differential diagnosis. Poorly differentiated adenocarcinoma can appear similarly, with numerous malignant cells containing eccentric nuclei. The dense cytoplasm seen in these cells is a feature of transitional cell differentiation. In cases of high-grade transitional cell carcinoma with cytoplasmic vacuolization, the distinction from adenocarcinoma cannot always be made using morphology alone (Papanicolaou-stained filter, × 250).

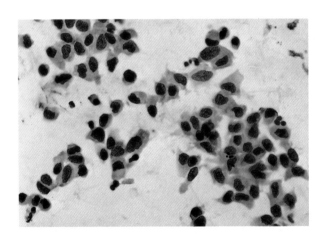

FIGURE 9–79. Vigorous bladder washing specimen containing cells derived from **Low-Grade Papillary Transitional Cell Neoplasm** (same case as shown in Fig. 9–78). The high cellularity and dispersed cell pattern result from the nature of the specimen. Individual cells are characterized by homogeneous cytoplasm and hyperchromatic nuclei with subtle nuclear membrane irregularities and granular, evenly dispersed chromatin without nucleoli (Papanicolaou-stained filter preparation, × 330).

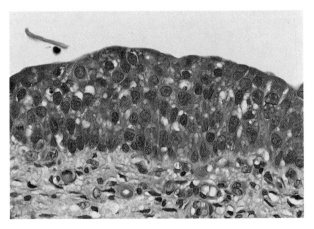

FIGURE 9–81. Carcinoma in Situ characterized by complete loss of polarity and composed of cells showing malignant nuclear features. Some cells contain macronucleoli, and many show cytoplasmic vacuolization (histologic section, × 132).

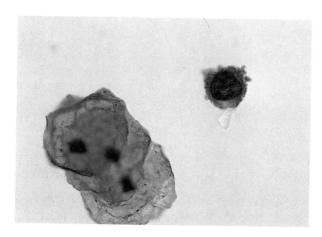

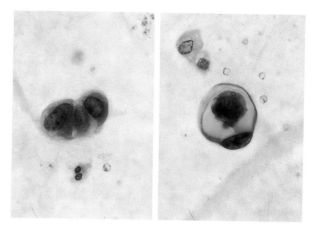

FIGURE 9–82. Single malignant cell originating from a **High-Grade Transitional Cell Carcinoma** with adjacent normal squamous cells (Papanicolaou-stained cytospin preparation, × 250).

FIGURE 9–84A. Group of malignant cells showing "Indian file" configuration exfoliated from a **High-Grade Transitional Cell Carcinoma.** Identical cell groupings can be seen in adenocarcinomas. The dense cytoplasm present in this group is a feature of transitional cell differentiation (Papanicolaou-stained filter preparation, × 250).

FIGURE 9–84B. Cell-in-cell grouping of malignant cells from a **High-Grade Transitional Cell Carcinoma.** The differential diagnosis includes other epithelial malignancies. A search for unequivocal transitional cell differentiation and clinical pathologic correlation can often allow distinction (Papanicolaou-stained filter preparation, × 250).

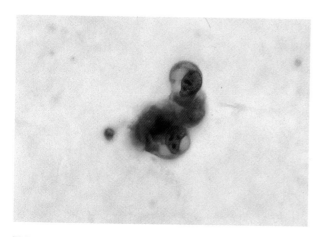

FIGURE 9–83. Three-dimensional group exfoliated from **High-Grade Transitional Cell Carcinoma.** These cells contain pleomorphic, malignant nuclei and vacuolated cytoplasm virtually indistinguishable from cells exfoliated from an adenocarcinoma. A mucin stain can sometimes provide the definitive diagnosis, since abundant mucin production is a feature of many primary and secondary adenocarcinomas seen in urine specimens (Papanicolaou-stained filter preparation, × 250).

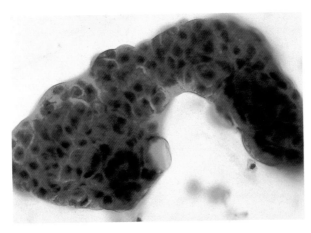

FIGURE 9–85. Papillary epithelial fragment exfoliated from an **Intermediate-Grade Transitional Cell Neoplasm**. Constituent cells show malignant nuclear features. The differential diagnosis includes a low-grade papillary urothelial neoplasm. The presence of many single cells in a voided specimen favors a higher-grade lesion (see Fig. 9–86) (Papanıcolaou-stained filter preparation, × 160).

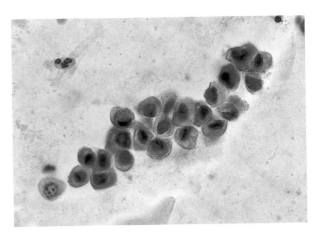

FIGURE 9–86. Intermediate-Grade Transitional Cell Carcinoma. Slide taken from same case shown in Figure 9–85 (Papanicolaou-stained filter preparation, × 250).

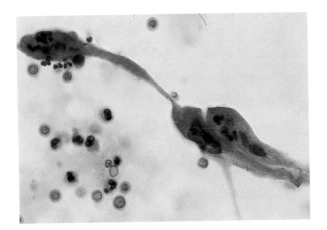

FIGURE 9–87. Keratinizing Squamous Cell Carcinoma of the urinary bladder. The differential diagnosis includes squamous dysplasia and squamous cell carcinoma of the genital tract. The presence of unequivocally malignant nuclei excludes the possibility of squamous dysplasia. The presence of the abnormal cells in a specimen without other evidence of genital contamination or in a catheterized specimen favors primary urothelial origin (Papanicolaou-stained cytospin preparation, × 250).

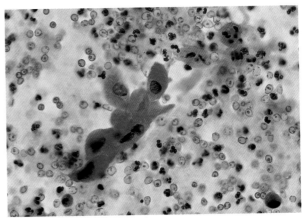

FIGURE 9–88. Keratinizing Squamous Cell Carcinoma of the urinary bladder (Papanicolaou-stained cytospin preparation, × 160).

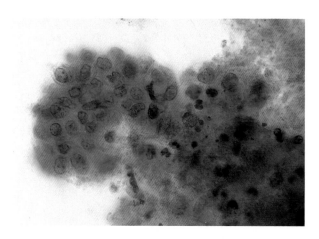

FIGURE 9–89. Three-dimensional group of cells exfoliated from a **Primary Adenocarcinoma** of the urinary bladder. Individual cells contain vesicular, hypochromatic nuclei, sometimes with prominent single nucleoli. Note abundant necrosis. The differential diagnosis includes benign endometrial cells and secondary adenocarcinoma, particularly from a colonic or rectal primary. Necrosis and malignant nuclear features exclude the possibility of a benign diagnosis. Furthermore, nuclear palisading is not seen in groups of endometrial cells. The distinction of primary adenocarcinomas from the more common secondary adenocarcinomas is made largely on clinical grounds (Papanicolaou-stained smear preparation, × 250).

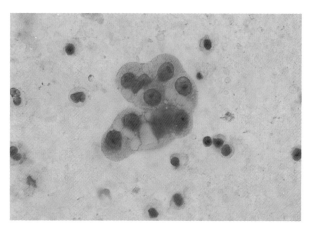

FIGURE 9–91. Cells exfoliated from **Colonic Adenocarcinoma** secondarily involving the urinary bladder. These cells have vesicular nuclei and prominent nucleoli. The differential diagnosis includes high-grade transitional cell carcinoma and primary adenocarcinoma. The three-dimensional and syncytial arrangement of malignant cells, prominent nucleoli, and vacuolated cytoplasm in this tissue fragment favor a diagnosis of adenocarcinoma. Abundant mucin secretion would be further evidence of glandular differentiation. The distinction from primary adenocarcinoma must be made on clinical grounds (Papanicolaou-stained filter preparation, × 250).

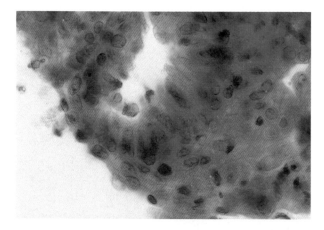

FIGURE 9–90. Primary Adenocarcinoma of the urinary bladder showing prominent nuclear palisading (Papanicolaou-stained smear preparation, × 250).

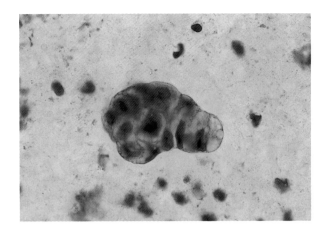

FIGURE 9–92. Cells from **Colonic Adenocarcinoma** appearing in urine show prominent cytoplasmic vacuoles. The differential diagnosis includes primary urothelial adenocarcinoma (Papanicolaou-stained filter preparation, × 250).

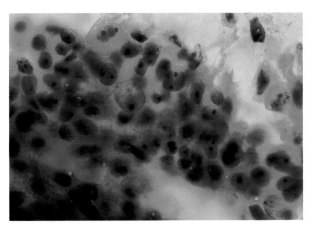

FIGURE 9–93. Cells exfoliated from **Prostatic Adenocarcinoma** secondarily involving the urinary bladder. Constituent cells show a characteristic appearance with finely granular chromatin and prominent macronucleoli. The differential diagnosis includes other adenocarcinomas and benign seminal vesicle epithelial cells, which characteristically have a powdery chromatin pattern. The nuclear crowding, pleomorphism, prominent nucleoli, and lack of cytoplasmic pigment distinguish these cells from benign seminal vesicle cells. Although these cells can be differentiated, on morphologic grounds, from most other adenocarcinomas, lack of mucin production and expression of prostate-specific antigen or prostatic alkaline phosphatase can help in determining the origin of less characteristic cases (Papanicolaou-stained filter preparation, × 250).

DIFFERENTIAL GROUPING

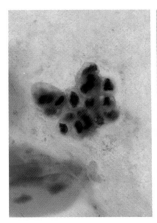
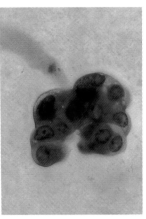

FIGURE 9–94A. Voided transitional cell fragment from patient with **Low-Grade Urothelial Neoplasm** (Papanicolaou-stained filter preparation, × 250).
FIGURE 9–94B. Voided transitional cell fragment from patient with **Renal Calculi**. Although an occasional prominent nucleolus favors a non-neoplastic diagnosis, fragments derived from neoplasms can appear virtually identical (Papanicolaou-stained filter, × 250).

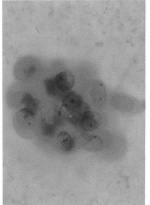
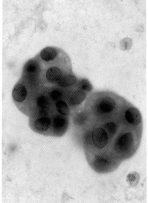

FIGURE 9–95A. **Fragment of Reactive Tubular Cells in Patient with Lupus Nephritis** closely resembling a transitional cell fragment (Papanicolaou-stained filter preparation, × 250).
FIGURE 9–95B. **Voided Transitional Cell Fragment from Patient with Renal Calculus** (Papanicolaou-stained filter preparation, × 250).

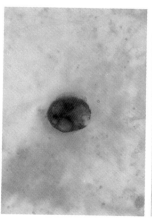
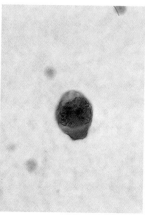

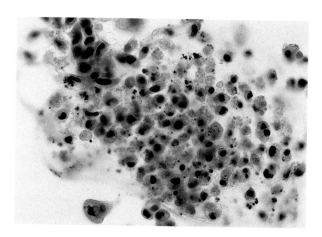

FIGURE 9–96A. Single cell showing **Cyclophosphamide Therapeutic Effect**. Note degenerated nucleus with peripherally displaced chromatin (Papanicolaou-stained filter, × 250).

FIGURE 9–96B. Single malignant cell exfoliated from a **High-Grade Transitional Cell Carcinoma**. Note malignant nuclear features with granular chromatin pattern (Papanicolaou-stained filter preparation, × 250).

FIGURE 9–97A. Necrotic Papillary Transitional Cell Neoplasm (Papanicolaou-stained cytospin preparation, × 160).

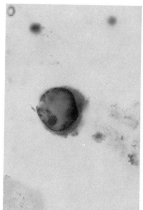
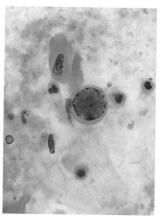

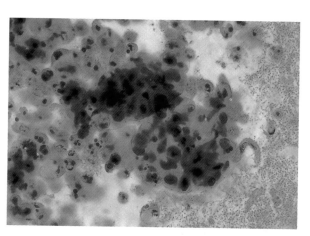

FIGURE 9–96C. Epithelial cell in urine from patient with **Polyoma Viral Infection**. This cell lacks a diagnostic intranuclear inclusion. Note similarity to the cell showing the cyclophosphamide therapeutic effect (see Fig. 9–96A) and the malignant cell (see Fig. 9–96B) (Papanicolaou-stained filter preparation, × 250).

FIGURE 9–96D. Epithelial cell containing intranuclear inclusion diagnostic of **Polyoma Viral Infection** (Papanicolaou-stained filter preparation, × 250).

FIGURE 9–97B. Ileal Conduit Specimen showing epithelial fragments and degenerated single cells resembling necrotic transitional cell neoplasm (Papanicolaou-stained filter preparation, × 160).

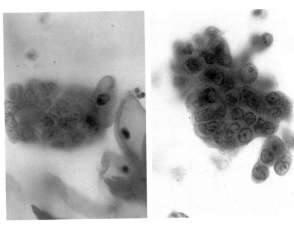

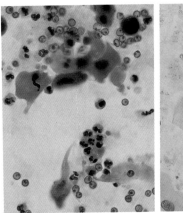

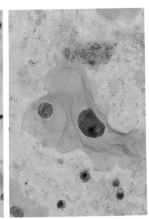

FIGURE 9–98A. Three-dimensional epithelial group of **Endometrial Cells** appearing similar to adenocarcinoma cells. The irregular nuclear borders are a result of degenerative wrinkling (Papanicolaou-stained filter preparation, × 250).

FIGURE 9–98B. Three-dimensional epithelial fragment derived from **Primary Urothelial Adenocarcinoma**. These hypochromatic cells show subtle malignant features, and rare cells contain prominent nucleoli (Papanicolaou-stained smear preparation, × 250).

FIGURE 9–99A. Cells derived from a **Primary Squamous Cell Carcinoma** of the urinary bladder. The hyperchromatic degenerated nuclei resemble those seen in a low-grade squamous intraepithelial lesion with features of human papilloma virus effect (Papanicolaou-stained cytospin preparation, × 160).

FIGURE 9–99B. Cells derived from a **Low-Grade Squamous Intraepithelial Lesion** (dysplasia with features of human papilloma virus effect) of the female reproductive tract contaminating a voided urine specimen (Papanicolaou-stained filter preparation, × 160).

C·H·A·P·T·E·R

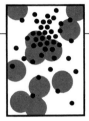

10

FINE NEEDLE ASPIRATION OF THE KIDNEYS, ADRENALS, AND RETROPERITONEUM

Barbara S. Ducatman

Fine needle aspiration (FNA) of the kidneys, adrenals, and retroperitoneum may be guided by computed tomography (CT), magnetic resonance imaging (MRI), or ultrasound. The principles of radiologic-guided FNA, as described in Chapter 8, apply. A pathologist should be present in the radiologic suite to ensure an adequate specimen, expedite the diagnosis, and triage material for further handling. Either air-dried (Romanowsky stains) or alcohol-fixed material (toluidine blue and eosin, hematoxylin and eosin, or rapid Papanicolaou stain) is used in this setting. The needle is flushed with 50% ethanol or a balanced electrolyte solution for cytocentrifugation, and any tissue chunks are placed in formalin and evaluated by histology. Cytospin material may be used for immunocytochemical studies.

FNA is used in this setting for the diagnosis of primary and metastatic disease and patient management. Primary neoplasms of the kidneys, adrenals, and retroperitoneum are often surgically excised or treated with radiation and/or chemotherapy. Histologic confirmation is less often obtained after a diagnosis of metastatic, inflammatory, or infectious diseases. A particular problem in this area is that the radiologist often cannot definitively pinpoint the site of a lesion (e.g., kidney versus adrenal); thus the differential diagnosis may be quite broad.

BENIGN DISEASES

Normal Kidneys and Adrenals

A normal kidney yields glomerular tufts and tubular epithelial cells on aspiration. Glomerular tufts have a characteristic lobulated appearance with spindle-shaped endothelial and mesangial cells (Fig. 10–1). Cells from the renal tubules are in sheets with well-defined cytoplasmic borders, abundant granular cytoplasm, and small, round, and regular nuclei (Fig. 10–1). The chromatin is finely granular; nucleoli are small and inconspicuous.

Cells aspirated from the adrenal cortex are in loosely arranged sheets and aggregates. Their cytoplasm is eosinophilic (pale gray on Diff-Quik) and may be finely vacuolated (Fig. 10–2). The nuclei are round and regular with finely granular chromatin and inconspicuous nucleoli. A mild degree of pleomorphism may be noted; such cells may resemble those from adrenal cortical adenoma and be difficult to distinguish from well-differentiated renal cell carcinoma. Cells of the adrenal medulla are more pleomorphic, with wispy granular cytoplasm, and are sometimes spindle-shaped (Fig. 10–3).

Renal Cysts

Cystic lesions in the kidney may represent either benign renal cysts or cystic degeneration of renal cell carcinoma. Benign renal cysts are generally hypocellular, with thin, clear fluid and rare macrophages and degenerating epithelial cells (Fig. 10–4). Benign renal cysts must be differentiated from cystic renal cell carcinoma, especially when the smears are more cellular (Table 10–1).

Inflammatory and Infectious Conditions

Abscesses of the adrenal and kidney present a similar appearance to those observed elsewhere. Numerous acute inflammatory cells and degenerating epithelial cells are seen. When this cytologic picture is seen during an immediate interpretation, material should be submitted for microbiology studies.

Granulomas also present a classic picture with clusters and single epithelioid histiocytes in a background of lymphocytes and plasma cells. The adrenals, in particular, often contain granulomas, especially in patients with acquired immunodeficiency syndrome (AIDS). In these cases, special stains (methenamine silver, periodic acid–Schiff, and acid-fast stains) are helpful.

Xanthogranulomatous pyelonephritis is a disease that may mimic renal cell carcinoma on radiologic, gross, and cytologic examination. Careful attention should be paid to the inflammatory background and the histiocytic nature of the cells (which is better appreciated on alcohol-fixed material).

Angiomyolipoma

Angiomyolipoma is a benign lesion, considered a hamartoma, composed of smooth muscle, blood vessels, fat cells, and fibrous tissue. The cytologic smear reflects this diversity. Benign-appearing spindle cells in sheets and syncytia are admixed with blood, hypocellular mesenchymal tissue, and fat vacuoles (Fig.

10–5). The spindle cells often have cigar-shaped nuclei, consistent with their smooth muscle origin and abundant dense cytoplasm.

MALIGNANT TUMORS

Kidneys

Renal cell carcinoma has a variable cytologic presentation owing to the diversity of its morphologic appearances. Well-differentiated renal cell carcinoma may be difficult to distinguish from either benign cells of proximal tubular or cystic origin. Aspirates are usually hypercellular, often with a background of old blood and necrotic debris. Cells are present in loosely cohesive sheets, clusters, papillae, syncytia, and singly (Figs. 10–6 to 10–8). Their cytoplasm is abundant, either granular or vacuolated, and the cells are round or spindled. The cytoplasm stains positive with oil red O stains for intracytoplasmic fat (Fig. 10–9). Nuclei are enlarged and pleomorphic with prominent nucleoli. Macronucleoli are often present. Renal cell carcinoma may be indistinguishable from adrenal cortical adenoma (Table 10–2). Sarcomatoid renal cell cancers must be distinguished from retroperitoneal sarcomas (Table 10–3).

Renal Oncocytoma. The renal oncocytoma is a rare, benign, and often asymptomatic neoplasm, apparently arising from the cells of the proximal convoluted tubules. Aspirates of oncocytomas show scant to moderate cellularity and sheets and single polygonal cells with abundant granular cytoplasm (Fig. 10–10). Nuclei are round and uniform and contain finely granular chromatin and small but prominent nucleoli.

Transitional Cell Carcinoma. Transitional cell carcinomas arising in the renal pelvis may give rise to masses in the kidney. Metastatic deposits from transitional cell carcinomas may also be aspirated from the retroperitoneum. The cells are large and present singly and in loose aggregates. Hyperchromatic nuclei, often eccentric in location, are a useful characteristic. These cells also have other obvious criteria of malignancy—anisonucleosis, irregular nuclear membranes, and prominent irregular nucleoli (Fig. 10–11). Poorly differentiated tumors may exhibit squamous differentiation or a sarcomatoid pattern.

Wilms Tumor. Wilms tumor is predominantly a tumor of infancy and childhood. Its bimodal nature is reflected in the cells aspirated, with a mixture of malignant epithelial and mesenchymal cells. Many dyshesive small, oval to fusiform cells with hyperchromatic nuclei and scant cytoplasm are noted in the background. It is easiest to diagnose Wilms tumor when epithelial cells in tight clusters and tubular-like structures are observed (Fig. 10–12). The mesenchymal cells are elongated and seen in clusters and singly. Wilms tumor must be differentiated from other small, blue, round cell tumors of childhood (Table 10–4).

Adrenals

Adrenal Cortical Adenoma and Carcinoma. Adrenal cortical adenomas cannot always be reliably distinguished from normal adrenal cortical cells or well-differentiated renal cell carcinoma on cytologic grounds alone. Therefore, a cytopathologist must rely on the radiologist's assurance that a mass in the adrenal was successfully aspirated. The cells are seen in loose sheets. Their cytoplasm may be granular or vacuolated and delicate; many naked nuclei and occasional binucleated cells are observed (Fig. 10–13). There may be no nuclear atypicality, with cells indistinguishable from normal cortical cells or marked atypicality with nuclear enlargement, pleomorphism, hyperchromasia, and prominent nucleoli.

The diagnosis of adrenal cortical carcinoma may rely on the presence of metastases and may not be diagnosed on morphology alone. Large tumor size (over 5 cm) also favors a malignant prognosis. The cytologic features most suggestive of carcinoma are marked cellular pleomorphism, dyshesion, abundant mitoses, and a necrotic background (Fig. 10–14).

Pheochromocytoma. Functioning pheochromocytomas are usually diagnosed on biochemical findings of increased blood and urinary catecholamines or their metabolites (such as vanillylmandelic acid). Fine needle aspiration is contraindicated in such cases as it may precipitate a hypertensive crisis. However, an occasional nonfunctioning and extra-adrenal pheochromocytoma (paraganglioma) may be aspirated.

Smears are usually cellular with loose aggregates and many single cells. There is often a marked cellular pleomorphism ranging from small polygonal cells with uniform, round to oval nuclei, granular chromatin, and inconspicuous nuclei to large myoid-like and spindle cells (Fig. 10–15). Nuclei are often pleomorphic and large or elongated. Nucleoli may be prominent, and intranuclear cytoplasmic inclusion may be seen. Such cells may be misdiagnosed as malignant. Cytoplasmic granularity, especially as distinct coarse red granules on Romanowsky-type stains and the "salt-and-pepper" nuclear chromatin pattern reminiscent of other neuroendocrine tumors, are useful diagnostic features.

Neuroblastoma. A neuroblastoma is another small blue-cell tumor of childhood (Fig. 10–16). Rosettes of tumor cells, when seen, are a useful distinguishing feature. However, diagnosis is often not possible by cytology; the characteristic biochemical features of increased urinary excretion of catecholamines and their derivatives is confirmatory in the appropriate clinical, radiologic, and cytologic setting.

Retroperitoneum

The retroperitoneum, the adrenals, and to a lesser extent the kidneys may be the recipient of metastases from diverse primary sites. The retroperitoneum may also be the site of origin of lymphomas and sarcomas, which are described in detail in other chapters of this book.

Bibliography

Hidvegi D, DeMay RM, Nunez-Alonso C, Nieman HL: Percutaneous transperitoneal aspiration of renal adenocarcinoma guided by ultrasound. Morphologic appearance of normal and malignant cells. Acta Cytol 23:467–470, 1979.

Katz RL, Patel S, Mackay B, Zornoza J: Fine needle aspiration cytology of the adrenal gland. Acta Cytol 28:269–282, 1984.

Orell SR, Langlois SLP, Marshall UR: Fine needle aspiration cytology in the diagnosis of solid renal and adrenal masses. Scand J Urol Nephrol 19:211–216, 1985.

Orell SR, Sterrett GF, Walters N-I, Whitaker D: Manual and Atlas of Fine Needle Aspiration Cytology. New York: Churchill Livingstone, 1986, pp 155–177.

Suen KC: Guides to Clinical Aspiration Biopsy. Retroperitoneum and Intestine. New York: Igaku-Shoin, 1987.

Table 10–1. DIFFERENTIAL DIAGNOSIS OF RENAL CYSTS

Feature	Benign Cyst (Fig. 10–17)	Cystic Renal Cell Carcinoma (Figs. 10–18 to 10–20)
Cyst fluid	Thin, clear, straw-colored	Degenerating blood, thick, red-brown
Background	Clean, bloody	Necrotic debris, old blood, inflammatory
Cellularity	Low to moderate	Low (with necrotic debris) to marked
Cellular arrangements	Predominantly single histiocytes; rare degenerating epithelial cells	Loose clusters, syncytia, or sheets; papillae; single cells
Nuclei	Histiocytic, bland	Pleomorphic; increased nuclear to cytoplasmic ratio
Nucleoli	Inconspicuous	Small but prominent to large irregular

Table 10–2. CELLS WITH ABUNDANT GRANULAR OR VACUOLATED CYTOPLASM

Feature	Benign Renal Tubular Cells	Benign Adrenal Cortical Cells	Renal Cell Carcinoma (Fig. 10–21)	Adrenal Cortical Neoplasm (Figs. 10–22 and 10–23)	Oncocytoma (Fig. 10–24)	Pheochromocytoma (Fig. 10–25)
Cellularity	Low	Low to moderate	Low to high	Moderate to high	Low to moderate	High
Cellular arrangements	Predominantly sheets; glomeruli present	Loose sheets and aggregates	Dyshesive sheets, syncytia, or papillae; many single cells	Loose sheets, single cells	Loose sheets, single cells	Loose aggregates, single cells
Cell shape	Round to oval, uniform	Round to oval, uniform	Variable, pleomorphic, polygonal to spindle-shaped	Round to oval, uniform	Polygonal, uniform	Variable; small, polygonal; pleomorphic; spindle-shaped
Cytoplasm	Granular; may contain lipofuscin	Granular and/or vacuolated, fragile	Granular and/or vacuolated; may contain hemosiderin	Granular and/or vacuolated, fragile	Granular	Granular, often with prominent reddish granules on Diff-Quik
Nuclei	Uniform, round, and regular	Uniform, round, and regular	Pleomorphic, enlarged	Uniform, pleomorphic; normal size to enlarged; naked	Slightly enlarged	Pleomorphic; small round to very large or spindle-shaped
Chromatin	Finely granular	Finely granular	Finely to coarsely granular to vesicular	Finely to coarsely granular	Finely granular	Coarsely granular, salt-and-pepper
Nucleoli	Inconspicuous	Inconspicuous	Small but prominent to macronucleoli	Inconspicuous to prominent	Inconspicuous	Inconspicuous to macronucleoli

Table 10-3. SPINDLE-SHAPED CELLS

Feature	Retroperitoneal Sarcoma (Figs. 10-26 and 10-27)	Sarcomatoid Renal Cell Carcinoma (Fig. 10-28)	Pheochromocytoma (Fig. 10-29)	Angiomyolipoma (Fig. 10-30)
Cellular constituents	Single population of single cells	Usually two: spindle-shaped and sheets and clusters of epithelial cells	Often three: polygonal, spindle, and myoid cells	Often four: spindle or round cells, fat vacuoles, blood, and hypocellular mesenchymal cells
Cytoplasm	Elongated, abundant to sparse	Abundant to sparse, finely granular or vacuolated	Abundant, reddish granules on Diff-Quik	Granular, dense
Nuclei	Finely to coarsely granular chromatin	Finely to coarsely granular chromatin, pleomorphic, macronucleoli, and intranuclear cytoplasmic inclusions	Coarsely granular, salt-and-pepper chromatin; small to macronucleoli; intranuclear cytoplasmic inclusions	Cigar-shaped, finely granular, regular

Table 10-4. SMALL ROUND-CELL TUMORS OF CHILDHOOD

Feature	Wilms Tumor (Fig. 10-31)	Neuroblastoma (Fig. 10-32)	Ewing Sarcoma (Fig. 10-33) and Embryonal Rhabdomyosarcoma (Fig. 10-34)	Lymphoma (Fig. 10-35)
Most common site of aspiration	Kidney	Adrenal medulla	Bone and soft tissue (Ewing sarcoma); urogenital tract (embryonal rhabdomyosarcoma)	Retroperitoneum
Cellular arrangements	Bimodal; epithelial cell clusters and single mesenchymal cells from tubules	Rosettes, loose clusters, single cells, neurofibrillar matrix	Loose clusters, single cells; pseudorosettes (Ewing sarcoma)	Single cells
Other		Increased urine catecholamine and vanillylmandelic acid; may differentiate to ganglioneuroblastoma or ganglioneuroma	PAS-positive cytoplasmic granules (Ewing sarcoma)	Lymphoglandular bodies (best on Diff-Quik)
Immunocytochemistry				
Neuron-specific enolase	−	+	−	−
Desmin	+/−	−	+ (embryonal rhabdomyosarcoma)	−
Vimentin	+/−	−	+	−
Leukocyte common antigen	−	−	−	+

NORMAL CELLS

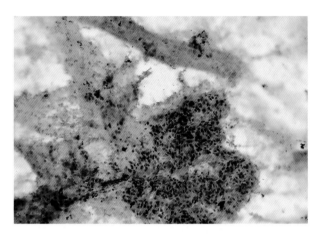

FIGURE 10–1. Normal Glomerulus. The aspiration of a glomerulus demonstrates a cohesive, three-dimensional grouping of benign-appearing spindle and round cells. The renal tubules are composed of cohesive cells with abundant eosinophilic cytoplasm and bland nuclei (toluidine blue and eosin stain, × 100).

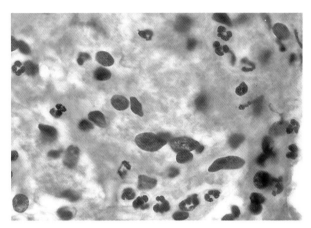

FIGURE 10–3. Normal Adrenal Medulla. Cells aspirated from the adrenal medulla have fragile cytoplasm, which often strips away, leaving a spindle-shaped, benign-appearing naked nuclei (Papanicolaou stain, × 250).

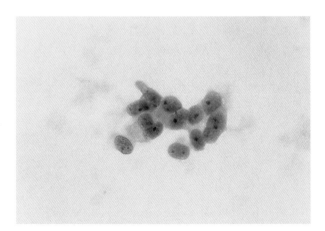

FIGURE 10–2. Normal Adrenal Cortex. These loosely cohesive cells with granular cytoplasm and benign nuclear features are characteristic of cells aspirated from the adrenal cortex. These cells lack any appreciable nuclear pleomorphism (Papanicolaou stain, × 250).

BENIGN CONDITIONS

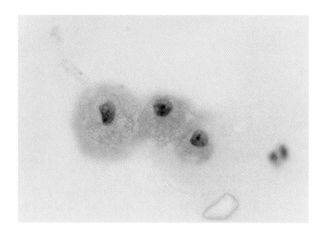

FIGURE 10–4. Renal Cyst. These cells, aspirated from a renal cyst, are often difficult to distinguish from those of a well-differentiated renal cell carcinoma. However, as demonstrated in this photograph, the specimen is hypocellular, with a clean, watery-proteinaceous background and an absence of necrotic cells or old blood. The nuclei are round and regular (Papanicolaou stain, × 250).

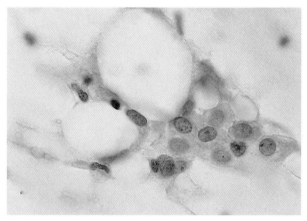

FIGURE 10–5. Renal Angiomyolipoma. Cells aspirated from this benign lesion may represent smooth muscle, blood vessels, fat cells, or fibrous tissue, and the appearance of the cytologic smear reflects the type of cells aspirated. In this picture, note the round and spindle-shaped cells, bland nuclei, and fat vacuoles (Papanicolaou stain, × 250). (Case courtesy of John Goellner, M.D., Mayo Clinic, Rochester, Minn.)

MALIGNANT TUMORS

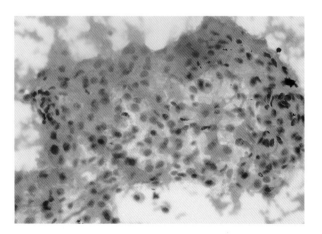

FIGURE 10–6. Cells Aspirated From a Renal Cell Carcinoma. The specimen is cellular, with cells arranged in loosely cohesive sheets. The background is bloody (Papanicolaou stain, × 100).

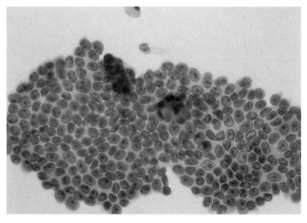

FIGURE 10–7. Renal Cell Carcinoma. These cells are arranged in a cohesive sheet and demonstrate minimal nuclear pleomorphism and atypicality. However, the remainder of the smear was very cellular, and numerous single cells were present. These features would all lead to the diagnosis of renal cell carcinoma (hematoxylin and eosin stain, × 100).

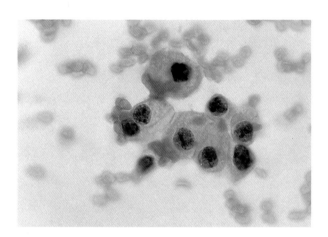

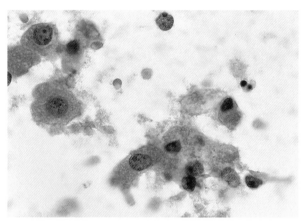

FIGURE 10–8. Renal Cell Carcinoma. Single cells are present in a background of blood. These cells are quite similar to those seen in Figure 10–4 (benign renal cyst). However, in contrast to those aspirates from benign lesions, the background shows old blood, and the specimen is hypercellular. Some of the cells demonstrate minor degrees of nuclear pleomorphism and irregularity. In addition, papillary, syncytial, and sheet-like arrangements of cells may be seen (Papanicolaou stain, × 250).

FIGURE 10–10. Renal Oncocytoma. Single cells from a renal oncocytoma demonstrate bland nuclear features and small, round nucleoli. The cytoplasm is abundant and exhibits a granular appearance. This tumor has to be differentiated from renal cell carcinoma. The cells are more likely arranged singly or in sheets. The nuclear uniformity and abundant granular cytoplasm help to differentiate this tumor from renal cell carcinoma (Papanicolaou stain, × 250). (Case courtesy of John R. Goellner, M.D., Mayo Clinic, Rochester, Minn.)

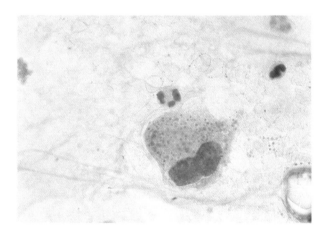

FIGURE 10–9. Renal Cell Carcinoma. The oil-red-O stain done on material from the previous figure demonstrates abundant intracellular fat (× 250).

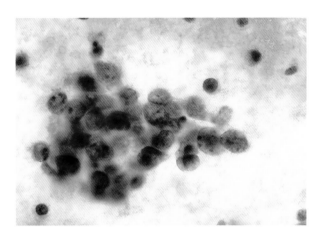

FIGURE 10–11. Transitional Cell Carcinoma Arising in the Renal Pelvis. The nuclei are quite hyperchromatic and eccentric in location, which is a useful feature in distinguishing them from other forms of malignancy. The cells also exhibit anisonucleosis and irregular nuclear membranes (Papanicolaou stain, × 250).

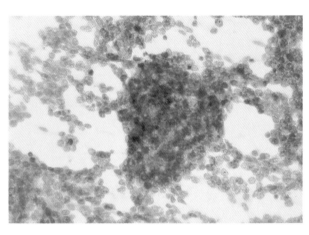

FIGURE 10–12. Wilms Tumor. A bimodal pattern often exists in this tumor, with cells present in both clusters and tubule-like structures and single cells. However, when prominent, single, small blue round cells are noted, immunocytochemical stains may be necessary to confirm the diagnosis (Papanicolaou stain, × 100). (Case courtesy of John R. Goellner, M.D., Mayo Clinic, Rochester, Minn.)

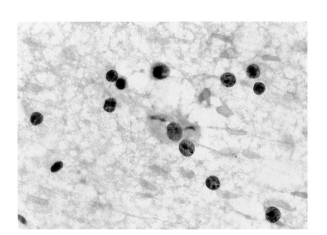

FIGURE 10–13. Adrenal Cortical Adenoma. Many of the nuclei are naked and small; however, note the centrally located cell with abundant granular or finely vacuolated cytoplasm and the mild nuclear enlargement. These cells may be difficult to distinguish from those of the normal adrenal cortex. Hypercellularity of the aspirate and a mild degree of nuclear enlargement and pleomorphism are useful differential features (Papanicolaou stain, × 100).

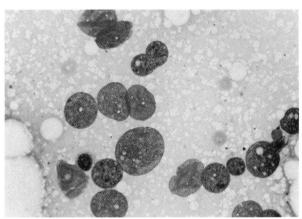

FIGURE 10–14. Adrenal Cortical Carcinoma. In contrast to the cells in the previous figure (adrenal cortical adenoma), the nuclei are much larger, and a marked degree of anisonucleosis is noted. Nucleoli are prominent. A diagnosis of carcinoma may not be present based solely on cytology; however, abundant mitoses and a necrotic background may suggest this diagnosis (May-Grunwald-Giemsa stain, × 250). (Case courtesy of John R. Goellner, M.D., Mayo Clinic, Rochester, Minn.)

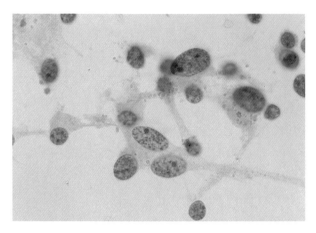

FIGURE 10–15. Pheochromocytoma. This aspiration is cellular, with many single spindle cells. Nuclear pleomorphism may be quite pronounced (Papanicolaou stain, × 250).

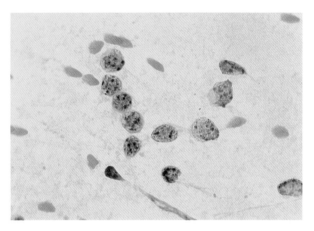

FIGURE 10–16. Neuroblastoma. This is another of the small, blue, round cell neoplasms of childhood. When rosettes of tumor cells or neurofibrillar material are present, they may help to suggest the diagnosis; however, immunocytochemical stains may be necessary (Papanicolaou stain, × 250). (Case courtesy of John R. Goellner, M.D., Mayo Clinic, Rochester, Minn.)

DIFFERENTIAL GROUPING

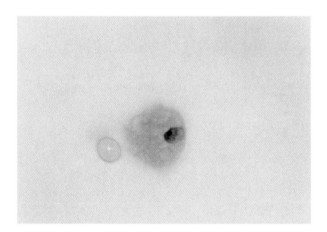

FIGURE 10–17. Renal Cyst. The background is clean, with very few cells. The cells present are predominantly histiocytic, with rare, degenerating epithelial cells. The nucleus here is bland and histiocytic in type (Papanicolaou stain, × 250).

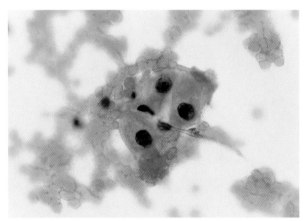

FIGURE 10–18. Cystic Renal Cell Carcinoma. The specimen is more cellular than that in a benign cyst. There is often degenerating blood in the background with necrotic debris. In occasional cases, with abundant necrotic debris, only a few cells may be seen. The nuclei are more pleomorphic and have a greater nuclear to cytoplasmic ratio than those observed from a benign cyst (Papanicolaou stain, × 250).

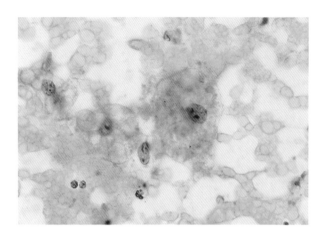
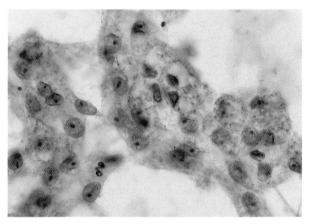

FIGURES 10–19 and 10–20. Cystic Renal Cell Carcinoma. Single cells with bland-appearing nuclei and hemosiderin are noted. However, the nuclei do show prominent nucleoli, and the specimen is hypercellular, with loose clusters and syncytia of cells, an increased nuclear to cytoplasmic ratio, nuclear pleomorphism, and small but prominent nucleoli (toluidine blue and eosin stain, × 250).

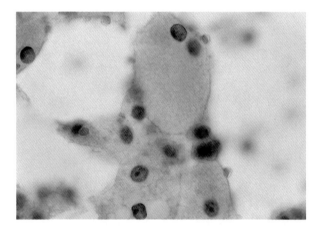

FIGURE 10–21. Renal Cell Carcinoma. Note the numerous cells with abundant, foamy, finely vacuolated cytoplasm. This specimen contained abundant lipid on electron microscopy (Papanicolaou stain, × 250).

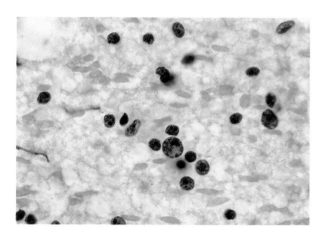

FIGURE 10–22. Adrenal Cortical Adenoma. The cytoplasm may be granular or vacuolated, but it is extremely fragile and strips away, often leaving naked nuclei. These show a mild degree of pleomorphism but no significant enlargement (Papanicolaou stain, × 250).

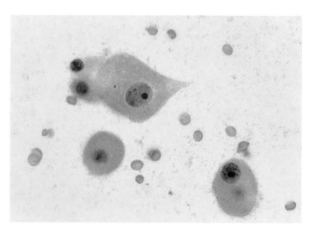

FIGURE 10–24. Renal Oncocytoma. Note the single cells with abundant granular cytoplasm, finely granular chromatin, and small but prominent nucleoli. Cells are present either singly or in loose sheets, and the cells are polygonal around and very uniform (Papanicolaou stain, × 250). (Case courtesy of John R. Goellner, M.D., Mayo Clinic, Rochester, Minn.)

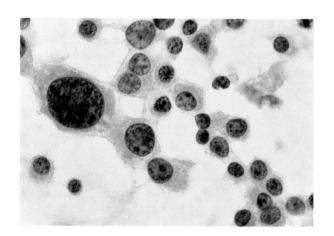

FIGURE 10–23. Adrenal Cortical Carcinoma. The specimen is hypercellular, with marked nuclear pleomorphism and very enlarged nuclei, suggesting the malignant nature of the tumor. Adrenal cortical adenoma and carcinoma may not be separable on cytology (Papanicolaou stain, × 250). (Case courtesy of John R. Goellner, M.D., Mayo Clinic, Rochester, Minn.)

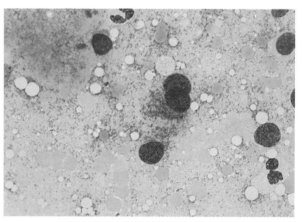

FIGURE 10–25. Pheochromocytoma. On Romanowsky-type stains, prominent reddish granules are often observed. These are a useful distinguishing feature. The cells are pleomorphic and range from small to very large or spindled (Diff-Quik stain, × 250).

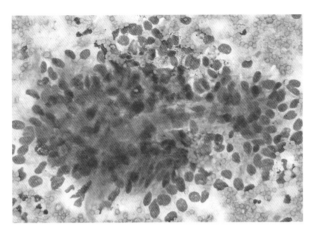

FIGURE 10–26. Pelvic Sarcoma. A loose cluster of spindle cells is arranged around a blood vessel. This may represent either a sarcoma or a sarcomatoid carcinoma; when epithelial-type cells are not seen, immunocytochemistry is necessary to make this distinction (Diff-Quik stain, × 250).

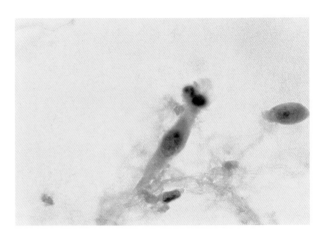

FIGURE 10–28. Sarcomatoid Renal Cell Carcinoma. A single spindle cell is noted, located in the center of the field. That more usual types of renal carcinoma cells are seen in the background leads to the proper diagnosis; however, if a pure population of spindle cells is noted, then immunocytochemical studies must be performed (Papanicolaou stain, × 250).

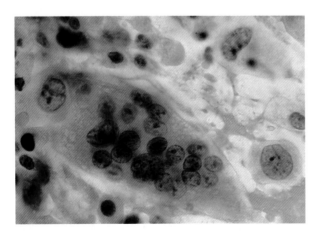

FIGURE 10–27. Osteogenic Sarcoma Aspirated From the Retroperitoneum. This patient had a history of primary osteogenic sarcoma arising in the bladder. Note the osteoclast-type giant cells and malignant single, round, and spindled cells in the background (Papanicolaou stain, × 250).

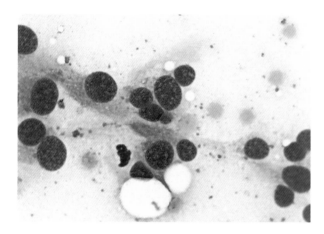

FIGURE 10–29. Pheochromocytoma. Cells from a pheochromocytoma may show prominent spindling. It is useful to look for reddish cytoplasmic granules on Romanowsky-type stains. Such cases often exhibit marked nuclear pleomorphism (Diff-Quik stain, × 250).

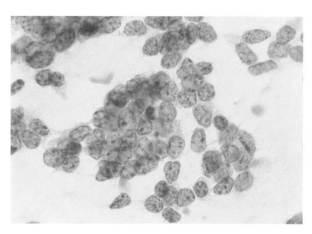

FIGURE 10–31. Wilms Tumor. A bimodal population of cells is often seen with tubules, epithelial cell clusters, and single mesenchymal cells. When only single blue round cells are noted, they must be distinguished from the cells of other small-cell tumors. A Wilms tumor originates in the kidney. When immunocytochemical stains are used, the diagnosis must be one of exclusion; see Table 10–4 (Papanicolaou stain, × 250). (Case courtesy of John R. Goellner, M.D., Rochester, Minn.)

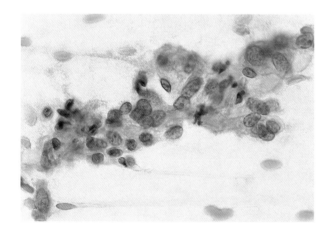

FIGURE 10–30. Renal Angiomyolipoma. A component of benign spindle cells is often noted, admixed with fat cells and hypocellular mesenchymal cells (Papanicolaou stain, × 250). (Case courtesy of John R. Goellner, M.D., Mayo Clinic, Rochester, Minn.)

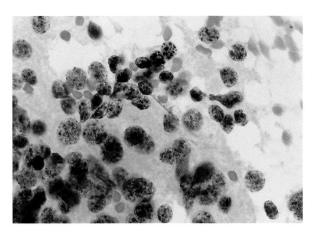

FIGURE 10–32. Neuroblastoma. These small blue round cells are arranged in neurofibrillar matrix. Rosettes may often be seen. The patient may have increased urinary catecholamines and vanillylmandelic acid, and immunocytochemical studies may be useful. Such cases may also show ganglion cells if maturation to ganglioneuroblastoma or ganglioneuroma has occurred (Papanicolaou stain, × 250). (Case courtesy of John R. Goellner, M.D., Mayo Clinic, Rochester, Minn.)

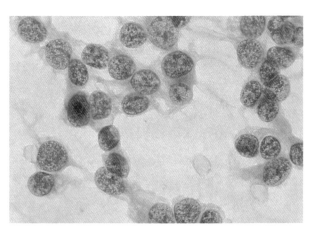

FIGURE 10–34. Embryonal Rhabdomyosarcoma. Another of the small, round, blue cell neoplasms of childhood; immunocytochemical markers to demonstrate the muscle origin may be useful. Such cases are often aspirated from the urogenital tract. (Papanicolaou stain, × 250). (Case courtesy of John R. Goellner, M.D., Mayo Clinic, Rochester, Minn.)

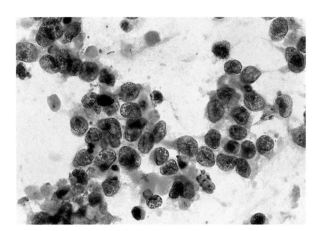

FIGURE 10–33. Ewing Sarcoma. The cells may be seen in loose clusters or with pseudorosettes. Material positive for periodic acid-Schiff stain may be present. These tumors most often are present in bone or soft tissue (Papanicolaou stain, × 250). (Case courtesy of John R. Goellner, M.D., Mayo Clinic, Rochester, Minn.)

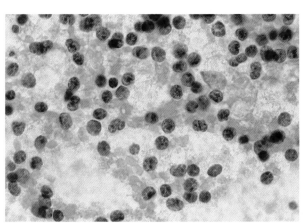

FIGURE 10–35. Lymphoma. Such cases are most commonly aspirated from retroperitoneal nodes. The cellular pattern is composed only of single cells. Lymphoglandular bodies may be noted on a Diff-Quik stain, and staining for leukocyte-common antigen is positive, whereas epithelial markers are negative (Papanicolaou stain, × 250).

C·H·A·P·T·E·R

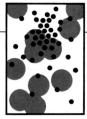

11

THIN NEEDLE BIOPSY OF THE PROSTATE

G. Fred Worsham

Russell Ferguson, a urologist at New York's Memorial Hospital, first reported the use of fine needle aspiration biopsy (FNAB) in 1930 and acknowledged Martin and Ellis at his institution for its development. The technique received relatively little interest until it was adopted by the Karolinska Institute in Sweden and subsequently modified by Sixten Franzen, who developed a finger guide and a flexible needle to sample the prostate transrectally. Enthusiasm for the procedure in this country increased in the late 1970s, as the efficacy of FNAB applied to other organs was shown. The substantial reduction in morbidity over traditional core biopsy, the high sensitivity and specificity in experienced hands, the convenience, and the relatively low cost of this office procedure promoted the use of the technique through the 1980s. In 1989, the Prostate Cancer Working Group of the National Cancer Institute, recognizing the progress made in this area of diagnosis, devoted its annual seminar at Prouts Neck, Maine, to a state-of-the-art review of cytopathology and related subjects, including flow cytometry and computer-aided image analysis.

It is probable that interest in FNAB of the prostate peaked in this country in the late 1980s and is now declining. While cytologic criteria for diagnosis of the prostate were being refined and disseminated, a competing technology was being developed in order to both image and sample the prostate. This technology employs prostatic ultrasound and ultrasound-directed thin-core (18-gauge) biopsy. Briefly, this newer technique involves the rectal insertion of an ultrasound probe, which contains a slot to hold and direct the biopsy device, which is

407

usually the Biopty gun (Bard) that obtains a 17 mm long core sample in approximately 1/10 of a second. Many urologists have purchased this equipment for office use; the technique has the advantage of recording an image of the prostate while the biopsy needle transfixes the abnormality. Other advantages include the ability to reassure the patient and the urologist that a specific abnormality has been sampled, morbidity approaching that of FNAB, brief patient discomfort, easier specimen handling for the urologist, and expertise of pathologists in all types of practices already trained and experienced in interpreting tissue sections of the prostate. Finally, the Gleason grading scheme has been widely advocated as the standard for use in prostate cancer so that interinstitutional data can be compared. Although there are correlations between the patterns in cytologic material and histologic material, Gleason's patterns are fundamentally architectural and not cytologic. These have all led to rapid acceptance and preference of this procedure over FNAB.

Indications dictating which of these procedures should be used in a given situation have not been clearly established. Neither one has proved useful for screening in the absence of a palpable abnormality. Both have been clearly shown to be of value in the diagnosis of clinically suspected prostate cancer, which in the United States affects approximately one in 11 men and claimed 30,000 lives in 1990, making it the second leading cause of death by cancer in men. Since there is a recent excellent monograph on the histology of the prostate by Epstein, this chapter emphasizes cytopathologic presentation, particularly in conditions that are diagnostically difficult. Histopathology is provided for selected correlations and to illustrate a few lesions that are not yet described cytologically but that could present diagnostic pitfalls.

TECHNIQUE

The procedure is performed in the office or at the bedside, usually without anesthesia or antibiotics. Clinicians usually prefer the patient to be in the knee-chest position, although the technique reportedly has been successful with the patient on his side or in the dorsal lithotomy position. We prefer to use the Franzen needle guide, a Cameco syringe holder or a control syringe, and a 22-gauge needle. The needle is 5 cm longer than the guide, giving an adequate operating distance for sampling most lesions, even in unusual areas such as the distal prostate. Adjusting the palm plate of the guide, so that the examining finger is comfortably positioned in the ring, will place the port of the guide at the fingertip. Vacuum should be applied only after the insertion of the needle to a 0.5 to 1.0 cm depth to avoid rectal contamination. The needle should be advanced slowly and repeatedly into the clinically suspicious area for distances up to 1.0 cm. Occasionally, unusually situated lesions require greater distances. Care should be used to avoid puncture of the bladder, since urine dilutes the specimen. Seminal vesicles may also contain fluid. When sampling has been thorough or if fluid appears in the hub of the needle, the aspiration is complete. Since there is subjectivity in localizing a lesion, we recommend four passes, including each side of the prostate, to ensure maximum diagnostic yield.

Once the aspirate is obtained, there are several technical options for preparation. Smears prepared in the usual manner at the time of aspiration may be air-dried or immersed in 95% ethanol (we add three drops of glacial acetic acid per Coplin jar for red cell lysis). Alternatively, some authors advocate rinsing of the needle after aspiration with a transport or preservative solution such as Saccomano carbowax fixative to relieve the clinician from slide smearing. After receipt of the specimen in the laboratory, filtration or centrifugation can be used to concentrate the specimen. This technique may result in increased efficiency in screening smears since direct smears from a four-pass FNAB may result in 16 to 20 slides with relatively widely dispersed cells. Good results have been reported with both methods. We use the former technique because of the internal laboratory simplicity and because we teach the clinicians and their office personnel the technique and assist during the procedures until they can consistently obtain abundant, well-fixed samples. Training, consistent feedback, and clear statements regarding the adequacy of sampling are necessary during this period, until the operator and staff are providing optimal diagnostic material.

Although many series have reported excellent results with air-dried smears and variants of May-Grunwald-Giemsa stains, Papanicolaou staining does offer an advantage in nuclear detail that is useful in the recognition of intra-acinar atypias (discussed later) and low-grade adenocarcinoma.

CYTOLOGIC FEATURES OF THE MAJOR DISEASES OF THE PROSTATE

Benign Aspirates

Most benign prostatic aspirations are from glands that have some degree of hyperplasia. Cellular material consists of variable amounts of prostatic acinar epithelium and stroma, albeit the stromal component is infrequently evident in FNAB material. Cases of predominantly stromal hyperplasia often yield cell-poor aspirates. There is no consensus on minimal numbers of cells for adequacy of interpretation, but generally, 10 to 20 fragments of prostatic epithelium on each of four slides are needed. Some judgment must be applied, since a cell-poor aspirate is more likely caused by stromal predominance when obtained by an experienced operator. Low to moderate cellularity at scanning power is an important initial feature in determining that an aspirate is benign.

Characteristics of prostatic epithelium in benign aspirates include the following:

1. Cells in sheets of variable size, sometimes three-dimensional, with larger fragments identifiable as portions of acini (occasionally, small acini may be evident within a large fragment).
2. Sharp cytoplasmic borders with evenly spaced nuclei, resulting in a honeycomb pattern.
3. Nuclei basally oriented away from the lumen in fragments where a luminal border is evident.
4. Prominent small spindle cells (basal cells) with scant cytoplasm and slightly hyperchromatic nuclei found at the periphery of sheets as well as occasionally on the surface of three-dimensional fragments.
5. Virtually no nucleoli but occasionally prominent chromocenters.
6. Pale cytoplasm, which may contain golden brown, relatively uniformly dispersed lipochrome granules.
7. Intra-acinar components: corpora amylacea; frequently fractured, foamy histiocytes; and lymphocytes.

8. Infrequently, small fragments of fibromuscular stroma with spindle-shaped nuclei and a uniform chromatin pattern.
9. Occasional fragments of basaloid epithelium with features similar to those described above, representing basal hyperplasia or atrophy.
10. Occasional clusters of transitional cells, from the periurethral prostatic ducts, from more peripheral acini with transitional metaplasia, or rarely from the urinary bladder or urethra.
11. Relatively clean background.

Cells of nonprostatic origin, found relatively frequently in benign aspirates, are of four types.

1. Adipose tissue. Adipose tissue is infrequently present in aspirates from experienced operators, and is usually obtained from a biopsy of the perirectal soft tissue.
2. Rectal mucosa. A frequent finding, rectal mucosa is usually present in small sheets but occassionally in larger sheets and disrupted fragments. When viewed on edge, the cells are columnar and have luminally oriented intracytoplasmic mucus vacuoles and prominent basal orientation of the nuclei. Nuclei are somewhat larger and more oval than the nuclei of prostatic epithelium. They also have a more open chromatin pattern and thicker nuclear membranes, prominent grooves, or distinct nuclear notches. These nuclear indentations often correlate with the intracytoplasmic mucus vacuole. Basophilic background mucus may be prominent and adjacent to the cell fragments.
3. Squamous cells. Squamous cells are frequently encountered, usually originating from the anal mucosa or less commonly arising from squamous metaplasia within the prostate.
4. Seminal vesicle cells. Seminal vesicle cells present a major problem in the differential diagnosis between benignancy and malignancy. Their origin must be recognized to prevent a false-positive diagnosis. The seminal vesicles are located somewhat laterally and cephalad to the prostate in the soft tissue between the posterior prostate and the anterior rectal wall. Occasionally, when the seminal vesicle is sampled, the clinician may give a history of the lesion being reduced in size as the sample was obtained. In other cases, seminal vesicle contamination occurs during movement of the needle, and the operator is unaware that the seminal vesicle has been sampled.

   When only the seminal vesicle is sampled, the character of the aspirate is usually moderately cellular with a dirty background of degenerated cells, histiocytes, sperm, corpora amylacea–like structures (usually of smaller and more uniform size than in prostatic aspirates), and seminal vesicle epithelium. The epithelial cells are arranged in small tubular formations, small fragments and groups, and as single cells. Cells in groups frequently have relatively scant cytoplasm and more oval and somewhat darker staining nuclei than those of prostatic epithelial cells. Cytoplasm is finely vacuolated, and lipochrome pigment may be prominent in many of the cells. Other cells may vary considerably in size, appear as single cells, and have marked nuclear irregularities including abnormalities of shape, intranuclear inclusions, and prominent hyperchromasia. Nucleoli are relatively uncommon in the nuclei of seminal vesicle epithelium. When only the seminal vesicle has been sampled, usually the diagnosis is not difficult. However, frequently seminal vesicle samples are mixed with prostatic epithelium and rectal epithelium. The mixture of these cytologically pleomorphic epithelial cells with the background prostatic material may cause diagnostic problems. Care should be taken to find the characteristic lipochrome pigmentation within some of the cells. Occasionally immunocytochemistry for prostate-specific antigen (PSA) may be useful, since seminal vesicle epithelium does not contain PSA.

If there is substantial seminal vesicle contamination, the question of adequacy of sampling may arise. We usually recommend repeat sampling if the majority of the specimen is from the seminal vesicle, unless the clinician believes the palpated abnormality was, in fact, seminal vesicle.

Prostatitis

Cellular characteristics of FNAB samples of prostatitis are usually striking at low power. These are very cellular to moderately cellular specimens. The low-power differential diagnosis often includes high-grade adenocarcinoma. Analysis at high power shows a mixture of cells, however, with a dirty inflammatory background of neutrophils, histiocytes, and giant cells. Degenerated cells are frequent, and if the prostatitis is associated with prostatic infarcts, necrosis may also be present. Epithelial cells are usually present in smaller groups than in other benign aspirates, and there may be some dyshesion, loss of polarity, nuclear crowding, and loss of distinct cytoplasmic borders in inflamed fragments, features that are worrisome for malignancy. Prostatic epithelial cells may show some nuclear enlargement and contain small nucleoli or chromocenters. Rarely, we have observed prominent nucleoli in sheets of cells associated with prostatitis and infarcts, changes resembling repair often seen in the uterine cervix. Basal hyperplasia, transitional metaplasia, and squamous metaplasia may be prominent in cases of prostatis or prostatic infarction.

A number of pitfalls are associated with the presence of prostatitis. First, there is the problem of differentiating the reactive changes noted above from adenocarcinoma. Well to moderately differentiated adenocarcinoma may be suspected when there is high cellularity, mild dyshesion, and variable nuclear atypia. High-grade adenocarcinoma may be in the differential diagnosis because of necrosis and atypical reparative change. In the author's experience, repair mimicking carcinoma is usually present only in rare fragments, whereas in high-grade adenocarcinoma, marked atypia is the rule in most of the fragments. Aside from this false-positive problem, there is the false-negative problem, e.g., cases in which both prostatitis and adenocarcinoma may be present in the same prostate. The atypia may then be ascribed only to prostatitis and the tumor not appreciated. Finally, there are problem cases in which prostatitis cannot be distinguished from carcinoma clinically. Urologists do not knowingly biopsy prostatitis because of the risk of sepsis. Small nodules of carcinoma may be masked by the general induration of prostatitis and therefore may not be sampled. Because of these problems inherent in aspirates of inflamed prostates, we recommend antibiotic therapy and repeat biopsy within three months. Ultrasound has not been useful in distinguishing prostatitis from adenocarcinoma, since both usually present as hypoechoic lesions of the prostate.

Atypical Hyperplasia

Atypical hyperplasia in the prostate can be categorized by atypia of either the epithelium or of the acinar architecture. The former is referred to as dysplasia (also known as large acinar atypical hyperplasia or prostatic intraepithelial neoplasia). Dysplasia can be divided into three grades. Histologically, there is an intra-acinar atypia characterized by increasing nuclear size, variability, and stratification within the prostatic acinus. The architectural pattern is usually not disturbed, but there is prominent tufting within the acini, unusual in simple prostatic hyperplasia. The stroma between the glands is not unusual, and, in general, there is a preserved basal layer in all grades of dysplasia. Nuclear abnormalities increase with the grade of dysplasia. Severe dysplasia is characterized by large vesicular nuclei with prominent eosinophilic nucleoli similar to those seen in carcinoma.

High-grade dysplasia, as defined above, has a definite association with invasive prostatic adenocarcinoma. A number of studies show a definite association between higher grades of dysplasia and adenocarcinoma of the prostate; however, there is controversy about whether dysplasia is only a cancer-associated lesion or is a precursor lesion for adenocarcinoma. There have been few studies addressing the significance of dysplasia identified histopathologically by needle biopsy and even fewer studies defining or attempting to report this lesion in FNAB material.

Because of the definite association of high-grade dysplasia with invasive carcinoma, the author attempts to recognize it in FNAB samples and report it. We have seen only rare examples in which it was the only finding in FNAB. Our working cytologic definition of dysplasia is essentially the same as the histologic definition of dysplasia. We require that the epithelial cells in question be configured in a pattern closely resembling a prostatic acinus. Nuclear stratification, crowding, and prominent tufting are features similar to those seen histologically. The cells are cohesive, generally show relatively sharp cytoplasmic borders except where crowding is evident, and may exhibit a gradation of atypia within the acinar fragment. The nuclei are larger than those of normal prostatic epithelium, more oval, have a vesicular chromatin pattern, and by definition have conspicuous nucleoli. Basal cells at the periphery and on the surface of a three-dimensional fragment are essential for distinction of this lesion from adenocarcinoma. We have not seen extensive examples of severe dysplasia unassociated with patterns of invasive carcinoma.

Until dysplasia becomes better defined clinically and cytologically, we have recommended close clinical follow-up of any patient in which this cytologic diagnosis is rendered. Specifically, we recommend ultrasound with biopsy of any visible lesion, or if no lesion is detected, blind biopsy by either repeat FNAB or core biopsy.

Atypical architectural patterns, including adenosis and sclerosing adenosis, have generally not been recognized cytologically. Since adenosis is characterized by lack of nuclear atypia and tends to be centrally located, it is unlikely to pose a problem in cytologic diagnosis. Sclerosing adenosis may show nuclear atypia, but, in the author's experience, it is also a central lesion characterized by prominent, spindle basal cells. Although this lesion has not been defined cytologically, the presence of the characteristic spindle basal cells may be useful in suggesting this diagnosis.

Adenocarcinoma of the Prostate

The author uses the criteria established by Kline for the diagnosis of malignancy. These include increased cellularity relative to benign aspirates, a general tendency for cells to be arranged in smaller groups, dyshesion, cellular and nuclear enlargement, anisonucleosis, the presence of macronucleoli, and nuclear membrane irregularities. There is increasing divergence from normal as grade increases.

Particular attention must be directed to distinguishing well-differentiated adenocarcinoma from benign conditions. Experience indicates that adenocarcinomas with a Gleason score of 4 or less tend to be arranged predominantly in small- to medium-sized groups of cells, which often have a tubular or microacinar configuration. Dyshesion is not a particularly prominent feature in adenocarcinomas with a Gleason score of 4 or less but more common for higher-grade tumors. The author has also found the presence of basal cells at the periphery and within groups of cells to be a useful criterion in distinguishing well-differentiated adenocarcinoma from dysplasia, since basal cells are present in dysplasia and not in carcinoma. A rare cytologic finding in well-differentiated adenocarcinoma is the presence of crystalloids similar to those described in tissue. These have been identified histopathologically in as many as 10% of adenocarcinomas and rarely in benign conditions.

A number of authors have attempted to correlate cytologic grade with histologic grade and have achieved variable success. Most studies show a tendency to undergrade adenocarcinoma of the prostate by any form of small biopsy relative to follow-up by radical prostatectomy or transurethral prostatectomy. This discrepancy probably reflects the natural tumor heterogeneity of prostate cancer, which is underestimated by the small sample size obtainable by any biopsy method. The criteria for relating cytologic findings to Gleason histologic score remain relatively subjective. Reported correlations have ranged from 67% to 96%, with higher degrees of correlation being obtained when core biopsy was the histologic standard rather than transurethral resection of the prostate (TURP) or radical prostatectomy. The photomicrographs illustrate exemplary cases and typical examples for delineation of these criteria. Well-differentiated adenocarcinoma with a Gleason score 4 or less is relatively uncommon in FNAB or core biopsy material and is more commonly encountered as small foci in TURP specimens. For practical reporting the author has classified adenocarcinoma into three Gleason groups: scores of 2 to 4, scores of 5 to 7, and scores of 8 to 10. These are clinically useful break points, since most practitioners make their clinical decisions at these points. Since Gleason's grading system is based on histopathology, the term "predicted Gleason score" is used.

In patients treated by irradiation, chemotherapy, or hormonal therapy, there has been interest in the assessment of tumor regression by FNAB. Although complex grading schemes have been established to assess the presence of regression, the literature suggests that a relatively simple approach achieves excellent prognostication. Recurrent neoplasm that either closely resembles the original neoplasm or is of higher grade closely correlates with progression. Hypocellular aspirates or specimens with cellular atypia of uncertain significance have low correlation with tumor progression.

Uncommon Malignancies

Variant Adenocarcinoma. The author has not seen cytologic examples of pure prostatic ductal adenocarcinoma. The few examples in which there has been an exophytic intraurethral presentation of papillary ductal adenocarcinoma have also had components of usual acinar adenocarcinoma. These cases have resembled adenocarcinoma of the cribriform type (Gleason pattern 3). Prostate-specific antigen (PSA) immunostaining is not useful in making this distinction since both acinar and ductal adenocarcinoma are reactive with PSA. We believe that this variant of adenocarcinoma represents the endometrioid variant described in the older literature. Mucinous adenocarcinoma, small-cell undifferentiated adeno-carcinoma, adenosquamous carcinoma, and basaloid carcinoma resembling adenoid cystic carcinoma have all been described in the prostate.

Transitional Cell Carcinoma. Transitional cell carcinoma usually involves the prostate by extension from a urinary bladder primary neoplasm. As many as 45% of patients undergoing cystectomy for bladder carcinoma have evidence of intraprostatic extension. This may be in situ, invasive, or a combination and is usually accompanied by transitional cell carcinoma in situ of the prostatic urethra, where it may occasionally arise. There is often extensive involvement of the intraprostatic ducts and acini. We have seen several examples of transi-tional cell carcinoma that was relatively easy to recognize by conventional cytologic features. Immunohistochemistry with PSA and prostatic acid phospha-tase (PAP) may be useful in some cases, but a negative result may not preclude the possibility of prostatic adenocarcinoma, since some poorly differentiated prostatic adenocarcinomas may be negative for these markers, particularly if the sample size is small or if there are problems with fixation.

Metastatic Adenocarcinoma. The most common metastatic lesion to the prostate in the author's experience is adenocarcinoma arising in the colon or rectum. The differential diagnosis with primary prostatic carcinoma may be difficult, and colonic adenocarcinoma may closely resemble poorly differentiated prostate adenocarcinoma with a Gleason pattern of 5. As noted above, PSA and PAP immunostaining may be helpful.

Mesenchymal Tumors. Leiomyomas, rhabdomyosarcomas, leiomyosarcomas, spindle-cell lesions resembling nodular fasciitis following operative procedures, cystosarcoma, and other very rare mesenchymal tumors have been described in the prostate. The most useful feature in their diagnosis is recognition that they may occur, since their cytologic appearances are not easily confused with adenocarcinoma.

Lymphoma. We have seen several examples of lymphoma presenting in the prostate. Two of these patients have had AIDS. Lymphoma occurring in this setting is usually of the diffuse aggressive type. Other lymphomas, Hodgkin disease, myeloma, and pseudolymphoma have also been reported involving the prostate.

PERFORMANCE CHARACTERISTICS AND SUMMARY

In most series, the performance of FNAB in identifying prostate carcinoma has been excellent, with a sensitivity equal to or superior to traditional core biopsy (80 to 96%), a substantially lower morbidity, usually less than 2% versus approximately 10% for traditional core biopsy, and at substantially reduced cost if the core biopsy is performed in a hospital setting. A risk factor for complications is the presence of prostatitis. Since FNAB is usually performed in the physician's office, we immediately notify the clinician in any case of prostatitis so that antibiotic therapy may be implemented quickly. The majority of cases with complications of fever and the only case of sepsis in the author's experience have occurred following FNAB in patients with prostatitis.

Ultrasound-directed biopsy, so far, has been intermediate in cost between traditional core biopsy performed in a hospital setting and FNAB. The complication rate with ultrasound-directed thin-core biopsy has been very low and comparable to the author's experience with FNAB. Despite the advantages associated with prostatic imaging and thin-core biopsy, there are no prospective data that show a substantial advantage of one technology over the other as documented by patient outcome. Whether or not the advantages are worth the extra cost is yet to be determined. A recent report suggests an additional problem with the Biopty gun, which has not been a problem with FNAB: tumor may involve the needle track of the 18-gauge needle.

In summary, FNAB is still being used by many urologists and has substantial cost advantages relative to other technologies. It has some definite theoretical advantages in assessing the putative precursor lesions of prostate carcinoma, since these lesions probably cannot be imaged reliably and since most of the studies on these conditions have used removal of substantial portions of the gland for their recognition.

FINE NEEDLE ASPIRATION BIOPSY OF THE TESTES AND TESTICULAR ADNEXA

Despite interest in FNAB of the testes in both the diagnosis of intrascrotal mass lesions and in the evaluation of infertility, there has been relatively little published experience on this technique in this country. Fine needle aspiration biopsy has successfully distinguished neoplasms from inflammatory conditions and has been used to assess spermatogenic activity. Since 1979 few reports of the use of FNAB have been published. The most complete illustrated reference on the testes and testicular adnexa remains Zajicek's monograph. A recent reference (Rajawanshi et al.) on the cytomorphology of infertility has excellent illustrations of these conditions.

Bibliography

Cavanna L, Fornari F, Civardi G: Extramedullary plasmacytoma of the testicle: Sonographic appearance and ultrasonically guided biopsy. Blut 6:328–330, 1990.
Epstein JI: Prostate Biopsy Interpretation, in Biopsy Interpretation Series, ed. Silverberg SG, New York, Raven Press, 1989.
Kline TS: Guides to Clinical Aspiration Biopsy: Prostate. New York, Igaku-Shoin, 1985.
Nagler HM, Kaufman DG, OToole KM, et al.: Carcinoma in situ of the testes: Diagnosis by aspiration flow cytometry. J Urol 143:359–361, 1990.
Nagler HM, Thomas AJ: Testicular biopsy and vasography in the evaluation of male infertility. Urol Clin North Am 14:167–176, 1987.
Nseyo UO, Englander LS, Huben RP, et al.: Aspiration biopsy of testis: Another method for histologic examination. Fertil Steril 42:281–284, 1984.
Perez-Guillermo M, Thor A, Lowhagen T: Paratesticular adenomatoid tumors. The cytologic presentation in fine needle aspiration biopsies. Acta Cytol 33:610, 1989.
Pettinato G, Insabato L, De Chiara A, et al.: Fine needle aspiration cytology of a large calcifying Sertoli cell tumor of the testes. Acta Cytol 31:578–582, 1987.
Rajawanshi A, Indudhara R, Goswani AK, et al.: Fine-needle aspiration cytology in azoospermic males. Diagn Cytopathol 7:3–6, 1991.
Sundqvist C, Lukola A, Parvinen M: Testicular aspiration biopsy in evaluation of fertility of mink (Mustela vison). J Reprod Fertil 531:5, 1986.
Zajicek J: Aspiration biopsy cytology. Part 2: Cytology of infradiaphragmatic organs. Monogr Clin Cytol 7:104–128, 1979.

EQUIPMENT

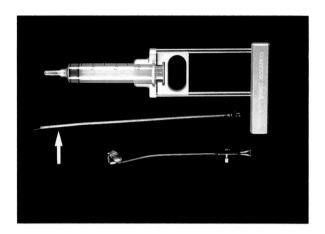

FIGURE 11–1. Cameco "gun" with syringe, 22-gauge needle in plastic sheath, and Franzen needle guide. Note palm plate (arrow) at trumpet end of needle guide.

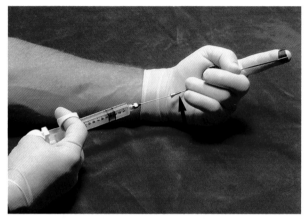

FIGURE 11–2. Operator with Franzen needle guide using control syringe. Note position of palm plate (arrow).

COMMON CONTAMINANTS IN PROSTATE FNAB

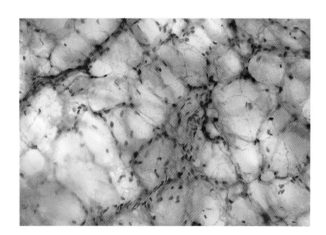

FIGURE 11–3. Fat from Periprostatic Soft Tissue. Fragments such as this are often seen in initial aspiration attempts. These consist of normal adipocytes associated with a delicate capillary network (Papanicolaou stain, × 200).

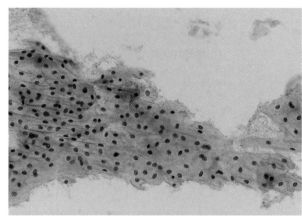

FIGURE 11–4. Squamous Cells of Anal Origin. These can be recognized by their association with rectal mucosa. They can be distinguished from squamous metaplasia associated with prostatic infarcts by the lack of background inflammation and necrosis. Squamous metaplasia associated with estrogen therapy may be more difficult to distinguish and may necessitate a clinical history (Papanicolaou stain, × 200).

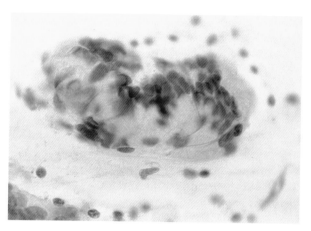

FIGURE 11–5. Fragments of Rectal Mucosa, Fecal Material, and Seminal Vesicle. The rectal mucosal fragments near the center show characteristic tubular colonic glands (arrow) viewed on end, with goblet cells visible even at scanning power. Dyshesive material from the seminal vesicle is in the portion of the smear at the double arrow (Papanicolaou stain, × 80).

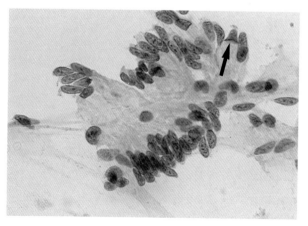

FIGURE 11–7. Rectal Mucosa. A single colonic gland has a three-dimensional appearance. Note prominent nuclear notches and cup-shaped indentations created by the mucus vacuoles, ovoid or slightly spindled nuclei, somewhat uneven nuclear membranes, and occasional small nucleoli (Papanicolaou stain, × 500).

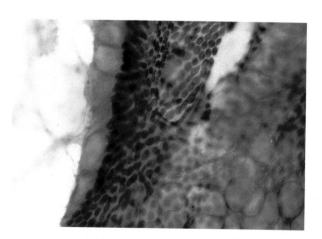

FIGURE 11–6. Rectal Mucosa. Note characteristic nuclear polarity, mucus within the cytoplasm at the edge of the fragment, and prominent "honeycombing" of the mucus-filled goblet cells on the surface of the fragment (Papanicolaou stain, × 200).

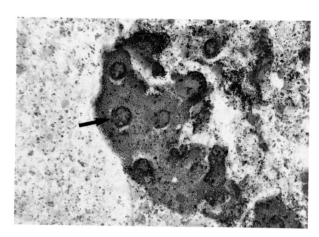

FIGURE 11–8. Rectal Mucosa. The fragment is two-dimensional because of smearing, and the goblet cell pattern is less apparent. Note the conspicuous nuclear polarity, pale cytoplasm, and cup-shaped nuclear indentations (arrow) previously seen (Papanicolaou stain, × 500).

NORMAL CELLS

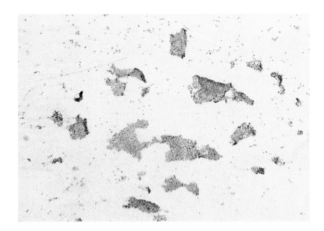

FIGURE 11–9. Prostatic Epithelium. This is a typical benign aspirate at the upper range of cellularity. There are variable-sized fragments and a relatively clean background containing only occasional histiocytes (Papanicolaou stain, × 40).

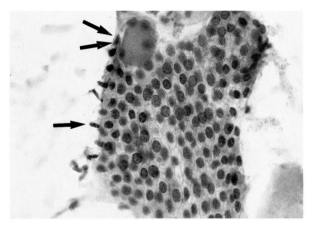

FIGURE 11–11. Prostatic Epithelium. This typical fragment of benign prostatic epithelium shows sharp cytoplasmic borders, pale, finely granular cytoplasm, which may occasionally contain very small lipochrome granules, round to oval nuclei with minimal anisonucleosis, and even chromatin patterns. Note the tufted basal cells at the periphery of the fragment (arrow). Intra-acinar corpora amylacea may be present (double arrow) (Papanicolaou stain, × 400).

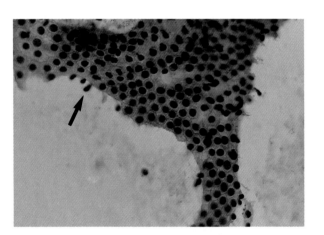

FIGURE 11–10. Prostatic Epithelium. Typical fragment of benign prostatic epithelium showing uniform nuclei, good cohesion, distinct honeycomb pattern with obvious cell borders, small acini within the fragment, and tufted basal cells at the periphery (arrow) (Papanicolaou stain, × 200).

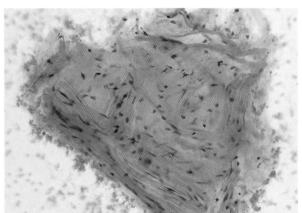

FIGURE 11–12. Prostatic Stroma. A small fragment contains spindle cells with indistinct cytoplasmic borders and bland, fusiform nuclei against a fibrillar background (Papanicolaou stain, × 200).

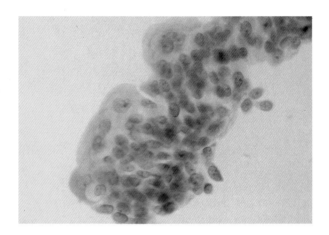

FIGURE 11–13. Transitional Cells. Transitional cells may be of a bladder or metaplastic origin. This fragment shows prominent surface polarity with umbrella cells. Note that transitional cell nuclei may be relatively atypical in metaplasia associated with reactive processes (Papanicolaou stain, × 400).

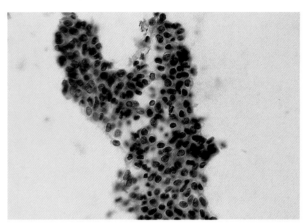

FIGURE 11–14. Basal Cells. Basal cell fragments are common in benign aspirates. The nuclei are somewhat more variable and hyperchromatic, and the nuclear to cytoplasmic ratio is higher than in usual prostatic epithelial cells (Papanicolaou stain, × 200).

PROSTATITIS

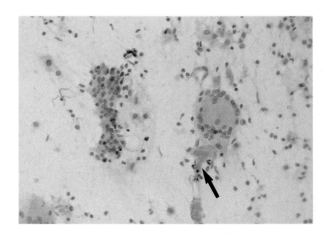

FIGURE 11–15. Prostatitis. The smear is cellular and has fragments of prostatic epithelium, fractured corpora amylacea (arrow), histiocytes and giant cells, and other inflammatory cells. The prominent histiocytes are characteristic of granulomatous prostatitis (Papanicolaou stain, × 200).

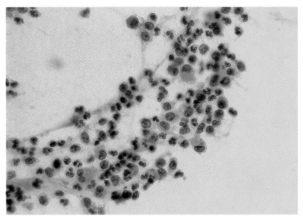

FIGURE 11–16. Prostatitis. The inflammatory cell infiltrate in usual cases is mixed with numerous neutrophils as well as some histiocytes. No epithelium is visible (Papanicolaou stain, × 400).

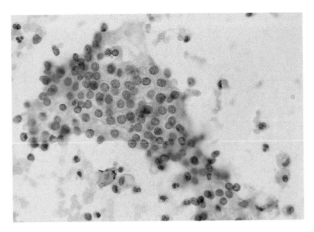

FIGURE 11–17. Prostatitis. The prostatic epithelium may be atypical in prostatitis, as seen here, with slight dyshesion (arrow), some anisonucleosis, and small nucleoli. Neutrophils are present within the fragments, a key feature in ascribing nuclear atypia to inflammation (Papanicolaou stain, × 400).

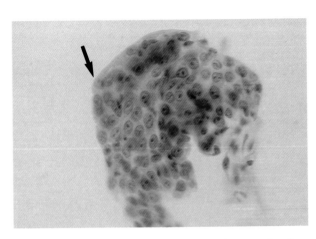

FIGURE 11–19. Prostatitis with Reparative Atypia. Occasional cases of prostatitis show striking nuclear atypia resembling cervical and endocervical repair. Note the relatively good cohesion, sharp border of the group, curving nuclear polarity, and the suggestion of transitional differentiation (arrow). The nuclear atypia is worrisome for carcinoma; however, elsewhere in the smears there was marked inflammation and a gradation of atypia characteristic of prostatitis. This patient had a transurethral resection of the prostate, which showed prostatic infarcts, a follow-up core biopsy, which confirmed prostatitis, and 5 years of clinical follow-up, with no evidence of malignancy (Papanicolaou stain, × 400).

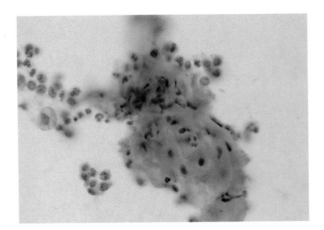

FIGURE 11–18. Prostatitis and Squamous Metaplasia. Prominent squamous metaplasia is seen in association with inflammation. Follow-up by transurethral resection of the prostate on this patient showed extensive prostatic infarcts, with squamous metaplasia and prostatitis. Note the abundant dense cytoplasm and small, pyknotic nuclei characteristic of squamous cells (Papanicolaou stain, × 400).

SEMINAL VESICLE

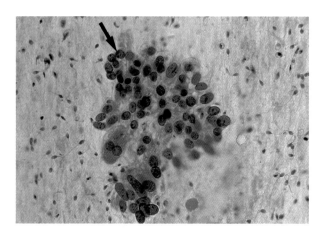

FIGURE 11–20. Seminal Vesicle. A group of seminal vesicle epithelial cells shows vague microacinar arrangements (arrow), and some individual cells have a basaloid appearance. Intracytoplasmic pigment and sperm in the background confirm the origin of these cells (Papanicolaou stain, × 400).

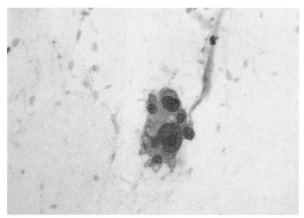

FIGURE 11–22. Seminal Vesicle. A fragment of seminal vesicle epithelium shows characteristic cytoplasmic vacuolation and lipochrome pigmentation. The large nucleolus is relatively unusual in seminal vesicle epithelium (Papanicolaou stain, × 400).

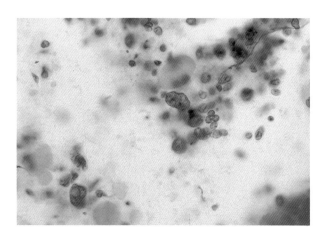

FIGURE 11–21. Seminal Vesicle. Marked nuclear atypia with naked nuclei, irregular nuclear borders, and prominent intranuclear inclusions. Note the "dirty" background and the prominent small corpora amylacea, the latter a characteristic feature of seminal vesicle origin. Intracytoplasmic pigment is easily seen in several of the cells (Papanicolaou stain, × 400).

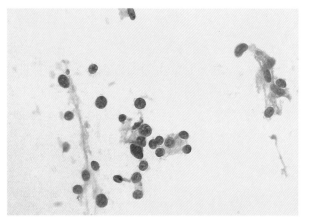

FIGURE 11–23. Seminal Vesicle. Atypical epithelium shows prominent loss of cohesion, naked nuclei, and cells with indistinct cytoplasm. Nuclei vary in shape from oval to spindle and often show dense nuclear hyperchromasia. As seen here, pigment is not always evident. The marked abnormalities of size and shape and characteristic nuclear hyperchromasia should suggest that this aspirate is from the seminal vesicle. Review of the remainder of the smear may be necessary to confirm the origin of cells with features such as these (Papanicolaou stain, × 400).

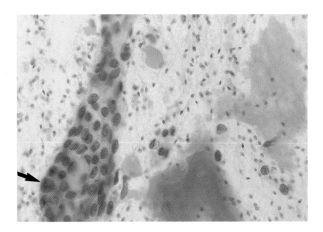

FIGURE 11–24. Seminal Vesicle with Adenocarcinoma of the Prostate. The more cohesive group of cells is from a moderately differentiated adenocarcinoma (arrow). It is present amid a background of sperm and pigmented seminal vesicle epithelium (Papanicolaou stain, × 400).

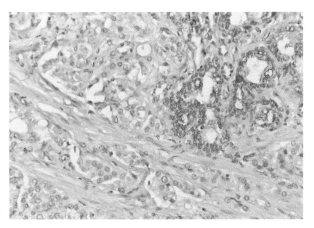

FIGURE 11–25. Adenocarcinoma Involving the Seminal Vesicle. Histologic follow-up confirms the diagnosis in Figure 11–24. It is possible that a single aspiration pass might contain cells from both the seminal vesicle epithelium and an adenocarcinoma, reflecting a combination of the cells in the aspiration process. Therefore, we have been reluctant to classify the seminal vesicle as "involved" by FNAB. Documentation by thin core biopsy is usually a more straightforward interpretation (hematoxylin and eosin stain, × 200).

DYSPLASIA

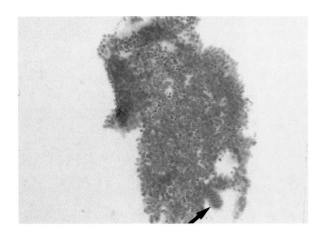

FIGURE 11–26. Dysplasia. A three-dimensional fragment at low power has the configuration of an acinar fragment but shows prominent nuclear crowding and a tufted appearance close to the acinar lumen (arrow), a characteristic feature also seen histologically (Papanicolaou stain, × 200).

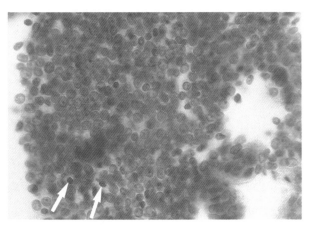

FIGURE 11–27. Dysplasia. A higher magnification of the fragment in Figure 11–26 confirms prominent nuclear crowding and prominent eosinophilic nucleoli. Note that numerous basal cells are evident throughout the fragment (arrows). The overall .features are characteristic of high-grade dysplasia. The differential diagnosis includes the intra-acinar extension of carcinoma. The large fragment size, good cohesion, and lack of other fragments with any of the patterns of invasive growth noted below would preclude a diagnosis of frank adenocarcinoma. This patient has had 6 years of clinical follow-up and three follow-up biopsies (FNAB and thin core) and has no clinical or pathologic evidence of malignancy (Papanicolaou stain, × 500).

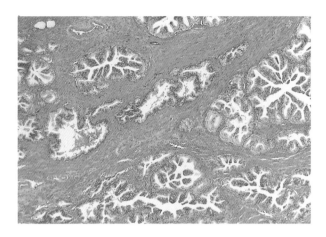

FIGURE 11–28. Dysplasia. Radical prostatectomy follow-up of a different case from that of Figures 11–26 and 11–27, with invasive carcinoma showing extensive dysplasia. Note prominent tufting within acini (hematoxylin and eosin stain, × 40). .

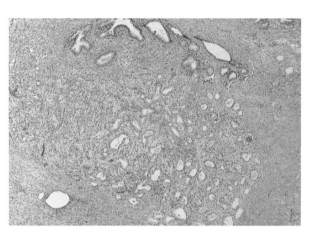

FIGURE 11–30. Sclerosing Adenosis. This lesion has not yet been defined cytologically. Closely packed tubular glands are associated with a cellular fibrous stroma. Lesions are often small and recognized only in transurethral resection specimens.

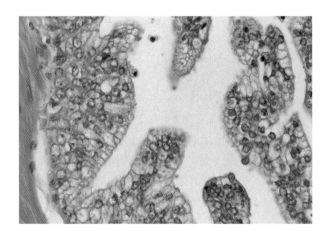

FIGURE 11–29. Dysplasia. Intra-acinar nuclear atypia is histologically similar to that noted cytologically and varies somewhat within the acinus (hematoxylin and eosin stain, × 400).

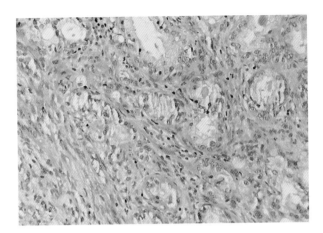

FIGURE 11–31. Sclerosing Adenosis. Higher power shows visible small nucleoli and somewhat irregular nuclei. The stroma is cellular (hematoxylin and eosin stain, × 200).

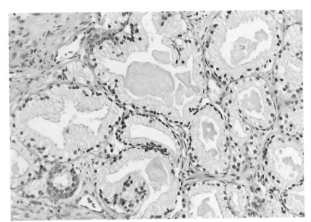

FIGURE 11–32. Adenosis. This lesion has also not yet been clearly identified in an FNAB specimen. Acini are relatively small and closely packed. Nuclear atypia is usually not significant (hematoxylin and eosin stain, × 200).

ADENOCARCINOMA

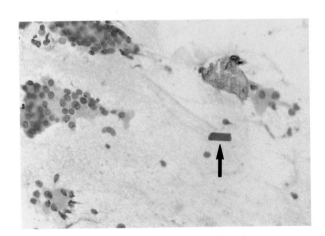

FIGURE 11–33. Well-Differentiated Adenocarcinoma (Gleason Scores of 4 or Less). The smear is cellular and composed of relatively small fragments of epithelium, which have tubular or microacinar configurations. Note that there is no significant inflammation in the background. A crystalloid (arrow) is present and is often seen in tissue sections of well-differentiated adenocarcinoma. Crystalloids are uncommon in aspirate smears and can rarely be seen within benign prostate (Papanicolaou stain, × 200).

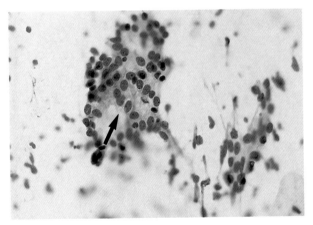

FIGURE 11–34. Well-Differentiated Adenocarcinoma. Note characteristic microacinar formations or microglandular complexes in the large fragment (arrow). The microacinar arrangement is characterized by nuclei distributed at the periphery of a small acinus. The cytoplasm of individual cells is often oriented toward the center of the acinus, giving a rosette appearance. Many fragments of this type should be required for an unequivocal diagnosis of adenocarcinoma (Papanicolaou stain, × 400).

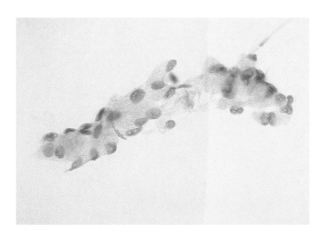

FIGURE 11–35. Well-Differentiated Adenocarcinoma. A tubular fragment is another common conformational pattern in well-differentiated lesions. Dyshesion is slight. Nuclei viewed on edge may resemble basal cells. Anisonucleosis is a prominent feature. Nucleoli are visible but small in most nuclei (Papanicolaou stain, × 500).

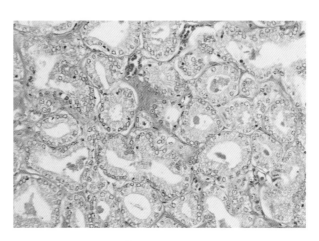

FIGURE 11–37. Well-Differentiated Adenocarcinoma. Radical prostatectomy, a follow-up of case seen in Figure 11–36, shows an adenocarcinoma with a Gleason score of 2 + 2 = 4 (hematoxylin and eosin stain, × 200).

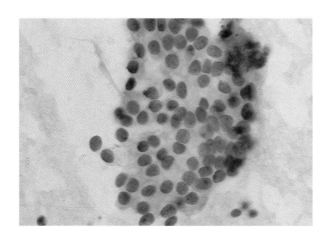

FIGURE 11–36. Well-Differentiated Adenocarcinoma. A relatively small fragment shows nuclear enlargement with mild anisonucleosis (up to twofold variation in nuclear diameter), some crowding, some nuclear contour irregularities, and prominent nucleoli. Cytoplasmic borders are visible, and microacini are again present (Papanicolaou stain, × 500).

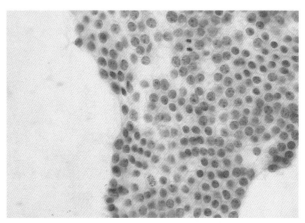

FIGURE 11–38. Dysplasia Versus Well-Differentiated Adenocarcinoma. A relatively large fragment shows no significant loss of cohesion. Preserved cytoplasmic borders and nuclear atypia are similar to features seen in the previous photomicrographs. Two mitotic figures are visible within this field, which would be unusual in benign prostate in the absence of inflammation (Papanicolaou stain, × 400).

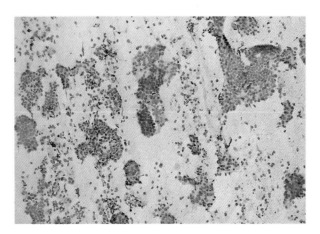

FIGURE 11–39. Moderately Differentiated Adenocarcinoma (Gleason Scores 5 to 7). Very cellular aspirate from moderately differentiated adenocarcinoma. There is a prominent mixture of variable-sized fragments, loosely cohesive cells, and single cells. At this power, these features are intermediate between well-differentiated adenocarcinoma and poorly differentiated adenocarcinoma (Papanicolaou stain, × 80).

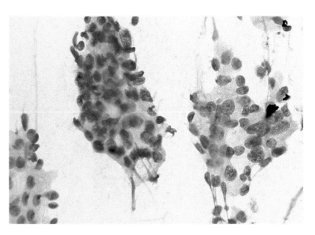

FIGURE 11–41. Moderately Differentiated Adenocarcinoma. Nuclear fragility, atypia, and dyshesion are all more prominent, as seen here (Papanicolaou stain, × 400).

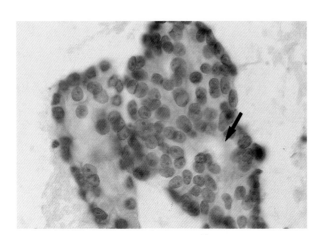

FIGURE 11–40. Moderately Differentiated Adenocarcinoma. Compared with the previous examples (Figures 11–33 through 11–36), there is increasing nuclear atypia, nucleolar prominence, and loss of polarity here. Microacinar configurations are less distinct, although still visible (arrow) (Papanicolaou stain, × 500).

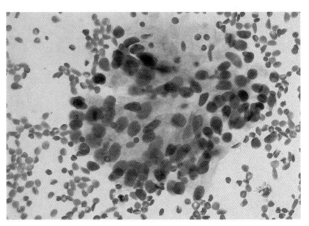

FIGURE 11–42. Moderately Differentiated Adenocarcinoma. This figure shows a hematoxylin- and eosin-stained cytospin preparation rather than a smear. Cellular and nuclear detail are not as sharp as in the Papanicolaou-stained preparation, but the diagnosis of adenocarcinoma is not difficult (hematoxylin and eosin stain, × 400).

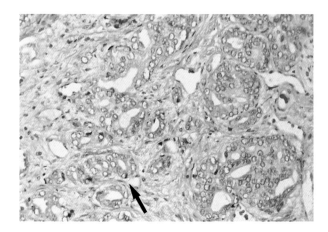

FIGURE 11–43. Moderately Differentiated Adenocarcinoma. Biopsy specimen follow-up of the examples seen in Figures 11–39 and 11–41 shows a moderately differentiated adenocarcinoma with a Gleason score of $3+4=7$. The dominant pattern was an infiltrating single gland pattern (arrow) (hematoxylin and eosin stain, × 200).

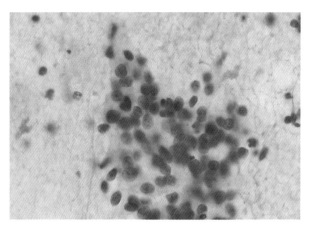

FIGURE 11–45. Moderately Differentiated Adenocarcinoma. Similar complex three-dimensional fragment, with more prominent loss of cohesion and dyshesive cells present in the background. Marked nuclear variability is evident. The absence of significant inflammation, particularly inflammatory cells within the fragment, and the complexity of this fragment exclude prostatitis (Papanicolaou stain, × 400).

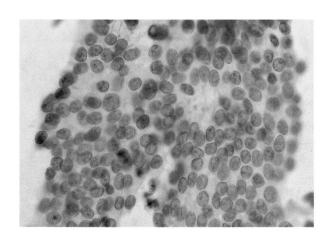

FIGURE 11–44. Moderately Differentiated Adenocarcinoma. Note this large, complex fragment with nuclear enlargement, some crowding, variably prominent nucleoli, and relatively evenly dispersed chromatin. In our experience, large, complex gland fragments correlate with the cribriform areas in Gleason's pattern 3 (Papanicolaou stain, × 400).

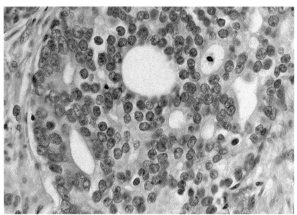

FIGURE 11–46. Moderately Differentiated Adenocarcinoma. Tissue follow-up of Figure 11–44 shows a dominant pattern of cribriform adenocarcinoma in contrast to the previous histopathologic photomicrograph, in which a small gland pattern is prominent (hematoxylin and eosin stain, × 400).

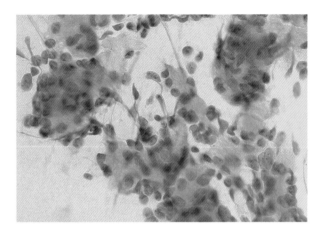

FIGURE 11–47. Moderately Differentiated Adenocarcinoma. Irregular tubular configurations show marked fragility, atypia, and loss of polarity. Abundant dense cytoplasm is present. There is enough evidence of acinar differentiation to keep this cytologic presentation in the moderately differentiated group. These configurations correlate with the fused gland areas seen in Gleason's pattern 4, and the abundant cytoplasm correlates with the "hypernephroid" appearance noted in the following figure (Papanicolaou stain, × 400).

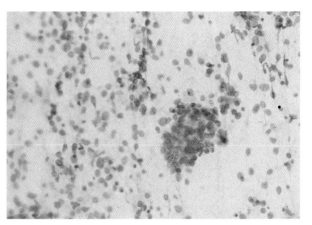

FIGURE 11–49. High-Grade Adenocarcinoma (Gleason Scores of 8 to 10). The differential diagnosis at this power includes prostatitis. Analysis at higher power of the loosely cohesive cells is necessary to differentiate histiocytes and inflammatory cells from the naked nuclei and cells with high nuclear to cytoplasmic ratios of poorly differentiated carcinoma (Papanicolaou stain, × 200).

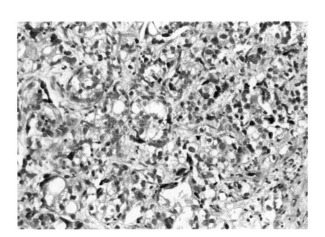

FIGURE 11–48. Moderately Differentiated Adenocarcinoma. Tissue follow-up shows a fused gland pattern with large cells having clear cytoplasm (hypernephroid) characteristic of Gleason pattern 4. The Gleason score on the tissue was 4 + 3 = 7 (Papanicolaou stain, × 200).

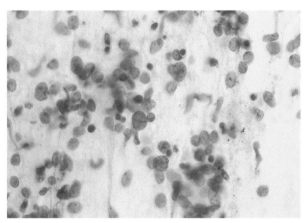

FIGURE 11–50. High-Grade Adenocarcinoma. Individual cells show indistinct cytoplasm, marked nuclear atypia with hyperchromasia, and prominent nuclear karyorrhexis. Although very large nucleoli are common in poorly differentiated adenocarcinomas, many neoplasms in this group show only marked nuclear hyperchromasia and nucleoli may be inconspicuous. There is only vague acinar differentiation. A diagnosis of prostatitis can be excluded at this power by distinguishing nuclear fragments from inflammatory cells (Papanicolaou stain, × 400).

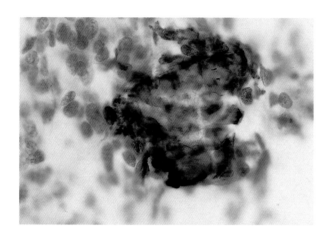

FIGURE 11–51. High-Grade Adenocarcinoma. Note the focus of necrosis in the center amid the abnormal cells. There is apparent dystrophic calcification, and this process can be easily distinguished from corpora amylacea, common in benign conditions, by the irregular character of dystrophic calcification and the abnormal cellular background (Papanicolaou stain, × 500).

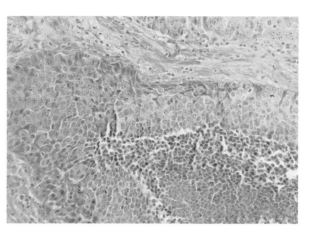

FIGURE 11–53. High-Grade Adenocarcinoma. Tissue follow-up on aspirate seen in Figure 11–51 showed an adenocarcinoma with a dominant Gleason pattern of 5 (comedo necrosis pattern) and a total score of 5+4=9 (hematoxylin and eosin stain, × 80).

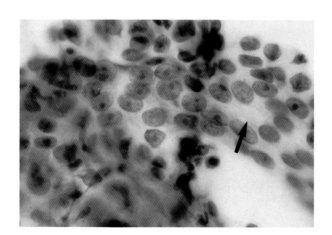

FIGURE 11–52. High-Grade Adenocarcinoma. Note the extremely large size of the cells. Nucleoli are very prominent. Vague acinar formation is evident (arrow) (Papanicolaou stain, × 500).

FIGURE 11–54. Prostate-Specific Antigen. The aspirate is from a patient with a bone lesion and an unknown clinical primary. An immunoperoxidase stain for PSA showed faint positivity within the neoplastic cells. Less differentiated tumors may show only relatively weak positivity (Papanicolaou stain, × 400, destained and reacted with antibody to PSA-immunoperoxidase).

OTHER TUMORS

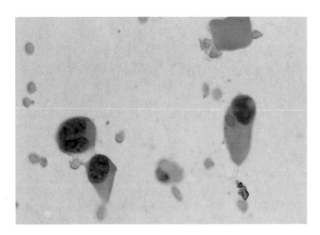

FIGURE 11–55. Transitional Cell Carcinoma. Highly pleomorphic dyshesive cells that have variable nuclear to cytoplasmic ratios and nuclear hyperchromasia are present. This case was diagnosed as a malignancy suggestive of a transitional cell carcinoma extending from a bladder primary, although the patient had no history of bladder cancer. Adenocarcinoma of the prostate was felt to be unlikely because of the dominant presentation as single cells, the nuclear characteristics, and the resemblance of some of the cells to transitional cell carcinoma (Papanicolaou stain, × 500).

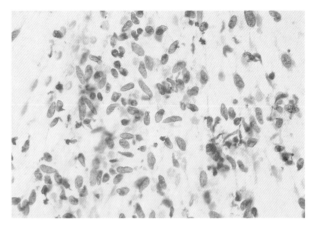

FIGURE 11–57. Leiomyosarcoma. This is an aspirate from a 46-year-old man with a large prostatic mass. The aspirate is very cellular. Most cells have spindle nuclei with some pleomorphism and indistinct cytoplasm. Nuclear karyorrhexis is conspicuous in this field. The cytologic diagnosis was spindle cell neoplasm, probably leiomyosarcoma. The differential diagnosis should include a cellular leiomyoma. The dense and relatively uniform cellularity of this aspirate would exclude the rare, reactive, nodular faciitis–like lesions reported in the prostate. Clinical features and immunocytochemistry could be used to further refine the differential diagnosis and exclude other spindle cell neoplasms (Papanicolaou stain, × 400).

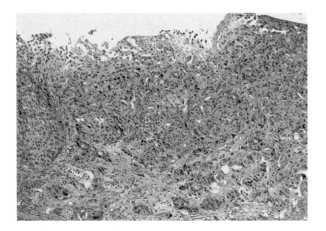

FIGURE 11–56. Transitional Cell Carcinoma. Follow-up biopsy shows a transitional cell carcinoma primary to the prostatic urethra. There was extensive intra-acinar extension and invasive carcinoma (hematoxylin and eosin stain, × 80).

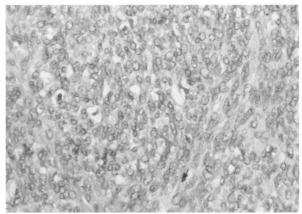

FIGURE 11–58. Leiomyosarcoma. Tissue obtained simultaneously shows a mitotically active, cellular smooth muscle tumor characteristic of leiomyosarcoma (hematoxylin and eosin stain, × 400).

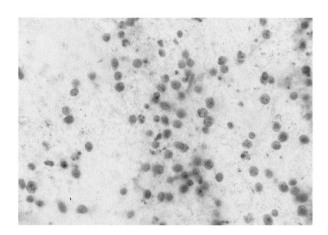

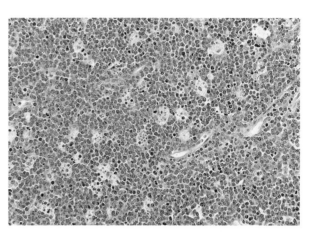

FIGURE 11–59. Malignant Lymphoma. A young man presented with a large prostatic mass. The aspirate is cellular and consists of small, loosely cohesive cells with scant cytoplasm and several small nucleoli within vesicular nuclei. Nuclear karyorrhexis is a prominent feature. The roundness of the nuclei and the uniform presentation as a single cell exclude the diagnosis of adenocarcinoma. The clinical presentation is also unusual for adenocarcinoma (Papanicolaou stain, × 400).

FIGURE 11–61. Malignant Lymphoma. Simultaneous tissue sample confirms a Burkitt lymphoma. Note classic "starry-sky" appearance. Subsequent follow-up showed that the patient had acquired immune deficiency syndrome (hematoxylin and eosin stain, × 200).

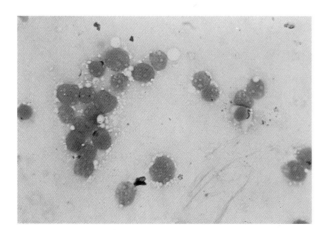

FIGURE 11–60. Malignant Lymphoma. Air-dried, Wright-Giemsa stain from the same case seen in Figure 11–59 shows the characteristic blue cytoplasm and intracytoplasmic lipid vacuoles of a Burkitt lymphoma (Wright-Giemsa stain, × 600).

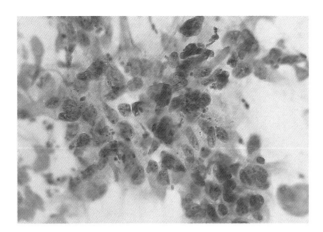

FIGURE 11–62. Adenocarcinoma of the Colon. An elderly man developed a vague prostatic mass following surgery for an unfavorable colon carcinoma. The aspirate shows very large, atypical cells and vague glandular configurations with prominent nuclear hyperchromasia and nuclear karyorrhexis. The differential diagnosis on the Papanicolaou-stained material included high-grade prostatic carcinoma (Papanicolaou stain, × 400).

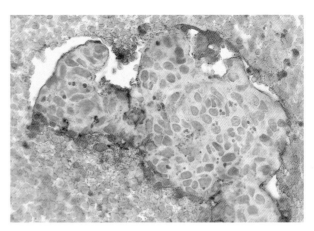

FIGURE 11–63. Adenocarcinoma of the Colon. Material for cell block was available, and a carcinoembryonic antigen stain shows prominent membrane and some intracytoplasmic positivity. A PSA stain was negative, and recurrent colon carcinoma was confirmed (carcinoembryonic antigen immunoperoxidase stain, × 200).

C·H·A·P·T·E·R

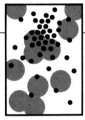

12

FINE NEEDLE ASPIRATION OF THE BREAST

Barbara S. Ducatman

PALPABLE MASSES

Fine needle aspiration (FNA) of the breast is a widely used diagnostic tool to evaluate the patient with a palpable breast mass. At some institutions, this technique has been used to triage the patient with a positive test result for immediate mastectomy, avoiding the need for an intervening biopsy. Over the past 10 years, both state laws and standards of care have changed to limit the use of the one-step surgical procedure in which a patient with a breast mass has a frozen section and further therapy (usually a mastectomy) as determined by the results. The use of FNA to supersede the traditional frozen section done on incisional biopsy, excisional biopsy, or core needle biopsy has made this a most challenging area; both high sensitivity and specificity of diagnosis are demanded.

However, evolution in the management of breast carcinoma by conservative treatment is changing the usefulness of breast aspiration cytology (Fig. 12–1). The use of lumpectomy followed by radiation treatment rather than mastectomy expands the options for a woman with breast cancer, but there may be further usefulness of FNA in this setting. A lumpectomy is usually done regardless of the FNA result. Further management decisions are based upon histologic factors, such as the status of microscopic margins and the extent of associated ductal carcinoma in situ, which must be assessed histologically and cannot be determined by cytologic examination. In this setting, FNA of the breast no longer abrogates the need for open biopsy; nevertheless, it may still play a useful, albeit more limited, role. In centers known for conservative treatment of breast carcinoma, there is a tendency to perform FNA in the following situations: (1) women with suspected malignancy who desire a mastectomy, (2) women with a large or advanced cancer not amenable to conservative treatment, and (3) women with presumably benign disease who are not good operative candidates or who are pregnant. In addition, FNA is often used as a means of expediting a diagnosis for social and psychologic reasons or in order to convince a patient who is reluctant to have a biopsy. Newer developments in the treatment of breast carcinoma, such as preoperative breast chemotherapy or radiation therapy, if proved efficacious, will undoubtedly expand the role of aspiration cytology.

NONPALPABLE LESIONS

Routine use of screening mammography has resulted in the detection of earlier and smaller breast cancers. However, only a minority of breast lesions excised because of mammographic suspicion are proved to be malignant on biopsy. Fine needle aspiration of nonpalpable lesions under conventional or stereotaxic mammographic or sonographic guidance offers the prospect of increasing the specificity of mammography. With conventional mammography, the breast is placed between two compression plates that have a localization grid. The needle is inserted using the x-y coordinates from a scout film, and the depth is checked on a second film taken perpendicular to the first. When the needle is in proper position, an aspiration is performed.

The stereotaxic device may be either a free-standing unit or an attachment added to a conventional mammographic machine. The breast is compressed between two plates. Two views, at 30 degrees to each other, are taken, and the Cartesian coordinates are translated into polar coordinates using a trigonometric program on an attached microprocessor. The needle is advanced at a precalculated angle and to a set depth, and an aspiration is performed.

In contrast to palpable cancers, those detected by mammography are often only in situ rather than infiltrating; a biopsy is usually required to adequately evaluate for most positive cytology diagnoses (Fig. 12–2). However, some investigators believe that a negative result combined with low mammographic suspicion may require only careful follow-up. Concerns over failure to diagnose a malignancy from a false-negative cytology may limit the utility of FNA in this setting.

GENERAL TECHNIQUES

Aspiration cytology of the breast may be evaluated by fixed and/or air-dried direct smears. Papanicolaou stain is best for evaluation of nuclear detail, and Diff-Quik is better for background material. Alternatively, aspirated material may be expelled in a preservative solution, such as Saccomano carbowax fixative, 50% ethanol, or a balanced electrolyte solution. The laboratory then centrifuges the specimen and prepares cytospin smears. This alternative is particularly useful when the aspiration is performed by a clinician in a private office and a cytotechnologist or pathologist is not present to make the direct smears. When immunohistochemical staining for estrogen receptors is requested, slides coated with an adhesive are required. These slides are fixed in picric acid paraformaldehyde.

CYTOLOGIC FEATURES OF MAJOR DISEASES OF BREAST

Benign

Fibrocystic Changes. Fibrocystic changes may show a spectrum of cytologic features akin to those seen in the corresponding histologic picture. Intraductal hyperplasia presents as a cohesive two-dimensional sheet of cells with distinct cell borders and admixed myoepithelial cells (Fig. 12–3). Nuclei are round to oval, regular and small, with a finely granular chromatin. Nucleoli, if present, are inconspicuous. Apocrine metaplastic cells are large with granular or foamy cytoplasm and round, distinct eosinophilic nucleoli (Fig. 12–4). These may be arranged loosely in papillary configurations, clusters, and sheets (Fig. 12–5). Rare, single apocrine cells and foamy macrophages are also found in a proteinaceous background and may be quite prominent in cystic lesions. A granular cell tumor may present a similar picture on aspiration. However, the cells are single with central, small, dark nuclei and a clean background; some investigators feel that positive results for staining with S-100 protein and periodic acid–Schiff with diastase are helpful to distinguish aspirated cells from a granular cell tumor.

Ductal proliferative lesions demonstrate a spectrum ranging from intraductal hyperplasia through atypical ductal hyperplasia to ductal carcinoma in situ. These may be difficult to separate even by histopathology. Since the diagnosis of atypical ductal hyperplasia on histologic sections is in part architectural, the cytologic differentiation of intraductal hyperplasia with and without atypia may not be possible by cytology. Most cytopathologists would only be able to diagnose a case of atypical ductal hyperplasia as atypical cells and/or groups with a recommendation for a surgical biopsy. Cells aspirated from atypical ductal hyperplasia demonstrate more nuclear enlargement and atypicality than normal epithelium or ductal hyperplasia without atypia. They are present in flat sheets; however, nuclear overlapping is more pronounced than in hyperplastic sheets. Cellular dyshesion is not noted; myoepithelial cells are present. Cell borders are distinct, nuclear spacing is regular, and the chromatin pattern is finely granular (Fig. 12–6). All the elements of fibrocystic change may be found together on a single aspiration. Markedly fibrotic lesions or sclerosing adenosis often presents as hypocellular aspirations, which are insufficient for diagnosis. If benign foam cells are present and there are few single cells, an unequivocal diagnosis of malignancy, based on atypical cells in clusters, should not be made.

Fibroadenomas. Fibroadenomas usually yield a cellular specimen. Cohesive sheets and clusters of epithelial cells, often with a classic staghorn appearance, are seen (Fig. 12–7). There may be considerable nuclear overlapping and a mild to moderate degree of nuclear atypicality with nuclear enlargement, finely granular chromatin pattern, and micronucleoli (Fig. 12–8). Occasionally, rare apocrine metaplastic cells are also noted. Many stripped nuclei and/or bipolar cells are seen in the background. In addition, stromal fragments may be present. These features help distinguish fibroadenoma from fibrocystic changes. When the cellularity is not high and the stromal and bipolar cells are not prominent, a differentiation from fibrocystic changes is not always possible.

Phyllodes Tumor. The phyllodes tumor is an uncommon lesion composed of benign epithelium disposed in a cellular stroma. The cytologic picture is similar to that of fibroadenoma; however, in general, the specimen is more cellular. This is particularly true for the stromal component, although both epithelial and stromal elements may contribute to this process. The epithelial cells may appear quite alarming, with a three-dimensional configuration and considerable nuclear atypicality (Fig. 12–9). An occasional mitosis and dyshesion may even be observed. The stromal component may be quite cellular with many elongated, enlarged nuclei and prominent blood vessels within the stroma; however, the diagnosis of malignant phyllodes tumor is usually not possible by cytology alone. The lesions need to have a surgical resection but should not be diagnosed cytologically as malignant. This tumor may be the cause of a false-positive diagnosis of carcinoma; careful attention should be paid to the variation in appearance of the epithelial cells, lack of single malignant cells, and the prominence of the stromal component (Fig. 12–10).

Pregnancy and Lactation. The breast aspirate during pregnancy and lactation often presents a "turned-on" appearance, which may easily be confused with neoplastic processes. The smear often has a proteinaceous background with many single cells. These cells have a delicate, foamy, or vacuolated cytoplasm that is quite fragile and easily stripped away, leaving many single naked nuclei (Fig. 12–11). Lobular structures may be preserved (Fig. 12–12). Large ductal sheets are unusual. The nuclei are regular and round to oval with very prominent round nucleoli. There may be some variation in nuclear size. Pregnancy and lactation always should be kept in mind when an aspirate of a woman of child-bearing age is examined, as the appropriate history may not be given. Of course, breast carcinoma may also be discovered during pregnancy; the presence of significant nuclear or nucleolar irregularity in single cells and groups of cells and a dirty or inflammatory (rather than proteinaceous) background are features suspicious for a malignant process. When in doubt, a surgical biopsy should be suggested.

Therapy-Induced Changes. The most common therapeutic effects that may impact on breast aspirate diagnosis are fat necrosis and radiation changes. These are particularly common in women who have chosen breast-conserving therapy for treatment of their cancer. Unfortunately, in such patients, the suspicion for recurrent carcinoma is also high. Fat necrosis is characterized by a hypocellular aspirate with predominantly single cells and finely to coarsely vacuolated cytoplasm (Fig. 12–13). The nuclei are round or oval, often with small but prominent nucleoli. Careful examination of nuclear detail helps disclose the histiocytic nature of the cells; in this setting, multinucleated cells are particularly useful. An aspiration showing radiation effect is also generally characterized by a poorly cellular specimen. Nuclei are enlarged and hyperchromatic, but the nuclear to cytoplasmic ratio is preserved. Bi- and multinucleated cells may be seen. Nucleoli, when present, are small and inconspicuous (Fig. 12–14). These cells may have vacuolated cytoplasm.

Inflammatory Lesions. Mastitis or breast abscesses may present clinically as a breast mass. The predominant cellular component is acute cellular inflammation; sparse, degenerate epithelial cells are also present. This combination should lead to this diagnosis (Fig. 12–15). Mastitis is commonly found in lactating patients, and in this instance, inflammatory cells are admixed with typical lactation changes.

Malignant Lesions

Ductal Carcinoma in Situ

Ductal carcinoma in situ (DCIS) is a difficult cytologic diagnosis. At one end of the spectrum, it may be difficult to separate noncomedo ductal carcinoma in situ from atypical ductal hyperplasia (ADH). At the other extreme, comedo types of DCIS may be difficult to distinguish from invasive cancers. However, there are several points of differentiation between ADH and DCIS. Although both have three-dimensional groupings with enlarged, hyperchromatic nuclei, only ductal carcinoma in situ also has many single malignant cells, an inflammatory background, and coarsely granular chromatin pattern (Fig. 12–16). Myoepithelial cells and cell borders are usually not noted within the cell groupings. On the other hand, it is not always possible to reliably separate ductal carcinoma in situ from infiltrating carcinoma. This is probably especially true for the comedo variant of in situ, which often has necrotic background with many single, very atypical epithelial cells (Figs. 12–17 and 12–18). Papillary carcinoma is characterized by many three-dimensional papillary groups of cells with a smooth, tight cellular configuration of the outside border of the group (Fig. 12–19). Nuclear atypicality is variable. Differentiation of papillary carcinoma from intraductal papilloma is often not possible (Fig. 12–20). In such instances, it is most prudent to diagnose "papillary lesion—recommend biopsy."

Infiltrating Ductal Carcinoma

The diagnosis of carcinoma is usually much easier than the diagnosis of preceding entities. Ductal cancer usually is characterized by a richly cellular aspirate with a background that is variable but can be either clean, bloody, inflammatory, or necrotic (Fig. 12–21). The best criteria are probably the many large and small, dyshesive, three-dimensional cellular groupings (Figs. 12–22 and 12–23) with a large proportion of single cells. The single cells are characteristic in appearance with abundant cytoplasm, and eccentric nuclei may appear to protrude out of the cytoplasm (Fig. 12–24). Classic nuclear features of malignancy that are often seen include nuclear pleomorphism, irregular nuclear membranes, and single or multiple irregular, prominent nucleoli (Fig. 12–25). In such a setting, a confident diagnosis of malignancy is easily made; however, such a diagnosis should be rendered only on a slide that is technically excellent—appropriately smeared, preserved or dried, and stained.

The most common variants of ductal carcinoma often present characteristic appearances by aspiration cytology. The mucinous background of colloid carcinoma is most easily appreciated on Romanowsky-type stains, where it is seen as metachromatic purple-to-pink material (Fig. 12–26A). Loosely or tightly cohesive clusters of tumor cells are often quite banal in appearance, with minimal nuclear atypicality (Fig. 12–26B). Thin, delicate branching capillary structures may also be noted (Fig. 12–27). Cells may also be seen singly or in sheets. This diagnosis is most easily appreciated on low-power examination where the aforementioned features are best seen. Mucinous carcinoma is often admixed with the more classic forms of in situ and infiltrating carcinoma; in such instances, the cytologic picture may reflect a mixture of features of each entity present.

Medullary carcinoma is cytologically characterized by many markedly enlarged atypical cells present in either dyshesive sheets or singly. Nuclei are large and pleomorphic and have clumped chromatin, irregular nuclear membranes, and macronucleoli (Fig. 12–28). Many bizarre naked nuclei and benign lymphoid cells are also present. Presence of the characteristic epithelial and lymphoid components is necessary to suggest this diagnosis.

Ductal carcinoma with apocrine features is similar in appearance to ordinary infiltrating carcinoma, but the cytoplasm is more abundant and granular. Nuclei often have central, large, prominent eosinophilic nucleoli. The cytoplasm is similar to that seen in apocrine metaplasia: dense green on Papanicolaou, eosinophilic on hematoxylin and eosin, and gray on Giemsa stains. As with typical ductal carcinoma, the nuclei are often protuberant and eccentrically placed (see Fig. 12–17).

Lobular Carcinoma

The diagnosis of lobular carcinoma in situ is often very difficult or impossible. Such lesions often appear as cohesive sheets of cells with some nuclear enlargement and overlapping (Fig. 12–29). The lack of cellular dyshesion or significant nuclear atypicality precludes a definite diagnosis. Nuclear chromatin is often hypochromatic in comparison to that of ductal type cells. The presence of signet-ring cells within groupings may prove useful; unfortunately, these cells are often not easily appreciated.

The smear of infiltrating lobular carcinoma generally has low to moderate cellularity with predominantly single cells and small groupings (Fig. 12–30). The presence of the classic "Indian files" may be especially helpful. The cells of lobular carcinoma have smaller and less atypical nuclei than ductal carinoma. These nuclei are round and eccentric and show chromatin clearing. When present, nuclear molding, or signet ring cells, are also particularly useful in identifying a case as lobular carcinoma rather than ductal carcinoma (Fig. 12–31).

Uncommon Variants of Breast Cancer

Adenoid cystic carcinoma of the breast has cytologic features identical to those seen in a salivary gland aspiration. Smears are cellular with a mucoid background and characteristic dense, round, pink-to-purple globules best appreciated on air-dried preparations. The cells, which may be arrayed around the globules, are small and regular and have scant cytoplasm.

Breast cancer that shows neuroendocrine differentiation is uncommon. Such lesions yield cellular aspirates, with many small cells present in loose clusters or singly. Nuclei are typically eccentric, with scant granular cytoplasm. The chromatin pattern shows the classic salt-and-pepper, coarse granularity with inconspicuous nucleoli. These tumors may demonstrate positive immunostaining for chromogranin. The differential diagnosis includes lobular carcinoma, lymphoma, and metastatic neuroendocrine tumor (Fig. 12–32).

Inflammatory carcinoma is a clinical diagnosis. The histologic picture of tumor within dermal lymphatics cannot be appreciated on cytology. A classic infiltrating ductal carcinoma is observed when such lesions are successfully aspirated. Secretory carcinoma presents a picture similar to typical infiltrating ductal carcinoma, but the cells contain clear or vacuolated cytoplasm. Dyshesive sheets of cells may be noted. The nuclei exhibit some anisonucleosis and nuclear irregularity. Tubular carcinoma in the classic case has small, cohesive, three-dimensional clusters of cells often with pointed ends and a comma-like configuration. These distinctions do not have to be made on FNA. It is sufficient to recognize such cases as suspicious or malignant.

Metaplastic carcinoma (e.g., carcinosarcoma or sarcomatoid carcinoma) may present with foci that have very dissimilar histologic appearances; the cytologic picture is likewise variable and often confusing. Certainly, malignant squamous cells and heterologous sarcomatoid elements (e.g., osteoclast giant cells and chondrocytes) should provide valuable clues to this diagnosis. These may not be present, and a pure population of malignant spindle cells (with or without an epithelial component) may be noted (Fig. 12–33). It may be necessary to use immunocytochemical markers to differentiate a metaplastic carcinoma from a primary sarcoma of the breast. Generally, the final diagnosis is not possible until surgical biopsy, although it may be suggested cytologically.

Nonepithelial Malignancies and Metastatic Carcinoma. The cytologic appearance of breast lymphoma and sarcoma is identical to that seen in other sites. A cellular smear of monomorphic, atypical lymphoid cells or malignant-appearing spindle cells should be judged in the same way as they would in a common location such as a lymph node or soft tissue. Metastatic carcinoma to the breast should be considered in all patients who have a history of prior malignancy or whenever the pattern and cytologic appearance of the aspirate do not conform to the typical appearance of the variants of breast carcinoma (see Fig. 12–32).

Male Breast. Aspiration of the male breast is uncommon. The major differential diagnosis is between gynecomastia and carcinoma. Gynecomastia has a cytologic appearance similar to that seen in fibroadenoma. There are variable-sized cohesive clusters and sheets of cells with regularly spaced nuclei. Nuclei are round or oval with a finely granular chromatin pattern. Stripped nuclei and bipolar stromal cells are present (Fig. 12–34). The cytologic appearance of carcinoma of the male breast is in most cases identical to that of infiltrating ductal carcinoma observed in the female breast.

Sensitivity and Specificity. The diagnostic accuracy of aspiration cytology has generally been quite good, with reported sensitivity of 85 to 90% and specificity of 98 to 100%.

PITFALLS

False-Negative Results. The most common cause of a false-negative result is failure to obtain the malignant cells during the aspiration. This may be due to operator inexperience or to the lesion itself. The lesions that most commonly provide scant or nondiagnostic cells include scirrhous, cystic, or necrotic carcinomas. A false-negative result from improper placement of the needle is a particular problem in aspiration of nonpalpable lesions. Inexperience on the part of the diagnosing pathologist may also lead to false-negative results. This is especially true for cases of well-differentiated carcinoma and noncomedo variants of ductal carcinoma in situ.

False-Positive Results. A common cause for a false-positive result is the overinterpretation of poorly made and/or preserved slides, especially smears that are too thick, too bloody, or partially air-dried (when they are supposed to be alcohol-fixed). A definitive malignant diagnosis should not be made on a hypocellular specimen. Since a mastectomy or definitive treatment may result from any positive diagnosis, it is most prudent to reserve a positive diagnosis for cases in which there is virtually no doubt of malignancy. In cases where there is some hesitancy, a suspicious diagnosis should be rendered and biopsy suggested.

Certain lesions, such as fibroadenoma, pregnancy, lactation, radiation changes, ADH, and fat necrosis, are notorious for causing false-positive results. It is important to keep these entities in mind when an FNA is examined. If there is any suspicion that one of these lesions has been aspirated, a clinical history must be obtained; unfortunately, historical data are often not submitted with the specimen.

INTERACTING WITH THE CLINICIANS

It is important that the pathologist reading the aspirate understand the implications of his or her diagnosis. It is equally important that the pathologist and clinician agree and communicate on the nomenclature. The pathologist should never make a positive diagnosis on less-than-definitive material with the assumption that a confirmatory biopsy will follow; this could lead to an unnecessary mastectomy. In addition, the pathologist should understand the limitations of the procedure and communicate these to the clinician. Particularly, it must be recognized that the absence of malignant cells on the cytology preparations does not necessarily imply that there is no malignancy within the patient. Cytologic features must be carefully considered in light of the clinical impression and mammographic findings. Nor is a positive result a guarantee of infiltrating carcinoma—it is not always possible to differentiate in situ from infiltrating ductal carcinoma. This is a particularly important factor when considering the use of preoperative adjuvant chemotherapy and in nonpalpable lesions. When there is doubt, a surgical biopsy is always a prudent procedure. Lastly, FNA is not as good as surgical biopsy in rendering a specific diagnosis, whether the differential is benign (e.g., fibroadenoma or fibrocystic changes), preneoplastic (e.g., atypical ductal hyperplasia or lobular carcinoma in situ), or malignant (e.g., infiltrating lobular carcinoma or specific subtypes of ductal carcinoma) cells.

Differential diagnoses are summarized in Tables 12–1 to 12–7.

Bibliography

Bell DA, Hajdu SI, Urban JA, Gaston JP: Role of aspiration cytology in the diagnosis and management of mammary lesions in office practice. Cancer 51:1182–1189, 1983.
Frable WJ: Needle aspiration of the breast. Cancer 53:671–676, 1984.

Kline TS, Joshi LP, Neal HS: Fine needle aspiration of breast: Diagnosis and pitfalls. A review of 3545 cases. Cancer 44:1458–1469, 1979.

Kline TS, Kline IK: Breast. In Kline TS (ed.): Guides to Clinical Aspiration Biopsy Series. New York: Igaku-Shoin, 1989.

Oertel YC: Fine Needle Aspiration of the Breast. Boston: Butterworths, 1987.

Oertel YC, Galblum LI: Fine needle aspiration of the breast: Diagnostic criteria. Pathol Annu 18:375–407, 1983.

Wang HH, Ducatman BS, Eick DM: Comparative features of ductal carcinoma in situ and infiltrating ductal carcinoma of the breast on fine needle aspiration biopsy. Am J Clin Pathol 92:736–740, 1989.

Table 12–1. DIFFERENTIAL DIAGNOSIS OF SINGLE EPITHELIAL CELLS

Cytologic Features	Ductal Carcinoma in Situ (Fig. 12–35A) and Infiltrating (Figs. 12–35B and 12–35C)	Lobular Carcinoma Infiltrating (Figs. 12–35D and 12–35E)	Pregnancy and Lactation (Figs. 12–35F and 12–35G)
Background	Inflammatory; dirty, bloody; clean	Clean	Watery, proteinaceous
Cellularity	Highly infiltrating Low to high in DCIS	Low to moderate	Low to high
Cellular arrangement	Dyshesive small and large clusters; irregular nuclear spacing	"Indian files"; small clusters with pronounced nuclear molding	Loosely and tightly cohesive lobules
Single cells	Numerous; large eccentric nuclei with abundant cytoplasm	Small cells with eccentric nuclei and scant cytoplasm; signet-ring cells	Many naked nuclei and cells with delicate wispy cytoplasm
Nuclear pleomorphism	Mild to pronounced	Mild	Minimal
Chromatin pattern	Finely to coarsely granular	Bland, hypochromatic, cleared	Bland, finely granular
Nucleoli	Variable	Inconspicuous	Prominent but small, round, regular

Table 12–2. DIFFERENTIAL DIAGNOSIS OF ATYPICAL APOCRINE CELLS

Cytologic Features	Apocrine Metaplasia and Cystic Lesions (Fig. 12–36A)	Apocrine Carcinoma (Figs. 12–36B and 12–36C)
Cellularity	Low to moderate	High
Background	Proteinaceous fluid and foamy macrophages in cystic lesions	Tumor diathesis; inflammatory
Cellular arrangement	Cohesive sheets, clusters, and papillary groupings	Dyshesive clusters and sheets
Single cells	Rare; central nuclei	Numerous; eccentric nuclei
Nuclear pleomorphism	Mild to moderate	Marked
Nucleoli	Small to large, regular	Small to very large

Table 12–3. DIFFERENTIAL DIAGNOSIS OF THREE-DIMENSIONAL CELL GROUPINGS WITH OVERLAPPING AND NUCLEAR ATYPICALITY

Cytologic Features	Fibroadenoma (Fig. 12–37A) and Phyllodes Tumor (Fig. 12–37B)	Atypical Ductal Cells (Atypical Ductal Hyperplasia) (Fig. 12–37C)	Lobular Carcinoma in Situ (Fig. 12–37D)	Ductal Carcinoma in Situ (Fig. 12–37E) and Infiltrating (Figs. 12–37F and 12–37G)
Cellularity	High—both stromal and epithelial in phyllodes tumor; high—predominantly epithelial in fibroadenoma	Low to moderate	Low to moderate	Low to high in in situ and high in infiltrating ductal carcinoma
Background	Clean; many stripped and bipolar cells	Clean	Clean	Inflammatory, bloody, dirty, clean
Cellular arrangement	Sheets; tight clusters often in staghorn configuration	Sheets with nuclear overlapping; cohesive clusters	Loose clusters and sheets; tight small clusters	Dyshesive sheets and clusters
Nuclear spacing	Regular	Regular	Regular	Irregular
Single cells	Numerous bipolar cells and stripped nuclei but no single epithelial cells	Few	Few	Many epithelial
Nuclear pleomorphism	Mild in fibroadenoma; mild to moderate in phyllodes tumor	Mild	Mild	Marked
Chromatin pattern	Finely granular; may be coarsely granular in phyllodes tumor	Finely granular	Bland; hypochromatic (washed out)	Finely to coarsely granular

Table 12–4. DIFFERENTIAL DIAGNOSIS OF PAPILLARY CONFIGURATIONS

Cytologic Features	Papillary Lesion, Favor Papilloma (Figs. 12–38A and 12–38B)	Papillary Lesion, Favor Papillary Carcinoma (Figs. 12–38C and 12–38D)
Cellularity	Low	High; many tall, columnar cells
Background	Clean; cystic-foam cells and apocrine metaplasia	Bloody, dirty
Single cells	Few	Few to many
Nuclear pleomorphism	Mild to moderate	Mild to marked
Nuclear membrane irregularity	Minimal	Mild to moderate
Nuclear shape	Round or oval	Tall, columnar

Table 12–5. DIFFERENTIAL DIAGNOSIS OF PROMINENT STROMAL COMPONENT

Cytologic Features	Fibroadenoma (Figs. 12–39A and 12–39B)	Phyllodes Tumor (Figs. 12–39C and 12–39D)	Metaplastic Carcinoma (Figs. 12–39E to 12–39G)	Primary Breast Sarcoma (Fig. 12–39H)
Cellularity	High	High	High	High
Types of cells	Predominantly epithelial	Both epithelial and stromal	Both epithelial and stromal	Stromal
Arrangement of stromal cells	Stripped nuclei and single bipolar cells; hypocellular stromal fragments	Many cellular stromal fragments; single bipolar cells and stripped nuclei	Dyshesive sheets and clusters; single atypical cells; osteoclast giant cells or chondrocytes may be visible	Dyshesive sheets and clusters; single, very atypical spindle cells
Atypicality	Epithelial—mild to moderate	Epithelial—mild to moderate; stromal—variable	Epithelial—minimal to marked; stromal—marked	Stromal—marked; epithelial, if present—minimal
Keratin	Not useful	Not useful	Positive; may be focal	Negative
Vimentin	Not useful	Not useful	+/−	Positive

Table 12–6. DIFFERENTIAL DIAGNOSIS OF MANY INFLAMMATORY CELLS

Cytologic Features	Intramammary Lymph Node (Fig. 12–40A)	Medullary Carcinoma (Figs. 12–40B and 12–40C)	Lymphoproliferative Lesion (Figs. 12–40D and 12–40E)	Mastitis (Fig. 12–40F)
Cellularity	High	High	High	Low to high
Inflammatory cells	Polymorphous lymphoid with tingible body macrophages	Polymorphous lymphoid with lymphocytes and plasma cells	Monomorphic lymphoid; atypical	Polymorphonuclear leukocytes; small lymphocytes and plasma cells
Epithelial component	None	Malignant single cells with macronucleoli; many bare nuclei	None	Benign, if present

Table 12–7. DIFFERENTIAL DIAGNOSIS OF VACUOLATED CELLS

Cytologic Features	Fat Necrosis (Fig. 12–41A)	Mucinous Carcinoma (Figs. 12–41B and 12–41C)	Lobular Carcinoma (Fig. 12–41D)	Pregnancy and Lactation (Figs. 12–41E and 12–41F)	Silicone Injection (Figs. 12–41G and 12–41H)	Secretory Carcinoma
Background	Clean, macrophages	Mucinous material; purple on Diff-Quik, greenish on Papanicolaou; prominent capillaries	Clean; rarely inflammatory	Watery, proteinaceous	Clean	Proteinaceous; inflammatory
Cellularity	Low	Low to high	Low to moderate	Low to high	Low to moderate	High
Cellular arrangement	Single cells	Tight balls and tight and loose clusters	Loose clusters; many single cells	Lobules; many single, naked nuclei	Tight clusters; single macrophages	Dyshesive clusters and sheets; many single cells
Nuclear pleomorphism	Minimal, histiocytic-type cells	Mild	Mild	Mild	Minimal	Moderate
Cytoplasm	Finely vacuolated	Large vacuoles	Small cells; single vacuoles	Finely vacuolated, wispy, delicate	Large vacuoles	Clear cytoplasm; signet ring cells

443

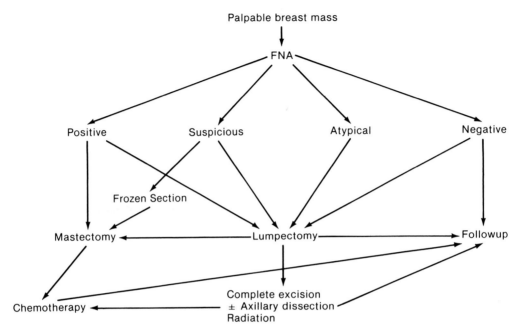

FIGURE 12–1. Decision-making based on FNA of palpable breast masses.

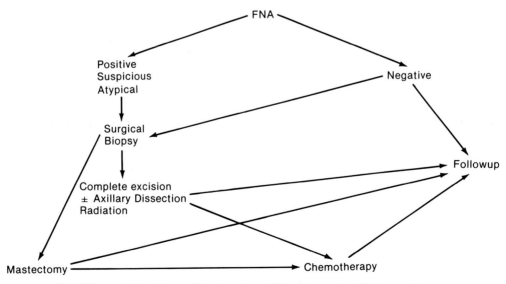

FIGURE 12–2. Decision-making based on FNA of nonpalpable breast lesions.

BENIGN LESIONS

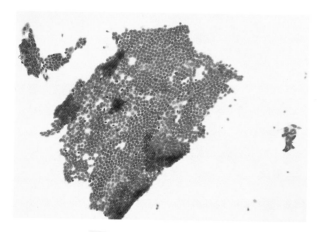

FIGURE 12–3. Intraductal Hyperplasia. The ductal cells are round, regular, and arranged in a tight sheet. Cytoplasmic boundaries are distinct. There is no appreciable atypicality. Such a picture may be noted with other fibrocystic changes (Papanicolaou stain, × 250).

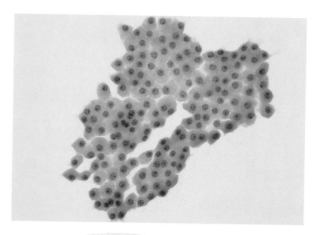

FIGURE 12–5. Apocrine Metaplasia. Here the cells are arranged in a cohesive sheet. These findings are common in aspirations of the breast with fibrocystic changes (Papanicolaou stain, × 100).

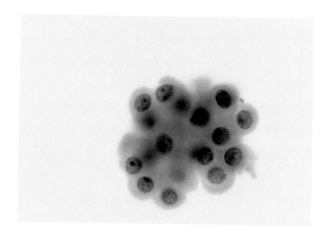

FIGURE 12–4. Apocrine Metaplasia. These cells are arranged in a papillary cluster. The cytoplasm is dense, granular, and green. Nuclei are small, round, and regular, with inconspicuous nucleoli, but these may occasionally be more prominent in apocrine metaplasia (Papanicolaou stain, × 250).

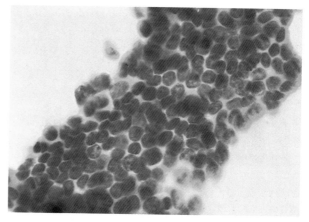

FIGURE 12–6. Atypical Ductal Hyperplasia. This picture may be difficult to differentiate from intraductal hyperplasia without atypia, non–comedo-type ductal carcinoma in situ, or a fibroadenoma. The benign features of this entity include the cohesion of the cellular groupings and the lack of significant nuclear atypicality, pleomorphism, or single cells (Diff-Quik stain, × 250).

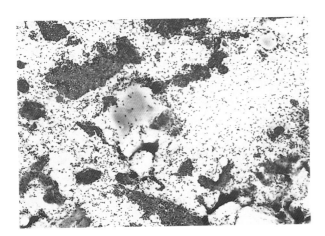

FIGURE 12–7. Fibroadenoma. This low-power picture demonstrates hypercellularity. Many of the cell groups are arranged in the classic staghorn configuration with single, stripped nuclei and bipolar cells in the background. Secretions are also present that stain purple to bright blue in the background (Papanicolaou stain, × 50).

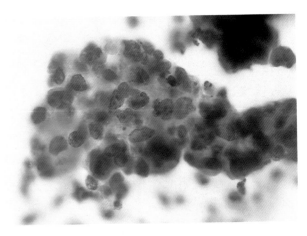

FIGURE 12–9. Benign Phyllodes Tumor. The epithelial component shows pronounced nuclear overlap with moderate atypicality and hemosiderin granules. Note the cellular cohesion similar to that seen in a fibroadenoma (Papanicolaou stain, × 250).

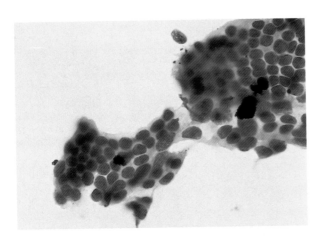

FIGURE 12–8. Fibroadenoma. Nuclei are enlarged, with overlap and mild pleomorphism. Care should be taken not to overdiagnose a fibroadenoma as malignant. Although the nuclear atypicality may be worrisome, the cells are cohesive. In addition, background often contains stromal fragments and single, stripped nuclei and bipolar cells. If the background is not well-appreciated, a fibroadenoma cannot always be distinguished from other entities (Papanicolaou stain, × 250).

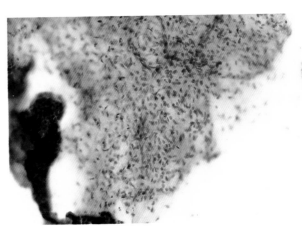

FIGURE 12–10. Benign Phyllodes Tumor. A prominent cellular stromal component with many cohesive spindled cell is present. These lesions cannot always be separated from those of a fibroadenoma, but the stromal component is often more pronounced (Papanicolaou stain, × 100).

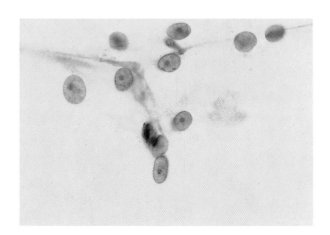

FIGURE 12–11. Pregnancy/Lactational Change. Many stripped nuclei with wispy, delicate cytoplasm are visible in the cells. The chromatin pattern is bland. Nucleoli are very prominent, but they are round, regular, and distinct (Papanicolaou stain, × 250).

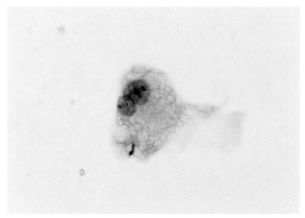

FIGURE 12–13. Fat Necrosis. Binucleate histiocyte with bland nuclei and vacuolated cytoplasm. The smear is usually hypocellular, with a clean background. Careful attention to the benign nuclear characteristics should help to separate this entity from malignant tumors (Papanicolaou stain, × 250).

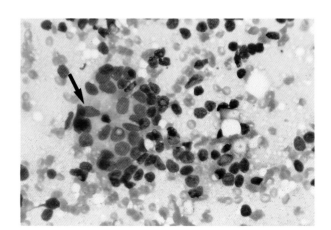

FIGURE 12–12. Pregnancy/Lactational Change. A lobule is present (arrow) with many single cells and proteinaceous debris in the background. The typical lobular formation with the watery, proteinaceous background and many stripped nuclei are features that should suggest this diagnosis (Diff-Quik stain, × 150).

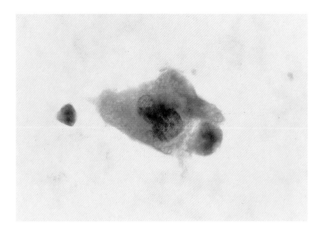

FIGURE 12–14. Radiation Change. This binucleate cell has a finely vacuolated cytoplasm, which is often polychromatic. The nuclear to cytoplasmic ratio is preserved, although the nuclei are enlarged. The nuclei lack a crisp chromatin pattern. A degenerating malignant cell is present in the background (Papanicolaou stain, × 250).

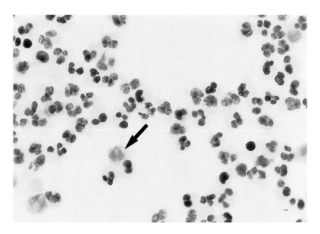

FIGURE 12–15. Acute Mastitis. Many acute inflammatory cells and rare degenerating epithelial cells (arrow) are noted in the specimen from this patient with acute mastitis (Papanicolaou stain, × 250).

ADENOCARCINOMA

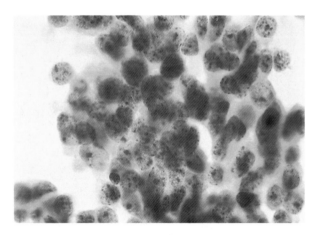

FIGURE 12–16. Ductal Carcinoma in Situ. This aspirate is from a patient with pure ductal carcinoma in situ. The cells are arranged in dyshesive clusters, with coarsely granular chromatin and irregular nuclear spacing. Nucleoli are present and are irregular and variable. The marked pleomorphism, coarsely granular chromatin, dyshesion, and irregular nuclear spacing help to differentiate this case from one of atypical ductal hyperplasia (see Figure 12–6). However, on the aspirate, a diagnosis of invasive carcinoma cannot be excluded (Papanicolaou stain, × 250).

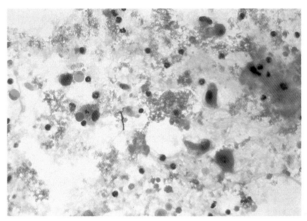

FIGURE 12–17. Comedo-Type Ductal Carcinoma in Situ. There are few pleomorphic single cells in a necrotic background, consistent with a tumor diathesis. This picture cannot be separated from one of infiltrating ductal carcinoma (Papanicolaou stain, × 100).

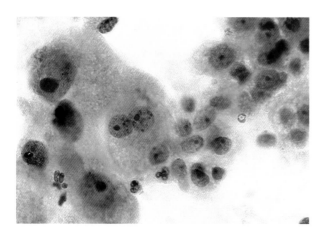

FIGURE 12–18. Comedo-Type Ductal Carcinoma in Situ with Apocrine Features. There is a group of large and highly atypical apocrine cells and loosely cohesive clusters of smaller cells with scant cytoplasm. Nuclei are eccentric and pleomorphic, with prominent macronucleoli, and the cytoplasm is granular. This picture could also represent an infiltrating ductal-type carcinoma with apocrine differentiation (Papanicolaou stain, × 250).

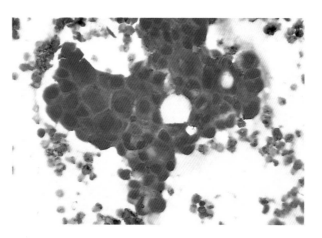

FIGURE 12–20. Intraductal Papilloma. A cohesive cluster of ductal cells is present, with a moderate amount of cytoplasm. Nuclei are slightly enlarged and vary in size and shape. The background is often hemorrhagic, with hemosiderin-laden macrophages. Note the cytoplasmic clearing (Diff-Quik stain, × 150).

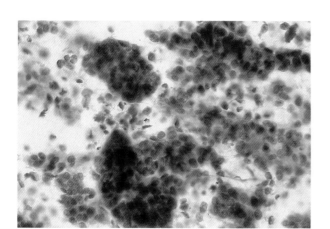

FIGURE 12–19. Papillary Ductal Carcinoma. This was diagnosed as a papillary neoplasm, favor papillary carcinoma. Nuclei are uniform and regularly spaced, and differentiation from a papilloma would be difficult. However, the specimen is cellular, and in the background are many single abnormal cells (Papanicolaou stain, × 100).

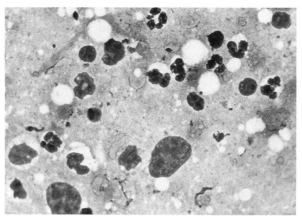

FIGURE 12–21. Infiltrating Ductal Carcinoma. Many single, very atypical, and pleomorphic cells are present in a background of blood, inflammatory cells, and necrotic debris (Diff-Quik stain, × 250).

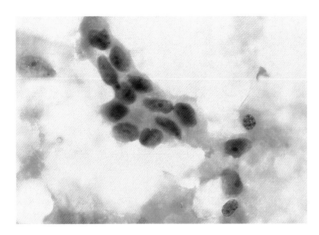

FIGURE 12–22. Infiltrating Ductal Carcinoma. Dyshesive cluster of cells with variation in the size and shape of the nuclei (Papanicolaou stain, × 250).

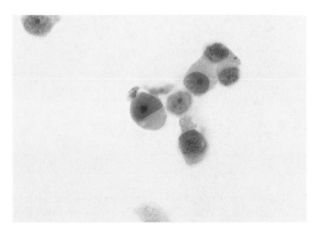

FIGURE 12–24. Infiltrating Ductal Carcinoma. Single atypical cells, some of which have protuberant nuclei, showing marked pleomorphism (Papanicolaou stain, × 250).

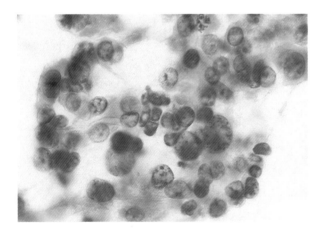

FIGURE 12–23. Infiltrating Ductal Carcinoma. Dyshesive cluster of cells with irregular nuclear spacing and dyshesion. The chromatin pattern is variable, with some degenerative changes, and ranges from cleared to finely granular and clumped (Papanicolaou stain, × 250).

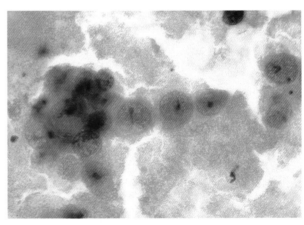

FIGURE 12–25. Infiltrating Ductal Carcinoma. Single cells are adjacent to a loose cluster. Note the bloody background and the markedly enlarged and pleomorphic nuclei with considerable nuclear atypicality and irregular nucleoli (Papanicolaou stain, × 250).

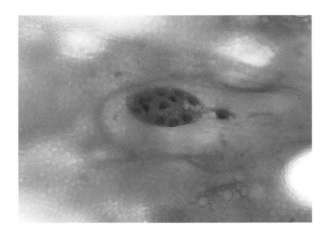

FIGURE 12–26A. Mucinous Carcinoma. Rare, tight clusters of cells with finely vacuolated cytoplasm interspersed in a mucinous matrix. Aspirates for a colloid carcinoma must be evaluated for cellularity, nuclear variability and irregularity, and proper background. A diagnosis of malignancy may not always be possible to make (Diff-Quik stain, × 100).

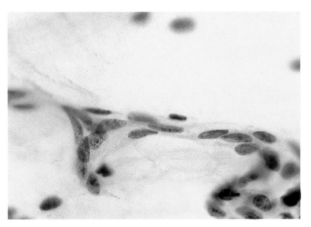

FIGURE 12–27. Mucinous Carcinoma. A characteristic feature of mucinous carcinoma is the presence of capillaries with plump, spindled endothelial cells. These are often present in a complex branching structure (Papanicolaou stain, × 250).

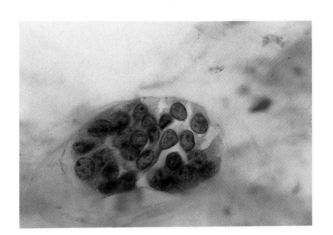

FIGURE 12–26B. Mucinous Carcinoma. This high-power view shows a tight cluster of cells with variably sized nuclei, some of which are irregular. Note that the mucin does not show as well as in the corresponding Diff-Quik preparation (Papanicolaou stain, × 250).

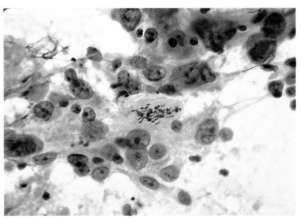

FIGURE 12–28. Medullary Carcinoma. Dyshesive sheets of cells with pleomorphic, large nuclei. These cells have abundant cytoplasm and prominent nucleoli. A mitosis is present in the center of the field, and a few lymphocytes are present (hematoxylin and eosin stain, × 250). (Courtesy of Edmund S. Cibas, M.D., Boston, Mass.)

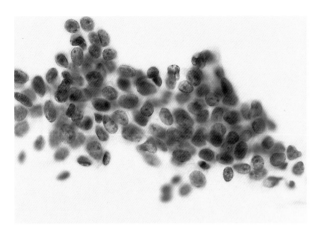

FIGURE 12–29. Lobular Carcinoma in Situ. Such a case would never be diagnosed as malignant but, rather, as atypical. The small cells are arranged in a loose cluster. Nuclei exhibit minimal anisonucleosis and a finely granular chromatin pattern. This picture may be difficult to distinguish from that of an atypical ductal hyperplasia or a fibroadenoma (Papanicolaou stain, × 250).

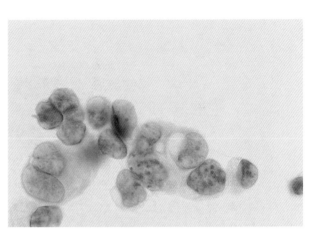

FIGURE 12–31. Recurrent Carcinoma (Primary Diagnosed as Lobular) with Lobular and Ductal Features. These cells are much larger than those of the typical lobular carcinoma; however, they show the characteristic intracytoplasmic vacuoles, pronounced nuclear molding, and bland chromatin pattern (Papanicolaou stain, × 250).

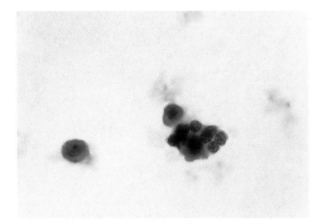

FIGURE 12–30. Infiltrating Lobular Carcinoma. The cells are the size of lymphocytes. They are present in one tight cluster with single, larger, and more pleomorphic cells. The nuclear to cytoplasmic ratio is high (Papanicolaou stain, × 250).

OTHER TUMORS AND CONDITIONS

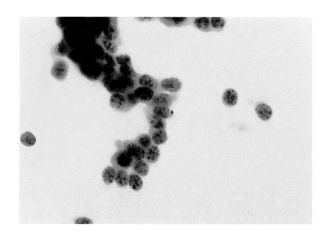

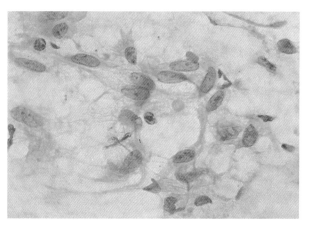

FIGURE 12–32. Metastatic Neuroendocrine Tumor to the Breast. Note the eccentric nuclei and coarsely granular chromatin. This pattern might also be consistent with that of a lobular carcinoma. This woman had a history of a prior mastectomy and a small bowel carcinoid. The aspirate was from the region of the mastectomy scar; she had other metastases. In this case, immunocytochemical stains were necessary. The cells stained positively for keratin and chromogranin. Stains for epithelial membrane antigen were negative, and the cells did not stain for estrogen receptors with the Abbott-ERICA reagents. This was presumed to represent metastatic carcinoid to the breast, but a breast cancer with neuroendocrine differentiation (argyrophilic carcinoma) would present an identical picture (Papanicolaou stain, × 250).

FIGURE 12–33. Metaplastic Carcinoma. Many loosely cohesive, atypical spindle cells are seen. This aspirate did not show any typical epithelial component and was not called malignant but, rather, atypical. The epithelial nature of the tumor was noted on the resection specimen only by the use of immunocytochemical stains and was positive for both vimehtin and keratin (hematoxylin and eosin stain, × 250).

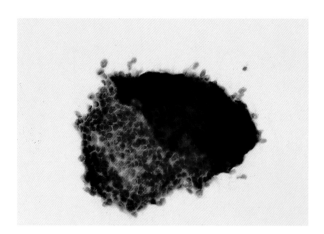

FIGURE 12–34. Gynecomastia. The cells are arranged in a large, cohesive sheet, which is flat and folded. The cells have a distinct, crowded, honeycomb appearance, with uniform spacing. There are a few myoepithelial cells falling away from the edges of the duct. However, this is not dyshesion because of the tightness of the rest of the border (Papanicolaou stain, × 100).

DIFFERENTIAL GROUPING

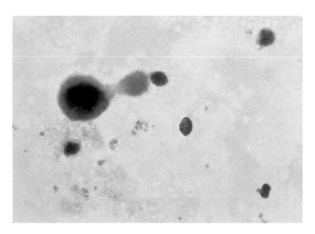

FIGURE 12–35A. Comedo-Type Ductal Carcinoma in Situ. A very large and abnormal single cell is present, with an eccentric nucleus in a background of inflammatory cells and proteinaceous debris. This case is easily diagnosed as malignant; however, it cannot be differentiated from that of an infiltrating ductal carcinoma (Papanicolaou stain, × 250).

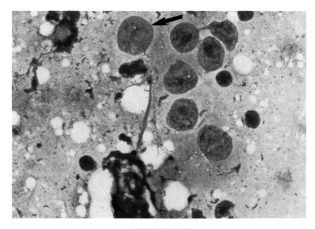

FIGURE 12–35C. Invasive Ductal Carcinoma. Dyshesive cells are visible, with eccentric cytoplasm and huge, irregular nucleoli (arrow) in a background of necrosis (Diff-Quik stain, × 250).

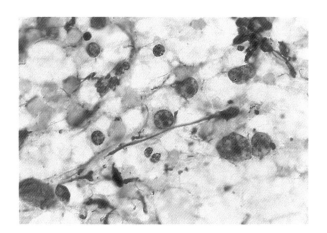

FIGURE 12–35B. Infiltrating Ductal Carcinoma. Many single cells are seen in the background of a tumor diathesis. The number of cells with prominent nucleoli and the cellular necrosis preclude a diagnosis of pregnancy or lactation (Papanicolaou stain, × 250).

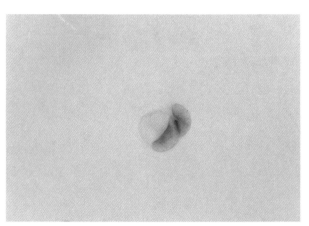

FIGURE 12–35D. Infiltrating Carcinoma with Ductal and Lobular Features. Note the signet-ring cells with bland chromatin. Based on these cells alone, a diagnosis of malignancy might be difficult. However, in the background there were many cells, both singly and in dyshesive clusters, demonstrating marked nuclear variability, molding, and signet-ring features (Papanicolaou stain, × 250).

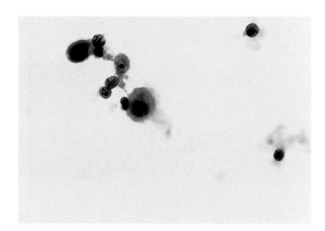

FIGURE 12–35E. Infiltrating Lobular Carcinoma. Note the small single cells with variable but generally high nuclear to cytoplasmic ratios. The nuclei are only slightly larger than those of lymphocytes. Note the difference in cytoplasm relative to Figure 12–35D (Papanicolaou stain, × 250).

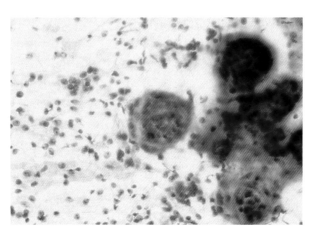

FIGURE 12–35G. Pregnancy/Lactational Changes. The corresponding Papanicolaou-stained smear shows hypercellularity. A tight cluster of cells in a lobular arrangement is noted, with a background of many single cells and stripped nuclei. The nuclei are round, regular, and uniform (Papanicolaou stain, × 150).

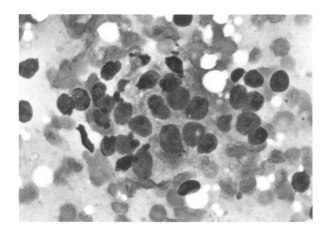

FIGURE 12–35F. Pregnancy/Lactation Effect. There are many stripped nuclei and single cells in a watery, proteinaceous background, which lacks necrotic nuclei. The naked nuclei are generally round and regular. These features would suggest pregnancy or lactational changes with the appropriate history (Diff-Quik stain, × 250).

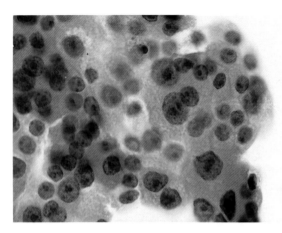

FIGURE 12–36A. Cyst Contents with Apocrine Cells. Variation in nuclear size and prominent nucleoli are seen. However, the cells are cohesive, and single cells are rare. Such atypical changes may occasionally be found in a cyst. It is important not to call such a case positive but, rather, atypical or suspicious and to suggest biopsy. When a cyst is aspirated, it should be completely drained, and any residual mass should be aspirated (Papanicolaou stain, × 250).

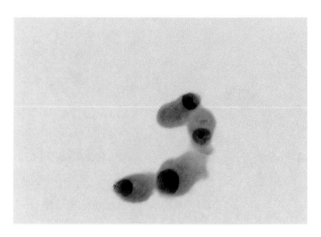

FIGURE 12–36C. Infiltrating Ductal Carcinoma with Apocrine Differentiation. Single cells with granular cytoplasm and eccentric nuclei are shown. The presence of such "protuberant nuclei" in single cells is a useful feature in that it suggests malignancy (Papanicolaou stain, × 250).

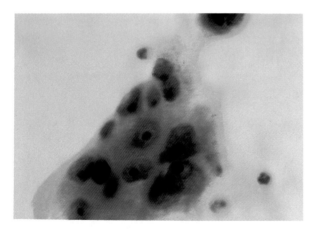

FIGURE 12–36B. Comedo-Type Ductal Carcinoma in Situ with Apocrine Differentiation. Nuclei are irregular and enlarged, with irregular nuclear spacing and macronucleoli. Although this picture is similar to the previous one (Fig. 12–36A), many single cells are present (Papanicolaou stain, × 250).

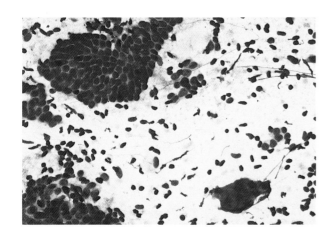

FIGURE 12–37A. Fibroadenoma. Cellular aspirate with many cohesive clusters of epithelial cells in a background of bipolar cells and naked nuclei. Cellular cohesion and background are necessary to make this diagnosis (Diff-Quik stain, × 100).

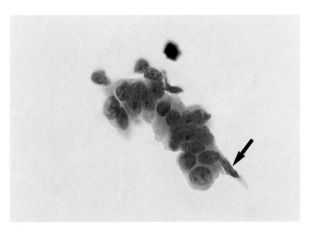

FIGURE 12–37C. Atypical Ductal Hyperplasia. Cohesive cluster of cells in a clean background, with mild nuclear enlargement and crowding. The cells maintain regular nuclear spacing, and myoepithelial cells are present (arrow) (Papanicolaou stain, × 250).

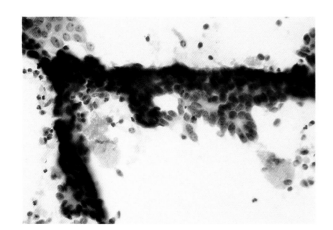

FIGURE 12–37B. Benign Phyllodes Tumor. Note the tight, cohesive cluster with epithelial atypia in a staghorn configuration similar to that of a fibroadenoma. This degree of epithelial atypicality may occasionally be noted in both fibroadenoma and benign phyllodes tumor and should not be overdiagnosed as malignant, given the proper background. Elsewhere in the slide, there was a prominent stromal background (Papanicolaou stain, × 150).

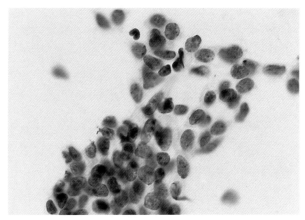

FIGURE 12–37D. Lobular Carcinoma in Situ. Dyshesion is minimal, nuclear spacing is regular, and the chromatin pattern is bland. This picture could not be separated on cytology from atypical ductal hyperplasia (see Fig. 12–37C) (Papanicolaou stain, × 250).

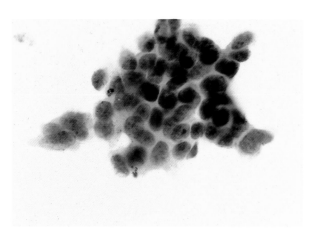

FIGURE 12–37E. Ductal Carcinoma in Situ. These very atypical ductal cells are arranged in a loose cluster, with irregular nuclear spacing and nuclear irregularity. In this case, there were no single cells and the background was clean. The nuclear atypicality should lead to a suspicious diagnosis. A biopsy specimen is needed to exclude a diagnosis of infiltrating carcinoma (Papanicolaou stain, × 250).

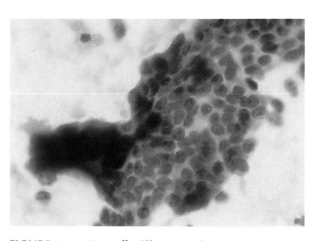

FIGURE 12–37G. Well-Differentiated Ductal Carcinoma. Although the cluster appears cohesive, there were single epithelial cells in the background and nuclear crowding. This case was originally diagnosed as atypical, and a biopsy was performed that led to the diagnosis of a well-differentiated infiltrating ductal carcinoma (Papanicolaou stain, × 250).

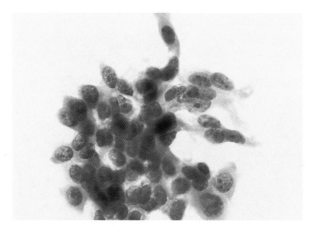

FIGURE 12–37F. Infiltrating Ductal Carcinoma. The dyshesive cluster of ductal cells shows marked nuclear pleomorphism and loss of nuclear polarity (Papanicolaou stain, × 250).

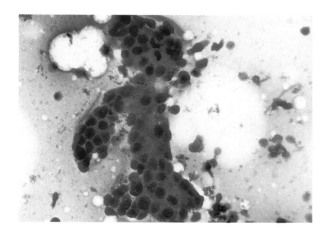

FIGURE 12–38A. Intraductal Papilloma. Tight cluster of cells with cytoplasmic clearing and small, regular nuclei (Diff-Quik stain, × 150).

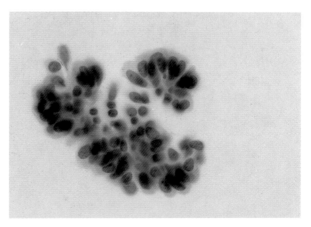

FIGURE 12–38C. Papillary Carcinoma. This should be diagnosed as papillary neoplasm, favor malignancy. The cells are in papillary groupings, which are three-dimensional, with a smooth boundary to the cluster. The nuclei are bland, but the tumor cells are tall and columnar, with elongated nuclei. There is a bloody background (Papanicolaou stain, × 250). (Courtesy of Edmund S. Cibas, M.D., Boston, Mass.)

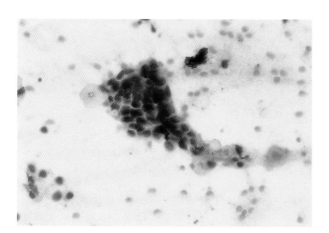

FIGURE 12–38B. Intraductal Papilloma. The corresponding Papanicolaou smear also shows a tightly cohesive cluster of cells (Papanicolaou stain, × 250).

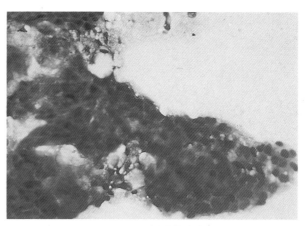

FIGURE 12–38D. Papillary Carcinoma. This Diff-Quik preparation corresponds with that shown in Figure 12–19. It was diagnosed as papillary neoplasm, favor malignancy, because of the hypercellularity and the bloody background (Diff-Quik stain, × 150).

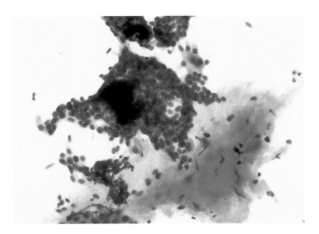

FIGURE 12–39A. Fibroadenoma. This low-power view demonstrates both the epithelial and hypocellular stromal components (Papanicolaou stain, × 100).

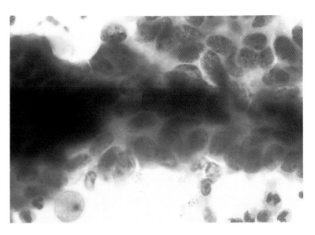

FIGURE 12–39C. Benign Phyllodes Tumor. The epithelial component shows marked nuclear atypicality, which leads to suspicion of malignancy. However, on review of the slides, a pronounced stromal component in the background was noted (Papanicolaou stain, × 250).

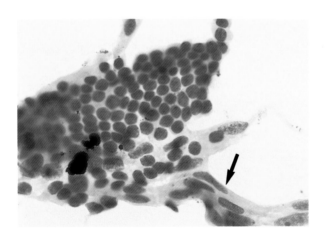

FIGURE 12–39B. Fibroadenoma. Note the epithelial sheet and adjacent spindled stromal cells (arrow) (Papanicolaou stain, × 250).

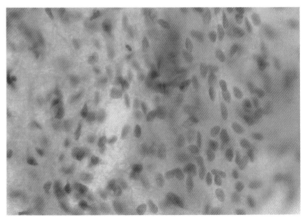

FIGURE 12–39D. Benign Phyllodes Tumor. The stromal component shows cohesive, three-dimensional stromal tissue fragments with bland nuclei. There were no mitoses in the stromal component (Papanicolaou stain, × 250).

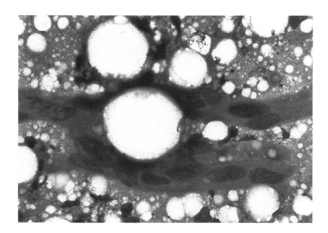

FIGURE 12–39E. Metaplastic Carcinoma. Spindle cells with elongated and enlarged nuclei are seen in a dirty background. A diagnosis of atypical spindle cells was made on the aspirate, and a biopsy was suggested. Keratin staining on the breast biopsy specimen was focally positive, which led to the diagnosis of metaplastic carcinoma. The stain for vimentin was also positive (Diff-Quik stain, × 250).

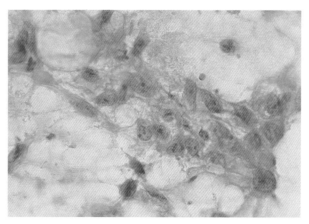

FIGURE 12–39G. Metaplastic Carcinoma. Corresponding alcohol-fixed material demonstrates dyshesive and pleomorphic spindle cells (hematoxylin and eosin stain, × 250).

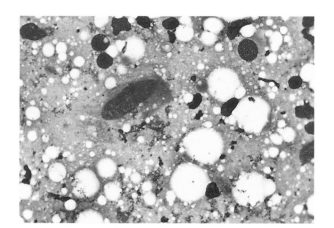

FIGURE 12–39F. Metaplastic Carcinoma. A single spindle cell demonstrates the pronounced nuclear enlargement (Diff-Quik stain, × 250).

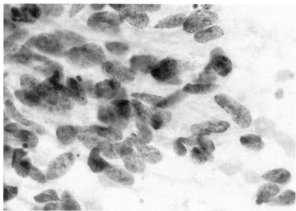

FIGURE 12–39H. Primary Sarcoma of the Breast. Very atypical spindle cells, suspect for malignancy. The spindle cells are pleomorphic and dyshesive, with coarsely granular chromatin. In contrast to the previous case (Figs. 12–39E through 12–39G), there was no staining with keratin (Papanicolaou stain, × 250).

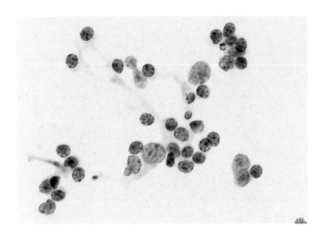

FIGURE 12–40A. Hyperplastic Lymph Node Within the Breast. The lymphoid population is polymorphous, with tingible-body macrophages (Papanicolaou stain, × 250).

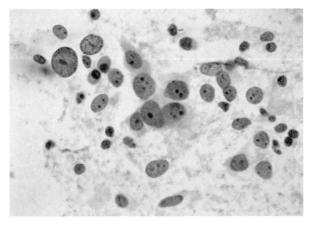

FIGURE 12–40C. Medullary Carcinoma. Note the plasma cells (hematoxylin and eosin stain, × 250). (Courtesy of Edmund S. Cibas, M.D., Boston, Mass.)

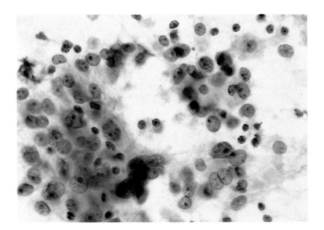

FIGURE 12–40B. Medullary Carcinoma. Dyshesive sheets of cells with pleomorphic nuclei are present in a background of lymphocytes and plasma cells (hematoxylin and eosin stain, × 250). (Courtesy of Edmund S. Cibas, M.D., Boston, Mass.)

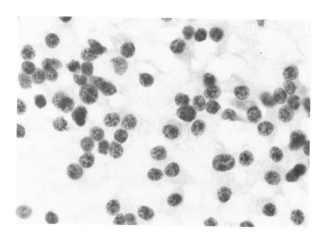

FIGURE 12–40D. Plasmacytoma of the Breast. The plasma cells have a clock-face chromatin pattern and small, round nucleoli. This aspirate from a breast mass was from a patient with known multiple myeloma (Papanicolaou stain, × 250).

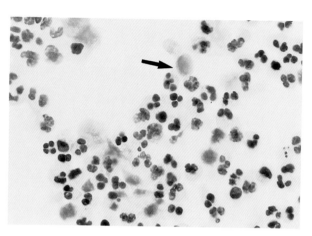

FIGURE 12–40F. Mastitis. Rare, degenerating epithelial cells (arrow) are interspersed in a background of acute inflammation (Papanicolaou stain, × 250).

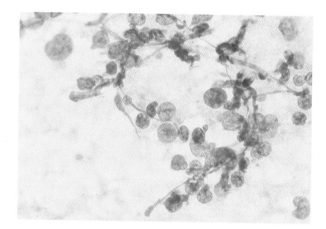

FIGURE 12–40E. Primary Lymphoma of the Breast. Only lymphoid cells are present. There is marked crush artifact, and the lymphoid cells are atypical (Papanicolaou stain, × 250).

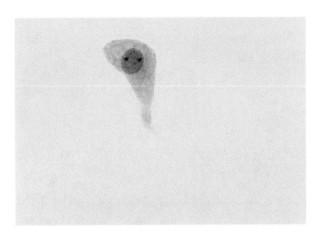

FIGURE 12–41A. Fat Necrosis. Rare single cell with a benign histiocytic nucleus and finely vacuolated cytoplasm (Papanicolaou stain, × 250).

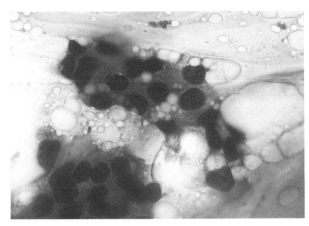

FIGURE 12–41C. Mucinous Carcinoma. The mucinous component is more prominent on Diff-Quik preparations (× 250).

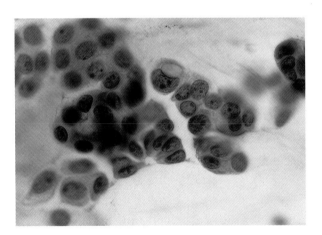

FIGURE 12–41B. Mucinous Carcinoma. There are cell clusters and a single cell with a large vacuole. The background is mucinous, but this is poorly appreciated on a Papanicolaou stain (Papanicolaou stain, × 250).

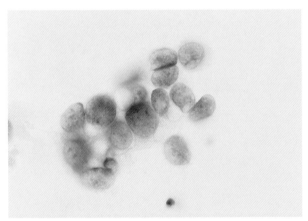

FIGURE 12–41D. Recurrent Carcinoma with Ductal and Lobular Features. The large cytoplasmic vacuoles are prominent. In contrast to the cells seen in pregnancy, in which the cytoplasm is fine and wispy, these cells show large vacuoles that displace the nucleus and form signet ring cells (Papanicolaou stain, × 250).

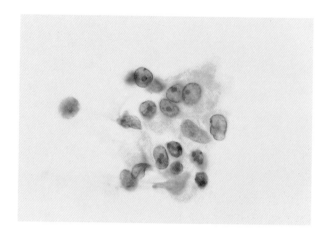

FIGURE 12–41E. Pregnancy/Lactation Effect. The cytoplasm is finely vacuolated. Nuclei are round and regular, with small, round, prominent nucleoli. Elsewhere in the smear, there were naked nuclei. No nuclear molding is seen (Papanicolaou stain, × 250).

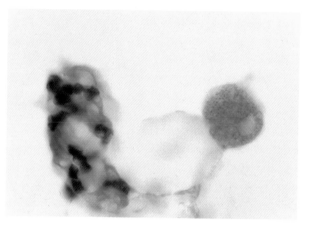

FIGURE 12–41G. Silicone. These coarsely vacuolated cells and a foamy macrophage containing foreign material were noted in the breast aspiration of a woman who had had a silicone breast augmentation 20 years prior to the aspiration (Papanicolaou stain, × 250).

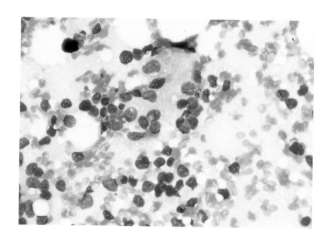

FIGURE 12–41F. Pregnancy/Lactation. This air-dried smear demonstrates both the finely vacuolated cytoplasm and the many single, naked nuclei. Nuclei are round and regular. The combination of a proteinaceous background, many single cells, naked, stripped nuclei, and cells with round, regular nuclei and wispy cytoplasm is characteristic of pregnancy-lactation effect (Diff-Quik stain, × 100).

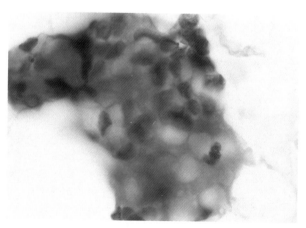

FIGURE 12–41H. Silicone. The cells are arranged in a tight, cohesive cluster in a clean background. The specimen was hypocellular and was diagnosed as atypical. The breast biopsy showed only silicone (Papanicolaou stain, × 250).

C·H·A·P·T·E·R

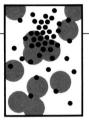

13

OVARIAN ASPIRATION CYTOLOGY

Ibrahim Ramzy

Mary R. Schwartz

Fine needle aspiration biopsy of the ovaries has not been widely accepted in the United States. This is due mainly to the fear of rupture and spread of tumor during aspiration, a generally held belief that any solid lesions should be surgically removed, and, to a lesser extent, to lack of experience with cytologic features of ovarian lesions. Aspiration biopsy is not considered the preferred technique for diagnosis of ovarian carcinoma in the postmenopausal patient unless the patient is a poor surgical candidate. However, aspiration is an excellent technique for examining cysts and other masses in the younger patient who desires preservation of fertility and ovarian function, since the risk of malignancy is relatively low in these patients (Ganjei and Nadji, 1984). When an ovarian tumor is found at surgery, ovarian aspiration can also be used for examining the contralateral ovary and determining if additional oophorectomy is necessary.

In this chapter, some aspects of the technique of aspiration are considered, followed by a discussion of the cytologic features of non-neoplastic cysts, primary ovarian neoplasms, and metastatic tumors. Finally, diagnostic accuracy and pitfalls are analyzed.

TECHNIQUE

Ovarian masses can be aspirated transvaginally, transrectally, transabdominally, during laparoscopy, or directly at exploratory laparotomy. Aspiration may be done under ultrasound guidance, with or without anesthesia. Ultrasound-guided transvaginal aspiration is the most common route for oocyte retrieval for in vitro fertilization. Transrectal aspiration is not generally recommended, except in solid neoplasms, because of the high risk of infecting a cystic lesion. Prophylactic antibiotic coverage is recommended before transrectal aspiration. The transabdominal approach is not widely used for aspiration of lesions suspected to be malignant because of concern of leaking neoplastic cells from a cystic tumor into the abdominal cavity. The transvaginal or transrectal route may be used for aspiration of masses fixed to the pelvic wall.

Most of the ovarian aspirates we see are obtained at laparoscopy or directly at surgery. Direct smears may be immediately alcohol-fixed and stained with Papanicolaou stain, or they may be air-dried and stained with Diff-Quik, May-Grunwald-Giemsa, or a similar stain. Aspirated fluid should be concentrated, usually by cytocentrifugation.

NON-NEOPLASTIC CYSTS

Follicular cysts, the most common type of non-neoplastic ovarian cysts, are lined by several layers of granulosa cells. Aspirates of such cysts are usually scant and contain follicular cells in a clear, proteinaceous, or occasionally bloody background. The follicular cells occur singly, in clusters, or as small sheets, with only rare rosette formation seen. They have uniform round or oval nuclei. The cytoplasm is usually scant with indistinct cell borders, although some cells have moderate amounts of foamy cytoplasm, giving the cells the appearance of histiocytes. Ova having a mantle of granulosa cells are rarely seen (Figs. 13–1 and 13–2). Selvaggi (1990) found nuclear grooves in several nuclei of two follicular cysts studied but distinguished them from granulosa cell tumors by the absence of Call-Exner bodies. Stanley et al. described three non-neoplastic cellular cysts, initially interpreted as low grade malignant neoplasms. The fluids were hypercellular and contained many groups of cells with a high nuclear to cytoplasmic (N/C) ratio, hyperchromatic nuclei, and prominent nucleoli. Call-Exner bodies were present in one aspirate. They were distinguished from granulosa cell tumors by the absence of hyperconvoluted nuclei with grooves. Distinction from well-differentiated serous carcinoma was felt not to be possible without histologic confirmation.

Aspirates from *corpora lutea and corpus luteum cysts* are more cellular than those from follicular cysts. They are composed largely of luteinized cells with abundant foamy or granular eosinophilic to cyanophilic cytoplasm, vesicular nuclei, and small, prominent nucleoli (Fig. 13–3). There is usually fresh or hemolyzed blood in the background. Cells intermediate between smaller non-luteinized and larger luteinized cells are also present and correspond to nonluteinized follicular cells or theca interna cells. Some spindled stromal cells may be found. Macrophages containing hemosiderin or hematoidin pigment are often found in hemorrhagic or regressing corpora lutea.

Ovarian, paraovarian, and paratubal serous cysts are cytologically indistinguishable. The aspirated fluid is clear and hypocellular, and the smear's background is clear or finely granular. The cells vary from cuboidal to low columnar (Fig. 13–4A, B), with occasional cilia (Fig. 13–4B). Cells are present in small clusters, small sheets, and occasionally as single naked nuclei. The low columnar cells have round nuclei and uniform chromatin and may have prominent nucleoli.

Some degenerated cells have pyknotic nuclei. The cuboidal cells have pyknotic round nuclei and minimal cytoplasm.

Endometriotic cysts are usually hemorrhagic with abundant fresh and hemolyzed blood in the background. Hemosiderin-laden macrophages compose the predominant nucleated cell type. There are few degenerated endometrial stromal, epithelial columnar, or cuboidal cells, which may be arranged in cell balls, clusters, or loose sheets (Fig. 13–5). These cells have round to oval nuclei with uniform chromatin and scant cytoplasm. Endometrial epithelial cells tend to be rounder and sometimes have small cytoplasmic vacuoles. The epithelial cells are occasionally atypical but can be distinguished from carcinoma by the absence of frank cytologic criteria of malignancy and relative paucity compared to the hypercellularity of most carcinomas. Endometrial stromal cells may occasionally be single and stripped of cytoplasm. A definitive diagnosis of endometriosis cannot be made without the presence of endometrial cells. The diagnosis may be suggested, but not rendered, when aspiration of a cyst yields abundant hemorrhagic material with hemosiderin-laden macrophages.

SEROUS TUMORS

Aspiration of *serous cystadenomas* and *serous cystadenofibromas* yields smears of low cellularity with epithelial and stromal cells in a pale eosinophilic granular background. The cuboidal to columnar epithelial cells are arranged in small clusters with occasional cohesive monolayered sheets or papillae (Fig. 13–6). The cytoplasm is scant, cyanophilic, or purple, and the taller columnar cells may have visible cilia. An occasional small single vacuole may be seen. The uniform oval or round nuclei have finely granular chromatin, inconspicuous nucleoli, and some nuclear molding. Spindled stromal cells have uniform oval nuclei and moderate to scant amounts of eosinophilic cytoplasm and are usually arranged in bundles. Stromal cells are relatively more abundant in cystadenofibromas. Histiocytes, including some multinucleated ones, and small, round, dark, naked nuclei of degenerated cuboidal cells may also be present.

Serous adenocarcinomas include borderline and frankly invasive types. The aspirates are usually cellular, with epithelial cells arranged in sheets, papillae, or isolated. The cells have large pleomorphic hyperchromatic nuclei, coarse irregular chromatin, prominent nucleoli, and frequent mitotic figures. The cytoplasm is cyanophilic and moderate in amount and may have an occasional single small vacuole. Necrotic debris, bare nuclei, foamy histiocytes, red blood cells, and psammoma bodies are also often present (Figs. 13–7 to 13–9). Stromal invasion cannot be assessed cytologically. Diagnosis of borderline serous tumors may not be feasible by cytology, but the tumors usually have increased N/C ratios and nuclear pleomorphism. They may have papillary fragments with cellular crowding. In some cases, aspirates show a mixed population of cells having features ranging from benign to malignant (Ramzy and Delaney, 1979).

MUCINOUS TUMORS

Aspirates from *mucinous cystadenomas* are usually abundant and grossly mucoid. The smears show numerous cells resembling endocervical epithelium, dispersed in large amounts of background mucin, which may be basophilic or amphophilic, granular to fibrillary (Fig. 13–10). Most of the epithelial cells appear as single cells that round up into oval cells with eccentric nuclei. There are occasional sheets of epithelial cells that maintain their tall columnar shape and have a honeycomb appearance when viewed en face. Vacuoles are prominent and may be either a single, large, hyperdistended vacuole surrounded by a thin cytoplasmic rim or multiple small vacuoles filling the cytoplasm. The oval to semilunar nuclei, which are compressed to the periphery by the cytoplasmic vacuoles, have finely granular chromatin and eosinophilic, indistinct nucleoli. As a result of distention and secondary flattening of the epithelial lining, large cysts are often lined by cuboidal or flat cells, and it may be difficult to recognize these as mucinous in type. Multinucleated giant cells may be seen in some cases. These tumors are cytologically distinguished from serous cystadenomas by greater prominence of vacuoles and the presence of mucin.

Borderline mucinous tumors usually result in aspirates with abundant mucin. The cells are single or in clusters of crowded cells and may show a range of cytologic features from benign to malignant. This dual population is helpful in the recognition of mucinous borderline tumors (Abrams and Silverberg, 1989). If cytologically benign cells predominate, the lesion may be difficult to distinguish from a mucinous cystadenoma because epithelial stratification and architectural complexity cannot be assessed cytologically. Recognition of cellular crowding within clusters may provide a clue. If atypical cells predominate in the aspirate, distinction from well-differentiated mucinous adenocarcinoma may not be possible because stromal invasion and epithelial stratification cannot be evaluated.

Mucinous cystadenocarcinomas produce aspirates with numerous epithelial cells and variable amounts of background mucin. In general, the amount of mucin is less than that seen in mucinous cystadenomas. The epithelial cells may appear as isolated cells or in loosely cohesive groups, sheets, papillary structures, and cell balls. Cytoplasmic mucin vacuoles may or may not be prominent. The nuclei are eccentric, a feature best seen at the edges of cell clusters. Well-differentiated mucinous adenocarcinomas have greater amounts of background mucin and more epithelial sheets of columnar or cuboidal cells and tend to have pale cytoplasm. The nuclei tend to be relatively uniform and have finely granular chromatin and macronucleoli. In some cases the nuclei may appear deceptively innocuous, and the lesion is difficult to distinguish from mucinous cystadenoma. Moderately and poorly differentiated mucinous adenocarcinomas have less background mucin but more single cells, cell balls, and papillary groups and tend to have less prominent cytoplasmic vacuolation (Figs. 13–11 and 13–12). The nuclei have more obvious malignant features, with pleomorphism, outline irregularity, hyperchromasia, unevenly distributed chromatin, and macronucleoli.

ENDOMETRIOID TUMORS

The majority of these neoplasms are carcinomas; benign and borderline tumors are uncommon. These tumors occur predominantly in women from 40 to 60 years of age. They tend to be cystic but may be solid. Microscopically, they resemble uterine endometrial adenocarcinomas. Smears show an eosinophilic mucoid or granular background containing red blood cells and hemosiderin-laden histiocytes with tumor cells arranged in sheets and clusters. Well-differentiated carcinomas are composed of columnar-shaped cells with moderate cytoplasm, finely granular chromatin, and prominent nucleoli. A squamous cell component may be encountered in endometrioid neoplasms. Cells of poorly differentiated endometrioid carcinomas have a high N/C ratio, hyperchromatic nuclei, thickened irregular nuclear membranes, and irregular chromatin distribution. Poorly differentiated endometrioid carcinomas may be difficult to distinguish from poorly differentiated serous carcinomas (Fig. 13–13).

OTHER SURFACE EPITHELIAL TUMORS

Malignant mixed müllerian tumors yield aspirates composed of malignant epithelial and mesenchymal cells. The epithelial cells resemble those of endometrial adenocarcinoma and are most commonly present in clusters and sheets. The mesenchymal component may be homologous or heterologous, and the cells tend to be noncohesive.

Clear cell tumors are mostly carcinomas, with rare borderline tumors occurring. Although they may be solid, they are usually cystic. These tumors, which are believed to be of müllerian origin, cytologically resemble clear cell tumors at other sites in the female genital tract. Fine needle aspirates are composed of large cells with abundant amounts of pale to clear cytoplasm and peripherally located pleomorphic nuclei that are frequently bi- or multinucleated (Nadji, 1985).

Brenner tumors are almost always benign and solid. Fine needle aspirates yield sheets of epithelial cells with moderate amounts of cytoplasm and uniform oval to round bland nuclei having fine chromatin. There may be folding of the nuclear membrane producing a nuclear groove and giving the nuclei a coffee-bean appearance. Globular or multilobulated hyaline-like bodies can be seen in the center of some of the epithelial islands or free in the background (Figs. 13–14 and 13–15). Occasional bare nuclei representing stromal cells may be found. Although this overall appearance is fairly characteristic, nuclear grooves may also be seen in granulosa cell tumors and less commonly in mesothelial cells (Fig. 13–16). Malignant Brenner tumors are rare, and a cytologic diagnosis beyond malignant epithelial neoplasm may not be possible. They may resemble transitional cell or nonkeratinizing squamous cell carcinomas. Aspirates show syncytial aggregates or papillary fragments of tumor cells with oval nuclei and coarse, irregular chromatin (Nadji, 1985).

SEX CORD/STROMAL TUMORS

Fine needle aspirates of sex cord tumors show an admixture of epithelial and mesenchymal stromal cells. The formation of trabeculae, acini, or rosettes suggests a sex cord tumor. Since the course of these neoplasms cannot be predicted with certainty by cytomorphologic features, clinical and biochemical evaluation is necessary, and laparotomy is needed to establish the diagnosis in most cases (Ramzy, 1989).

Granulosa cell tumors usually occur in adults. Presenting symptoms are often related to the large amounts of estrogen the tumor may produce. The natural history is that of a tumor of low-grade malignancy with a 60 to 90% five-year survival rate. Fine needle aspirates of granulosa cell tumors yield cellular aspirates of uniform oval cells arranged in sheets, singly, or in trabeculae. Some of the cells may form round acinar or rosette-like structures with central homogeneous eosinophilic material, reminiscent of Call-Exner bodies. The pale-staining cytoplasm is scant and ill-defined. The small round to oval nuclei are centrally located and have finely granular, evenly distributed chromatin; small, single nucleoli; and only rare mitotic figures. While the nuclei may have a characteristic longitudinal groove giving them a coffee-bean appearance, this is often not seen in cytologic preparations (Fig. 13–17). There may be a few admixed stromal cells in the form of elongated bare nuclei.

Juvenile granulosa cell tumors are rare variants that usually occur in the first two decades of life. They differ cytologically from the more common adult granulosa cell tumors by having no or only rare nuclear grooves, absence of Call-Exner bodies, and focal mucin associated with granulosa cells.

Sertoli-Leydig cell tumors are difficult to differentiate from granulosa cell neoplasms. They may show acini or trabeculae and also have uniform oval nuclei (Fig. 13–18). The neoplastic cells are admixed with fibroblast-like stromal cells.

Sex cord tumors with annular tubules are rare neoplasms that usually follow a benign course but may occasionally behave malignantly. One third of the cases have been associated with Peutz-Jeghers syndrome and in this setting are usually multiple and small. Tumors unassociated with the syndrome are usually solitary and larger. Yazdi (1987) described findings of an intraoperative fine needle aspiration of this type of tumor. The cellular smears contained numerous single, uniform, small to medium-sized neoplastic cells as well as cells arranged in follicles, solid sheets, and a trabecular pattern. In the solid sheets there were occasional homogeneous hyaline bodies rimmed by palisaded nuclei forming rosette-like structures. Similar free ring-like structures with central hyaline were also present. The small nuclei were oval to round and contained evenly distributed chromatin and small nucleoli. An occasional grooved nucleus was seen, raising a diagnostic consideration of granulosa cell tumor.

Sex cord tumors with annular tubules should be differentiated from adenocarcinoma and carcinoid tumor. Adenocarcinomas have larger, more pleomorphic, more hyperchromatic nuclei than sex cord tumors with larger nucleoli. They are more often mucin-positive. Carcinoid tumors tend to have smaller nuclei than sex cord tumors and lack nuclear grooves. Immunocytochemical or histochemical silver-staining neuroendocrine markers may be helpful. The presence of nuclear grooves would raise a consideration of Brenner tumor and mesothelial cells. The latter generally have more cytoplasm than granulosa cell tumors and lack Call-Exner bodies.

Fibromas and thecomas yield material of scant cellularity. The oval to spindle-shaped cells have elongated hyperchromatic nuclei and minimal, if any, cytoplasm. When there is cystic degeneration, the background may show areas of finely granular blue to purple matrix on Papanicolaou-stained smears.

Signet ring cell tumor, a benign tumor arising from ovarian stroma, produces cells with large vacuoles that push the nuclei to the side (Ramzy, 1976). These vacuoles are mucin-negative, unlike malignant signet ring cells constituting Krukenberg tumors (Fig. 13–19).

GERM CELL TUMORS

Benign cystic teratomas are the most common germ cell tumors of the ovary. Aspirates show abundant purple to cyanophilic finely granular background material in which there are anucleated, superficial, and scant intermediate squamous cells. Amorphous amphophilic material, presumably representing sebaceous material, is also seen. Hair shafts, ciliated columnar and mucinous cells, and mesodermal cells are uncommon in fine needle aspirates (Fig. 13–20). Histiocytes, including multinucleated foreign-body type giant cells, may be seen. Malignant transformation within a benign cystic teratoma is rare and, when it occurs, is most often squamous cell carcinoma. Aspiration of such malignant neoplasms yields components of a benign cystic teratoma as well as cells having typical cytologic features of squamous cell carcinoma.

Dysgerminomas account for approximately 50% of all malignant germ cell tumors of the ovary. Most occur in women under the age of 30. Aspiration yields cellular material composed of tumor germ cells admixed with lymphocytes and often with plasma cells, histiocytes, and giant cells. The large germ cells are predominantly in sheets and loose syncytial aggregates with some single cells. They have a high N/C ratio, round to oval large pleomorphic nuclei, irregular distribution of chromatin, prominent single or multiple nucleoli, and increased mitoses (Fig. 13–21). The cyanophilic cytoplasm varies in amount and may contain vacuoles composed of glycogen (Akhtar et al., 1990).

Dysgerminomas should be differentiated from malignant lymphoma and other rarer germ cell neoplasms, such as embryonal carcinoma and yolk sac tumor. The two latter tumors tend to show more cohesiveness and lack the lymphoid background of dysgerminomas. Alpha-fetoprotein is commonly found in yolk sac tumors and sometimes embryonal carcinomas, but it is absent in dysgerminomas. Malignant lymphoma usually has a more monomorphous population than dysgerminomas and has noncohesive cells rather than sheets of tumor cells. Immunostaining for common leukocyte antigen may be helpful in difficult cases.

Carcinoid tumors may be primary in the ovary, a component of teratoma, or metastatic to the ovary. One third of primary ovarian carcinoids are associated with carcinoid syndrome. Aspirates are cellular and composed of monotonous, generally single or loosely cohesive cells, with occasional sheet or rosette formation. Nuclei are oval with finely granular, evenly distributed chromatin; nucleoli, when present, are small. Histochemical silver staining for argentaffin or argyrophil granules, ultrastructural examination for neurosecretory granules, or immunocytochemical staining for neuroendocrine markers such as chromogranin, neuron-specific enolase, or serotonin may be helpful.

LYMPHOMA AND LEUKEMIA

Malignant lymphoma may present as an ovarian mass, occasionally as the first manifestation of the disease. Most ovarian involvement by lymphoma represents secondary involvement by more generalized disease, with rare primary ovarian lymphomas. Fine needle aspiration yields cellular smears of noncohesive, generally uniform cells. The exact cytomorphology depends on the subtype of lymphoma. Most lymphomas involving the ovary are non-Hodgkin lymphomas. Burkitt lymphoma predominates in childhood, whereas small cleaved cell lymphoma and, to a lesser extent, large cell lymphoma are most frequent in adults.

Leukemias may also involve the ovaries. The absence of cellular cohesion or clustering would aid in the differentiation from poorly differentiated carcinoma and granulosa cell tumor, whereas the absence of two distinct populations would be against dysgerminoma. In contrast to the relatively uniform population of most lymphomas, a chronic inflammatory process would have a polymorphous population of variably sized lymphocytes admixed with histiocytes and possibly polymorphonuclear leukocytes. Immunocytochemical staining or flow cytometry for lymphoid markers may be helpful.

TUMORS METASTATIC TO THE OVARY

The most common primary site of metastases to the ovary is to the breast or gastrointestinal tract, with stomach predominating over colon. Most metastatic tumors are adenocarcinomas and, without appropriate history, may be difficult to distinguish from a primary ovarian adenocarcinoma. Metastatic signet ring cell adenocarcinoma needs to be differentiated from signet ring cell tumor, a benign primary tumor of ovarian stroma. The latter lacks nuclear features of malignancy and does not contain cytoplasmic mucin.

Adjuvant Techniques

Analysis of DNA ploidy by flow cytometry or image cytometry may be helpful in the future to help distinguish between benign and malignant ovarian masses. Pinto and associates (1990) described the measurement of CA-125, carcinoembryonic antigen (CEA), and alpha-fetoprotein (AFP) in ovarian cyst fluid as a diagnostic adjunct to cytology. All three tumor markers were low in follicular and luteinized cysts. Very high levels of CA-125 and low levels of CEA and AFP were found in both benign and malignant serous tumors. Elevated levels of CEA and CA-125 were found in benign and malignant mucinous tumors, whereas colonic carcinoma metastatic to the ovary had elevated CEA with low CA-125. Thus, whereas in most cases non-neoplastic cysts could be separated from neoplastic epithelial cysts, this method was not useful in distinguishing benign from malignant neoplasms.

EVALUATION OF PERITONEAL METASTASIS OF OVARIAN CARCINOMA

Examination of pelvic washings and peritoneal fluid is important for staging, estimating prognosis, and deciding on subsequent therapy at the time of initial surgery for ovarian carcinoma. It is especially useful in the assessment of residual ovarian cancer at second-look operations. Positive peritoneal fluid after therapy, even without macroscopic disease, has been correlated with a worse prognosis. Many patients with ovarian carcinoma unfortunately present with malignant ascites, and examination of the fluid may help to point to the ovaries as the primary. In addition to spontaneous effusions and washings, direct peritoneal smears obtained at laparoscopy or laparotomy by brushing or scraping have been reported to have similar sensitivity to peritoneal wash fluids. Peritoneal dialysate removed during instillation of chemotherapeutic agents for advanced ovarian carcinoma can also be examined cytologically.

Although the differentiation between ovarian borderline tumors and well-differentiated invasive carcinomas can be made with certainty only in histologic material, the cytologic appearance of these tumors in peritoneal fluids differs. Positive fluids from borderline tumors contain small to large cohesive papillary fragments, most of which have smooth borders; single tumor cells are few (Figs. 13–22 and 13–23). Invasive carcinomas tend to have small dyscohesive papillary fragments with numerous single cells. There is greater variation in cell size and shape, greater nuclear irregularity, more prominent nucleoli, and more prevalent cytoplasmic vacuolation in cases of invasive carcinomas. Psammoma bodies may be found with either type of tumor. Unlike invasive carcinomas, positive peritoneal washings in patients with serous borderline tumors have not been found to correlate with survival (Bell et al., 1988).

The differentiation of carcinoma cells from reactive mesothelial cells can be difficult, especially after chemotherapy. Histochemical staining for neutral mucins using the mucicarmine stain is helpful when the results are positive but not helpful in over half the cases when the results are negative. Immunocytochemistry can be very helpful. In the authors' experience, immunostaining using monoclonal antibodies B72.3 and for carcinoembryonic antigen have been most efficacious to identify carcinoma cells. No staining of mesothelial cells was found. DNA analysis of fluids and washings using flow cytometry or image cytometry may also be used to try to differentiate malignant epithelial cells from reactive mesothelial cells. They are helpful only when an aneuploid population is identified, indicating the presence of a malignant population, but they are not helpful when only diploid cells are found.

The presence of psammoma bodies is helpful but not pathognomonic for metastatic ovarian carcinoma (Fig. 13–24). CA-125, a monoclonal antibody directed against antigens primarily on nonmucinous epithelial ovarian carcinomas, is helpful.

ACCURACY AND RESULTS

As is the case with fine needle aspiration of other parts of the body, accuracy is related to the skill of the aspirator and to the expertise of the interpreter. Kjellgren and Angstrom (1979) reported diagnostic accuracies of 85.5% for benign ovarian lesions and 90% for malignant lesions, with a false-positive rate of 4.3%. Nadji and Sevin (1989) reported a diagnostic accuracy of 94.5% for fine needle aspiration of all benign and malignant gynecologic lesions. The specificity of aspiration of malignant gynecologic tumors was 97.9%.

Diagnostic pitfalls and causes of false-negative results include failure to accurately hit the lesion in question, inadequate sampling, and the overeagerness of an accommodating cytopathologist to render diagnoses on insufficient or poorly prepared material.

The technique used and type of lesions influence the accuracy of cytologic examination. Ultrasound-guided cyst aspiration appears to be a reasonable alternative to surgery, especially when the cyst is thought to be nonbloody. De Crespigny and colleagues (1989) aspirated 100 cysts in 88 patients under ultrasound guidance. Most patients were premenopausal. Cysts were aspirated only if larger than 10 cm. Seventy-two aspirates were acellular or showed only blood and/or histiocytes and thus could not be further cytologically subclassified. Twenty aspirates showed cells compatible with follicular or luteal cysts. Four aspirates showed blood and macrophages suggestive of endometriosis, and another four aspirates contained epithelial cells from a mucinous cystadenoma, endometriotic cyst, or cystic fallopian tube remnant. Although the accuracy was low, cytology could be combined with estradiol assay of the cyst fluid.

SUMMARY

Despite the rapidly growing rate of the use of fine needle aspiration for examining multiple organs and tissues in the United States in the last several years, ovarian aspiration is not widely accepted. Many feel that any solid ovarian lesion should be resected regardless of preoperative diagnosis, thus diminishing the role of fine needle aspiration for these types of masses. Because patients with ovarian carcinoma generally undergo a staging laparotomy, fine needle aspiration does not spare them a procedure. Other concerns about ovarian aspiration include sampling errors, as in mucinous or serous neoplasms where part of the tumor may be cytologically benign and other parts frankly malignant. Furthermore, stromal invasion, so important in distinguishing between borderline tumors and well-differentiated carcinomas, cannot be assessed cytologically.

There are limited but valid uses for ovarian fine needle aspiration (Ramzy, 1989). The most important of these is the examination of cysts in young patients where preservation of ovarian function is desired. The overall risk of carcinoma in this age group is low, making the use of ovarian aspiration fairly safe. Probably, only large symptomatic or persistent cysts need to be evaluated in most circumstances. Cysts may also be encountered while ova are being retrieved for in vitro fertilization using transvaginal ultrasound-guided aspiration. Examination of cyst aspirates in such cases is probably of limited value for cancer diagnosis, unless the fluid is of unusual volume or appearance (Greenebaum et al.). Another use for ovarian aspiration is during surgery to examine the contralateral ovary, when one ovary is resected for tumor, in order to determine if bilateral oophorectomy is necessary. This is of most value for the premenopausal patient.

Cytology can also be used as an adjunctive technique with frozen section for the intraoperative examination of specimens from the ovary. The advantages are preservation of small amounts of tissue, if needed, for permanent sections, hormone receptor analysis, or DNA studies and greater sampling capacity than frozen section alone (Abrams and Silverberg, 1989). Needle aspiration has been used in pelvic inflammatory disease. Ovarian aspiration may be used for the patient in poor medical condition who cannot tolerate surgery. The major use of cytologic examination of ovarian lesions, however, is for the evaluation of recurrent or metastatic disease. Fluids, washings, and aspirations of solid masses can all be examined cytologically, providing valuable staging, prognostic, and therapeutic information.

Bibliography

Abrams J, Silverberg SG: The role of intraoperative cytology in the evaluation of gynecologic disease. Pathol Annu 24(Part 2):167–187, 1989.

Akhtar M, Ali MA, Huq A, et al.: Fine-needle aspiration biopsy of seminoma and dysgerminoma: Cytologic, histologic, and electron microscopic correlations. Diagn Cytopathol 6:99–105, 1990.

Bell DA, Weinstock MA, Scully RE: Peritoneal implants of ovarian serous borderline tumors: Histologic features and prognosis. Cancer 62:2212–2222, 1988.

De Crespigny LC, Robinson HP, Davoren RAM, Fortune D: The "simple" ovarian cyst: Aspirate or operate? Br J Obstet Gynaecol 96:1035–1039, 1989.

Ewing TL, Buchler DA, Hoogerland DL, et al.: Percutaneous lymph node aspiration in patients with gynecologic tumors. Am J Obstet Gynecol 143:824–828, 1982.

Ganjei P, Nadji M: Aspiration cytology of ovarian neoplasms. A review. Acta Cytol 28:329–332, 1984.

Greenebaum E, Mayer JR, Rojas P, Stangel JJ: Aspiration cytology of ovarian cysts in *in vitro* fertilization patients (abstract). Acta Cytol 33:711, 1989.

Kjellgren O, Angstrom T: Transvaginal and transrectal aspiration biopsy in diagnosis and classification of ovarian tumours. In Zajicek J (ed.): Aspiration Biopsy Cytology. Part 2. Cytology of Infradiaphragmatic Organs. Basel: Karger, 1979.

Moriarty AT, Glant MD, Stehman FB: The role of fine needle aspiration cytology in the management of gynecologic malignancies. Acta Cytol 30:59–64, 1986.

Nadji M: Aspiration cytology in the diagnosis and assessment of ovarian neoplasms. In Roth LM, Cxernobilsky B (eds.): Tumors and Tumorlike Conditions of the Ovary. New York: Churchill Livingstone, 1985, pp. 153–173.

Nadji M, Sevin B-U: Pelvic fine needle aspiration cytology in gynecology. In Linsk JA, Franzen S (eds.): Clinical Aspiration Cytology. Philadelphia: J. B. Lippincott, 1989, pp 261–282.

Pinto MM, Bernstein LH, Brogan DA, et al.: Measurement of CA-125, carcinoembryonic antigen, and alpha-fetoprotein in ovarian cyst fluid: Diagnostic adjunct to cytology. Diagn Cytopathol 6:160–163, 1990.

Ramzy I: Signet-ring stromal tumor of ovary: Histochemical, light and electron microscopic study. Cancer 38:166–172, 1976.

Ramzy I: The value and limitations of aspiration cytology in the diagnosis of primary tumors. A symposium. Acta Cytol 33:741–790, 1989.

Ramzy I, Delaney M: Fine needle aspiration of ovarian masses. I. Correlative cytologic and histologic study of celomic epithelial neoplasms. Acta Cytol 23:97–104, 1979.

Ramzy I, Delaney M, Rose P: Fine needle aspiration of ovarian masses. II. Correlative cytologic and histologic study of nonneoplastic cysts and noncelomic epithelial neoplasms. Acta Cytol 23:185–193, 1979.

Selvaggi SM: Cytology of nonneoplastic cysts of the ovary. Diagn Cytopathol 6:77–85, 1990.

Stanley MW, Horowitz CA, Frable WJ: Cellular follicular cyst of the ovary: A cause of false-positive fluid cytology (abstract). Acta Cytol 34:733, 1990.

Yazdi HM: Fine needle aspiration cytology of ovarian sex cord tumor with annular tubules. Acta Cytol 31:340–344, 1987.

NON-NEOPLASTIC CONDITIONS

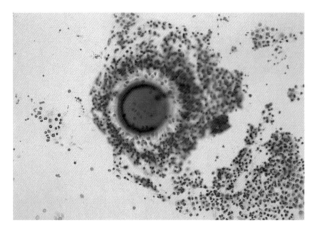

FIGURE 13–1. Cystic Follicle With Ovum. The central ovum with abundant eosinophilic cytoplasm is surrounded by a mantle of follicular cells (Papanicolaou stain [throughout unless otherwise indicated], × 160).

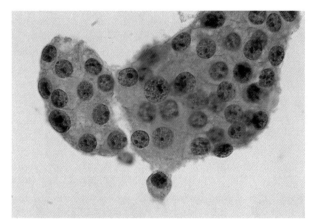

FIGURE 13–3. Corpus Luteum Cyst With Luteinized Cells. Compare the abundant granular and foamy cytoplasm to that of the nonluteinized follicular cells in Figure 13–2 (× 400).

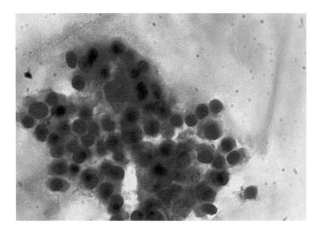

FIGURE 13–2. Granulosa Cells in a Nonluteinized Follicular Cyst. The cells are clustered and have round, uniform nuclei and a minimal amount of cytoplasm (× 225).

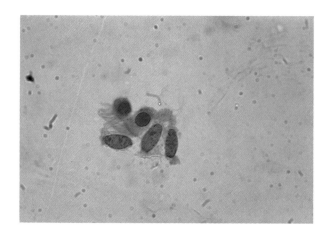

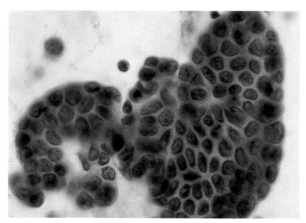

FIGURE 13–4. Simple Paratubal Serous Cyst. (Fig. 13–4A) Only a few ciliated low columnar, and often cuboidal, cells are present; they form a single layer. (Fig. 13–4B) The low columnar epithelial cells form a cohesive sheet with a papillary configuration. Note the square or angulated outlines of some nuclei and the occasional micronucleoli (× 400).

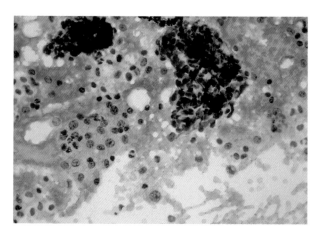

FIGURE 13–5. Endometriotic Cyst. The crowded cluster of endometrial cells is not unlike cells seen in cervicovaginal smears. They are small, with nuclear overlapping and angulation and minimal amounts of cytoplasm. These cells are surrounded by a hemorrhagic background with histiocytes (× 225).

NEOPLASTIC CONDITIONS

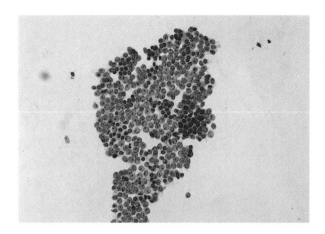

FIGURE 13–6. Serous Cystadenoma. The uniform neoplastic cells have round or slightly oval nuclei with micronucleoli, but they exhibit cellular monotony. The neoplastic cells form a sheet; papillae are not commonly seen in aspirates (× 160).

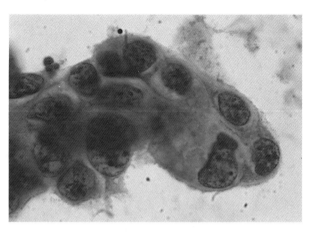

FIGURE 13–8. Serous Cystadenocarcinoma. Cells of this neoplasm, seen at a higher magnification than in Figure 13–7, have a high N/C ratio. The chromatinic rim is thick, and in some nuclei it shows some folds. Note the coarse granularity of the chromatin (× 400). (From Ramzy I, Delaney M: Fine needle aspiration of ovarian masses. I. Correlative cytologic and histologic study of celomic epithelial neoplasms. Acta Cytol 23:97–104, 1979.)

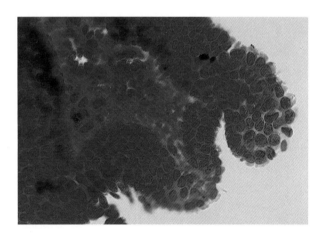

FIGURE 13–7. Serous Tumor of Borderline Group. A papilla reveals a connective tissue core surrounded by three to eight layers of epithelium. Although by definition borderline neoplasms should not have more than three layers of epithelium, the large number of layers may be a result of viewing the papilla en face. This illustrates the difficulty in separating borderline from frankly malignant tumors by cytomorphology, particularly in view of the similarity in nuclear atypia (× 225).

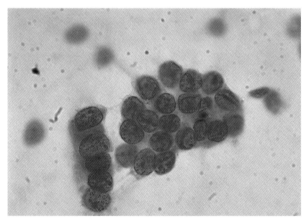

FIGURE 13–9. Serous Adenocarcinoma. These cells show marked nuclear atypia, with pleomorphic outlines and disrupted polarity. High-grade tumors usually do not present a diagnostic problem in establishing their malignant nature (× 400).

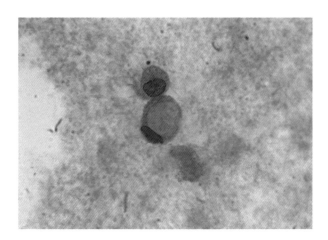

FIGURE 13–10. Mucinous Cystadenoma. The scant cellularity is not unusual, against an abundant granular or homogeneous mucinous background material. The tall, mucin-producing columnar epithelial cells often acquire a more round or oval shape when seen isolated in such a fluid background (× 630).

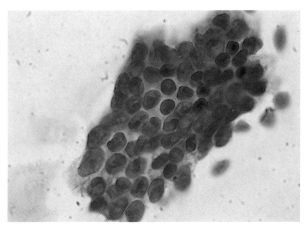

FIGURE 13–12. Mucinous Adenocarcinoma. Although these cells were cohesive, they show nuclear pleomorphism with irregularity in size and chromatin distribution. Careful examination may be necessary before the mucinous nature can be detected, since only a few cells may show evidence of such secretion, as illustrated at the upper edge of this sheet (× 400).

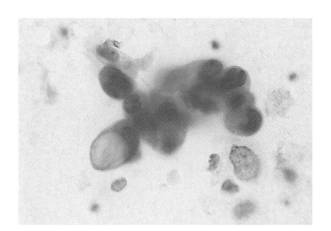

FIGURE 13–11. Mucinous Adenocarcinoma. Malignant tumors usually produce more cellular specimens than benign lesions (× 630).

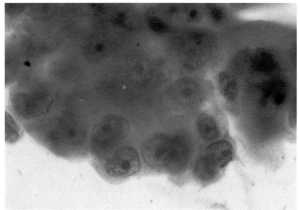

FIGURE 13–13. Poorly Differentiated Carcinoma with highly abnormal nuclei and prominent nucleoli. Such tumors show no evidence of serous, mucinous, or endometrioid differentiation (× 630).

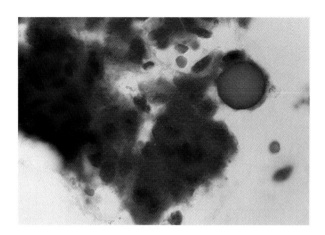

FIGURE 13–14. A Brenner Tumor. Sheets of squamous-like epithelial cells similar to parabasal cells are seen. The round, brightly eosinophilic body is derived from cysts that appear in the center of the epithelial nests (× 400).

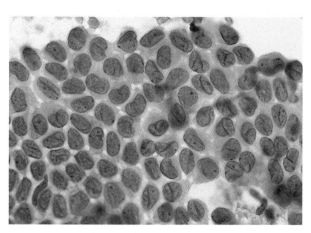

FIGURE 13–16. An aspirate from a patient presumed to have an adnexal mass. The coffee bean foldings in these nuclei suggested a Brenner tumor or a granulosa cell tumor. Laparotomy revealed a large uterine subserous leiomyoma and no adnexal mass. These cells are probably of mesothelial origin (× 630).

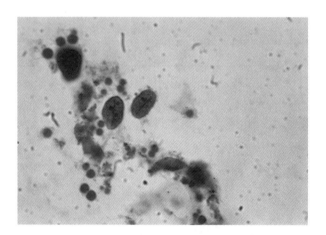

FIGURE 13–15. Brenner Tumor Epithelial Cells with the characteristic coffee bean nuclear folds (× 630).

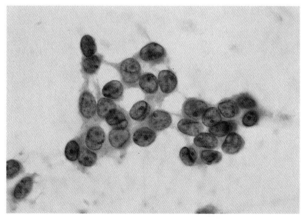

FIGURE 13–17. Granulosa Cell Tumor. The uniform cells have a moderate to scant cytoplasm. Note the fine chromatin, the uniform but well-defined nucleoli, and the presence of folds in the nuclear membranes. Call-Exner rosettes are fairly characteristic, but are rarely seen in aspirates (× 630).

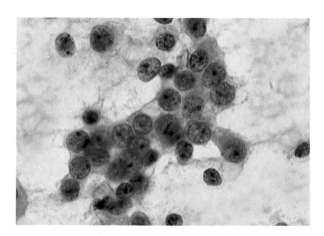

FIGURE 13–18. Sertoli-Leydig Cell Tumor. These cells may be similar to granulosa cells, as evident by a comparison with Figure 13–17. In some cases, spindled cells dominate the aspirate (× 630).

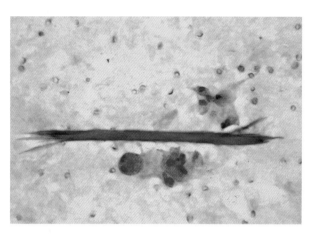

FIGURE 13–20. Mature Teratoma. In the ovary, most teratomas are cystic and contain this granular sebaceous material and anucleated squamous cells. A fragment of a hair shaft is seen in the center (× 225).

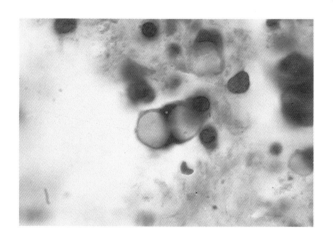

FIGURE 13–19. Benign Signet Ring Cell Tumor. These rare tumors consist of signet ring cells, but the nuclei are fairly bland. Unlike mucinous and Krukenberg tumors, the vacuoles in signet ring cell tumors do not contain mucin. They differ from other ovarian stromal tumors by the lack of lipids in these vacuoles (× 630).

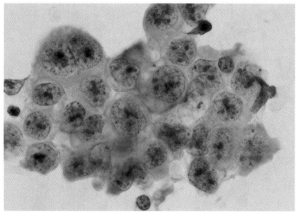

FIGURE 13–21. Germinoma. The neoplastic cells are quite large, with large, pleomorphic nuclei that exhibit coarse granularity of chromatin. The delicate cytoplasm is lacy or vacuolated because of its rich glycogen content, and it often ruptures. A sprinkling of lymphocytes may be seen in the background (× 630).

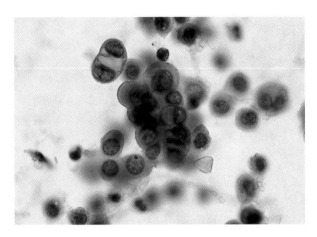

FIGURE 13–22. Serous Adenocarcinoma in Peritoneal Fluid. The presence of an occasional vacuolated cell does not exclude the diagnosis of a serous tumor (× 400).

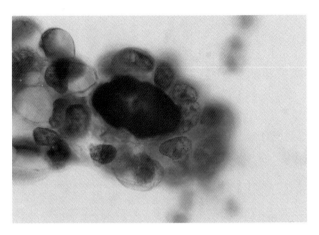

FIGURE 13–24. Serous Adenocarcinoma in Peritoneal Fluid. A brown psammoma body is surrounded by a mass of malignant cells. It is important to establish the diagnosis of malignancy on the basis of the nuclear features and not because of the presence of psammoma bodies. The latter occur in benign cysts, on the surface of normal ovaries, and in primary serous tumors of the peritoneum, among others (× 630).

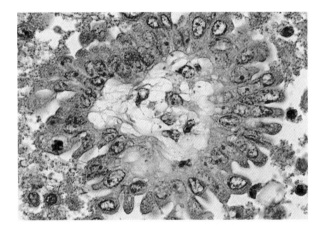

FIGURE 13–23. Serous Adenocarcinoma in a cell block preparation from the same case illustrated in Figure 13–22. The papillary nature of this tumor is clearly seen (hematoxylin and eosin stain, × 400).

C·H·A·P·T·E·R

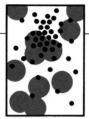

14

ASPIRATION BIOPSY OF LYMPH NODES: REACTION AND PRIMARY NEOPLASIA

Michael D. Glant

Douglas E. King

Fine needle aspiration (FNA) of lymph nodes has been a controversial topic since it was first used to evaluate lymphadenopathy in the early 1900s. Most of the early reports and much of the current literature describe and correlate the cytomorphologic patterns in malignant lymph node aspirates, whether from primary or metastatic disease. In the early to mid-1940s there finally appeared in the Scandanavian literature several descriptions of reactive lymph node hyperplasia (RLNH) or "nodes within normal limits." This spawned more interest in non-neoplastic lymph node aspiration, and the American literature over the past 10 years or so reflects this renewed interest.

Despite this new-found support for using needle aspiration for evaluating unexplained lymphadenopathy, there remains resistance to this application from both pathologists and clinicians. This is related to:

1. Lack of clinician understanding regarding the application of FNA in the management of lymphadenopathy.

2. Inexperience on the part of the pathologists who interpret lymph node aspirates (resulting in both false-negative and false-positive interpretations).
3. The relative paucity of reliable, well-founded cytomorphologic criteria for the evaluation of these specimens.
4. A failure to obtain and accurately correlate clinical data with cytologic findings when making the final diagnosis.

In the authors' experience and as the recent literature suggests, when these factors are controlled, the sensitivity and specificity of lymph node aspiration diagnoses are dramatically improved.

There are several advantages to using FNA in the evaluation of unexplained lymphadenopathy:

1. It is an easy, reliable office procedure.
2. It is cost-effective and safe.
3. It helps distinguish benign from malignant disease.
4. It assists in patient management.
5. It reduces patient anxiety.
6. It provides material for additional studies (e.g., surface markers, special stains, culture, and flow cytometry).
7. It provides data for appropriate therapy.
8. It eliminates the need for open biopsy in most cases of RLNH.

Remember, however, that RLNH is a heterogeneous process composed of several sets and subsets of reactive patterns. Because of this it may be difficult or impossible to distinguish some reactive patterns from primary neoplasia. Application of appropriate clinical data and special techniques minimizes the differential diagnostic problems.

Clearly, while it is necessary to have adequate patient information in all areas of diagnostic cytology, it is essential in the interpretation of lymph node aspirate specimens. It is also critical to obtain an adequate and representative sample and prepare exquisite smear preparations. In some cases cell suspensions for immunologic studies may be needed.

What are the expectations of the clinician who refers the patient? The clinician expects the pathologist to distinguish between a benign and a malignant process (whether primary or metastatic). Usually, this is as much as most clinicians expect, especially if the node is benign. But the clinician must be confident that this benign diagnosis is accurate so that he or she can plan appropriate management for the patient.

What is the predictive value of a benign diagnosis determined by FNA, and is it possible to further define the process involving the node using cytology? In the authors' experience for cases in which follow-up has been obtained, the predictive value of a negative diagnosis in a lymph node is about 98%. With this degree of certainty, the clinician is comfortable with merely observing most patients with RLNH and prescribing the appropriate treatment (such as antibiotics). Usually, the patient has already been taking antibiotics for several weeks prior to aspiration with little or no resolution in the size of the node. With persistence or increase in size of the node after aspiration, excision and histologic examination may be indicated to rule out occult neoplasm.

When appropriate, the authors try to provide the clinician with a more definitive interpretation than just benign versus malignant by:

1. Attempting to clarify the etiology of the reactive hyperplasia. In most cases a range of possibilities may exist, given the clinical data and morphologic pattern seen on the aspirate, and sometimes a more specific etiology can be established.
2. Correlating the cellular pattern in the node aspirate with the sequential events that occur in immune reactions to antigens. By knowing the duration of the palpable node, the approximate onset of any infectious process (e.g., influenza), and other pertinent clinical data (e.g., age, recent vaccinations, and serology), the authors indicate to the clinician the presumptive time frame for resolution of the palpable node. This gives the patient and the clinician a reference point by which time resolution is likely to occur, given normal resolution patterns. Thus, we designate whether the RLNH is an early phase, a mid-phase, or an end stage pattern and suggest an approximate time frame for resolution of the mass.
3. Attempting to be as definitive as possible in subtyping the lymphoma. The use of correlating immunologic surface markers (by flow cytometry or immunocytochemistry on air-dried cytospin preparations) can allow highly specific classification in many cases.

It is important to use a *systematic approach* when evaluating patients with palpable lymph nodes. The role of clinical information cannot be overemphasized, whether trying to distinguish RLNH from malignant neoplasia or attempting to specify the etiology or clinical stage of the reactive process. The physical characteristics of the node—shape, size, location, rapidity of onset, and extent of adenopathy—are important for correct evaluation. The most critical factor is the shape of the node. A spherical node is abnormal despite its size, and a spherical node larger than 2 cm is very likely to be a malignancy.

Serologic testing may also be important and should be performed either prior to aspiration or subsequent to aspiration as a follow-up to confirm the interpretation. Marker studies using immunocytochemical stains can be performed on properly collected and processed aspirate samples. The authors' preference is to procure extra samples in addition to needle and syringe rinsing and holding them in RPMI 1640 cell culture media for flow cytometry.

SPECIMEN PROCUREMENT

One of the authors (M.D.G.) has been involved in the procurement and processing of aspiration biopsies for over 10 years and has systematically studied a variety of techniques. The following approach is generally used in aspiration biopsies of most palpable masses.

1. Minimal anesthesia with 2% lidocaine is instilled as a pathway from the skin surface to the edge of, but not into, the lesion.
2. Multiple samples are taken with a 25-gauge 1.5-inch venipuncture needle via the puncture site made for anesthesia.
3. Four to six samples are taken using a fresh needle for each pass. Firm digital pressure using a clean gauze pad is applied to the puncture site between each sample and after the last for 3 to 5 minutes.
4. The samples are taken using a 10 ml syringe with a pistol grip (DLP, Inc., Grand Rapids, MI) with limited negative pressure and using a short (about 5 mm) vibratory needle motion once the needle tip is within the mass. All

negative pressure is discontinued when blood begins to fill the needle hub or after 20 to 25 vibratory reciprocations.

5. Smears are made by placing one to three drops of material onto the center of a plain glass slide (do not use frosted-surface slides in lymph node aspirates because severe crush artifact is likely). Then a second slide is placed face-to-face with the first, and the specimen pool is allowed to spread *without* applying pressure on the slides. Once the pool has nearly stopped spreading, the slides are gently pulled sideways rather than lengthways so that the smear is made with a very short stroke distance (which reduces trauma and limits the area required for microscopic review).

6. One slide is rapidly immersion-fixed by plunging it into 95% ethanol for Papanicolaou stain. The other is allowed to air-dry for rapid Romanovsky stain.

7. Each needle and any syringe containing material are rinsed in a true balanced salt solution (such as Ringer's lactate), 5 ml in a 50 ml centrifuge tube. If flow cytometry, multiple cytospin preparations, or cell blocks (metastatic lesions) are anticipated, several extra aspirations are usually placed entirely in the rinse solution. RPMI 1640 (10 ml) is added to the rinse if flow cytometry is to be done.

MORPHOLOGIC CHARACTERISTICS OF LYMPH NODE ASPIRATES

The maximum amount of morphologic information that is possible by routine light microscopy is gained by using Romanovsky and Papanicolaou-stained preparations in tandem. Evaluating lymph node samples in primary processes is similar to bone marrow aspiration. It is the mixture of the cellular population that is important rather than the atypia of individual cells. Therefore, understanding the spectrum of morphology seen with reactive (transforming) lymphocytes and their ratios is crucial for accurate diagnosis by FNA. The following are useful features when evaluating aspirations of lymph nodes.

The single most important feature in lymph node interpretation is the pattern of lymphoid elements present on the smear. Since both T and B lymphocytes undergo functional changes when stimulated that produce morphologically distinct cell types of varying maturities, reactive nodes usually contain a mixed or polymorphous population of cells. It is the relative proportion of these cells in the overall pattern that gives one of the best criteria for benignity. This population pattern can best be visualized on Romanovsky-stained slides on low power because of the flattening of the cells during air-drying. In a benign population, expect a greater percentage of small round lymphocytes (either mature mantle B cells or paracortical T cells) than follicular center cells (small cleaved, and large noncleaved) or immunoblasts and plasmacytoid cells. This ratio, however, is dependent upon the stage of the reaction. In other patterns of reactive lymph node hyperplasia there is a greater relative proportion of immunoblasts and plasma cells and a smaller relative proportion of small round and small cleaved lymphocytes. Accurately characterizing this lymphoid population and determining the relative mix of these cells is the first critical step in interpreting lymph node aspirates. As with *all* cytologic specimens, this feature is *not absolute*, and utilizing this criterion out of context without considering other morphologic features may lead to inaccurate interpretations.

The presence of lymphohistiocytic aggregates (LHAs) is also a significant diagnostic feature when defining reactive lymph node hyperplasia. These aggregates are actually fragments of hyperplastic follicles that are held together by dendritic and fibroblastic reticular cells. This reticulin network is a connective tissue framework that provides both structural support for lymph nodes and a site for the attachment of fixed macrophages and subsequent B-cell activation in the sinusoids. These reticular cells have oval, histiocyte-like nuclei with micronucleoli and long fragile cytoplasmic processes. Another component of LHAs is the tingible body macrophage (TBM). These phagocytic mobile histiocytes generally have cell debris in their cytoplasm, are easily recognized in lymph node aspirates, and are usually but *not always* associated with benign nodes. Scattered in the LHAs is a mixed population of lymphoid cells, usually follicular center cells varying in size from small round to large noncleaved cells and (rarely) plasmacytoid cells. Although LHAs usually indicate a benign follicular hyperplasia, they are sometimes associated with some lymphomatous processes (e.g., Burkitt lymphoma), especially in partially involved nodes.

Background changes in lymph node aspirates are helpful when evaluating reactive processes because they may assist in further defining both the type of reaction occurring and the causative agent. Identifying a background of neutrophils suggests a suppurative process perhaps from the microabscesses seen in cat-scratch disease or the abscesses associated with an unidentified bacterial infection. The presence or absence of caseating necrosis, with or without giant cell formation and epithelioid cells, is associated with a panorama of granuloma-producing processes, including tuberculosis, sarcoidosis, toxoplasmosis, and tularemia. Culture and special stains are indicated when either of these background patterns predominates. Lymphoglandular bodies (fragments of lymphocyte cytoplasm) are seen in nearly every Romanovsky-stained aspirate containing lymphocytes and are useful in distinguishing malignant epithelial from lymphoid (benign or malignant) processes.

It is important to be able to recognize and distinguish other nonlymphoid and lymphoid cell types in lymph node aspirates since they help distinguish benign from malignant processes and assist in specifying the etiology of RLNH. These cell types include epithelioid histiocytes, giant cells (e.g., Warthin-Finkeldey and Langhans), eosinophils, plasmacytoid cells, and mast cells.

SPECIFIC PATTERNS IN REACTIVE LYMPH NODE HYPERPLASIA

There are a limited number of histologic patterns in lymph node hyperplasia that involve to varying degrees the different compartments of a lymph node: follicles, paracortical zone, and sinuses. There is a great deal of overlap between these reactive histologic patterns and even with some malignant lymphomatous processes. So much overlap occurs at times that, without immunocytochemical stains or other sophisticated techniques, differential diagnoses are nearly impossible to make. Histologically, one looks at flat B5-fixed tissue sections with some relative perspective as to where these compartments are. In fine needle aspirates from lymph nodes the authors obtain random cellular samples from different areas of a node and then mix them all up on a slide. Hopefully, with four or six needle passes and with paired Papanicolaou- and Romanovsky-stained slides, we have adequately sampled all diagnostically significant areas so that the predictive value of our interpretation is high. Usually, only a presumptive interpretation regarding specific etiology can be rendered.

The literature on FNA cytology of RLNH is rather limited. There are case reports, however, that illustrate the cytologic patterns in specific types of node reactions: tuberculosis, viral change, toxoplasmosis, infectious mononucleosis, giant lymph node hyperplasia (angiofollicular lymphadenopathy), lymphangiography adenopathy, sarcoidosis, cat-scratch disease, abscess, postvaccinial lymphadenopathy, anticonvulsant adenopathy, and leishmaniasis.

The normal morphology of lymphoid cells in various stages of transformation must be understood. The following paragraphs summarize their characteristics in the order of cellular proliferation and transformation.

Small round cells (SRC) are the mature or mitotically inactive cells that may be programmed (memory cell) to make antibody or are yet uncommitted to antibody production and awaiting transformation. On a Romanovsky-stained slide, the SRC is the smallest lymphoid cell and has a dense smudged chromatin. The cytoplasm is scant and no nucleoli are present. On a Papanicolaou-stained slide, the SRC has a condensed to coarse clumped chromatin and a round nucleus. The cytoplasm is scant, but sometimes a small comet-like tail of light blue cytoplasm may be seen.

Small cleaved cells (SCC) are in the mantle zone, follicle, or medullary areas (T cells) and represent the first change in transformation. A spectrum in size is seen from that of the SRC to just less than the size of a large cell (with the diameter of a normal histiocyte nucleus). A Romanovsky-stained slide shows a round to cleaved nucleus with a lighter chromatin than the SRC and cytoplasm that is pale blue and scant. On a Papanicolaou-stained slide, the chromatin is a regular coarse clumped pattern without obvious nucleoli; however, a chromocenter may mimic a nucleolus. As the SCC reaches its largest size, the chromatin granules may appear more widely dispersed. On a Papanicolaou-stained slide, the SCC may have a grooved or angulated nuclear membrane, but it is not as prominent as seen on B5 histology.

Large cleaved cells (LCC) are in the follicle and less often in the medullary area (T cells). The LCC has the nuclear size of a normal histiocyte or slightly larger and scant cytoplasm. Otherwise, the chromatin, nuclear membrane characteristics, and cytoplasm on Romanovsky- and Papanicolaou-stained slides are similar to the SCC.

Small noncleaved cells (SNCC) are rarely found in nodes because of their rapid mitotic activity and progression to the next phase. If found, they have a round regular nucleus just below the size of a large cell (intermediate size), and the chromatin is finely granular (almost clear). One to three small nucleoli are usually present. The cytoplasm is a deeper blue than is seen in LCCs and often contains vacuoles on Romanovsky-stained slides.

Large noncleaved cells (LNCC) are mainly in the follicles and have a nuclear size of a histiocyte or larger. The Romanovsky stain characteristics are very similar to the LCC, with the exception of visible nucleoli and a more abundant cytoplasm that varies from light to deeper blue. On Papanicolaou-stained slides, the chromatin is like an SNCC, very finely granular to clear. Prominent, usually multiple, round and bar-like nucleoli are present, some appearing bound to a nuclear membrane, which is often folded or grooved. A rim of pale blue cytoplasm is present on Papanicolaou-stained slides.

Immunoblasts (IMB) are in the follicle and interfollicular zones. Like the SNCC, they are very mitotically active and, if they are of B-cell origin, produce immunoglobulin. On Romanovsky-stained slides, the nucleus is larger than a large cell with one or two prominent nucleoli, often central. The cytoplasm of

B-cell IMBs is more abundant than a large cell and deep blue. On Papanicolaou-stained slides, the pattern is similar, with finely granular chromatin, large central nucleoli, and a rim of well-defined blue-green cytoplasm. T-cell IMBs are rare and have a pale blue to clear cytoplasm on either stain.

Plasmacytoid lymphocytes (B cells only) are seen as a spectrum of cells that vary from the size of large cells (plasmablasts) to that of an SRC. Their chromatin becomes progressively more coarse and dense as they become smaller. They have a deep blue cytoplasm that is relatively abundant. They are frequent in early reactions and rare later on unless recurrent stimuli trigger their production.

There is usually much confusion about the terms "cleaved" and "noncleaved" in descriptions of lymphocytes, mainly because both cleaved and noncleaved cells have nuclear convolutions and folds. In fact, on cytologic preparations the LNC cells are the most likely to show folds and cleaves in the nuclear membrane. It is easier to relate the morphology to mitotic potential or metabolic activity. Cleaved cells have very limited metabolic or mitotic activity and therefore have a coarse, denser chromatin and no nucleoli (from increased heterochromatin). In contrast, the noncleaved cells are very metabolically or mitotically active and therefore have an open chromatin with prominent nucleoli.

Follicular hyperplasia is the most common type of lymph node hyperplasia and is especially common in children. It represents a B-cell response to antigen, usually of nonspecific etiology. Cytologically, one sees a mixed population of lymphocytes of varying maturities with a relative increase in the number of large cleaved and large noncleaved cells, immunoblasts, and plasmacytoid cells in early reactions. Larger relative numbers of mature lymphocytes and small cleaved cells are present as the reaction approaches resolution. It is usually in this type of reaction that the cytologic picture can be correlated best with the phase or duration of the reaction. This can be differentiated from a "pure" interfollicular hyperplasia only by the presence of lymphohistiocytic aggregates. Since most reactive hyperplasias are actually a mixture of follicular and interfollicular hyperplasia, it is generally of little or no help to issue a diagnosis of either type. It is very helpful to diagnose the temporal phase of the reaction and give a presumptive etiology. This allows the clinician to follow the patient with an expected period of resolution of the adenopathy or to perform further testing to confirm the presumed etiology if needed. Regardless of follicular or interfollicular proliferations, the temporal patterns are the same.

Early Phase Reactive Pattern

The early phase reactive pattern is seen during the first 10 to 14 days of a reaction, with the length varying with intensity, duration, and type of antigenic stimulus. The ratios of the cell types are as follows:

$$SRC + SCC > LC, LNC > IMB, PC$$

There is an increased relative proportion of immunoblasts and plasmacytoid cells and a decreased relative proportion of small round or cleaved lymphocytes. At the peak of this phase, the large cells may almost equal the small cells. This is the reaction phase that simulates an immunoblastic lymphoma. Since most early immune responses generate increased numbers of IgM-producing plasma cells, one would expect to see abundant plasmacytoid cells, immunoblasts, and a smaller relative proportion of small cleaved and small round cells in these early reactions. Fortunately, such reactions are rarely seen in needle aspirates, since the nodes may be small or biopsy deferred until after a 7- to 10-day course of antibiotics. Mononucleosis and other intense stimuli can cause prolonged early phase reactions. Other etiologies include herpes zoster infection, postvaccinial lymphadenitis, and reactions to anticonvulsant medication (diphenylhydantoin).

Mid-Phase Reactive Pattern

This reactive pattern is seen 10 to 28 days following the antigenic stimulus, and this is the most common pattern encountered. The ratios of the cell types are as follows:

$$SRC + SCC >> LC, LNC > IMB, PC$$

There is approximately a 50:50 ratio between small round and small cleaved cells. Large cells, immunoblasts, and plasmacytoid cells are about half as frequent as small cells. Aspirates from mid-phase reactive lymph nodes are composed of a mixed lymphoid population: declining numbers of plasmacytoid cells and immunoblasts and a relative increase in the number of mature lymphocytes (memory cells: mantle zone and paracortical lymphocytes) compared with early reactions.

End Stage Reactive Patterns

Assuming no further antigenic stimulation, progression to the end stage pattern occurs in another one to two weeks. Clinically, this is typically a node that decreased in size after observation or antibiotic therapy but did not disappear. The patient may be more concerned about the node than the physician. The aspirate is more likely to be bloody, and the node may feel firm or rubbery on aspiration. The cell ratios are as follows:

$$SRC + SCC >>> LC, LNC >> IMB, PC$$

There is a complete dominance of small round and small cleaved cells over large cells, and very few immunoblasts or plasmacytoid cells are seen. In the end stage and resolution phase, the mixed smear pattern consists primarily of mature lymphocytes and greatly reduced numbers of large cleaved and large noncleaved cells. Rare immunoblasts, plasmacytoid cells, and LHAs may be seen in the early phase of an end stage reaction.

Recurrent Antigenic Stimulation

If there is a second or third antigenic challenge, e.g., a viral infection superimposed on the existing reaction, the pattern gets even more complicated. Most often, many mature lymphocytes suggesting a mid-phase to end stage reaction are mixed with a lesser number of plasmacytoid lymphocytes. Scattered immunoblasts and fairly typical plasma cells may also be present (which are generally not seen this late in single antigenic stimuli). In children, this usually indicates a recurrent antigenic stimulation that is virally induced.

In adults, rheumatoid arthritis and syphilis are rare examples of chronic disease processes that recurrently stimulate and induce follicular hyperplasia in nodes. In general, these are both characterized by intense interfollicular plasma cell reactions adjacent to transformed follicles (follicular center cells). With the appropriate clinical and serologic data, a presumptive diagnosis of these two entities may be made in lymph node aspirates.

Giant lymph node hyperplasia (Castleman disease) is also an example of a chronic follicular hyperplasia that can be suggested by the cytologic pattern in node aspirates. It is characterized by a mixed population of cells (small round and cleaved cells > large cleaved, large noncleaved cells > immunoblasts), LHAs, and numerous branching vascular structures. Hyalinization of the vessel walls can also be appreciated in cytologic samples. The plasma cell variant of GLNH is indistinguishable from the pattern seen in rheumatoid arthritis. Clinically, GLNH is seen in enlarged mediastinal nodes, although it may be observed in other sites, including cervical and axillary nodes. Many hyperplasias other than GLNH are characterized by vascular proliferation, especially of postcapillary venules, and these are commonly seen in node aspirates.

Granulomatous Patterns in Lymphadenopathy

Toxoplasmosis and cat-scratch disease are common infectious processes in lymph node aspirates. They are both examples of a mixed type of lymph node hyperplasia with different cytologic and histologic patterns.

Lymphadenitis caused by *Toxoplasma gondii* usually affects cervical lymph nodes unilaterally (in the posterior triangle) and results from contact with contaminated cat feces (e.g., dust from cat litter) or by eating infected raw meat. The cytologic pattern is phase-specific but is most often dominated by small lymphocytes with fewer numbers of immunoblasts and plasma cells (follicular hyperplasia). Tingible body macrophages are frequent, as are LHAs. Also seen are numerous histiocyte aggregates that are *not* TBMs but represent epithelioid histiocytes. Giant cells are uncommon. It is significant to remember that the dominant cellular population in toxoplasmosis is lymphoid rather than epithelioid. This closely mimics the histologic picture that features follicular hyperplasia with interfollicular epithelioid histiocytes, some of which may impinge upon follicles. Distended sinusoids with monocytoid histiocytes are also seen.

Cat-scratch disease is self-limiting and may be chlamydial in origin. It does, however, have a relatively distinct and well-documented cytologic picture as long as the clinical picture fits. During the first two to three weeks, lymph node aspirates contain aggregates of spindle epithelioid cells, which are in palisade arrangement at the periphery of these groups, giving them a stellate appearance. The background is composed of a mixture of lymphoid elements, including mature lymphocytes, immunoblasts, plasma cells, and occasional eosinophils. A characteristic feature in cat-scratch disease is the presence of numerous neutrophils, which is suggestive of microabscess formation in the node. This pattern correlates with the histologic picture of suppurative granulomas with stellate abscesses surrounded by palisading rows of epithelioid histiocytes and fibroblasts. Necrosis is usually minimal unless the lesion is advanced (three to four weeks), at which time there is abundant necrosis and neutrophilic infiltration. Culture and special stains should always be performed on the aspirated material in this latter pattern to rule out mycobacteria, fungus, and other bacteria, since it is identical to any other acute adenitis.

Other granulomatous processes that may mimic the pattern seen in cat-scratch disease are tuberculosis, sarcoidosis, and tularemia. Although their cytologic patterns are not distinct (giant cells, epithelioid histiocytes, and mixed lymphoid population), caseation necrosis is usually associated with tuberculosis, whereas the granulomas seen in sarcoid are of the noncaseating type.

PRIMARY NEOPLASIA IN LYMPH NODES

Hodgkin Disease

Hodgkin disease (HD) is a malignancy of lymphoid tissue characterized by the Reed-Sternberg (R-S) cell or a variant of the R-S cell. Usually, a background of reactive lymphoid cells, granulocytes (especially eosinophils), and histiocytes is present. The R-S cell is of unknown origin, but some data suggest origin in the dendritic reticulum cell. The patients usually present with painless lymphadenopathy (supradiaphragmatic in 90%, cervical > > mediastinal > axillary). They may have fever, night sweats, pruritus, malaise, or weight loss (B symptoms). Later in the course, many patients have retroperitoneal lymph node, spleen, liver, and/or bone involvement. About 50% of cases occur in patients between 20 and 40 years of age. Less than 10% of cases occur before age 10 and less than 10% after age 60. The male to female ratio is 4:3 (males also have a worse prognosis). HD accounts for 30 to 40% of all lymphomas.

The four histologic types of Hodgkin disease by the Rye classification system cannot be definitively diagnosed by FNA alone. However, when correlated with clinical findings, the subtype is often apparent. The general pattern of HD and a short discussion of the subtypes follow. Recently, oncologists have not relied on histologic typing of HD as much as on the clinical stage. This has resulted in frequent staging laparotomies or treatment without node excision in cases diagnosed by FNA.

In FNA the diagnosis of HD requires the presence of classic R-S cells in the appropriate background of reactive cells, just as in histology. If R-S cells are not frequent or "classic," a definitive diagnosis should be avoided, and an Epstein-Barr virus infection should be excluded. In many cases FNA samples processed with Romanovsky stain are the easiest and most rapid approach to diagnose HD. This may be particularly true in the lymphocyte predominant type, which is difficult to diagnose by histology. In air-dried Romanovsky-stained smears, the flattening of the R-S cells accentuates their size as compared to the reactive background. In addition, the cells appear much different than the immunoblasts that mimic them on histology. The R-S cell is usually 40 to 100 μ in greatest dimension, so that on a 7 μ tissue section it is difficult to cut a perfect central portion of the R-S cell to include both nuclei and nucleoli. In early stage reactions with numerous immunoblasts, two large immunoblasts may be adjacent and appear as one cell on histology. On FNA smears, every R-S cell and immunoblast is "whole-mounted," allowing a complete analysis of each, and on a Romanovsky-stained slide, the R-S cells may flatten to reach nearly 150 μ. Immunoblasts are rarely binucleate and do not have features typical of R-S cells on a Romanovsky-stained slide. They are more difficult to differentiate with Papanicolaou stain.

With Romanovsky stain, immunoblasts have deeper blue cytoplasm, round nuclear contour, fine even chromatin, more regular nucleoli, and a paranuclear cytoplasmic hof. Reed-Sternberg cells have gray cytoplasm without the hof, irregular lobulated nuclei, coarse chromatin, and irregularly shaped nucleoli. It is also helpful to evaluate these cells in the context of the mixed plasmacytoid cells and numerous large cells in the background. This spectrum of transformation is usually not seen in Hodgkin disease. Always beware of a node that has a Hodgkin disease pattern and associated early phase hyperplastic changes. It may represent a reactive node that has been only partially replaced by Hodgkin disease.

In lymphocyte predominant HD, the patient is generally a child with a single large spherical node and no other symptoms. The aspirate contains a background of an end stage reaction with a scattering of typical R-S cells. The FNA diagnosis is usually fairly easy, but confirmatory histology is not. If R-S cells are less frequent, the pattern of small round cell lymphoma would need to be considered because of the very large node. It would, however, be inconsistent with the patient's age.

Nodular sclerosing HD often causes densely fibrotic tissue in larger nodes or masses, which are scantily cellular in aspirates (very rubbery to woody at aspiration). Multiple samples and additional sampling of smaller adjacent soft nodes is often required to obtain an adequate sample (smaller nodes show the cellular phase). In this type of HD there are many typical R-S cells and mononuclear variants. The latter are similar to typical R-S cells except for the lack of nuclear bilobation. In fibrotic areas the fragile R-S cells often lose their cytoplasm and may present as bare nuclei. The background is usually a population of lymphocytes similar to a mid-phase reactive node often with eosinophils and plasma cells. Occasional cases have areas of suppurative necrosis.

Mixed cellularity HD is the most readily diagnosed type of Hodgkin disease because of the presence of numerous R-S cells and their variants. One variant, the popcorn cell, is a polylobed R-S cell that has been described in all types but is uncommon in nodular sclerosing HD. Mixed cellularity HD can have any background but typically has abundant eosinophils. Because it lacks the fibrosis seen in nodular sclerosing HD, the nodes are clinically soft and the aspirates are very cellular.

Lymphocyte depleted HD is the least common type and may be fibrotic or cellular. It is characterized by very pleomorphic R-S cells in a limited lymphoid background. The authors have seen this type of Hodgkin disease only in patients with recurrent HD many years after initial therapy. The aspirates from these cases showed extremely large, bizarre polylobed R-S cells with rare small lymphocytes.

At times HD has a granulomatous or histiocyte-rich reaction in the background. This can be particularly prominent in some cases of lymphocyte predominant HD. In addition, a reactive node draining an area of active HD can have such a reactive pattern. This must be kept in mind in patients with diffuse adenopathy and clinical symptoms suspicious for HD. Repeat or multiple site aspirates can be used to locate the best site for subsequent excision in such cases.

Non-Hodgkin Lymphoma

Lymphocytic lymphomas compose the vast majority of the remaining primary malignancies of lymphoid tissue and arise from the lymphocytic stem cell. Rarely, a malignancy of true histiocytic cell line is found.

Clinically, non-Hodgkin lymphoma (NHL) is observed more often in the older patient. About 25% of cases are in patients between 50 and 59 years old, with maximal risk in the seventh decade. The male to female ratio is 4:1. Early involvement of oropharyngeal lymphoid tissue, skin, gastrointestinal tract, and bone is common. In children, about one third present with abdominal manifestations. About 13% of lymphocytic lymphomas (especially small cleaved cell type) are leukemic. NHL may be accompanied by an immune deficiency, which is usually humoral (e.g., hypogammaglobulinemia or poor antibody formation). Multiple myeloma rarely affects lymph nodes and has an incidence nearly equal to that of all NHL cases combined. Although it is a well-differentiated B-cell neoplasm, multiple myeloma is generally not included in the classification of NHL (abbreviated NCI-NHLC) since it is usually based in bone marrow.

The National Cancer Institute's Working Formulation for clinical grading of NHL (abbreviated NCI-NHLC) has recently replaced the Rappaport classification system and is utilized in the following discussion (Table 14–1).

The histologic classification of NHL is based on the predominant cell population, which is often a monomorphic or dimorphic pattern of lymphoid cells. This seems to illustrate a block in the transformation sequence of these cells. Lymph node architecture is variably altered, usually with effacement of cortical and medullary structures with an outpouring of cells through the capsule. A vague or obvious nodular (follicular) pattern at low-power microscopy may mimic reactive germinal cells and is a critical prognosticator for many subtypes (with a good prognosis). Increased mitotic activity correlates to poor prognosis.

The histopathology of the spectrum of NHL is beyond the scope of this discussion, and the authors assume that the reader has an understanding of histology. The FNA features in most cases of NHL are distinctly different from reactive lesions, but others are difficult to differentiate without experience using exquisite preparations. It is important to correlate clinical findings and to use immunologic studies when questionable or suspicious patterns are encountered.

With experience, the initial diagnosis of lymphoma can be accurate in most cases (85 to 90%). Subtyping of a lymphoma is reliable in up to 75% (using NCI-NHLC), if surface markers for kappa and lambda light chains, pan–B-cell antigen, pan–T-cell antigen, CD5 (Leu-1) and CD10 (CALLA) are utilized.

Cellular patterns may be monomorphic or polymorphic (usually dimorphic), but the normal lymphoid proliferative population distribution of mature forms > immature forms > blasts must be absent (excluding infiltration of reactive cells, such as macrophages and granulocytes). Virtually all cases of lymphoma have a small population of benign cells integrating with the neoplastic population. This is often up to 2 to 5% of the cells in the FNA. This is particularly true in the small celled lymphomas.

FNA of nonlymphoid tissue infiltrated with lymphoma (e.g., muscle and soft tissue) often contains clusters of cells that mimic the cohesive and molding patterns seen in carcinomas. Although uncommon, this may cause a major classification error. Romanovsky-stained smears (if not blood diluted) are invaluable because of the presence of characteristic lymphoglandular bodies virtually diagnostic of lymphoid cells.

Low-Grade Lymphomas

Data on low-grade lymphomas show that this type of lymphoma has a survival rate after treatment equal to the survival rate in untreated patients. Both groups also have approximately a 30% incidence of progression to a higher grade lymphoma and about a 20 to 25% rate of spontaneous complete regression. There are three types of low-grade lymphoma (Table 14–2).

In the small round cell lymphoma (or chronic lymphocytic leukemia in a lymph node), a cellular smear shows over 80% small round lymphocytes with rare or no mitoses. The cells are small and round but appear in many cases larger than normal SRC and have a more open chromatin. In fact, on Romanovsky-stained slides, they usually have a chromatin more like normal SCC. On Papanicolaou-stained slides, the chromatin may be smudged or plasmacytoid (coarse clumped chromatin). The pattern in chronic lymphocytic leukemia may be similar but often has a subpopulation of larger cells with chromocenters using Papanicolaou stain. These apparently come from the proliferation centers often present in lymph node infiltrates of this neoplasm. Waldenström macroglobulinemia and the plasmacytoid variant of small round cell lymphoma contain a clearly plasmacytoid population, often with multinucleated forms. Surface markers show a monoclonal population of B cells in most cases but weak marking for light chains. In the B-cell types there is a paradoxical T-cell antigen (CD5), which is helpful diagnostically.

In the small cleaved cell, follicular lymphomas the aspirate sample is usually cellular with more than 80% small cleaved lymphocytes of variable sizes with limited mitotic activity. The cells are small, but in some cases the population varies within a limited range of cell sizes. On Romanovsky-stained slides, the cells often appear similar to the cells of a small round cell lymphoma, so Papanicolaou stain is more helpful in classifying the cell type. However, the monotony of the population in most cases is more striking with Romanovsky than with Papanicolaou stain. Papanicolaou stain shows cells similar to normal SCC except for a more open chromatin and in some cases prominent nuclear clefts and grooves. Some cases can be difficult to distinguish from an end stage reaction if a significant population of normal cells is present. Surface markers are usually monoclonal for one of the light chains in B-cell neoplasms or for a T-cell antigen. Most of these will also be positive for CD10. Since nodular and diffuse growth cannot be discerned on FNA, this neoplasm often requires surgical excision for grading (see the section on "Intermediate-Grade Lymphomas").

In the mixed small cleaved, large cell, follicular lymphoma, there is usually a cellular smear with a mixture of small and large cells and a paucity of small round lymphocytes and immunoblasts. Because of the mixture, this lymphoma is most likely to be classified as reactive (see the section on "Ambiguous Patterns"). Generally, the large cells compose about 10 to 25% of the population with the small cleaved cells. The SCC are similar to those of the small cleaved cell, follicular lymphomas. The large cells can be either LNCC or LCC and are similar to benign cells of those types. Surface markers may indicate either a B-cell or T-cell neoplasm, and if the T-cell type exists, then diffuse growth is present. In B-cell neoplasms, histology is required to determine growth pattern for grading.

Intermediate-Grade Lymphomas

Data on intermediate-grade lymphomas continue to support the notion that this category has a more aggressive course than low-grade NHL. This grade is generally aggressively treated with chemotherapy. The four types of intermediate-grade lymphoma are listed in Table 14–3.

The small cleaved cell and mixed lymphomas are similar in the low and intermediate grades (see previous descriptions). Markers may be used to differentiate the various grades if a T-cell neoplasm is found, since these always have a diffuse growth pattern.

In large-cell lymphomas the smears are usually cellular and composed of over 80% large cells, which makes diagnosis relatively simple in most cases. On Romanovsky and Papanicolaou stains, the cells are similar to normal large cells but may be larger or show bizarre forms. In most cases the vastly dominant morphology is of an LNCC type. Necrosis and cell fragility (crush artifact) are not uncommon. Surface markers most often show a B-cell neoplasm.

High-Grade Lymphomas

Data on high-grade lymphomas continue to support the notion that this category has a more aggressive course than intermediate-grade NHL. This grade is generally treated very aggressively with chemotherapy.

The three types of high-grade NHL are listed in Table 14–4.

In immunoblastic lymphoma the smears are usually cellular and composed of a spectrum of cells, mostly immunoblasts with fewer numbers of large and small plasmacytoid cells. The large cells are similar to normal IMB but with more pleomorphism. Mitoses are frequent, and surface markers rarely indicate a T-cell neoplasm.

In lymphoblastic lymphoma the smears are cellular with a monotonous population of more than 90% medium-sized lymphoblasts with or without prominent convolutions. Mitoses are frequent in most cases, and there may be necrosis and tingible body macrophages. These neoplasms are composed of T cells and generally arise in the thymus. They are identical to many of the populations seen in childhood acute lymphocytic leukemia. On smears, two morphologic patterns are seen. Uniform, even chromatin (blastic on Romanovsky stain and dusty on Papanicolaou stain) with small nucleoli and scant pale cytoplasm is typical of the nonconvoluted type. Dense or coarse chromatin (smudged on Romanovsky stain and coarsely granular on Papanicolaou stain) with scant pale cytoplasm is seen in the convoluted type. Nucleoli may be seen but are less prominent. Cytospin preparations can be used for terminal deoxynucleotidyl transferase (Tdt) marking by cytochemistry, which is characteristic of this lymphoma.

In undifferentiated lymphoma (Burkitt and non-Burkitt lymphoma), the smear is usually cellular and composed of cells intermediate in size. Cells from this type of lymphoma are similar to the SNCC with uniform open chromatin and multiple small nucleoli in the more monotonous Burkitt type. The cytoplasm is typically deep blue and vacuolated on Romanovsky stain. These vacuoles contain lipid that stains with oil red O or Sudan black. These B-cell neoplasms usually express IgM heavy chains. The non-Burkitt type is similar except for a wider spectrum of cell size and more prominent nucleoli.

Ambiguous Patterns in Non-Hodgkin Lymphoma of the Lymphocytic Type

Cellular smears with mixed populations may be difficult to classify as reactive or malignant. In lymphomas of mixed type with abundant histiocytes and other reactive forms (e.g., Lennert lymphoma), this is particularly difficult. Suspect lymphoma if:

1. Normal SRC forms are lacking in the smear (less than 5%).
2. Many LCC forms with few or no LNCC/IMB are seen.
3. Histiocytes are not tingible body type and many are seen in a background of numerous SCC.
4. Numerous eosinophils and plasma cells are present.
5. Cellular pattern is composed of greater than 80% SCC + LCC.
6. Large cells show marked pleomorphism even if they compose less than 5% of the population.

In mixed lymphomas it is often difficult to exclude a large cell lymphoma, since the latter may have a significant number of small cells in the smear. Favor a mixed lymphoma if (1) the vast majority of large cells are LCC type or (2) there is a broad spectrum of anisonucleosis on Papanicolaou stain with no greater than 25% large cells.

In general, favor a large cell lymphoma if (1) the majority of large cells are of the LNCC type or (2) nuclei are monotonous in size on Papanicolaou stain and contain nucleoli.

The following NHL lymphocytic neoplasms are infrequent in lymph nodes but may be seen. Grades are not established for:

1. Mycosis fungoides, a T-cell lymphoma composed of smaller hyperconvoluted lymphocytes. Skin involvement is typical.
2. Plasmacytoma (extramedullary), an atypical plasma cell population with variable numbers of plasmablasts. Immunoglobulin monoclonality may be demonstrated.
3. Multiple myeloma, a marrow-based plasma cell neoplasm typically associated with a monoclonal serum immunoglobulin (some only have light chains in urine) and lytic bone lesions. Nodal or soft tissue infiltrates may be secondarily seen.

True Histiocytic Lymphoma

Rarely, a neoplasm of true histiocytic origin is encountered in aspirates of lymph nodes. Experience has shown that this is frequently initially misdiagnosed as a large-cell lymphoma but fails to respond well to chemotherapy. Clinically, patients are often febrile and pancytopenic, suggesting sepsis. However, testing for an infectious process is negative. Sampling palpable nodes or bone marrow may lead to the correct diagnosis, especially in the latter if erythrophagocytosis is present.

On FNA the cellular pattern depends on the differentiation of the lesion. If well differentiated, the features are characteristic, and enzyme or immunologic stains will confirm the histiocytic or monocytic nature of the neoplasm. The well-differentiated form is morphologically identical to lymph node infiltrates from monocytic leukemia. These neoplasms have several interesting morphologic features to watch for:

1. Pseudopodia-like cytoplasmic extensions, especially if well differentiated.
2. No lymphoglandular bodies despite high cellularity.
3. Cohesive on Papanicolaou-stained preparations and noncohesive on Romanovsky-stained slides.

Metastatic Carcinoma

Since clinical enlargement of a lymph node by a metastasis usually invokes more than a fourfold increase in mass, the majority of the node is replaced by metastatic carcinoma when it presents as lymphadenopathy. The basic cytomorphology of small cell groups and isolated cells is similar in FNA and exfoliative cytology. Large three-dimensional groups in FNA are not often seen in exfoliated samples and show many tissue patterns similar to surgical pathology.

Generally, the finding of cohesive cells with typical patterns of epithelial differentiation allows a confident diagnosis of carcinoma. A problem in an initial patient diagnosis is the definition of possible primary sites. The nearly endless spectrum of metastatic carcinoma to lymph nodes is not covered in this chapter. Virtually all cases of metastasis are similar to the primary site on FNA.

Bibliography

Cardoza PL: The cytologic diagnosis of lymph node punctures. Acta Cytol 8:194–205, 1964.

Feldman P, Covell J, Kardos T: Fine Needle Aspiration Cytology: Lymph Node, Thyroid and Salivary Gland. Chicago: ASCP Press, 1989.

Jaffe ES: Surgical Pathology of the Lymph Nodes and Related Organs. Philadelphia: W. B. Saunders, 1985.

Linsk JA, Franzen S: Fine Needle Aspiration for Clinicians. Philadelphia: J. B. Lippincott, 1986.

Qizilbash AH, Young JE: Guide to Clinical Aspiration Biopsy: Head and Neck. New York: Igaku-Shoin, 1988.

Rosenberg SA, et al: National Cancer Institute Sponsored Study of Classifications of Non-Hodgkin's Lymphoma: Summary and description of a working formulation for clinical usage. Cancer 49:2112–2135, 1982.

Stani J: Cytologic diagnosis of reactive lymphadenopathy in fine needle aspiration biopsy specimens. Acta Cytol 31:8–13, 1987.

Tani EM, Christensson B, Powit A, Skoog L: Immunocytochemical analysis and cytomorphologic diagnosis on fine needle aspirates of lymphoproliferative disease. Acta Cytol 32:209–215, 1988.

Table 14–1. NATIONAL CANCER INSTITUTE'S WORKING FORMULATION
FOR CLINICAL GRADING OF NON-HODGKIN LYMPHOMA*

Grade	Clinical Remission	Median Time to Relapse	Median Survival	Five-Year Survival
Low	61–73%	5 → 5.5 years	5.1–7.2 years	50–70%
Intermediate	56–69%	2 → 8 years	1.5–3.4 years	33–45%
High	48–69%	1.1 → 7.7 years	0.7–2 years	23–32%

*From Rosenberg SA, et al.: National Cancer Institute Sponsored Study of Classifications of Non-Hodgkin's Lymphoma: Summary and description of a working formulation for clinical usage. Cancer 49:2112–2135, 1982.

Table 14–2. TYPES OF LOW-GRADE LYMPHOMA

Type	Dominant Cell(s)	Tissue Growth Pattern
Small round cell lymphocytic	SRC	Diffuse
Small cleaved cell, follicular	SCC	Nodular
Mixed small cleaved, large cell, follicular	SCC/LCC–LNCC	Nodular

Table 14–3. TYPES OF INTERMEDIATE-GRADE LYMPHOMA

Type	Dominant Cell(s)	Tissue Growth Pattern
Small cleaved cell, diffuse	SCC	Diffuse
Mixed small cleaved, large cell, diffuse	SCC/LCC–LNCC	Diffuse
Large cell (cleaved or noncleaved), follicular	LNCC–LCC	Nodular
Large cell (cleaved or noncleaved), diffuse	LNCC–LCC	Diffuse

Table 14–4. TYPES OF HIGH-GRADE NON-HODGKIN LYMPHOMA

Type	Dominant Cell(s)	Tissue Growth Pattern
Immunoblastic	IMB	Diffuse
Lymphoblastic	Lymphoblast	Diffuse
Undifferentiated, Burkitt or non-Burkitt	SNCC	Diffuse

MORPHOLOGY OF NORMAL LYMPHOID CELLS

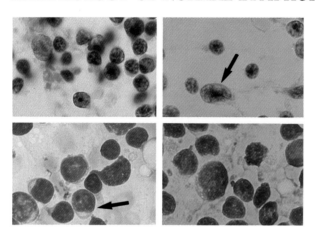

FIGURE 14–1A. Small Round and Small Cleaved Lymphocytes are shown stained by both air-dried Romanovsky stain and wet, fixed Papanicolaou stain methods. On the Papanicolaou stain, a histiocyte is seen with numerous small round and small cleaved lymphocytes. On the Romanovsky stain below is a similar population showing the small, round lymphocytes with dense chromatin, and at the arrow, a small cleaved cell. On the other Papanicolaou stain, small round and small cleaved cells are seen with a large cleaved cell (arrow). In the corresponding Romanovsky stain, small round and small cleaved cells are seen with a large cleaved cell (× 330).

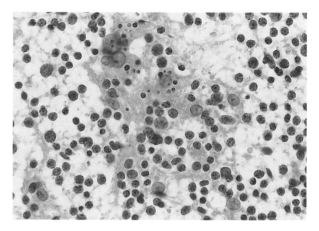

FIGURE 14–1C. Lymphohistiocytic Aggregate. A mixture of lymphocytes is seen, with histiocytes showing phagocytosis of debris (tingible body macrophages) (Papanicolaou stain, × 150).

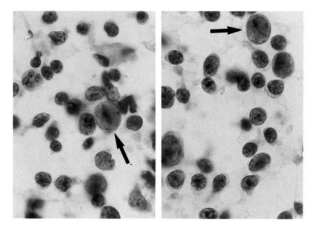

FIGURE 14–1B. Two fields with the Papanicolaou stain show a mixture of **Small and Large Lymphoid Cells with Large Noncleaved Cells** (arrows) seen in small numbers. Note the open chromatin and bar-like nucleoli of the large noncleaved cell (× 330).

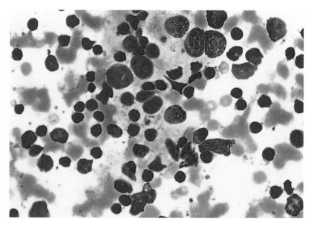

FIGURE 14–1D. Lymphohistiocytic Aggregate. The same spectrum on the Romanovsky stain is seen as compared to Figure 14–1C (× 198).

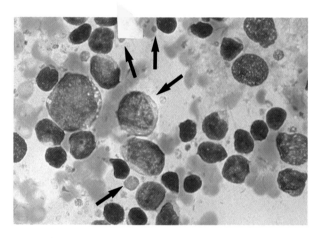

FIGURE 14–2A. Spectrum of **Lymphoid Cells** in a benign lymph node on Romanovsky stain. Note the background of small blue fragments (arrows), which originate from lymphoid cytoplasm, the so-called "lymphoglandular bodies" (× 330).

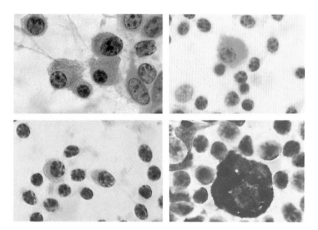

FIGURE 14–2C. Plasma Cells and Mast Cells. The left two Papanicolaou stains show typical plasma cells from a case of rheumatoid arthritis on the top and from a case of chronic viral adenitis (plasmacytoid lymphocytes) on the bottom. In the right upper field is a mast cell on a Papanicolaou stain with a more granular and abundant cytoplasm than the typical plasma cell. On the Romanovsky stain in the lower panel are the typical deep purple granules of the mast cell obscuring the nucleus (× 330).

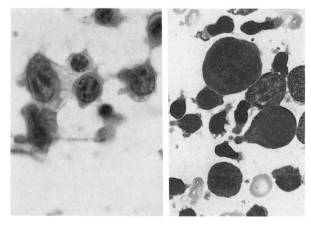

FIGURE 14–2B. Immunoblasts. A Papanicolaou and Romanovsky stain showing the large immunoblastic cells, which are the least common cells in a reactive lymph node. Note the deep blue cytoplasm on the Romanovsky stain and the large nucleoli on the Papanicolaou stain (× 330).

IMMUNOBLASTIC REACTION (EARLY-STAGE LYMPH NODE HYPERPLASIA)

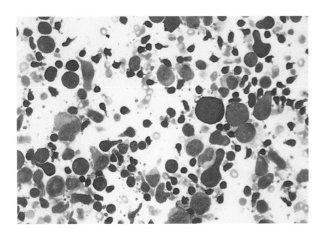

FIGURE 14–3A. Early Reaction, Secondary to Antigenic Stimulation from Tumor Necrosis in a Patient Who Had Radiation Therapy for Small Cell Carcinoma of the Lung. This Romanovsky stain shows the spectrum of proliferating lymphocytes with numerous immunoblasts that is typical in the first week of an intense lymph node reaction. See the diagram on cell populations in Figure 14–4C. Despite numerous large cells, the small lymphoid cell population is still dominant in this reaction (× 132).

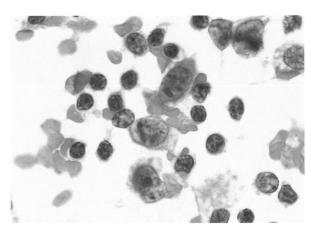

FIGURE 14–3C. Early Reaction Caused by Epstein-Barr Virus. Note the numerous large immunoblasts in this mononucleosis-induced hyperplasia (Papanicolaou stain, × 330).

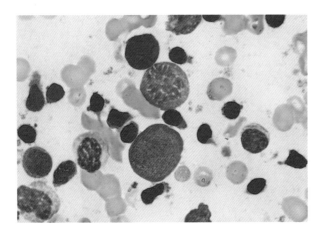

FIGURE 14–3B. High power of immunoblasts and other cells in an **Early Viral Reaction** (Romanovsky stain, × 330).

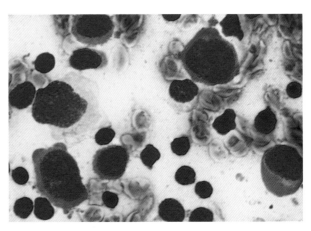

FIGURE 14–3D. Early-Stage Reaction from Epstein-Barr Virus. This photo corresponds to the Papanicolaou on Figure 14–3C. Note numerous large immunoblasts (Romanovsky stain, × 330).

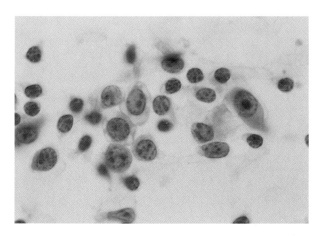

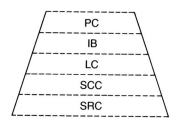

EARLY-PHASE PATTERN

FIGURE 14–4A. Early-Stage Reaction Caused by Nonspecific Viral Response. Note one immunoblast and other large cells. This is the Papanicolaou stain of the case seen in Figure 14–3B (× 330).

FIGURE 14–4C. Diagram of Early-Phase Reaction. Note how the population of lymphoid cells has shifted more to the proliferative forms (immunoblasts, large cells), yet the small cells still predominate when cell counts are done. Also in these reactions, the large cells, such as immunoblasts and differentiating plasmablasts, show deep blue cytoplasm. These reactions must be distinguished from immunoblastic lymphoma and lower-grade plasmacytoid lymphomas. The former generally shows a lack of many small cells and the latter shows an unusual dominance of small plasmacytoid forms without the immunoblast population and other large cells.

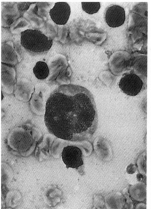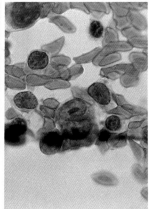

FIGURE 14–4B. Reed-Sternberg–like Cells in Early-Stage Reaction. Rarely, binucleate immunoblasts are seen in a reactive node, particularly in an early-stage reaction. These are generally not identical to typical Reed-Sternberg cells. Reed-Sternberg cells typically do not have deep blue cytoplasm, are usually fairly frequent, and are often associated with a background of a minimally reactive lymphoid population (× 330).

MID-PHASE LYMPH NODE REACTION

In the second to fourth week of reaction, the following patterns are seen.

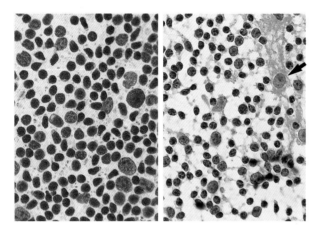

FIGURE 14–5A. Lower-power view of Midphase Reaction. The Romanovsky stain shows the dominance of small cells with an equal balance of small round and small cleaved cells and a smaller percentage of large cells with rare immunoblasts. The adjacent field shows the Papanicolaou stain with a similar population and a histiocyte at one edge (arrow) for size comparison (× 150).

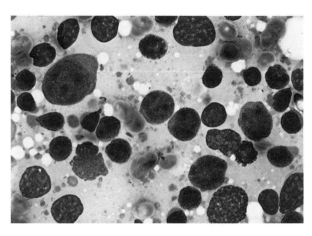

FIGURE 14–5C. Mid-phase Reaction showing a field with a proportionately increased number of large cells on Romanovsky stain. The distribution of lymphoid cells on aspirates varies throughout the slide. One has to get a mental picture of the overall population and realize that areas have increased numbers of large cells when they represent tissue aspirates from germinal centers. Note the background of numerous lymphoglandular bodies (× 330).

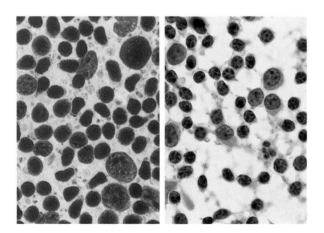

FIGURE 14–5B. Mid-phase Reaction. Comparison of Romanovsky and Papanicolaou stains showing the admixture of small cells, which dominate over the larger cells (× 250).

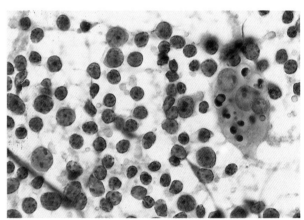

FIGURE 14–5D. Mid-phase Reaction. This Papanicolaou stain shows a comparison of a tingible body macrophage with a population of lymphoid cells. This area probably represents cells collected from a germinal center (× 250).

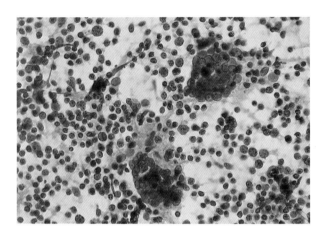

FIGURE 14–6A. Warthin-Finkeldey Cells. These large, multinucleate forms are rarely encountered in aspirates of lymph nodes. On the Papanicolaou stain the large cells with tightly packed nuclei have a vaguely defined cytoplasm and lie in a background of typical mid-phase reactive node. Such cells are described histologically in measles adenitis but apparently can be seen in other viral reactions. This aspirate is from a patient without clinical evidence of measles who did have a viral syndrome (× 132).

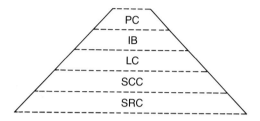

MID-PHASE PATTERN

FIGURE 14–6C. Diagram of a Mid-phase Reactive Node. Note the population distribution in a mid-phase reactive node. Mid-phase reactive nodes are seen in about the second to fourth week after a stimulus. At this point, many of the proliferating cells have formed more small round and cleaved cells and the reaction is subsiding. Therefore, there is an accumulation of small cells and a diminution in the number of larger cells. Generally, with a single stimulus, very few plasmacytoid cells, if any, are seen this late in the lymphoid population. With recurrent stimulation, more plasmacytoid cells are expected.

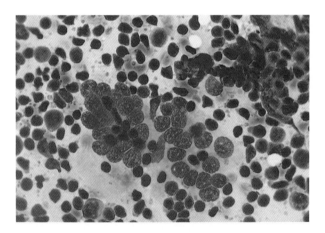

FIGURE 14–6B. Warthin-Finkeldey Cells in a Reactive Lymph Node. This is the Romanovsky stain of the same case as Figure 14–6A (× 198).

END STAGE LYMPH NODE REACTION

This pattern is generally seen in the last several weeks of the reaction.

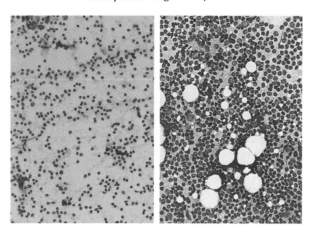

FIGURE 14–7A. Low-power view of **End Stage Reaction.** A Papanicolaou stain is on one side and a Romanovsky stain is on the other. Note the dominant pattern of small cells, mainly small round cells, with less frequent small cleaved cells (× 66).

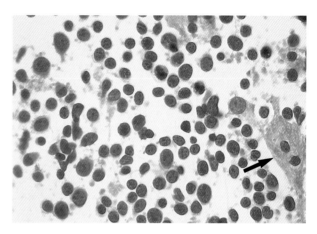

FIGURE 14–7C. End Stage Reaction on high power. This Papanicolaou stain shows the dominant pattern of small lymphocytes with a few large cells and a histiocyte (arrow) for comparison. This field was picked to demonstrate numerous large cells (× 280).

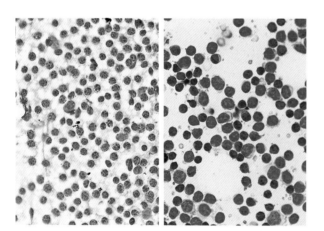

FIGURE 14–7B. End Stage Reaction. Papanicolaou and Romanovsky stains show a dominant pattern of small lymphocytes with almost an equal mixture of small round and small cleaved cells. These reactions have to be differentiated from a small round cell lymphoma (× 150).

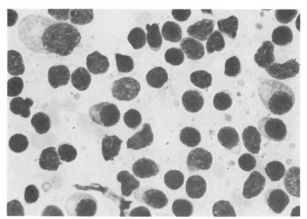

FIGURE 14–7D. End Stage Reaction in a patient with a history of recurrent viral infections. Note on this Romanovsky stain a pattern of small lymphocytes, some with fairly abundant blue cytoplasm (plasmacytoid lymphocytes). This pattern is often an indication of recurrent viral stimulation (× 240).

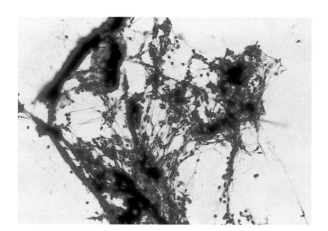

FIGURE 14–8A. End Stage Reaction with crush artifact. This shows the crushing effect often seen in a regressing lymph node that has increased stromal tissue. End stage reactions can cause an increased vascularization of lymph nodes, which may be reflected in fragments of blood vessels with associated crush artifact (Papanicolaou stain, × 150).

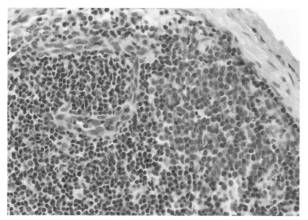

FIGURE 14–8B. Histology of **End Stage Reaction**. Beneath the capsule of this end stage reactive node there is a dominant pattern of small lymphocytes and a thick-walled vessel. This is the population of cells that would be expected in the aspirates of nodes at this stage (hematoxylin and eosin stain, × 100).

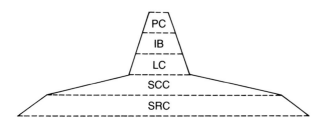

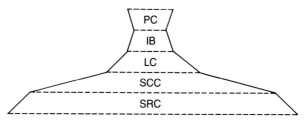

END-STAGE/RESOLUTION
PHASE PATTERN

RECURRENT ANTIGENIC
STIMULATION

FIGURE 14–8C and 14–8D. Diagram of Reaction. Note the population distribution in an end stage reaction. At this point in time, nearly all the proliferating cells have subsided and have formed a residual population of small cleaved and small round cells. Should this reaction occur in a node that has recurrent viral stimulation, there will be scattered residual plasmacytoid forms in the node. This reaction is referred to as "end stage reaction with recurrent stimulation." Typically this correlates clinically with a patient's long history of mild, recurrent stimuli. It is not uncommon for these patients to have numerous small nodes in the region where the node has been biopsied. End stage reactions in adults over age 50 have to be distinguished from small round cell lymphoma.

CAT-SCRATCH DISEASE

This reactive pattern must be distinguished from toxoplasmosis and resolving bacterial infection in a lymph node with microabscesses (partially treated with antibiotics).

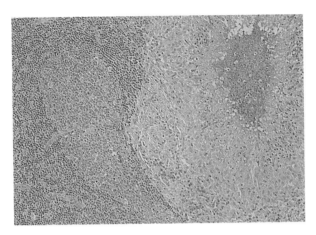

FIGURE 14–9A. Histology of **Cat-Scratch Disease**. Note the microabscess with adjacent follicular hyperplasia in this tissue section (hematoxylin and eosin stain, × 33).

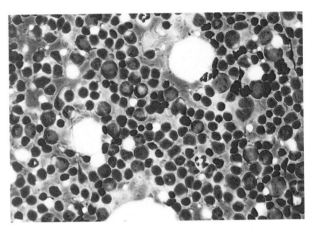

FIGURE 14–9C. Cat-Scratch Disease. Cytology on a Romanovsky stain shows a mid-phase reactive node in most areas of the smear (× 150).

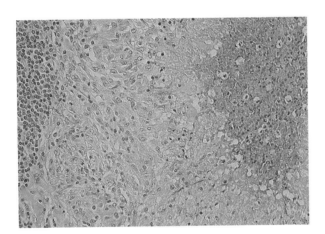

FIGURE 14–9B. Histology of **Cat-Scratch Disease**. Note the edge of a microabscess showing epithelioid histiocytes adjacent to the sterile abscess (hematoxylin and eosin stain, × 66).

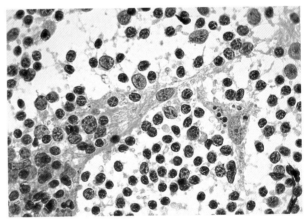

FIGURE 14–9D. Early Cat-Scratch Disease on a Papanicolaou stain. A mid-phase reactive node with lymphohistiocytic aggregates, reflecting the follicular hyperplasia (× 240).

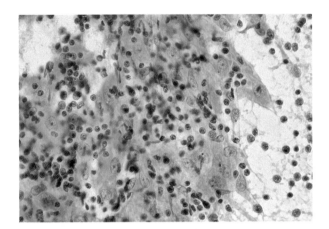

FIGURE 14–10A. Epithelioid Histiocytes in **Cat-Scratch Disease**. These cells come from the wall of the microabscesses and are scattered around in some smears. Note the abundant cytoplasm and the elongated shape of the histiocytes, with pale, oval nuclei and small nucleoli. In the smears these are often adjacent to or admixed with neutrophils and other abscess-associated debris (Papanicolaou stain, × 132).

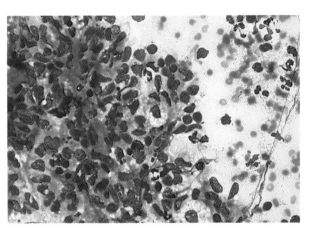

FIGURE 14–10C. Early Cat-Scratch Disease with material from microabscess. This Romanovsky stain shows epithelioid cells, neutrophils, and strands of nuclear debris typical of the microabscess material from cat-scratch disease in its early stages (× 198).

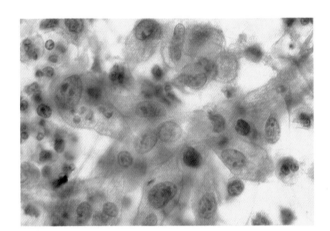

FIGURE 14–10B. Area from a microabscess in **Cat-Scratch Disease**. This Papanicolaou stain shows typical histiocytes with neutrophils from an area of microabscess (× 330).

COMMENT: Early cat-scratch disease must be distinguished from toxoplasmosis and resolving (usually partially treated) bacterial infection in lymph nodes. Toxoplasmosis generally shows clusters of histiocytes that are in smaller aggregates than seen in cat-scratch disease and that are not associated with the abscess debris or neutrophils.

   In bacterial infection, the pattern may be very similar; however, clinical history is often helpful. The exposure to cats with a scratch in the region of the lymph node is useful but is not always found. Most bacterial infections are associated with prior injury: either a skin wound with extreme tenderness or a head and neck infection with cervical lymphadenopathy. In addition, bacterial infections may progress to complete necrosis of the node unless an antibiotic has been intensively used.

ACUTE ADENITIS (LARGE ABSCESS OF LYMPH NODE) VERSUS LATE CAT-SCRATCH DISEASE

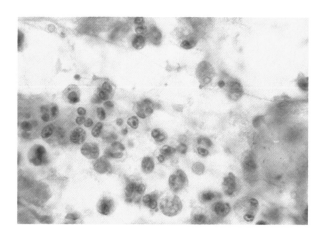

FIGURE 14–11A. Late Cat-Scratch Disease. On a Papanicolaou stain many neutrophils with necrotic debris and occasional histiocytes are seen. The specimen is grossly purulent but usually thick rather than watery. The patient has a long history of lymphadenopathy with limited antibiotic treatment and an exposure to cats. This is likely end-stage cat-scratch disease. Cultures should be performed to exclude active bacterial infection (× 330).

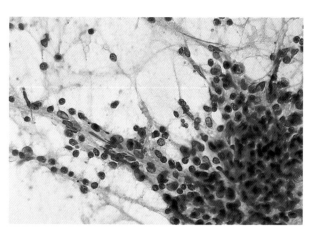

FIGURE 14–11C. Late Cat-Scratch Disease. In smears from this process, rare fragments of lymphocytes or epithelioid histiocytes can be found. If only a single sample is taken, this is less likely observed. With multiple samples, particularly if taken from the margin of the lesion, these aggregates are more likely to be found. This slide depicts a fragment of histiocytes with lymphocytes in a background of necrotic debris (Papanicolaou stain, × 132).

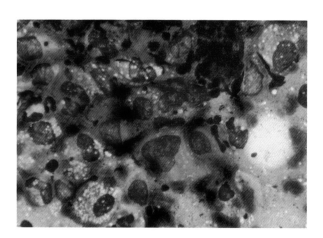

FIGURE 14–11B. Late Cat-Scratch Disease. A Romanovsky stain shows granular debris, histiocytes, and neutrophils typical of an abscess (× 330).

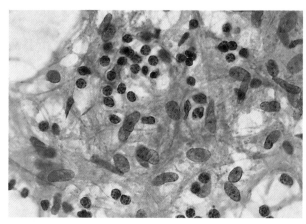

FIGURE 14–11D. Aggregate of epithelioid histiocytes with a few lymphocytes in **Late Cat-Scratch Disease**. This is seen only in rare foci in an otherwise purulent aspirate (Papanicolaou stain, × 240).

COMMENT: Late cat-scratch disease is clinically a liquefactive necrosis of a lymph node without bacteria. This is seen 6 to 8 weeks after the onset of adenopathy. This cannot be differentiated from an end-stage abscess, except by clinical criteria. If the patient has had intensive antibiotic treatment and no exposure to cats, it is likely that such an abscess results from a bacterial infection. In all cases, gram stains and aerobic as well as anaerobic cultures should be performed on the aspirate material. If giant cells are seen (which are uncommon in cat-scratch disease), culture for atypical tuberculosis should be performed.

GIANT LYMPH NODE HYPERPLASIA VERSUS LONG-TERM CHRONIC STIMULATION

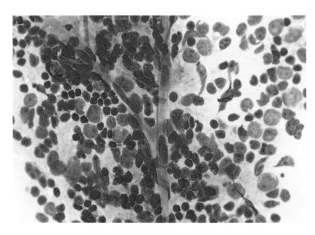

FIGURE 14–12A. Giant lymph node hyperplasia. The hyaline vascular type shows numerous vessels with a background of a mid-phase reactive lymph node. In this example, the Romanovsky stain shows the thick-walled capillary structures admixed with a reactive lymph node. Such a pattern cannot be differentiated from a recurrent chronic stimulation (Romanovsky stain, × 150).

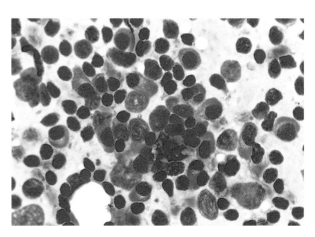

FIGURE 14–12C. Giant Lymph Node Hyperplasia with numerous plasmacytoid lymphocytes, a hallmark of chronic recurrent stimulation (Romanovsky stain, × 250).

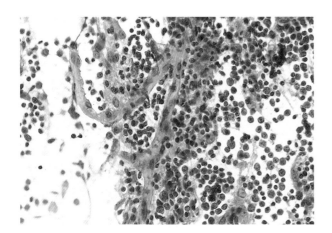

FIGURE 14–12B. Giant Lymph Node Hyperplasia showing numerous thick-walled vascular structures in a mid-phase reactive node (Papanicolaou stain, × 100).

TOXOPLASMOSIS

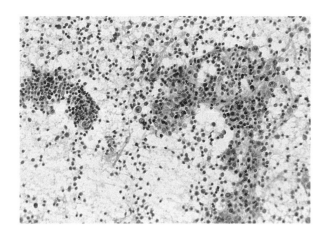

FIGURE 14–13A. Low-power view of **Toxoplasmosis**. This Papanicolaou stain shows some clusters of histiocytes admixed with a mid-phase reactive node pattern. Tingible body macrophages are absent or are very few in number (× 66).

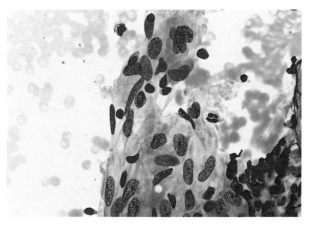

FIGURE 14–13C. Epithelioid histiocyte cluster in **Toxoplasmosis**. This Romanovsky stain shows the abundant cytoplasm and oval nuclei of epithelioid histiocytes. If an aspirate contains numerous small clusters of histiocytes and lymphohistiocytic aggregates, it is more likely a chronic restimulated lymph node with areas of histiocyte proliferation than toxoplasmosis (× 150).

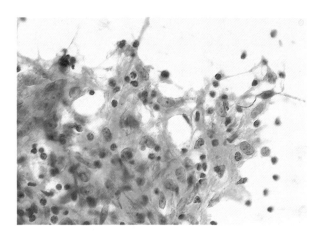

FIGURE 14–13B. Toxoplasmosis. High-power view of a cluster of epithelioid histiocytes. These cells look very similar to those seen around the wall of the microabscesses in cat-scratch disease. In toxoplasmosis, the abscesses are not seen, and these histiocyte clusters are scattered throughout the slide, either in small or large aggregates. There is usually a lack of typical lymphohistiocytic aggregates (Papanicolaou stain, × 150).

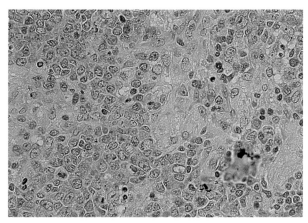

FIGURE 14–13D. Histology of **Toxoplasmosis**. This intermediate power shows the histiocyte clusters seen in a pattern of interfollicular hyperplasia secondary to toxoplasmosis (hematoxylin and eosin stain, × 160).

SARCOIDOSIS

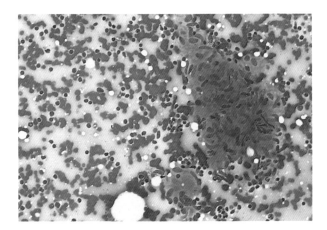

FIGURE 14–14A. Sarcoidosis. This photograph depicts a pattern of lymphocytes with a discrete cluster of epithelioid histiocytes and a single multinucleated giant cell in a Romanovsky-stained smear (× 66).

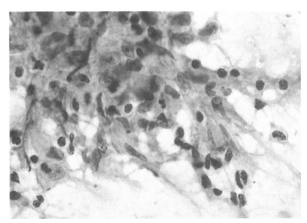

FIGURE 14–14C. Sarcoidosis. This Papanicolaou stain shows an area very similar to Figure 14–14B illustrating the histiocyte clusters in this noncaseating granuloma (× 198).

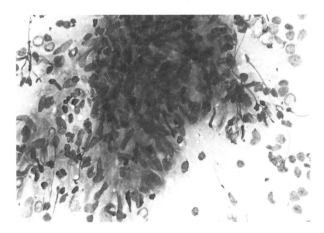

FIGURE 14–14B. Sarcoidosis. This Romanovsky stain shows a very tight cluster of histiocytes with a scattering of lymphocytes in the background. In sarcoidosis, these clusters of histiocytes are often observed in a scanty background of lymphocytes. The lymph node is usually quite firm at aspiration (× 132).

COMMENT: Sarcoidosis must be differentiated from a fungal or mycobacterial infection. Generally, special stains are used on smears to identify these organisms. Typically, in fungal or mycobacterial infections there is greater cellularity, areas of tissue necrosis, and a history more suggestive of active infection (tender nodes or clinical signs of infection such as fever or weight loss). In cases of sarcoidosis, the nodes are often asymptomatic but easily palpable. They are quite firm and yield a scanty sample with limited lymphoid material in association with histiocyte clusters and occasional giant cells.

SMALL ROUND CELL LYMPHOMAS (INCLUDING CHRONIC LYMPHOCYTIC LEUKEMIA)

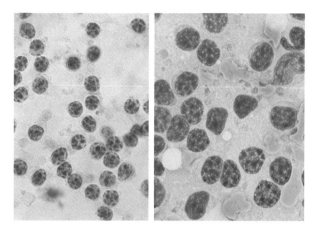

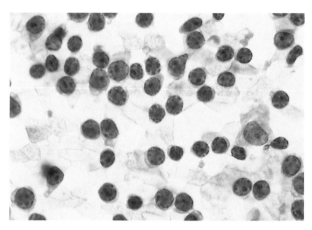

FIGURE 14–15A. Small Round Cell Lymphoma (Well-Differentiated Lymphocytic Lymphoma). These photographs compare the Romanovsky stain and Papanicolaou stain findings of a typical small round cell lymphoma composed of monotonous small round lymphocytes. On Papanicolaou stain, the chromatin is similar to that of a plasma cell, and on Romanovsky stain, the cells appear larger and have a more open chromatin than a normal small round cell (× 330).

FIGURE 14–15C. Small Round Cell Lymphoma. This Papanicolaou stain is from the same case as Figure 14–15B and shows a slightly more variable population than that seen in Figure 14–15A. A histiocyte is included for size comparison (× 330).

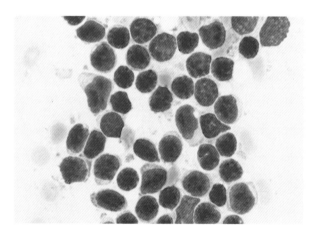

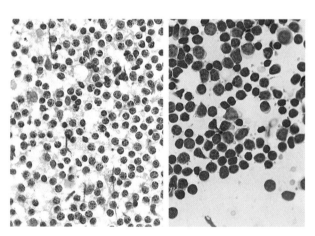

FIGURE 14–15B. Small Round Cell Lymphoma. This case shows a slightly smaller population of cells on Romanovsky stain. Usually, on Romanovsky stains it is difficult to tell small round cell lymphoma from small cleaved cell lymphoma. The Papanicolaou stains are more helpful in differentiating these two entities (Romanovsky stain, × 330).

FIGURE 14–15D. This is a low-power photograph of an **End Stage Reactive Node**. It may be impossible in aspirate specimens alone to differentiate this from small round cell lymphoma unless the pattern is similar to Figure 14–15A. Also compare with Figure 14–16C (Papanicolaou/Romanovsky stain, × 150).

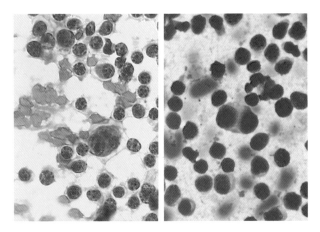

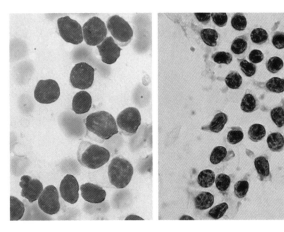

FIGURE 14–16A. Waldenström Macroglobulinemia. This slide compares the Papanicolaou and Romanovsky stains of a small round cell lymphoma with plasmacytoid features with an aspirate from a patient with Waldenström macroglobulinemia. Note how the population contains plasmacytoid lymphocytes as well as some larger multinucleated plasmacytoid cells. This biopsy specimen is from a patient who had diffuse adenopathy with Waldenström macroglobulinemia that had been followed for many years. A large axillary node was also biopsied and was found to contain a large cell lymphoma (× 198).

FIGURE 14–16C. End-Stage Reactive Node at high power. Note how the monotony of an end-stage reactive node is quite similar to many of the cases of a small round cell lymphoma. Surface markers for monoclonality and other antigens typical of small round cell lymphoma are quite helpful in differentiating these two entities. Additionally, the finding of a large, spherical lymph node is quite typical in a small round cell lymphoma, as opposed to the discoid nodes seen with most end-stage reactive patterns (Papanicolaou/Romanovsky stain, × 330).

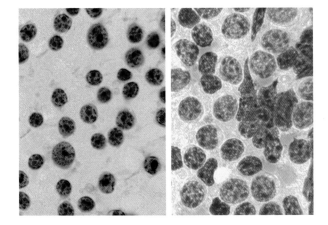

FIGURE 14–16B. Chronic Lymphocytic Leukemia. This figure compares the Papanicolaou and Romanovsky stains from a patient with lymph node involvement late in the course of chronic lymphocytic leukemia. The biopsy was performed to exclude progression to a higher-grade lymphoma. Note the fairly uniform small cells with occasional larger cells. These larger cells have "chromocenters," which are apparent on the Papanicolaou stain. These larger cells correspond with the large cells seen in the lymph node in "proliferation centers" when chronic lymphocytic leukemia involves nodes (× 330).

SMALL CLEAVED CELL LYMPHOMA (POORLY DIFFERENTIATED LYMPHOCYTIC LYMPHOMA)

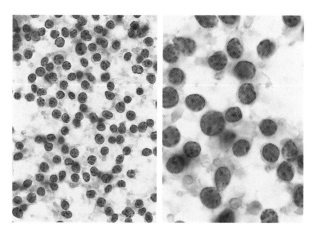

FIGURE 14–17A. Small Cleaved Cell Lymphoma. This photograph of a Papanicolaou stain shows the low- and high-power appearance of a typical small cleaved cell lymphoma population. Note the monotonous small cells, which show a more open chromatin pattern than normal small cleaved cells on high power, with subtle nuclear clefts and nuclear grooving. It is typical for a small cleaved cell lymphoma not to have obvious nuclear convolutions, as is typically seen in histologic specimens (Papanicolaou stain, × 150 and × 330).

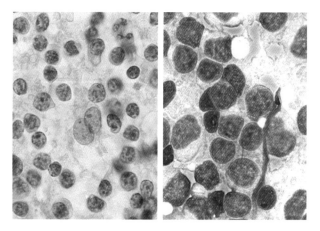

FIGURE 14–17C. Small Cleaved Cell Lymphoma. Small cleaved cell lymphomas can vary in size from case to case and at times may demonstrate substantial variability within the small cleaved cell population. This photograph shows a small cleaved cell lymphoma with cells in the smaller size range. On the Papanicolaou stain, the presence of nuclear convolutions is helpful in defining these as small cleaved cells. Note the histiocyte depicted in the center of the field in the Papanicolaou stain. On the Romanovsky stain, very few small lymphocytes with dense chromatin are seen (these are either normal cells or degenerated lymphoma cells) (× 330).

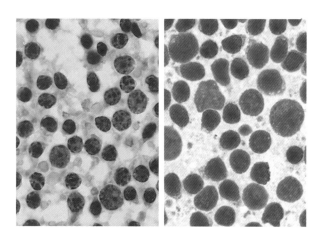

FIGURE 14–17B. Mid-phase Reactive Lymph Node. These Papanicolaou and Romanovsky stains are shown for comparison with a small cleaved cell lymphoma. Generally, in mid-phase reactions, the large number of small cleaved cells with fewer large cells can closely mimic some cases of small cleaved cell lymphoma or mixed lymphoma. Generally, the number of immunoblasts and small round cells can allow the differentiation from a small cleaved cell lymphoma (× 330).

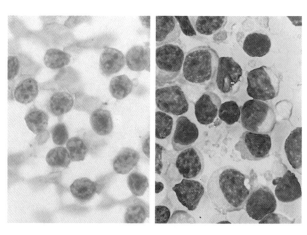

FIGURE 14–17D. Small Cleaved Cell Lymphoma. This case shows a slightly larger nuclear size than the example in Figure 14–17C. Note on the Papanicolaou stain a more open chromatin pattern and nuclear angulation (× 330).

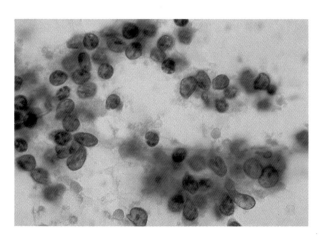

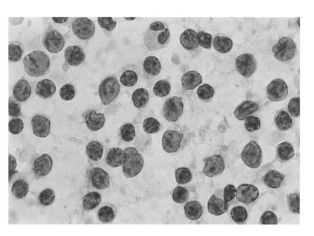

FIGURE 14–18A. Small Cleaved Cell Lymphoma, T-Cell Type, arising in skin. Lymphomas in nonlymphoid organs, such as skin or soft tissues, often show cell "cohesion," which closely mimics a poorly differentiated carcinoma in aspirate specimens. This example on Papanicolaou stain shows how the clustering of the angulated small lymphocytes could be mistaken for a cohesive fragment from a poorly differentiated carcinoma (Papanicolaou stain, × 252).

FIGURE 14–18C. Small Cleaved Cell Lymphoma. This Papanicolaou stain depicts a small cleaved lymphoma, with larger small cleaved cells and some larger cells making the differential from a mixed lymphoma difficult. Generally, large cells occupy more than 20% of the population in a mixed lymphoma and the large cells are distinctly larger than the small cleaved cell population (Papanicolaou stain, × 330).

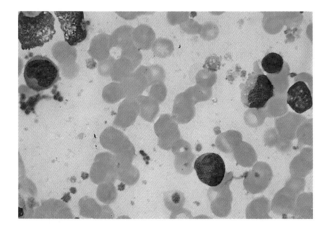

FIGURE 14–18B. Small Cleaved Cell Lymphoma, T-Cell Type. This is the air-dried smear from the case in Figure 18–1 illustrating the advantage of a Romanovsky stain in aspiration biopsy. The numerous small fragments of cell cytoplasm (lymphoglandular bodies) are easily seen and delineate the population as lymphoid (× 252).

MIXED LYMPHOMA (SMALL CLEAVED CELL AND LARGE CLEAVED MIXED TYPE)

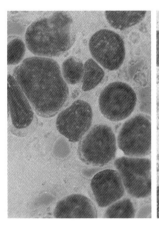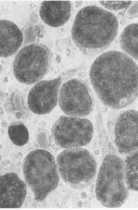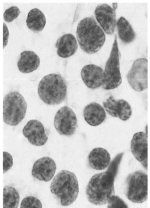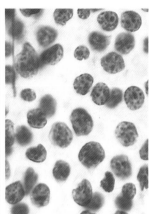

FIGURE 14–19A and 14–19B. These two sets of photographs are from the same case and show the Romanovsky and Papanicolaou stains from a **Mixed Lymphoma**. This pattern is the classic appearance of a mixed lymphoma: the small cleaved and large cleaved cells are virtually identical in chromatin pattern and can be distinguished only by size. Note how the population shows a broad spectrum of size yet lacks a significant number of large noncleaved or immunoblastic cells and small round cells. At times it is difficult to tell a mixed lymphoma from a lymphoma with transformation to large cell lymphoma. In this particular pattern it is rare that the lymphoma is a transformation to a large cell type because the large cells are generally of the noncleaved type, which is absent in this population (× 330).

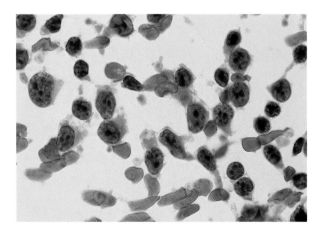

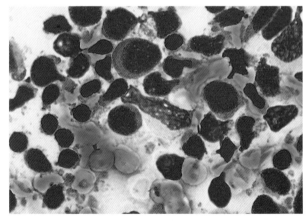

FIGURE 14–19C. Mixed Lymphoma. This Papanicolaou stain shows a mixed lymphoma with a greater range in size of lymphoid cells: large cells are of the non-cleaved variety. The helpful feature in this case is the pleomorphism of the nuclear shapes seen in the Papanicolaou stain. Such nuclear angulation, large numbers of nucleoli, and lack of small round cells are unexpected in any reactive pattern. This must be differentiated from the immunoblastic reaction, which should have more classic immunoblasts, with single, large nucleoli (× 330).

FIGURE 14–19D. Mixed Lymphoma. This is a Romanovsky stain of the same case as Figure 14–19C and illustrates again the broad spectrum in size seen in this mixed lymphoma. The Papanicolaou stain makes this case easier to designate as a lymphoma than does the Romanovsky stain (× 330).

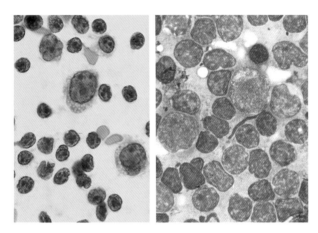

FIGURE 14–20A. Mixed Lymphoma. This mixed lymphoma shows an unusual dimorphic population, making it very difficult to differentiate from small cleaved cell lymphoma. There are very small, angulated, cleaved forms with few large noncleaved cells and virtually no other cell types in this population. Note the extreme angulation of the small cells on the Papanicolaou stain, some of which can also be seen on the Romanovsky stain. This was initially thought to be a small cleaved cell lymphoma but on biopsy was a mixed lymphoma. Such a pattern makes it difficult to exclude a diagnosis of small cleaved cell lymphoma with transformation to large cell lymphoma, particularly if more of the large cell forms are present (× 330).

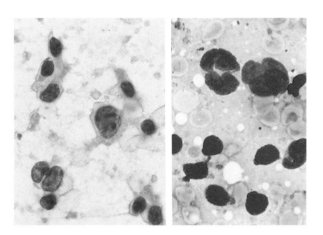

FIGURE 14–20C. Mixed Lymphoma, T-Cell Type. These Romanovsky and Papanicolaou stains show a dimorphic population, with the large cells showing extreme pleomorphism. Although T-cell lymphoma is often considered when the cells are pleomorphic, this can also be seen in B-cell lymphomas. Lymphoid populations with this degree of pleomorphism have always proved to be malignant (× 330).

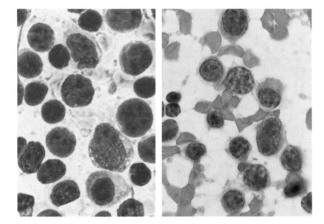

FIGURE 14–20B. Mixed Lymphoma. These Romanovsky and Papanicolaou stains show a mixed lymphoma with a spectrum of cell sizes. The fairly uniform chromatin pattern across the population of cells is helpful in making the correct diagnosis, since the large cells from a reactive process would be expected to have a more open chromatin pattern. This can be compared with Figure 14–19B, in which a similar chromatin pattern is seen in the Papanicolaou stain (× 330).

LARGE-CELL LYMPHOMA (HISTIOCYTIC LYMPHOMA)

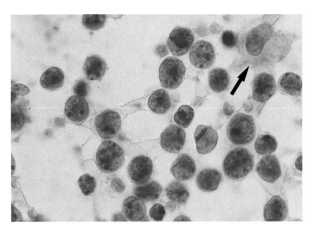

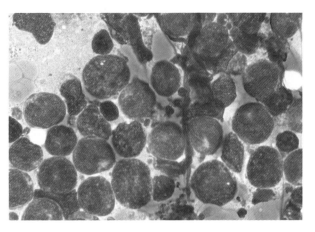

FIGURE 14–21A. Large-Cell Lymphoma. This Papanicolaou stain shows a classic large cell lymphoma composed of a monotonous population of noncleaved large cells. Such a pattern is easily diagnosed as a lymphoma, with excellent cell-typing correlation. Note the histiocyte in the upper corner (arrow) (× 330).

FIGURE 14–21B. Large-Cell Lymphoma. This Romanovsky stain shows the companion smear to Figure 14–21A, with the large cells showing some crush artifact and very few small cell forms in the background (× 330).

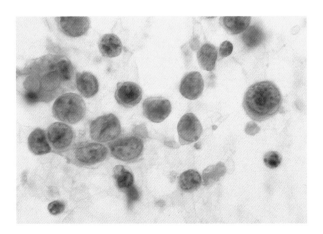

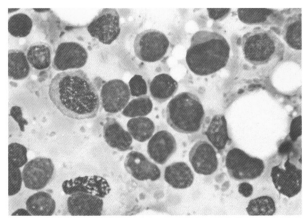

FIGURE 14–21C and 14–21D. These Papanicolaou- and Romanovsky-stained fields show another **Large-Cell Lymphoma** with a wider spectrum of small cells (probably benign cells in the population) (× 252).

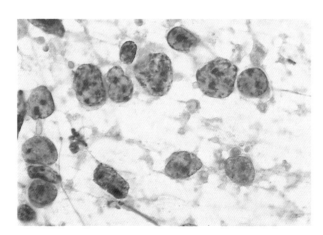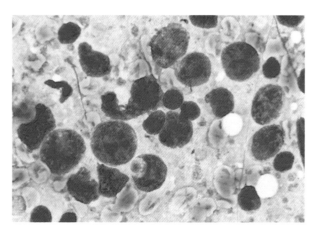

FIGURE 14–22A and 14–22B. These fields show Papanicolaou and Romanovsky stains of a **Large-Cell Lymphoma** with much greater nuclear size than that seen in Figure 14–21A. In some areas there is angulation and compression of adjacent cells suggestive of molding. Lymphoglandular bodies on the air-dried smear are helpful at defining this as a lymphoid population ($\times$ 330).

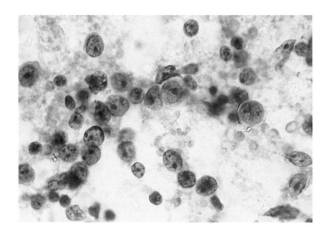

FIGURE 14–22C. Large-Cell Lymphoma. This lymphoma was sampled from the abdomen; the specimen was grossly bloody. However, it is easy to see the monotonous large-cell population. The difficulty in this case is differentiating it from an immunoblastic lymphoma. Note that the large cells have single, large nucleoli and a spectrum in size from large to relatively small cells with virtually identical morphology. If more plasmacytoid cells were present, then an immunoblastic lymphoma would be a prime consideration (Papanicolaou stain, $\times$ 160).

LYMPHOBLASTIC LYMPHOMA

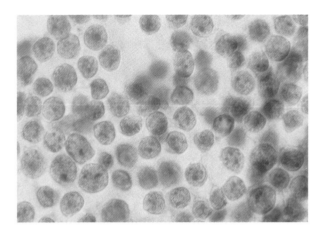

FIGURE 14–23A. Lymphoblastic Lymphoma. This Papanicolaou stain shows the uniform intermediate size and chromatin pattern in a lymphoblastic lymphoma of the nonconvoluted type. The cells are fairly uniform in size, with a very fine chromatin pattern and single nucleoli (× 330).

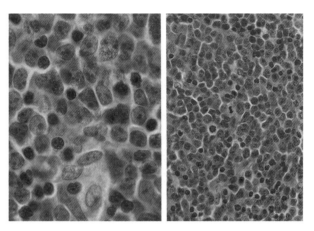

FIGURE 14–23C. Lymphoblastic Lymphoma. This is a low- and high-power view of lymphoblastic lymphoma on tissue section illustrating the uniform intermediate size of the neoplastic population. Scattered normal small round cells are present for size comparison. Note the mitoses on the lower power photograph (hematoxylin and eosin stain, × 80/× 160).

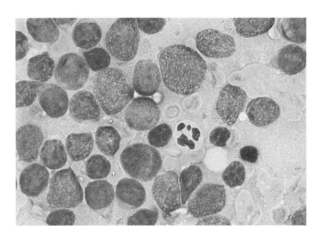

FIGURE 14–23B. Lymphoblastic Lymphoma, Nonconvoluted Type. This Romanovsky stain shows the "blastic" nature of the lymphoid population. Mitoses are frequently seen in this lymphoma (× 330).

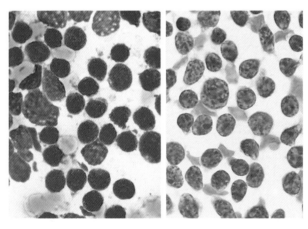

FIGURE 14–23D. Lymphoblastic Lymphoma, Convoluted Type. These photos depict the Romanovsky and Papanicolaou stain characteristics of a lymphoblastic lymphoma when it has a convoluted cell pattern. Note on the Romanovsky stain the smaller cells with more condensed chromatin pattern. On the Papanicolaou stain, the chromatin is more coarse, and nuclear size and pleomorphism are more pronounced. Note the prominent nucleoli on the Papanicolaou stain. The Papanicolaou stain in this case could be difficult to differentiate from small cleaved cell lymphoma (× 330).

UNDIFFERENTIATED LYMPHOMA (BURKITT AND NON-BURKITT LYMPHOMA)

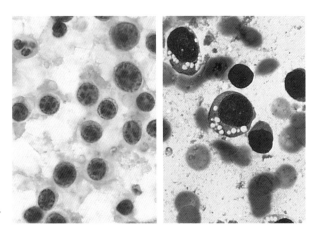

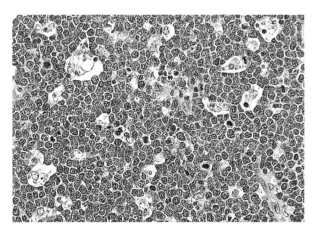

FIGURE 14–24A. Undifferentiated Lymphoma, non-Burkitt Type. These photographs show the Papanicolaou and Romanovsky stains of this lymphoma in an older adult. Note the spectrum in size from cells that are slightly smaller to slightly larger than histiocyte nuclei on the Papanicolaou stain. The chromatin pattern on the Papanicolaou stain is coarse in this case, with some larger forms showing a more open chromatin and prominent nucleoli. The Romanovsky stain is the most helpful in this type of lymphoma, demonstrating the cells having a deep blue cytoplasm and numerous vacuoles characteristic of this type (× 330).

FIGURE 14–24C. Burkitt Lymphoma. This histology shows the "starry-sky" pattern of a Burkitt lymphoma, in which histiocytes are phagocytizing cellular debris from the rapidly dividing population of undifferentiated lymphocytes (hematoxylin and eosin stain, × 80).

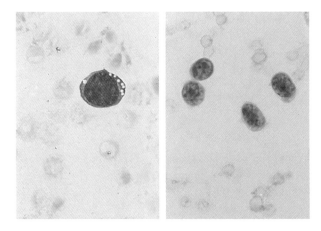

FIGURE 14–24B. Undifferentiated Lymphoma, Burkitt Type. This figure depicts cells from an abdominal aspirate in a pediatric patient with Burkitt lymphoma, illustrating the characteristic Romanovsky and Papanicolaou stain patterns. Note the uniform cell size on the Papanicolaou stain (× 330).

IMMUNOBLASTIC LYMPHOMA

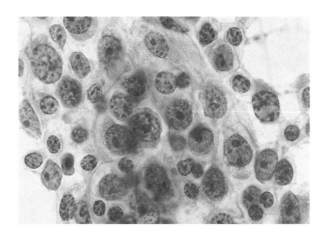

FIGURE 14–25A. Immunoblastic Lymphoma. This Papanicolaou stain shows the typical large cells of immunoblastic lymphoma with abundant cytoplasm and cells with obvious plasmacytoid differentiation. The cytoplasm of adjacent cells is often confluent, giving a syncytial look to the cells (× 330).

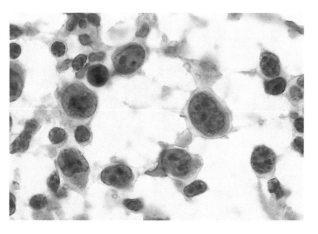

FIGURE 14–25C. Immunoblastic Lymphoma. This Papanicolaou stain shows a more pleomorphic immunoblastic lymphoma, in which the plasmacytoid cells are much less common. This makes it difficult to differentiate from a pleomorphic large-cell lymphoma (× 330).

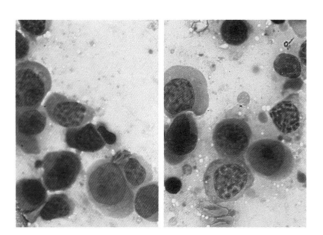

FIGURE 14–25B. Immunoblastic Lymphoma. This Romanovsky stain shows a typical immunoblastic population with a full range of sizes and plasmacytoid features (× 330).

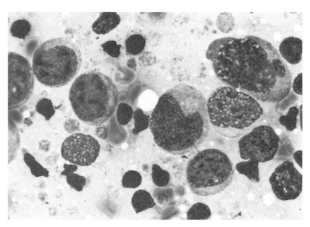

FIGURE 14–25D. Immunoblastic Lymphoma. This Romanovsky stain is the counterpart to Figure 14–25C and depicts cells with fairly abundant cytoplasm that have stained less deeply blue than would be expected for most cases of immunoblastic lymphoma. Pale cytoplasm may indicate a T-cell immunoblastic lymphoma. In this case, the surface markers were not obtained (× 330).

TRUE MALIGNANT HISTIOCYTIC LYMPHOMA

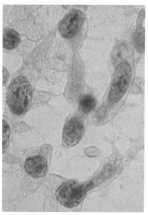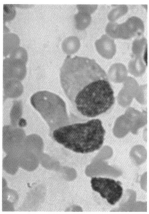

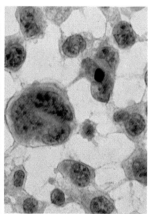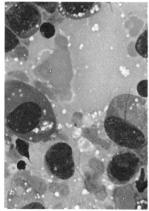

FIGURE 14–26A. True Malignant Histiocytic Lymphoma. This lymph node–based neoplasm was originally diagnosed as large-cell lymphoma but did not respond to treatment. On aspiration, the cells have an amoeboid appearance and lack lymphoglandular bodies on the Romanovsky stain, which is typical of a non-lymphoid neoplasm. Special stains shown in Figure 14–26B help define this as a histiocytic lesion (Papanicolaou/Romanovsky stain, × 252).

FIGURE 14–26C. Malignant Histiocytic Lymphoma, Pleomorphic Type. This lesion was a lymph node–based disease with rampant progression. The biopsy specimen did not definitively differentiate sarcoma from carcinoma or lymphoma. On aspiration, the cells appeared to be isolated, as in lymphoma, but on Romanovsky stain did not display lymphoglandular bodies. On the Papanicolaou stains, the pleomorphic malignant cells often showed cohesion and some amoebic shapes. The nonspecific esterase stain was positive in most of the cells, and other special stains confirmed a true histiocytic lesion. The patient did respond to a chemotherapy protocol for malignant histiocytic lymphoma (× 252).

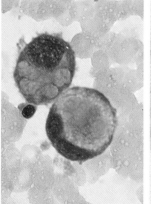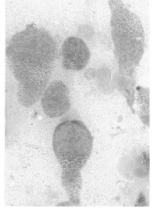

FIGURE 14–26B. True Malignant Histiocytic Lymphoma. These two slides depict a Romanovsky stain from the bone marrow of the patient in Figure 14–26A, in which abundant erythrophagocytosis was found. The other photograph is that of an air-dried nonspecific esterase, illustrating histiocytic enzymes in the neoplastic population. Muramidase and alpha-1-antitrypsin were also positive on tissue samples (× 252).

COMMENT: Recently, the immunologic definition of Ki-1 lymphoma has been noted. Some researchers have suggested that pleomorphic large-cell lymphomas are often of this type. Others have shown that a monotonous uniform large-cell lymphoma as well as a pleomorphic large-cell lymphoma can mark for Ki-1. Although initial studies indicated a poor prognosis in Ki-1 lymphoma, more recent work suggests that they may actually respond better to chemotherapy than do other large cell lymphomas. Some cases that may show the pleomorphism associated with some true malignant histiocytic lymphomas are thought to be the Ki-1 lymphoma. We have not seen the lack of lymphoglandular bodies in any large-cell lymphoma, a pattern that has been observed in all of our cases of true malignant histiocytic neoplasia. This is why our personal opinion is that the true malignant histiocytic lesions are properly classified and are not Ki-1 lymphomas.

HODGKIN DISEASE

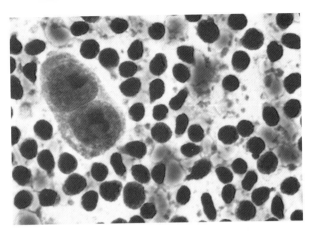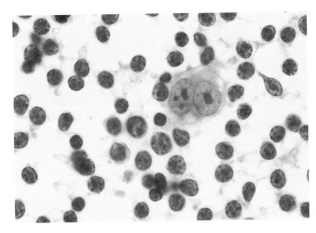

FIGURE 14–27A and 14–27B. These two photographs show the Romanovsky and Papanicolaou stains of **Hodgkin Disease, Lymphocyte-Predominant Type,** in a young child. Often, this type of Hodgkin disease is extremely difficult to diagnose from histologic specimens. We have found this not to be difficult in most cases when using aspiration biopsy, particularly on the Romanovsky stain. The very large binucleate Reed-Sternberg cells are easily identified, both because of their large size and because of their contrast to the monotonous small cell population of attending lymphocytes. Unlike tissue section, whole-mount cytology displays every Reed-Sternberg cell in the population (× 330).

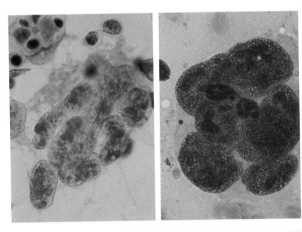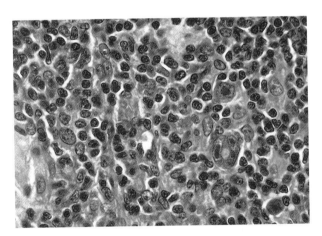

FIGURE 14–27C. Hodgkin Disease, Mixed-Cellularity Type. These Papanicolaou and Romanovsky stains show the polylobated "popcorn" type Reed-Sternberg cell. This type of cell is described as a hallmark for the lymphocytic and histiocytic types of Hodgkin disease. However, we have also commonly seen this in the mixed-cellularity type. In mixed-cellularity Hodgkin disease, numerous eosinophils generally are seen in the aspirate (× 330).

FIGURE 14–27D. Hodgkin Disease, histiologic specimen. This case of Hodgkin disease shows a typical reactive background and some mononuclear and binucleate Reed-Sternberg cells (× 160).

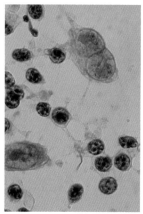
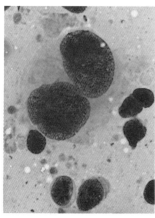

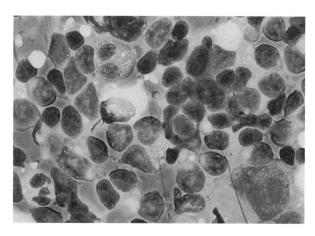

FIGURE 14–28A. Hodgkin Disease, Nodular Sclerosing Type. These photographs show the Papanicolaou and Romanovsky stains of typical Reed-Sternberg cells. Note the pale cytoplasm, bilobed nucleus, and nucleoli, which exceed the size of the adjacent small round lymphocytes. Note the mononuclear Reed-Sternberg cell in the Papanicolaou stain (× 330).

FIGURE 14–28C. Hodgkin Disease, Nodular Sclerosing Type. This figure shows the typical reactive background, including an eosinophil and a neutrophil with a mononuclear Reed-Sternberg cell in one corner (× 330).

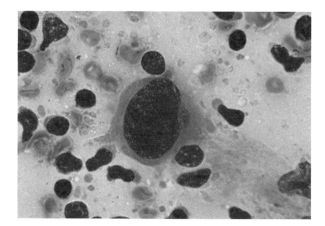

FIGURE 14–28B. Mononuclear Reed-Sternberg Cell from Hodgkin Disease. This Romanovsky stain shows a mononuclear form typical of the dominant variant of the Reed-Sternberg cell in nodular sclerosing Hodgkin disease (× 330).

C·H·A·P·T·E·R

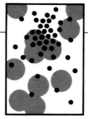

15

THYROID ASPIRATION CYTOLOGY

Carolyn Ernst Grotkowski

Fine needle aspiration (FNA) of the thyroid may be performed by a pathologist, endocrinologist, radiologist, or surgeon. The patient should be in the supine position with the neck hyperextended. If the lesion is cystic, as much fluid as possible is removed. The patient should be reexamined for any residual lesion, and aspiration is repeated for any remaining solid areas. The material in the syringe may be flushed into a centrifuge tube containing carbowax fixative or smeared directly onto the slide. Direct smears should be fixed in alcohol for Papanicolaou staining or air-dried for Wright staining. Cytospins and a cell block are prepared on material that is submitted in carbowax.

One of the primary indications for FNA of the thyroid is to assist in the selection of patients with thyroid nodules who require surgery; the goal is to reduce the number of open biopsies and to increase the specificity of surgical biopsy. The incidence of thyroid carcinoma is much less than the frequency of thyroid nodules. Theoretically comparing the frequencies of these disorders, a carcinoma would be found only once in every 1500 nodules surgically removed. Selectivity is therefore needed to prevent unnecessary thyroid surgery. Clinical presentation and the methods used to evaluate thyroid nodules do not differentiate benign from malignant lesions with any degree of certainty.

FNA is indicated for the evaluation of the solitary cold nodule, i.e., nodules that show no uptake or a relative lack of uptake of radionuclides on a thyroid scan. A solitary nodule typically causes concern because of the possibility of malignancy. In general, FNA is not done as a part of the evaluation of a hot or functioning nodule. The criteria for each specific diagnosis are given in the relevant section that follows.

It is first essential to evaluate the adequacy of the specimen. Specimens that are technically poor and acellular or do not contain sufficient numbers of follicular cells are considered unsatisfactory. Defining an adequate number of follicular cells may be difficult but is aided by clinical correlation and the other material present on the aspirate. In general, at least six groups of follicular epithelium should be identified. Some specimens may contain abundant colloid and numerous macrophages but have only rare or scattered follicular cells. In this situation, a descriptive diagnosis of the material with a qualifying statement about the scant amount of follicular epithelium may be given. Clinical correlation is done, and judgment is then exercised. If the clinical picture is compatible with cystic degeneration of nodular goiter, the patient may require follow-up only. The clinician, however, must be aware of the possibility of cystic degeneration of a papillary carcinoma; if there is any clinical reason for suspicion, repeat aspirate and/or surgical biopsy is indicated.

The first step in the evaluation of a thyroid nodule may be FNA. If FNA reveals a diagnosis of cyst or colloid nodule, the patient typically does not require surgical evaluation. These patients are often given thyroxine and seen in follow-up to evaluate reduction in size of the nodule. If the nodule is unresponsive, repeat FNA and/or surgical biopsy may be performed. Another group of patients for whom surgery may be avoided or is not indicated are those with anaplastic carcinoma, metastatic carcinoma, lymphoma, or thyroiditis; each of these can be diagnosed by FNA. A suspicious or unequivocal diagnosis of papillary or medullary carcinoma helps in preoperative planning.

Fine needle aspiration with a diagnosis of atypical follicular epithelium can be the most difficult to categorize with respect to recommendations for surgery or follow-up. If the atypia is felt to be related to a benign process, clinical follow-up after suppression or other treatment may be all that is required. Reaspiration and/or surgical biopsy is indicated if there is no change in the nodule or a clinical suspicion remains. Atypical follicular epithelium considered to represent a follicular lesion (adenoma versus carcinoma) must be managed surgically.

There are no contraindications to performing needle aspiration of the thyroid; caution is indicated in general in patients with a bleeding diathesis. Fine needle aspiration is a safe procedure, and complications are quite rare. Some have reported necrosis, increased mitotic activity, and even focal papillary changes following aspiration. There are no reports of tumor implants following aspiration. Some individuals have expressed concern about the possibility of dragging follicular cells into a capsule during FNA and the subsequent difficulty in evaluating a surgically removed encapsulated follicular lesion. This has not been a problem in the author's experience.

Correlation with tissue diagnosis is good with nonfollicular lesions, i.e., papillary, medullary, and anaplastic carcinoma, lymphoma, and thyroiditis. False-negative rates are low, with those reported ranging from 0.3 to 6%. The most common problem is differentiating follicular lesions of nodular goiter, adenoma, and follicular carcinoma. Criteria for each of these are described in depth in the following sections, but remember that the features that distinguish follicular adenoma from minimally invasive follicular carcinoma are vascular or capsule invasion. These features are not evident on FNA, and, therefore, surgical removal is required to evaluate these lesions. Establishing the degree of correlation of tissue diagnoses with cytologic diagnoses of follicular lesions may be quite difficult. A significant problem is the variability in criteria and terminology of follicular lesions by biopsy; correlation therefore may not seem precise.

NORMAL THYROID

The normal thyroid is divided into lobules composed of follicles. Each follicle is lined by epithelial cells that surround colloid. The follicles range in size from small to large (Fig. 15–5). The follicular cells also vary in size; some show a definite polarity with an apical cytoplasm directed toward the lumen of the follicles. Others appear small and attenuated or stretched. The interfollicular stroma is highly vascularized. Parafollicular or C cells are difficult to identify without special stains. Nests of cells (solid cell nest [SCN]) may be seen in the lateral lobes of the thyroid. An aspirate of a normal thyroid would be expected to contain follicular cells and colloid. The relative amounts of these components vary.

Follicular cells must be identified in an aspirate to consider it satisfactory for evaluation. In general, a minimum of six groups are required. The follicular cells are most often seen as small groups or clusters of cells, but they may occur as single cells (Fig. 15–1). Monolayered sheets without follicle formation may be seen; a honeycomb pattern may be appreciated; however, cell borders are often indistinct (Fig. 15–2). Three-dimensional clusters with colloid in whole follicles may also be seen. Colloid may or may not be present within the lumen of small clusters. Tissue fragments are more common from direct smears. The cells are uniform in size. There is an abundance of pale greenish blue cytoplasm. The nuclei are round with a fine chromatin. Nucleoli may be present in hyperplastic cells but are generally not prominent. The follicular cells may be small with pyknotic nuclei, presumably derived from a more flattened epithelium lining a large involuted follicle. Single cells may be difficult to differentiate from lymphocytes; the chromatin is less coarse in follicular cells, which are usually larger than lymphocytes. The use of specific markers (leukocyte common antigen [LCA] and thyroglobulin) in an immunoperoxidase assay may be helpful in distinguishing these cell types.

The identification of colloid is very helpful in the evaluation of thyroid aspirates. The appearance of colloid varies considerably. Colloid may appear as a thick amorphous material with sharply circumscribed edges or as thin translucent material in the background. In thick smears, colloid is pink-orange; it may be pale green on smears that have less blood. With Wright-Giemsa stain, colloid is violet-blue. Colloid has a tendency to crack in a linear fashion if it dries on the slide (Fig. 15–3). Colloid must be differentiated from muscle and amyloid (Fig. 15–35). Inspissated colloid may be confused with a psammoma body. The presence of a large amount of colloid is presumed to indicate a benign process since the majority of macrofollicular lesions are benign; this must be correlated with the clinical presentation, however.

Red blood cells are common owing to the vascularity of the gland. The number of inflammatory cells is variable. Some represent contamination from venipuncture. A large number or a predominance of lymphocytes suggests the possibility of thyroiditis.

CYSTS

Cysts of the thyroid may occur owing to degenerative changes in nodular goiter or a neoplastic process or as the result of a thyroglossal duct remnant. The vast majority of aspirated cysts are from nodular goiter. The amount of fluid aspirated varies; the color may be yellow, brown, or bloody. Smears from a benign cyst usually contain numerous macrophages. Hemosiderin may be present. The number of follicular cells varies; if follicular cells are not found, the aspirate is described but considered inadequate to exclude cystic papillary carcinoma.

Thyroglossal duct cysts are remnants of the thryoglossal duct. They usually are in the midline of the neck near the hyoid bone. Microscopically, they are lined by stratified squamous epithelium or columnar, ciliated epithelium (Fig. 15–14). The cysts commonly undergo secondary inflammatory changes. Aspirates from a thyroglossal duct cyst may show numerous benign squamous cells or columnar cells that may or may not be ciliated (Fig. 15–13).

THYROIDITIS

Granulomatous Thyroiditis

Synonyms of granulomatous thyroiditis include giant cell, de Quervain, and subacute thyroiditis. The inflammation is thought to be in response to a viral infection, most likely systemic. Epidemiologic studies show an association of the mumps virus with episodes of subacute thyroiditis. Other viruses have also been implicated.

Several stages are recognized. Initially, the patient may be hyperthyroid during active destruction of the gland with release of the hormone. A hypothyroid phase follows after sufficient destruction of the gland. Recovery is the final stage and is the rule. The disease usually lasts two to five months. The patient may present with a nodule if the disease focally involves part of the thyroid. Generally, the entire gland is involved. Pain usually makes the patient seek medical attention, although painless subacute thyroiditis may occur. Diagnosis in this situation may rest with FNA or biopsy. The involvement of the gland is characterized by an acute inflammatory response with microabscesses followed by an infiltration of plasma cells, lymphocytes, macrophages, and multinucleated giant cells. Eventually, affected areas undergo fibrosis. Aspirates may show a mixed inflammatory response with polymorphonuclear leukocytes, eosinophils, giant cells, and macrophages; if fibrosis is extensive, the aspirate may be relatively acellular or contain fragments of connective tissue (Fig. 15–15).

Chronic Lymphocytic Thyroiditis

In classic autoimmune (Hashimoto) thyroiditis, the thyroid is infiltrated by lymphocytes and plasma cells; formation of follicular centers may be prominent (Fig. 15–17). Normal thyroid follicles are destroyed, and fibrosis may occur. Antithyroid and antimicrosomal antibodies are found in 70% of patients with Hashimoto thyroiditis. The classic form is much more common in women; the degree of hypothyroidism may vary from subclinical to severe. At the end stage, extensive fibrosis and hypothyroidism are marked. A fibrosing variant is also seen in men. Classic autoimmune thyroiditis is the lesion most often seen in patients who are hypothyroid.

Lymphocytes are typically associated with chronic thyroiditis. Note, however, that lymphocytes may be seen in a variety of disorders, including goiter, Graves disease, and inflammatory lesions and as a component of drug reaction. Therefore, the presence of lymphocytes alone is not diagnostic of thyroiditis.

Microscopically, this disease is characterized by diffuse infiltration by lymphocytes and plasma cells with formation of follicular centers. Changes within the follicular epithelium include oxyphilic change, significant cytologic atypia, and presence of Hürthle cells. The follicular epithelium may be hyperplastic with papillary change. Fibrosis is variable.

Aspirates show a varying proportion of inflammatory cells and epithelial components. The cellularity is variable and depends on the stage of development. Lymphoid cells are usually quite numerous, with a range of sizes; nuclear crush or stretched lymphocytes are common (Fig. 15–16). Small fragments that represent follicular centers may be seen either on a smear or cell block. The epithelial cells may show considerable cytologic atypia. In general, a high degree of atypia is accepted as a component of Hashimoto thyroiditis. Therefore, a diagnosis of Hürthle cell tumor or follicular lesion is rarely made in the face of a clinical or cytologic picture compatible with chronic lymphocytic thyroiditis (Fig. 15–36).

Another difficulty is differentiating papillary hyperplasia from a potential concurrent papillary carcinoma. The hyperplasia associated with thyroiditis can be distinguished by the lack of vascular core, the less complex papillary structures, and the lack of characteristic nuclear features. Quite clearly, however, papillary carcinoma may occur in association with Hashimoto thyroiditis, and caution is warranted in ignoring papillary features. Later in the disease, with increasing fibrosis, the aspirate may yield very little material.

Differential diagnosis of a prominent lymphocytic infiltrate should include malignant lymphoma. The lymphoid population is heterogeneous in thyroiditis, whereas that in malignant lymphoma is a monomorphic population of abnormal lymphocytes (Fig. 15–44). If no follicular epithelium is identified but a population of lymphocytes is seen, two other nonthyroidal lesions should be considered: reactive lymph node or thymoma with extension to the neck.

NODULAR GOITER

Synonyms for nodular goiter include "adenomatous goiter," "colloid nodule," "nontoxic nodular goiter," and "multinodular goiter." This is a very common disorder, and most aspirates represent material from a dominant nodule of nodular goiter. The components present in a FNA from nodular goiter depend on the stage of the disease and any associated changes (Fig. 15–6). In the early stages there is diffuse enlargement of the thyroid, which is usually nonuniform with the development of nodules. Aspirates from nodular goiter contain some combination of colloid and follicular cells. The relative amount of these components is quite variable. There may be an abundance of colloid with scant cellularity, particularly in the hyperinvoluted stage.

Follicular cells must be identified, however, to consider the smear adequate. Alternatively, there may be relatively little colloid, and the cellular components may predominate. Although the cellularity of the specimen may be a useful criteria, there is considerable variability, depending on the experience of the operator and the number of aspirations made. The hyperplastic phase of nodular goiter may yield very cellular specimens; the differential diagnosis includes follicular adenoma or follicular carcinoma. Rarely, a papillary configuration may be seen in adenomatous hyperplasia (Figs. 15–40 and 15–41). The papillary fragment derived from a carcinoma may be distinguished from a hyperplastic lesion by a true fibrovascular core and characteristic nuclear features.

Secondary changes in nodular goiter are quite common and include infarction, hemorrhage, necrosis, cyst formation, fibrosis, and calcification. Cystic degeneration is seen most commonly. The fluid aspirated is brown and varies in amount. Smears contain abundant macrophages, which may contain hemosiderin or colloid. Cells with foamy vacuolated cytoplasm may also represent degenerating follicular cells. Multinucleated giant cells may also be seen. Some aspirates contain macrophages as the predominant cell type, with little or no follicular epithelium (Fig. 15–7), although this commonly represents cystic degeneration of a nodular goiter. One must consider the possibility of cystic papillary carcinoma that may not have been adequately sampled.

Stromal cells may be seen in association with hemorrhage, granulation tissue, infarction, or fibrosis (Fig. 15–9). They are usually seen as isolated single cells with a spindle-shaped cytoplasm and large nuclei. The differential diagnosis should include the stromal component of medullary carcinoma, anaplastic carcinoma, or a nonthyroid malignancy such as leiomyosarcoma. As a component of a benign inflammatory process, stromal cells are typically seen in small numbers, and there are other features of nodular goiter, such as macrophages, colloid, benign follicular epithelium, or hemosiderin in the background (Fig. 15–46).

Squamous metaplasia may be seen, especially in long-standing lesions. Hürthle cell change is common. Hürthle cells are large polygonal or oval shaped. Their cytoplasm is granular, dense, and eosinophilic. Nuclei are frequently eccentric and may by hyperchromatic or have prominent nucleoli (Fig. 15–11). Transitional forms with oncocytic dense cytoplasm without prominent nuclear changes share features of both Hürthle and follicular cells. Absolute categorization as one or the other may not be possible. Hürthle cells are a type of follicular cell and do not have different biologic properties. Hürthle cells may occur in nodular goiter, Hashimoto thyroiditis, or in Hürthle cell tumors. In general, when seen as a component of nodular goiter, they appear either singly or admixed in small groups with follicular epithelium (Fig. 15–12). Abundant colloid is more likely seen in nodular goiter. One should consider the possibility of a Hürthle cell lesion if the population is monomorphic or if architectural features, such as a trabecular or microfollicular pattern, are present. The Hürthle cell change that occurs in association with thyroiditis is usually seen on the background of a prominent lymphocytic infiltration. Calcific debris may be seen. Occasionally, psammoma bodies are seen in aspirates of nodular goiter.

FOLLICULAR LESIONS

The lesions characterized by a predominantly follicular pattern include nodular goiter, true follicular adenoma, atypical adenoma, and follicular carcinoma. The follicular variant of papillary carcinoma may have a prominent follicular pattern. The features most useful in the diagnosis of this lesion are discussed under papillary carcinoma. The primary difficulty is in differentiating nodular goiter, follicular adenoma, and follicular carcinoma.

Follicular Adenoma

A follicular adenoma is defined as an encapsulated mass of follicles that usually have a relatively uniform pattern throughout the nodules. If there are multiple nodules within the thyroid, one should consider the diagnosis of nodular goiter with adenomatous change. The features used to distinguish the lesions of adenoma from adenomatous hyperplasia are usually not seen in a FNA. These include solitary versus multiple nodules, encapsulation, uniformity within the adenoma from surrounding thyroid, and compression of the surrounding gland by the capsule. A variety of classifications of follicular adenomas have evolved based primarily on the architectural patterns that may be seen. These include macrofollicular, microfollicular, fetal, embryonal, and trabecular adenomas. Although these patterns have no clinical significance, the prominent architectural features seen on a cytology aspirate are useful in separating adenoma from adenomatous hyperplasia or nodular goiter. Thus, cytologic features that suggest adenoma rather than nodular goiter include a microfollicular or trabecular pattern (Fig. 15–23). Other features include increased cellularity (Fig. 15–18), syncytial groups, crowded and overlapped nuclei, ill-defined cell borders, altered polarity of the nuclei, enlargement of the cells, increased nuclear to cytoplasmic ratio (Fig. 15–19), and the absence of colloid. Nucleoli may be quite prominent, but this is not a consistent feature. Distinguishing a macrofollicular or colloid adenoma from nodular goiter may not be possible because they are cytologically and architecturally so similar. Microfollicular adenomas are characterized by small follicles with cuboidal lining cells (Figs. 15–20 and 15–22). Embryonal adenoma has a trabecular pattern, with enlarged cells having a dense cytoplasm (Fig. 15–21).

Hürthle Cell Adenoma

Hürthle cell adenomas are a type of follicular neoplasm composed predominantly or exclusively of Hürthle cells (Fig. 15–36B). The same criteria of invasion must be used to make a diagnosis of malignancy. Hürthle cell change in nodular goiter is quite common; therefore, features that suggest adenoma should also be present before considering Hürthle cell neoplasm. The architectural pattern is most often microfollicular or trabecular (Fig. 15–37B). Specimens in which these patterns are evident should always be biopsied in order to make a diagnosis of adenoma versus carcinoma.

Atypical Adenoma

Atypical adenomas include lesions that are cytologically worrisome but without demonstrable capsular or vascular invasion. These lesions often show numerous mitoses, considerable cytologic atypia, bizarre cells, and pleomorphic hyperchromatic nuclei. The secondary changes that occur in nodular goiter may also be seen in follicular adenomas.

Follicular Carcinoma

Follicular carcinoma is usually a solitary mass that presents as a nodule. Occult carcinoma is rare. Intralymphatic metastases are unusual. Follicular carcinoma has a tendency for vascular invasion, and the pattern of metastasis is therefore hematogenous spread to the bone, brain, lung, and liver. Widely invasive follicular carcinoma is readily recognized as a carcinoma clinically and surgically. These tumors tend to be very cellular and often have a microfollicular pattern. The role of an aspirate or tissue sample in this situation is to confirm the primary origin as thyroid.

Minimally invasive carcinoma, on the other hand, is a pathologic diagnosis. The features that distinguish follicular adenoma from minimally invasive follicular carcinoma are vascular or capsular invasion (Fig. 15–25). These features are rarely evident on needle aspirate, and therefore, a definitive diagnosis of carcinoma usually requires surgical removal of the lesion. Exceptions to this include situations in which the clinical presentation is compatible with malignant behavior (e.g., widely invasive follicular carcinoma) or in which the features of capsular or vascular invasion are demonstrated in a cell block preparation. Follicular carcinomas tend to be surrounded by a thick capsule. Degenerative changes are less common than with papillary carcinoma.

Aspirates from follicular adenomas and well-differentiated follicular carcinomas demonstrate very similar findings: increased cellularity, three-dimensional clusters with a microfollicular or trabecular pattern, scant colloid, and some atypia in follicular cells (Fig. 15–24). There is considerable controversy over differentiating follicular adenomas and follicular carcinomas based on differences in nuclear size and nuclear pleomorphism. The literature is mixed on this issue, with some studies showing an overall increase in size in malignant lesions and other studies indicating greater size variation in adenomas. Cytologic features that are more worrisome for and increase the likelihood of carcinoma include mitosis, marked architectural crowding, marked cellular atypia, pleomorphism, hyperchromatic nuclei, and prominent and variable nucleoli (Figs. 15–38 and 15–39). Adenomas very rarely contain mitoses; lesions that have been previously aspirated, however, may show an increased number of mitoses. One should be convinced that the mitosis is in a follicular epithelial cell and not in a macrophage. The presence of a mitosis is an indication for surgical removal of the lesion.

PAPILLARY LESIONS

Papillary Hyperplasia (Graves Disease)

The diagnosis of Graves disease is rarely made by needle aspiration because the clinical presentation is so characteristic. It should, however, be considered in the differential diagnosis of any papillary lesion, and the results of serum hormone levels and radioisotope scan should be reviewed. Papillary hyperplasia in Graves disease is distinguished from papillary carcinoma based on the lack of a true fibrovascular core and the nuclear features characteristic of carcinoma. Although there may be a piling up or infolding of the epithelium, there is no central core (Fig. 15–40). It is important to distinguish edema and colloid from a vascular core. A central core has small vascular structures.

If there are clinical features to suggest a hyperthyroid state (a hot nodule or a history of Graves disease that has been treated), hyperplasia should be excluded before a diagnosis of papillary carcinoma is given.

Papillary Carcinoma

Papillary carcinoma is the most common malignant tumor of the thyroid. Approximately 80% of thyroid malignancies can be classified as papillary. The key feature of papillary carcinoma is the papillae. These have a central fibrovascular core and a lining of cells that may be single or multiple (Fig. 15–40). The cells are crowded and have characteristic nuclear features.

The nuclei are described as pale, clear, or having a ground-glass chromatin. The chromatin is hypodense and the nuclear membrane thickened. Although it is debatable whether this represents an artifact, the presence of ground-glass chromatin may be quite useful to categorize the lesion as papillary when an architectural pattern is predominantly follicular. A small nucleolus may be seen. Another finding is the nuclear groove. This represents a line of hemotoxylin through the longitudinal axis of the nucleus. Intranuclear inclusions that represent an invagination of the cytoplasm into the nucleus are also frequently seen in papillary carcinoma (Fig. 15–26). Although both are a frequent finding in papillary carcinoma, they may be seen in benign lesions and are therefore not diagnostic of malignancy.

Psammoma bodies are a frequent and useful finding (Fig. 15–27). They must be distinguished from inspissated colloid and dystrophic calcification. The psammoma bodies are usually seen in the papillary core or associated with a papillary group; they may also appear isolated from cells. Rarely, they are found in benign conditions and have been reported in Graves disease, papillary hyperplasia, and thyroiditis. The presence of psammoma bodies in a needle aspiration is a very suspicious finding, however, and requires further evaluation.

Aspirates from papillary carcinoma tend to be cellular and have papillary fragments or large monolayered sheets (Fig. 15–28). The cells may be seen in small groups, however. The nuclei typically have the characteristic features of ground-glass chromatin, small nucleoli, nuclear grooves or intranuclear inclusions, and psammoma bodies. An unequivocal diagnosis can be made readily if papillary fragments and nuclear features are present. If the specimen is scant or only one of these features is present, a suspicious diagnosis is advisable. Some sclerotic papillary carcinomas are acellular; papillary carcinomas with extensive cystic change may show only macrophages if the solid areas are not aspirated.

In contrast to follicular carcinoma, papillary carcinoma frequently invades lymphatics. Multifocal intrathyroidal lesions and metastases to regional lymphatics are quite common.

Follicular Variant of Papillary Cancer

The follicular variant of papillary carcinoma is characterized by an architectural pattern that may be almost entirely follicular but which has definite features of papillary carcinoma. These features include psammoma bodies, clear nuclei, fibrosis, and focal papillary growth (Fig. 15–29).

Other Variants

The tall cell variant of papillary carcinoma is characterized by a tumor made up of cells that may be quite tall, with frequent mitoses and eosinophilic cytoplasm similar to Hürthle cell. These tend to be extrathyroidal and have a poorer prognosis. There is a rare variant composed of tall columnar cells with very clear cytoplasm, which may be confused with metastatic renal cell carcinoma.

ANAPLASTIC CARCINOMA

Anaplastic carcinoma is a tumor of the elderly, more frequent in women, and it usually presents with the rapid increase in size of a preexisting goiter. At the time of diagnosis, most have extended into surrounding neck tissue.

These tumors are characterized by marked pleomorphism with giant cell, spindle cell, and squamoid features. Mitoses are numerous. FNA reveals a cellular specimen with large bizarre pleomorphic cells. There may be considerable necrosis and secondary inflammation (Fig. 15–34).

Most often, the differential diagnosis includes metastatic lesions such as renal cell carcinoma or melanoma; malignant fibrous histiocytoma and other sarcomas should be considered. Spindle cells of a medullary carcinoma are more uniform in size and shape. If squamous features are prominent, this may be confused with squamous cell carcinoma. Large multinucleated giant cells may also be seen.

MEDULLARY CARCINOMA

Medullary carcinomas are derived from calcitonin-producing C cells. The tumor may occur sporadically or in a familial pattern. It accounts for 3 to 10% of thyroid malignancies. Approximately 10 to 20% of patients with medullary carcinoma have one of the multiple endocrine neoplasia (MEN) syndromes.

Most patients present with a painless firm thyroid nodule. Patients may have nodal metastases at the time of diagnosis. The tumor is usually in the lateral upper two thirds of the gland. Multiple nodules are not infrequent. Most tumors are well circumscribed but without a true capsule.

The microscopic appearance of medullary carcinoma is quite variable; this variability is recapitulated in FNA from this lesion. Tumor cells are arranged in nest-like patterns associated with a delicate vascular pattern. The tumor cells vary from round and epithelial to spindle-shaped (Figs. 15–31 and 15–32). Typically, the cells are uniform and somewhat bland. Interspersed among the nest of tumor cells is a variable amount of homogeneous eosinophilic material (Fig. 15–30). This material stains as amyloid and shows reactivity with antibodies against thyrocalcitonin (Fig. 15–33). Reports indicate that perhaps 20 to 40% of medullary carcinomas do not contain amyloid.

Classic medullary carcinoma has a combination of round eosinophilic cells and spindle cells with some amyloid material. The tumor, however, may be composed predominantly of epithelial-like cells or spindle cells. The diagnosis can be confirmed by immunoperoxidase localization of calcitonin-positive cells or elevated serum thyrocalcitonin.

METASTASES TO THE THYROID

Metastases to the thyroid are probably more common than they are believed to be. Autopsy series report 9.5% of patients with cancer may have metastatic foci in the thyroid. The neoplasms most frequently metastasizing to the thyroid include melanoma and breast, renal, and lung carcinoma. The appearance of a thyroid nodule in a patient with disseminated disease or with a known malignancy following a long disease-free interval may be helpful to determine whether the nodule represents a primary thyroid lesion or metastasis from another source. The cytologic features should be comparable with the primary tumor and dissimilar to features of a thyroid lesion to make a diagnosis of metastatic disease. Another tumor may involve the thyroid by direct extension, such as laryngeal or esophageal lesions. The author has seen both leiomyosarcoma and squamous cell carcinoma of the esophagus invade the thyroid.

LYMPHOMA

Malignant lymphoma of the thyroid may be either a primary or secondary involvement. In most patients with secondary involvement, one or more discrete nodules of lymphoma are surrounded by normal-appearing thyroid tissue. The thyroid is a relatively uncommon focus for extranodal or primary lymphoma; however, the frequency varies somewhat with the relative frequency of lymphoma. Usually, primary lymphoma arises in a thyroid with chronic lymphocytic thyroiditis. Women are affected more often than are men, and most patients are elderly. A diffuse pattern is more common than a nodular pattern. Areas of necrosis and follicles stuffed with malignant cells are common histologic findings. Invasion beyond the thyroid is seen in over half of the cases. The most common histologic type is large-cell lymphoma (Fig. 15–42). Differential diagnosis includes anaplastic carcinoma and florid thyroiditis (Figs. 15–43 and 15–44). Immunohistochemistry and/or lymphocyte phenotyping may be very helpful in defining the lesion.

NORMAL CELLS

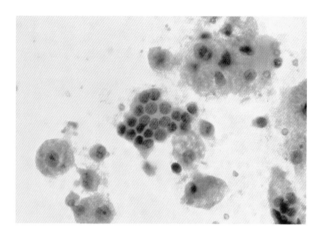

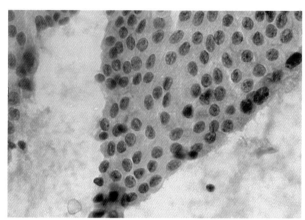

FIGURE 15–1. Normal Thyroid. A number of different cells are seen in this photograph. A small group of follicular cells is seen in the center of the field. They are arranged as a flat sheet and are uniform in size and shape. The nuclei are round, with a fine chromatin. Nucleoli are not seen. The follicular cell is approximately the same size as a normal lymphocyte, although they vary somewhat in size. Several macrophages are also present. Macrophages may contain either hemosiderin or colloid. Cells with vacuolated cytoplasm may also be degenerating follicular cells. A small amount of colloid is present. This is seen as the homogenous, opaque, greenish-blue material in the corner. Colloid may be seen freely or in association with follicular cells (cytospin, Papanicolaou stain; carbowax fixative, × 400).

FIGURE 15–2. Normal Thyroid. The follicular cells are seen as a sheet of cells with a honeycomb arrangement. Cell borders are indistinct. The cells are uniform in size. The sheet appears as a monolayer; follicle formation is not apparent. Although most often seen as small groups of cells, follicular cells may also be single (cytospin, Papanicolaou stain, × 400).

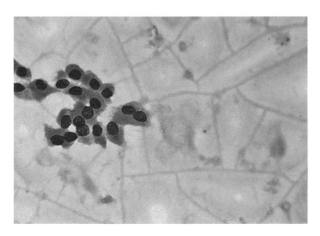

FIGURE 15–3. Normal Thyroid. Note the appearance of the follicular cells and colloid when prepared in a direct smear with a Wright-Giemsa stain. The features of the follicular cells are similar to those described above; the cytoplasm is more readily seen, and colloid is abundant. Colloid is identified as the purple-blue material in the background. Colloid has a tendency to crack in a linear fashion when it dries on the slide. The presence of abundant colloid is often taken as an indication of a macrofollicular or benign process (alcohol-fixed smear, Wright-Giemsa, × 225).

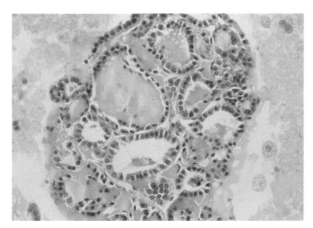

FIGURE 15–5. Normal Thyroid. A cell-block preparation often provides small tissue fragments that are quite informative. Thyroid aspirates are frequently quite bloody owing to the vascularity of the gland. Although blood may cause some problems with a smear, the preparation of a cell block is facilitated by the blood, which provides a clot and yields small tissue fragments. Note the variation in follicle size. Some of the follicles are lined by thin attenuated cells; the epithelium lining the smaller follicles are somewhat larger but are within normal size range (cell block, hematoxylin and eosin stain, × 100).

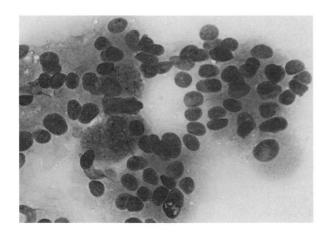

FIGURE 15–4. Normal Thyroid. In comparison with the cells seen on a Papanicolaou stain, these cells have been air dried and a Wright-Giemsa stain has been used. Note the increase in size, the differences in nuclear detail, and the appearance of colloid in the macrophage (air-dried smear, Wright-Giemsa, × 400).

NON-NEOPLASTIC CONDITIONS

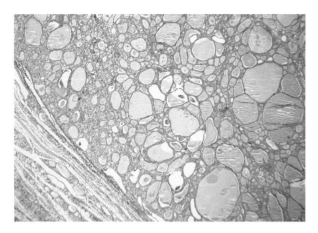

FIGURE 15–6. Nodular Goiter. In this low-power view of a surgical biopsy specimen, note the expanded area with follicles of varying sizes. A small amount of normal-appearing thyroid is seen compressed in the corner of the field. Secondary changes are not present in this field. No capsule is seen (tissue section, hematoxylin and eosin stain, × 60).

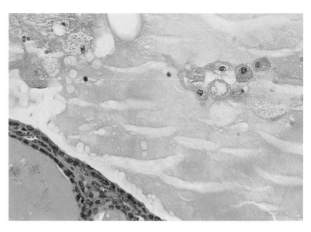

FIGURE 15–8. Nodular Goiter. Note the macrophages in center of the follicule. The origin of vacuolated cells may be degenerating follicular epithelium or monocyte-derived macrophages (cell block, hematoxylin and eosin stain, × 225).

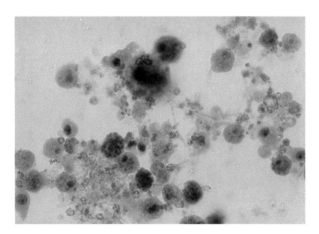

FIGURE 15–7. Nodular Goiter With Cystic Degeneration. Secondary changes in nodular goiter are common and include cyst formation. Aspirates from this lesion may contain numerous macrophages and little follicular epithelium or colloid. Of concern is the possibility of cystic degeneration of a papillary carcinoma. A minimum number of follicular cells or groups is required to consider an aspirate satisfactory (cytospin, Papanicolaou stain × 400).

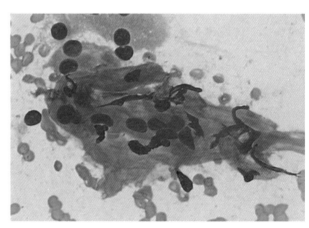

FIGURE 15–9. Nodular Goiter With Secondary Changes. Note the sheet of spindle-shaped cells surrounded by dense connective tissue. It may difficult to distinguish portions of capsule from secondary fibrosis. Interpretation rests with evaluation of other components that may be present (air-dried smear, Wright-Giemsa, × 400).

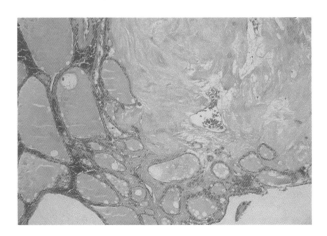

FIGURE 15–10. Nodular Goiter with Fibrosis. This low-power view of a tissue section shows an area of dense fibrosis within a nodular goiter (tissue section, hematoxylin and eosin stain, × 125).

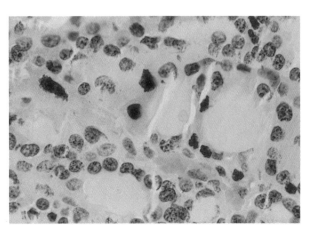

FIGURE 15–12. Nodular Goiter with Hürthle Cell Change. In this section, the focal scattered distribution of Hürthle cells within nodular goiter is seen (tissue section, hematoxylin and eosin stain × 400).

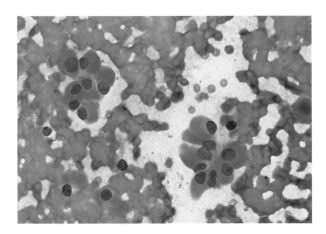

FIGURE 15–11. Nodular Goiter with Hürthle Cell Change. Hürthle cell change in nodular goiter is quite common. Hürthle cells are typically large, with polygonal- or oval-shaped cytoplasm. The cytoplasm is quite dense and may stain deep blue to eosinophilic. Nucleoli may be quite prominent and are typically uniform and single. Hürthle cells may be quite variable; some have nuclei that are hyperchromatic, quite bizarre, and irregular (air-dried, Wright-Giemsa stain, × 225).

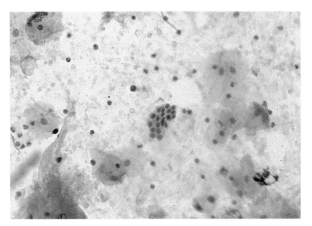

FIGURE 15–13. Thyroglossal Duct Cyst. Note the squamous cells, one group of follicular epithelium, and inflammatory cells in the background. Most thyroglossal duct cysts are in the midline and may be confused with a thyroid nodule. The presence of squamous cells and columnar epithelium are helpful features; an inadvertent aspirate of the trachea may also yield similar material (cytospin, Papanicolaou stain × 225).

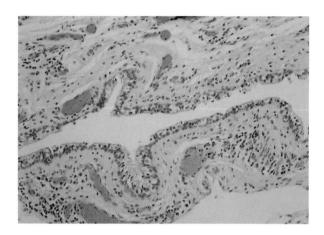

FIGURE 15–14. Thyroglossal Duct Cyst. In this resected specimen, the lining of the cyst is composed of stratified columnar epithelium. Approximately one third of these lesions may have thyroid tissue as a component (tissue section, hematoxylin and eosin stain, × 100).

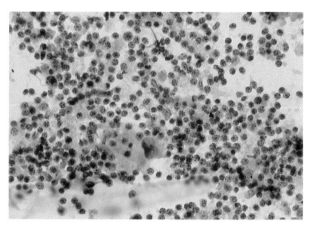

FIGURE 15–16. Hashimoto Thyroiditis. Note the prominent number of lymphocytes, which are heterogenous and show a range in size. This heterogeneity helps to distinguish this from lymphoma. A follicular cell with considerable atypia is also present. Cytologic atypia and Hürthle cell change are frequent findings in Hashimoto thyroiditis (smear, Papanicolaou stain, × 400).

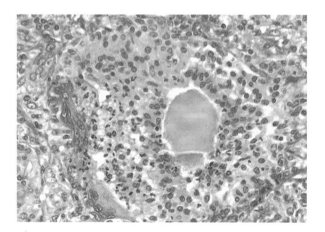

FIGURE 15–15. Granulomatous Thyroiditis. Note the necrosis and abscess formation with a small amount of residual colloid in this tissue section. Fine needle aspiration from this lesion shows a mixed inflammatory response with lymphocytes, polyps, eosinophils, and multinucleated giant cells (tissue section, hematoxylin and eosin stain, × 225).

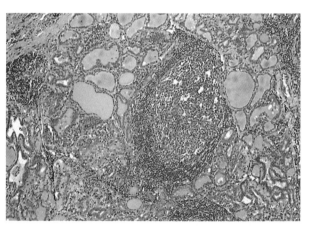

FIGURE 15–17. Hashimoto Thyroiditis. Formation of germinal centers may be prominent in chronic lymphocytic thyroiditis (tissue section, hematoxylin and eosin stain, × 100).

FOLLICULAR TUMORS

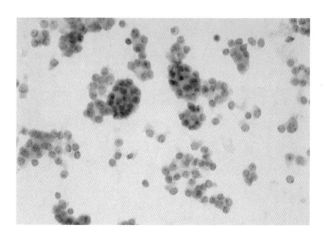

FIGURE 15–18. Follicular Adenoma. Note the increased cellularity, lack of colloid, and follicular arrangement of the cells. Differential diagnosis includes hyperplastic phase of nodular goiter, follicular adenoma, and follicular carcinoma. One must judge cellularity based on expertise and usual cellularity obtained by the particular aspirator (cytospin, Papanicolaou stain, × 225).

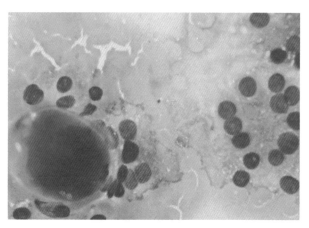

FIGURE 15–20. Follicular Adenoma. Microfollicular pattern. Compare features of a microfollicular adenoma in this Wright-Giemsa-stained smear. The colloid is seen as the violet material. Note the uniformity of the follicular cells (air-dried Wright-Giemsa stain, × 400).

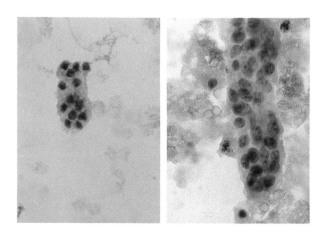

FIGURE 15–19. Comparison of Normal Follicular Cells and Atypical Follicular Cells. Note the increase in size of the follicular cells, the crowding, and the increased number of cells in the group derived from a follicular adenoma. The N/C ratio is also increased (cytospin, Papanicolaou stain, × 400).

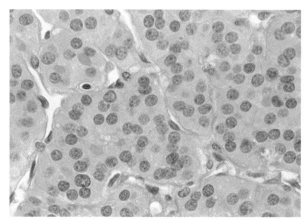

FIGURE 15–21. Follicular Adenoma. High-power view of tissue section demonstrates lack of colloid, increase in cell size, but relative uniformity of the cells (hematoxylin and eosin stain, × 400).

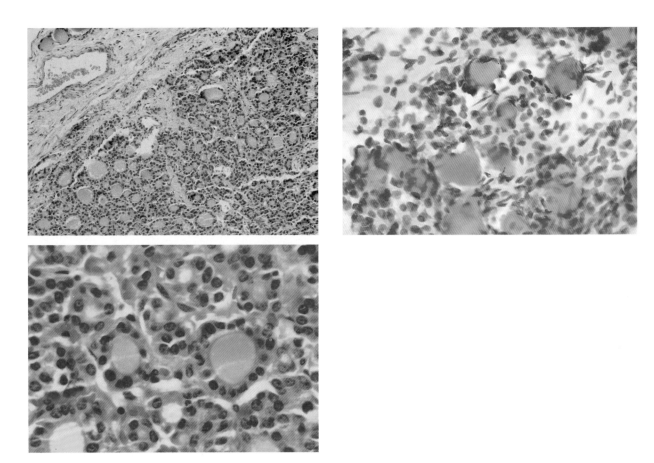

FIGURE 15–22. Follicular Adenoma. Microfollicular pattern. **Figure 15–22A.** Note the encapsulated lesion composed of uniformly small follicules. The capsule must be carefully examined to exclude minimally invasive follicular carcinoma (cell block, hematoxylin and eosin stain, × 60). **Figure 15–22B.** Higher magnification shows small follicules, some cytologic atypia, and relatively scant colloid (cell block, hematoxylin and eosin, × 125). **Figure 15–22C.** Direct smear shows microfollicular pattern. Colloid is seen as small spheres of orangophilic densely stained material. The follicular cells lining the colloid are relatively uniform in size (smear, Papanicolaou stain, × 100).

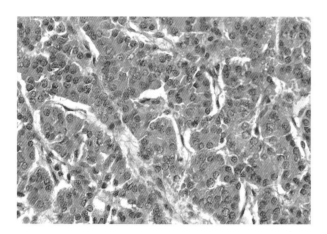

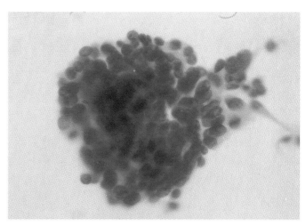

FIGURE 15–23. Follicular Adenoma. The trabecular pattern of the lesion is clearly demonstrated on the cell block from the above case. Although the architectural patterns seen in follicular lesions are of no biologic or clinical significance, a definite pattern seen on an FNA specimen is very helpful in distinguishing adenoma/carcinoma from nodular goiter (cell block, hematoxylin and eosin stain, × 400).

FIGURE 15–24. Follicular Carcinoma. Aspirates from follicular adenomas and minimally invasive well-differentiated follicular carcinomas show very similar findings. Cytologic features that are more indicative of carcinoma include marked architectural crowding, which is shown in this figure. The size of the group and the number of cells within the group are increased. At times it may be difficult to distinguish crowding from papillary groups. Note that there is some pleomorphism of the cells and that the nuclei are hyperchromatic. Nucleoli are not prominent in this field (cytospin, Papanicolaou stain, × 400).

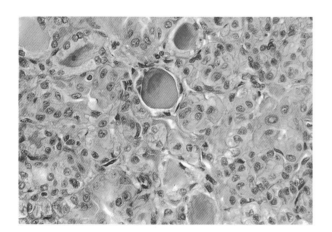

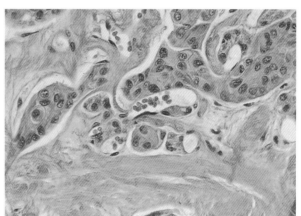

FIGURE 15–25. Follicular Carcinoma, Minimally Invasive. Figure 15–25A. Note the follicular pattern, scant colloid, and moderate cytologic atypia. Differentiation from an adenoma necessitates vascular or capsular invasion. The cytologic features of the follicular lesion shown here correspond to those seen on the FNA (tissue, hematoxylin and eosin stain). **Figure 15–25B.** Multiple sections of the capsule from the above lesion reveal areas of capsule invasion (tissue section, hematoxylin and eosin stain, × 400).

PAPILLARY CARCINOMA

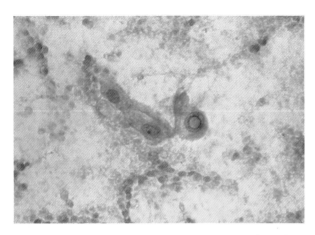

FIGURE 15–26. Papillary Carcinoma. The nuclei of these cells show a characteristic and frequent feature of papillary carcinoma, i.e., pseudoinclusion. They may be found in a variety of other malignancies and benign thyroid lesions and therefore are not exclusive to papillary carcinoma. Another characteristic feature of papillary carcinoma is the clearing of the nucleoplasm with margination of the chromatin. This gives the impression of ground-glass chromatin (cytospin, Papanicolaou stain, × 400).

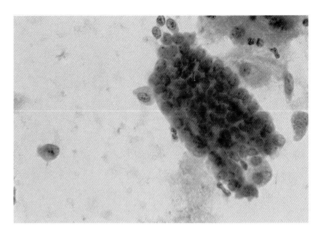

FIGURE 15–28. Papillary Carcinoma. A papillary cluster of cells is seen in this field. Features which characterize a papillary group include a "community border," crowded and overlapped cells with nuclei at all levels of focus. Characteristic nuclear features may be more difficult to appreciate because of the nuclear overlapping (smear, Papanicolaou stain, × 400).

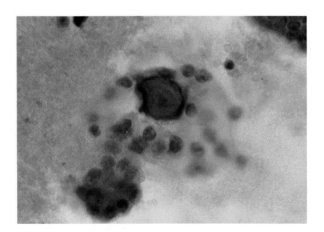

FIGURE 15–27. Papillary Carcinoma. Note the psammoma body in the center of the field. The presence of psammoma bodies in an FNA specimen raises the level of concern for papillary carcinoma considerably. Although very infrequent, psammoma bodies have been described in benign lesions such as nodular goiter. Identification of a psammoma body is an indication for further evaluation. Psammoma bodies must be distinguished from inspissated colloid and concentric calcification related to secondary changes (cytospin, Papanicolaou stain, × 400).

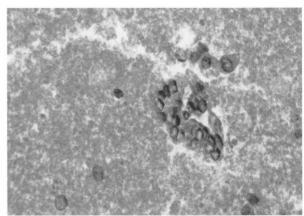

FIGURE 15–29. Papillary Carcinoma, Follicular Variant. This cell block shows a small group of cells with a follicular pattern, but nuclear features of papillary carcinoma are evident. Note the clearing of the chromatin (cell block, hematoxylin and eosin stain, × 400).

OTHER TUMORS

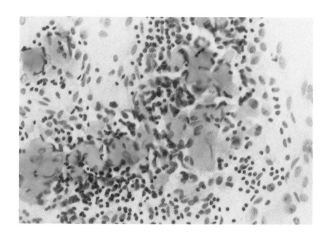 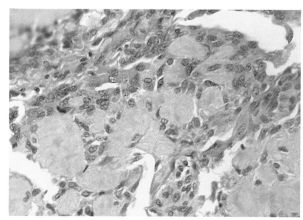

FIGURE 15–30. Medullary Carcinoma. Figure 15–30A. A direct Papanicolaou-stained smear shows abundant amyloid as pale blue-green material. The spindle cell component is prominent, although scattered epithelial cells were also seen (cytospin, Papanicolaou stain, × 225). **Figure 15–30B.** Note the similarities of the amyloid and cellular components with that seen in the direct smear (cell block, hematoxylin and eosin stain, × 225).

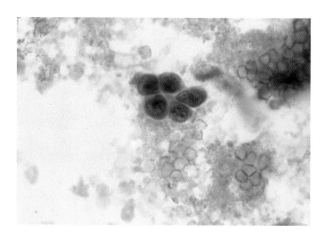

FIGURE 15–31. Medullary Carcinoma. The epithelial component from a medullary carcinoma may be quite atypical, as seen in this slide (cytospin, Papanicolaou stain, × 400).

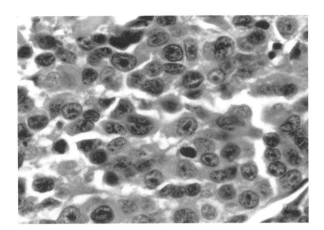

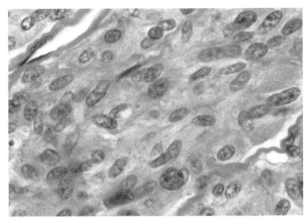

FIGURE 15–32. Medullary Carcinoma. Resection specimen shows the epithelial **(Figure 15–32A)** and spindle-cell **(Figure 15–32B)** components of the lesion seen in Figure 15–31 (tissue section, hematoxylin and eosin stain, × 400).

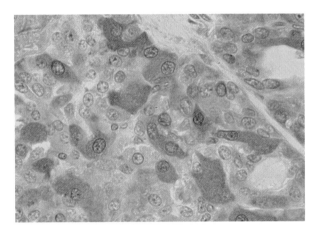

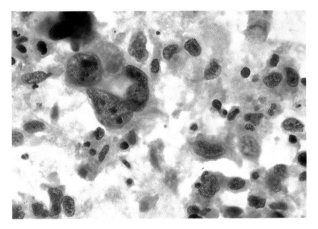

FIGURE 15–33. Medullary Carcinoma. An immunoperoxidase stain for thyrocalcitonin shows strong focal positivity. Demonstration of thyrocalcitonin may be necessary in some lesions to categorize as a medullary carcinoma (see Figure 15–45) (tissue section, immunoperoxidase stain, × 400).

FIGURE 15–34. Anaplastic Carcinoma. Note large pleomorphic and bizarre-shaped cells. At the time of diagnosis, most anaplastic carcinomas have extended beyond the thyroid, and surgery is considered palliative. A definitive diagnosis of anaplastic carcinoma on FNA may obviate surgery and lead to earlier radiation or chemotherapy (smear, Papanicolaou stain, × 400).

DIFFERENTIAL GROUPING

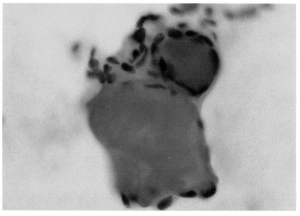

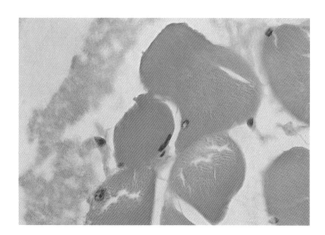

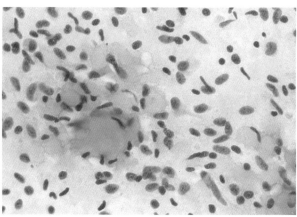

FIGURE 15–35. Colloid Versus Amyloid Versus Muscle. Figure 15–35A. High-power view of colloid and follicular cells. Note the sharp border and dense eosinophilia of the colloid. The appearance of colloid is quite variable; staining ranges from pale green to orange. It may be difficult to distinguish from amyloid. Occasionally, inspissated colloid may appear laminated and may be confused with a psammoma body (cytospin, Papanicolaou stain, × 225). **Figure 15–35B.** Amyloid is noted as the amorphous pale blue-green material in this smear of a medullary carcinoma (cytospin, Papanicolaou stain, × 225). **Figure 15–35C.** Muscle can be distinguished from colloid by identifying striations, the nuclei on the periphery, and the arrangement in bundles (smear, Papanicolaou stain, × 225).

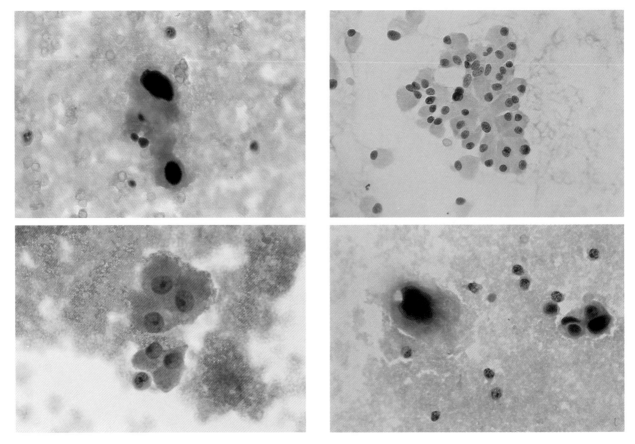

FIGURE 15–36. Hürthle Cells. Figure 15–36A. Nodular goiter with Hürthle cells. Bizarre-appearing Hürthle cells were seen individually on the background of nodular goiter, i.e. colloid and follicular epithelium (cytospin, Papanicolaou stain, × 400). **Figure 15–36B.** Hürthle cell lesion. A monomorphic population of Hürthle cells with a lack of colloid and an abnormal architecture characterize Hürthle cell lesions (adenoma vs. carcinoma) (cytospin, Papanicolaou stain, × 400). **Figure 15–36C.** Hürthle cell adenoma. Note the monomorphic population of cells with features of Hürthle cells: abundant cytoplasm, eccentric nucleus, and dense cytoplasma (cytospin, Papanicolaou stain, × 225). **Figure 15–36D.** Hürthle cells in Hashimoto thyroiditis. Note the lymphocytes in the background (cytospin, Papanicolaou stain, × 400).

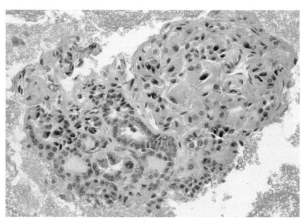

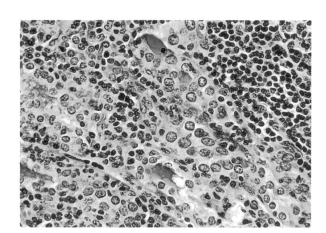

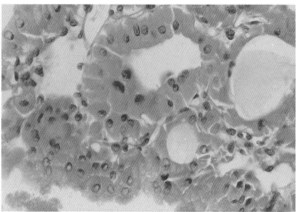

FIGURE 15–37. Hürthle Cells. Figure 15–37A. Nodular goiter with Hürthle cell change. In this cell block, the focal collection of Hürthle cells are noted. Hürthle cells may occur in nodular goiter, Hashimoto thyroiditis, or as tumors. In general, those seen in association with nodular goiter appear as single cells admixed with follicular epithelia and are not the dominant population. Other features should also be present (cell block, hematoxylin and eosin stain, × 225). **Figure 15–37B. Hürthle cell lesion.** A cell block from a Hürthle cell adenoma shows the monomorphic population of Hürthle cells in a microfollicular pattern. The same criteria must be applied to Hürthle cell lesions with respect to making a distinction of adenoma versus carcinoma; i.e., demonstration of capsular or vascular invasion (cell block, hematoxylin and eosin, × 225). **Figure 15–37C. Hürthle cells in Hashimoto thyroiditis.** Note the atypical follicular cells associated with a prominent lymphocyte background (cell block, hematoxylin and eosin stain, × 225 and 400).

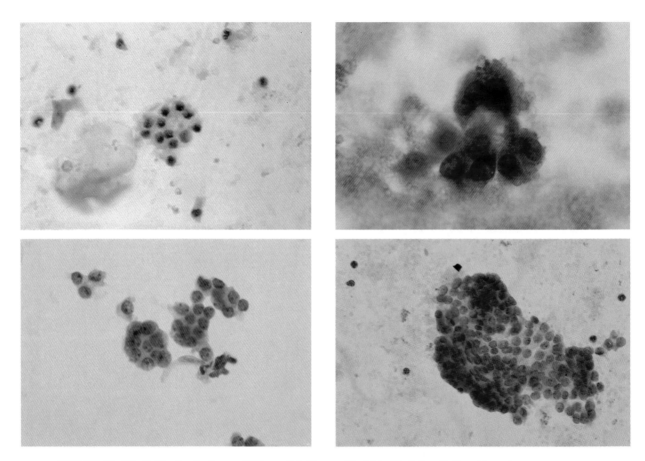

FIGURE 15–38. Follicular Lesions—Differential. Figure 15–38A. Nodular Goiter. Note the colloid in the background. The small group of follicular cells lacks cytologic atypia and has a follicular arrangement. **Figure 15–38B. Follicular Adenoma.** Higher magnification of the aspirate shown in Figure 15–18 shows the crowding and enlargement of the cells and a high N/C ratio. Nucleoli are also seen (smear, Papanicolaou stain, × 200). **Figure 15–38C. Follicular Carcinoma.** The cells depicted in this slide are pleomorphic, with hyperchromatic nuclei. There is a marked increase in N/C ratio. The cytoplasm is scant. The group is discohesive. Colloid is not present (cytospin, Papanicolaou stain, × 400). **Figure 15–38D. Papillary Carcinoma-Follicular Variant.** A monolayered sheet of cells with nuclear features of papillary carcinoma. The differential diagnosis also includes a follicular lesion (adenoma/carcinoma) and medullary carcinoma. Follicular variant of papillary carcinoma may be a difficult lesion to recognize from an FNA specimen because characteristic papillae features are absent or rare, psammoma bodies are rare, and the nuclear features are not exclusive to papillary carcinoma (cytospin, Papanicolaou stain, × 225).

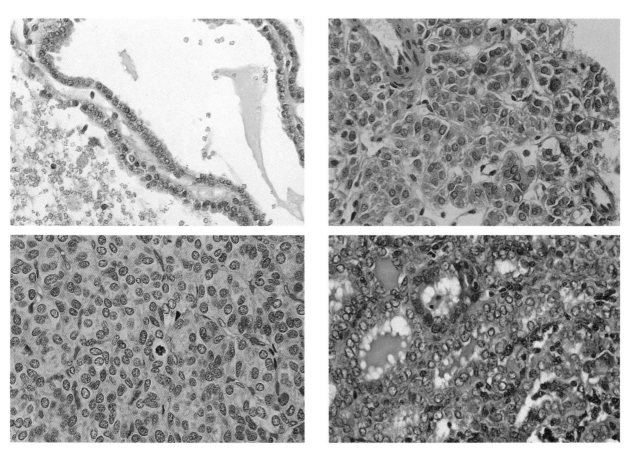

FIGURE 15–39. Follicular Lesions—Differential. Figure 15–39A. Nodular Goiter. Note the large follicle lined by a single layer of cells. A small portion of colloid remains in the center of the follicle (cell block, hematoxylin and eosin, × 225). **Figure 15–39B. Follicular Lesion.** Note the mitosis in the center of the lesion. The remainder of the lesion is characterized by a monotonous population of cells, which are uniform in size with a follicular pattern. Colloid is not seen. The presence of a mitosis is quite worrisome; it is unusual to see a mitosis in normal follicular epithelium or in adenomas. Previous aspiration may cause an increase in mitotic activity. Mitoses may be seen in a normal macrophage; therefore, in evaluating the significance of a mitosis it is essential to identify the cell properly. The presence of a mitosis in a follicular cell is a strong indication for further evaluation (cell block, hematoxylin and eosin, × 225). **Figure 15–39C. Follicular Carcinoma.** The cell block from the lesion shown above is composed of cells with a sheet-like arrangement. Follicle formation is poor. There is some pleomorphism and no colloid. A blood vessel is seen in the corner; follicular carcinomas tend to invade blood vessels, although no clear-cut invasion is demonstrated in this field. This FNA is from a widely invasive follicular carcinoma with clinical involvement outside the thyroid. An FNA from widely invasive follicular carcinoma may be performed to confirm the origin as thyroid (cell block, hematoxylin and eosin, × 225). **Figure 15–39D. Papillary Carcinoma, Follicular Variant.** Note the prominent nuclear clearing in the tumor arranged in a definite follicular pattern (tissue, hematoxylin and eosin stain, × 225).

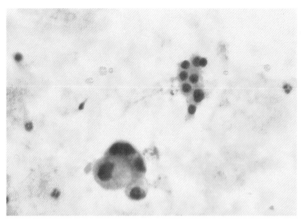

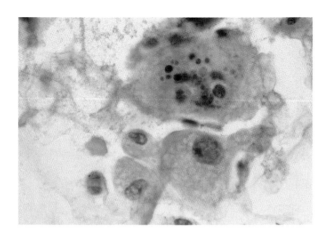

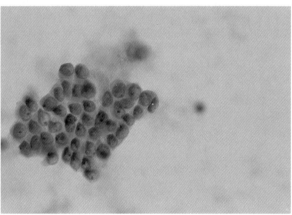

FIGURE 15–40. Papillary Hyperplasia Versus Papillary Carcinoma. Figure 15–40A. Nodular Goiter, Hyperplastic Phase. Note the relatively normal-size epithelium as compared with the small group of cells with vacuolated cytoplasm and nuclear atypia. In the hyperplastic phase, the cellularity may be increased, papillary like groups may be present, and the cells may exhibit some cytologic atypia (cytospin, Papanicolaou stain, × 225). Figure 15–40B. Papillary Carcinoma. Monolayers of cells may also be seen in papillary carcinoma. The nuclear features may be more readily seen when the cells are in a flat sheet. These include ground-glass chromatin, small nucleoli, and nuclear grooves. Nuclear grooves are the result of infolding of the nuclear membrane and are seen as a line of hematoxylin through the long axis of a nucleus. Although a frequent finding, nuclear grooves are also nonspecific; the finding of numerous grooves is perhaps more significant (smear, Papanicolaou stain, × 225). Figure 15–40C. Graves Disease. Note the nuclear atypia in loosely cohesive cells. The cytoplasm is prominent. Although not prominent in this field, papillary structures may be seen in Graves disease. The differential diagnosis includes papillary carcinoma. The clinical presentation is so characteristic that a diagnosis of papillary carcinoma should not be made in a patient with diffuse enlargement of the thyroid and hyperthyroidism (smear, Papanicolaou stain, × 400).

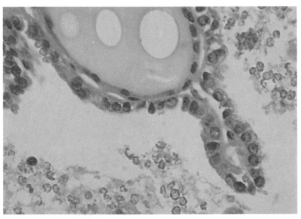

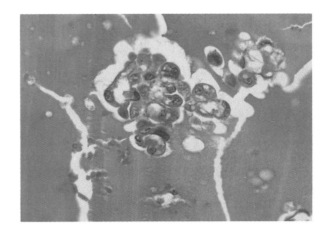

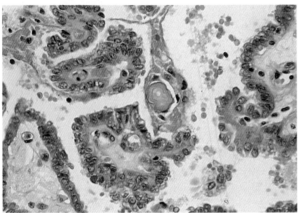

FIGURE 15–41. Papillary Hyperplasia Versus Papillary Carcinoma. Figure 15–41A. Nodular Goiter, Hyperplastic Phase. Note the cytologic atypia and folded epithelium. Note the lack of connective tissue and vessels in the area between follicular cells. This represents an area of minimal follicular atypia in the hyperplastic phase of nodular goiter (cell block, hematoxylin and eosin stain, × 225). Figure 15–41B. Papillary Carcinoma. The hallmark of papillary carcinoma is the identification of papillae with fibrovascular stalk. The cell block shown here demonstrates the vascular core of several papillae. A psammoma body is also noted (cell block, hematoxylin and eosin stain, × 125). Figure 15–41C. Graves Disease. Note the cluster of cells with vacuolated, clear cytoplasm. Vacuoles vary from small to large. Differential diagnosis includes clear cell carcinoma of the thyroid and metastatic carcinoma (cell block, hematoxylin and eosin stain, × 225).

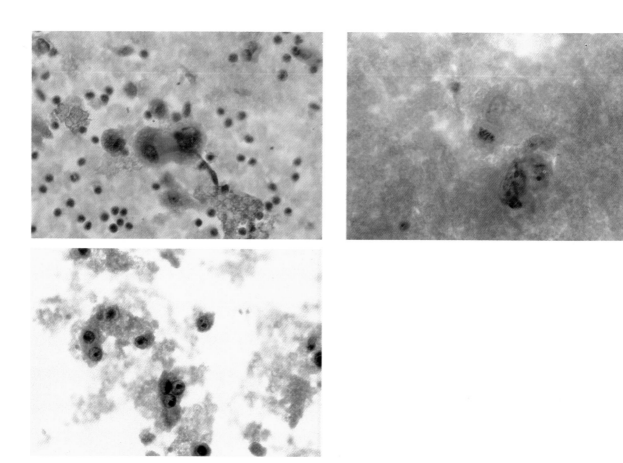

FIGURE 15–42. Thyroiditis Versus Lymphoma Versus Anaplastic Carcinoma. Figure 15–42A. Hashimoto Thyroiditis. Note the atypical follicular cells, macrophages, red blood cells, and numerous lymphocytes. Considerable cytologic atypia may be seen. The background, composed of numerous lymphocytes, suggests chronic lymphocytic thyroiditis (cytospin, Papanicolaou stain, × 400). **Figure 15–42B. Malignant Lymphoma.** Prominent nucleoli and small clusters of cells are seen. The differential diagnosis would include lymphoma, poorly differentiated carcinoma, and melanoma. Immunoperoxidase markers are helpful in distinguishing poorly differentiated lesions (cytospin, Papanicolaou stain, × 400). **Figure 15–42C. Anaplastic Carcinoma** (cytospin, Papanicolaou stain, × 400).

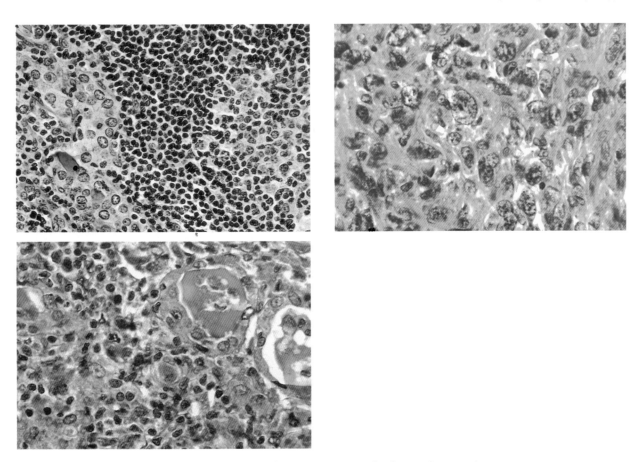

FIGURE 15–43. Thyroiditis Versus Lymphoma Versus Anaplastic Carcinoma. Figure 15–43A. Hashimoto Thyroiditis. Note the follicular atypia associated with thyroiditis in this section (tissue section, hematoxylin and eosin, × 225). **Figure 15–43B. Malignant Lymphoma.** The difficulty in distinguishing the malignant lymphoid from the follicular atypia associated with the process is demonstrated in this photograph. Note residual colloid. **Figure 15–43C. Anaplastic Carcinoma.** (cell block, hematoxylin and eosin, × 225).

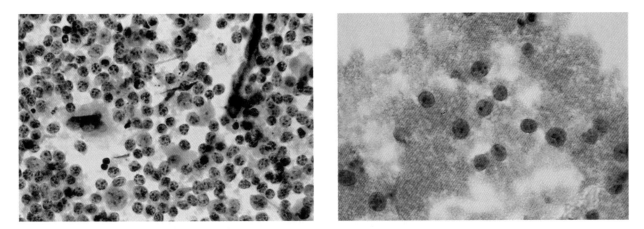

FIGURE 15–44. Hashimoto Thyroiditis Versus Lymphoma. Figure 15–44A. Hashimoto Thyroiditis. Note the heterogeneous population of lymphocytes. An atypical follicular cell is also present (cytospin, Papanicolaou stain, × 225). **Figure 15–44B. Malignant Lymphoma.** Monotonous population of malignant-appearing lymphocytes. In contrast to the infiltrate associated with thyroiditis, the population depicted is homogeneous (cell block, hematoxylin and eosin stain, × 400).

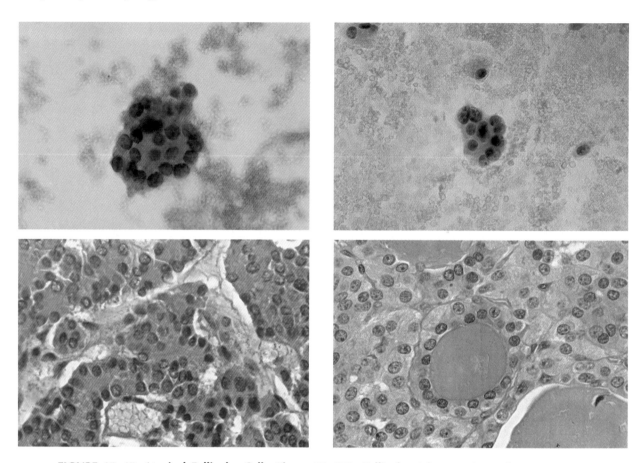

FIGURE 15–45. Atypical Follicular Cells. Figure 15–45A. Follicular Adenoma. Note the crowding of the cells within the group illustrated. The N/C ratio is somewhat increased, as is the size of the cells. Cytoplasmic features are not well seen. Although these cells would be considered atypical based on these features alone, it would be difficult to render a specific diagnosis. Evidence to support a diagnosis of follicular lesion includes a lack of colloid and a predominance of these cells. In many instances, architectural features are more readily seen on the cell block and a more specific diagnosis is given. The cellularity and the architectural features were more readily seen on the cell block belonging to this particular patient (cytospin, Papanicolaou stain, × 400). **Figure 15–45B. Follicular Adenoma.** Note the trabecular pattern; the follicular cells share similarities with Hürthle cells such as abundant eosinophilic cytoplasm. There may be considerable overlap in the cellular features of follicular cells and Hürthle cells, which accounts for some of the difficulty in categorizing these lesions (cell block, hematoxylin and eosin stain, × 400). **Figure 15–45C. Medullary Carcinoma.** The epithelial component of a medullary carcinoma may be very similar to that of cells from an adenoma (cytospin, Papanicolaou stain, × 400). **Figure 15–45D. Medullary Carcinoma.** A diagnosis of follicular adenoma, was originally made based on the microfollicular pattern but since stains for thyrocalcitonin revealed striking positivity (see Figure 15–33) a diagnosis of medullary carcinoma was made. (smear, Papanicolaou stain, × 400).

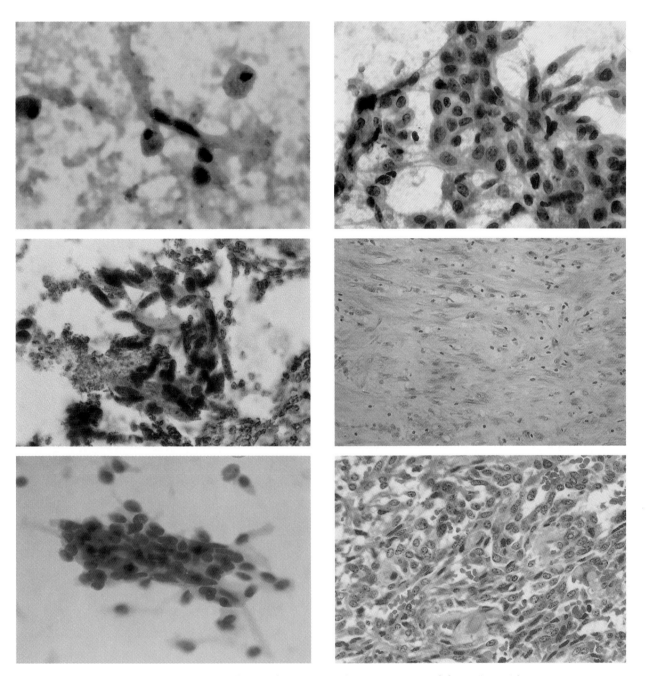

FIGURE 15–46. Spindle Cells—Differential Diagnosis. Figure 15–46A. Nodular Goiter with Secondary Changes. Note the spindle-shaped cell and several macrophages. The differential diagnosis of spindle cells in a thyroid aspirate includes secondary changes in nodular goiter, anaplastic carcinoma, the spindle-cell component of medullary carcinoma, and nonthyroid lesions, such as sarcoma. The secondary changes in goiter include infarction, hemorrhage, and necrosis. The cell depicted in this slide was associated with previous infarction, organization, and areas of dense fibrosis (cytospin, Papanicolaou stain, × 400). **Figure 15–46B. Leiomyosarcoma.** Note the hyperchromatic nuclei with coarsely clumped chromatin. The nuclear membrane is thickened and the N/C ratio is increased (cytospin, Papanicolaou stain, × 400). **Figure 15–46C. Medullary Carcinoma.** The presence of an epithelial component and/or amyloid would suggest the source of these cells (cytospin, Papanicolaou stain, × 400). **Figure 15–46D. Thymoma.** A prominent lymphocytic infiltrate associated with stromal cells should raise the possibility of a non-thyroidal lesion such as thymoma (cytospin, Papanicolaou stain, × 400). **Figure 15–46E. Fibrosis.** Note that fibroblasts are relatively scarce among the dense collagen (cell block, hematoxylin and eosin, × 225). **Figure 15–46F. Medullary Carcinoma.** Contrast the obviously increased cellularity of this lesion with that seen with benign fibrosis (cell block, hematoxylin and eosin, × 225).

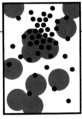
SALIVARY GLANDS, HEAD AND NECK, AND SKIN ASPIRATION CYTOLOGY

Michael D. Glant

Douglas C. King

There are four types of salivary glands: three are paired, encapsulated collections of glandular tissue (major salivary glands) and one is composed of small, diffusely scattered glands (minor salivary glands). The parotid glands (14 to 28 gm) are located in the cheek just in front of and partially below each ear. The secretions empty by single ducts (Stensen ducts) through the buccal mucosa. The facial nerve that supplies motor function to the facial muscles of expression passes through the parotid. The submandibular glands (5 to 7 gm) are approximately the size of a walnut and are located under the mandible. They empty by a single duct (Warthin duct), which opens into the floor of the mouth under the tongue. The sublingual glands (1 to 3 gm, almond-sized) are under the tongue and run parallel to its long axis. They empty by a separate row of ducts and one large duct (Bartholin duct) into the floor of the mouth on the sides of the tongue attachment (frenulum).

The minor salivary glands are composed of many tiny glands beneath the oral mucosa of the palate, side walls and floor of the buccal cavity, and tongue.

These glands are compound branching tubuloalveolar structures. The major salivary glands are lobulated and separated by fibrovascular investments that contain abundant fat.

The salivary ducts have three portions:

1. Excretory ducts, which are larger and have more distal portions lined by pseudostratified columnar epithelium and an occasional mucus goblet cell.
2. Striated ducts, which are so named because of the striations barely seen by light microscopy in the basal aspects of the duct-lining cells. These striations are manifestations of parallel rows of mitochondria that are found in the basal portion of these cuboidal to columnar cells arranged perpendicular to the basal lamina.
3. Intercalated ducts, which are lined by low cuboidal or somewhat flattened cells, connect the striated ducts to the acinar units. The intercalated portion is believed to be the site of regeneration of both adjacent ductal and acinar cells and is the origin of most neoplasms. Myoepithelial cells line the intercalated ducts and adjacent acini but not the striated ducts.

The acinar units are grape-like clusters of two types of secretory cells, serous or mucous. Serous cells are roughly cuboidal in shape with an eccentric nucleus and bluish gray, granular cytoplasm. Nuclei are regular and round. The cells form a spherical cluster. The parotid gland is composed of this secretory cell type. Mucous cells are cuboidal in shape with an eccentric nucleus that is flattened toward the basal portion. The cytoplasm contains pale blue droplets of mucin (red with mucicarmine stain), which are difficult to visualize by light microscopy. They form spherical clusters with more visible lumina than in serous clusters. The sublingual glands are composed of this secretory cell type.

The submandibular glands are mixed serous and mucous glands. The acini are organized so that the serous cells are farthest from the ducts, usually forming caps or serous demilunes on the mucinous acinar structures. The minor salivary glands may be pure serous, pure mucous, or mixed.

The aspiration technique used by the authors is the same as the one described in Chapter 14.

CYTOLOGY

Normal salivary gland tissue is aspirated with relative ease because of the intermingled fat within the gland. Generally, large fragments of intact tissue are obtained.

The acinar portions are surrounded by fat cells and capillaries. On Papanicolaou-stained material, the acinar cells form spherical clusters of uniform cells with finely vacuolated cyanophilic cytoplasm and basal nuclei. The nuclei are round and uniform. The lumina of acini are small and difficult to visualize. On Romanovsky-stained material, the pattern is similar, with purple nuclei and blue granular cytoplasm in acinar cells.

The ductal portions are less frequently observed in aspirates and are usually intact branching structures. The larger ducts are so cohesive and cellular that individual cells may be difficult to discern, but orderly uniform nuclei are usually visible. In some areas, their columnar nature is evident. The smaller ducts (striated and intercalated) are usually lined by cuboidal or flattened cells, and myoepithelial cells can be seen on intercalated ducts.

NON-NEOPLASTIC SALIVARY GLAND DISEASES

Cystic Lesions

True cysts are small (usually about 1 cm) intraglandular lesions often lined by stratified squamous epithelium. Most "cysts" in these major glands are duct ectasias caused by obstruction. Sialometaplasia usually results in a squamous lining if the cysts are long-standing. When inflammation coexists with such cysts, cellular atypia may be present that must be differentiated from a squamous carcinoma.

"Ranula" is a loosely used term for cysts or pseudocysts of the floor of the mouth caused by obstruction of a major salivary gland, usually the sublingual gland. Mucoceles of the sublingual glands are included.

Mucoceles are not true cysts because the majority are not lined by epithelium. They represent the extravasation of mucus into the surrounding tissues by excretory duct obstruction of a minor salivary gland often as a result of trauma. They are lined by granulation tissue and inflammatory cells, which follow the spillage of mucus into the connective tissue. Aspirates generally contain foamy histiocytes in a background of mucus with or without an inflammatory infiltrate (usually minimal). Epithelial cells are usually not seen.

Inflammatory Lesions

Acute Sialadenitis

Acute parotitis or acute sialadenitis may follow reduced salivary flow because of dehydration (e.g., fever, diuretics, or starvation) since bacteria (usually *Staphylococcus aureus*) can ascend Stensen duct and infect the glands. Acinar destruction and fibrosis follow. Duct dilitation and lymphoplasmacytic infiltration are late, secondary changes.

Patients have diffuse, painful, and tender swelling with erythema and warmth in the overlying skin. Fevers and leukocytosis are often present. The etiologic agent, its route of entry, the individual's immune status, and antibiotic therapy all influence the degree and distribution of the acute (neutrophilic leukocyte) infiltrates and degree of abscess formation.

Aspirates are usually composed of purulent material with neutrophils, necrotic debris, groups of histiocytes, and reparative ductal epithelium. Degenerated acini, fat, or ductal elements may be present. Gram stains and culture for microorganisms are key studies that should be performed on this material. Anaerobic cultures are important since *Actinomyces* sp. and *Phycomycetes* sp. may be present.

Sialolithiasis and Chronic Obstructive Sialadenitis

Sialolithiasis (with or without inflammation) is the formation of a calculus in the gland ducts that is uncommon in the minor salivary glands and sublingual glands. The submandibular and parotid glands are the most common sites, especially in the main ducts. Retrograde infection may follow. At times, stricture may have a similar presentation.

Chronic obstructive sialadenitis (COS) of undetermined etiology is one of the most common lesions requested for aspiration. This is sampled either to exclude a neoplastic origin of obstruction in a larger soft gland (with or without a focus of firmer tissue), to exclude a neoplasm in more firm discrete masses, or to evaluate the possibility of a benign lymphoepithelial lesion.

Patients with calculi have diffuse soft to firm swelling in a main duct obstruction. Acute infection commonly results in a painful and extremely tender gland with overlying erythema. If the gland is not infected, mild tenderness is typical, and more intense pain may be felt while eating because increased saliva flow increases the swelling. When there is no infection, the typical COS pattern is seen. In some patients with calculi, a localized nodule may be seen in a smaller duct obstruction. The history is usually that of a persistent nodule following antibiotic therapy for a previously more diffuse swelling associated with symptoms of inflammation. The histologic pattern is a combination of a stone within a duct, sometimes associated with a cystic area from a small duct ectasia and an adjacent chronic obstructive sialadenitis. There have been cases in which the ductal epithelium around the stone displayed goblet cell hyperplasia and squamous metaplasia (both with cytologic atypia) that closely mimicked the epithelial features of a low-grade mucoepidermoid carcinoma.

Many times the cause of an obstruction is unknown, but plugs of inspissated secretions or a stricture secondary to stone development may be the cause. Often, clinical data suggest local obstruction from significant lymphadenopathy, which may have resolved prior to the request for biopsy. Many times a discrete palpable nodule with adjacent gland swelling in the parotid tail area is from a persistent reactive lymph node.

Most patients do not complain of significant pain or tenderness in COS, especially when only a small or very peripheral portion of the parotid or submandibular gland is involved. Usually, the mass slowly shrinks from fibrous involution.

The posterior aspect of the submandibular gland is more likely to show COS and is more likely to be painful than the parotid. Regional swelling, usually in the tail of the parotid with a soft to firm texture is observed in obstruction of smaller duct radicals. These rarely become infected. If infection does occur, a secondary cyst may be a sequela.

With chronic obstruction the interstitial fat in the gland atrophies around the swollen acini and fibrosis ensues. As with all chronic obstructions, the greater the degree and duration of obstruction, the more widespread is glandular atrophy with subsequent fibrous involution.

The presentation of chronic obstructive sialadenitis in aspirates varies with the phase of the disease. However, regardless of the phase, a characteristic feature is that the smears processed for air-dried Romanovsky stains are usually more diagnostic than their wet-fixed counterparts stained by either Papanicolaou or hematoxylin and eosin (H and E). In obstruction the acinar cells are swollen and fragile. As they air-dry, they rupture, releasing many bare nuclei that closely mimic small round lymphocytes. These same acini have a different reaction to wet fixation because the alcohol stabilizes the acinar cells and inhibits cell rupture. This results in intact, minimally altered acinar structures in many cases.

However, if tissue fragility is marked, then the wet-fixed smears contain bare acinar nuclei that may be indistinguishable from lymphocytes.

This has led to two major misconceptions in this diagnostic category. First, the literature's description of mature lymphocytes in aspirates of COS is misleading because in most cases these are bare acinar nuclei and *not* lymphocytes. A few cases of chronic obstruction contain lymphocytes with plasma cells, but this is the exception rather than the rule. Secondly, this is why COS without inflammation is usually classified as normal salivary gland tissue when only Papanicolaou or H and E smears are used.

Fibrous involution of the gland in chronic obstruction results in a loss of fatty tissue in the aspirate, which produces decreased cellularity and a cellular pattern similar to earlier obstructive changes. Again, the Romanovsky stains are the most sensitive to early periacinar fibrosis. A band of pink stromal material can be seen surrounding acinar clusters. In more advanced fibrosis, the hyalinized collagen and acinar atrophy are easily seen even in the wet-fixed preparations. As fibrosis becomes more predominant, the acini are lost, and samples contain many more ductal structures relative to the acinar tissue, unlike what is seen in earlier phases. Fibrosis may be so advanced that it results in an inadequate aspirate despite vigorous repeat samplings.

Duct ectasia can generate a cystic fluid that may vary from tan and mucoid to clear and yellow. The former is usually the end phase of an infectious process showing some neutrophils and may have stone fragments, mucus goblet cell hyperplasia, and squamous metaplasia. These latter two components often show mild atypia and the exclusion of a low-grade mucoepidermoid carcinoma may be difficult. The stone is represented by irregularly shaped, refractile to opaque particles seen free-floating and entangled with tissue and cells on the smears. These particles appear red on Papanicolaou or H and E and purple or unstained (refractile) with Romanovsky stains.

Benign Lymphoepithelial Lesion and Reactive Lymph Node Hyperplasia

Frequently, lymph nodes are located adjacent to or within the capsule of the parotid gland or at the edge of the submandibular gland. Most often, the reactive nodes are sampled to exclude a primary or metastatic neoplasm (see Chapter 10). Sjögren syndrome is the complex of destructive lymphoid salivary gland inflammation with involvement of the lacrimal glands. Patients complain of dry eyes and dry mouth (sicca syndrome). Incomplete expression of this syndrome includes only portions of the symptom complex.

In Sjögren syndrome the inflammation is autoimmune; however, in some cases chronic obstruction can cause florid chronic inflammation that is morphologically similar. In both instances, the histologic lesion is called benign lymphoepithelial lesion (BLEL), or Mikulicz disease. Patients with Sjögren syndrome present with bilateral diffuse enlargement with firm, variably tender glands on palpation. Initially, acinar destruction begins in the center of the lobule and progresses to the periphery with lymphoreticular infiltrates and germinal center formation. With advanced involvement only ductal elements remain as islands that show myoepithelial cell proliferation and are called myoepithelial islands. BLEL without the full Sjögren complex can be a more localized process. Recent reports have shown an increased incidence of BLEL and benign lymphoepithelial cysts in patients with human immunodeficiency virus (HIV) infection.

Cytologically, the typical reactive lymph node is a nearly pure population of lymphocytes in a reactive, polymorphous pattern. If salivary gland tissue is seen, it may show the pattern of COS with the lymphoid cells showing no infiltration of or tropism for the epithelial component.

In early BLEL, glandular structures with adherent and infiltrating lymphocytes are seen. This is an example of the tropism that is commonly seen between the epithelial and lymphoid cells in BLEL. Clusters of degenerating ductal or acinar cells in a background of polymorphic lymphoid cells similar to reactive lymphoid hyperplasia are observed. In advanced BLEL, the pattern is predominantly lymphoid with rare myoepithelial islands seen as tightly cohesive groups of cells with high nuclear to cytoplasmic (N/C) ratios. The lymphoid cells have normal morphologic features except that they occasionally cluster into aggregates that may mimic epithelial groups. Myoepithelial islands can be distinguished both on Romanovsky and Papanicolaou stains by the intense molding and definite cytoplasmic continuity at the edge of the tissue fragments.

NEOPLASTIC SALIVARY GLAND DISEASES

Benign Neoplasms

Hemangioendotheliomas and lymphangiomas (cystic hygromas) occur mainly in children. Hemangiomas are vascular lesions that yield a very bloody sample with rare fragments of tissue composed of tightly coiled small vascular structures. Many samples may be devoid of material other than peripheral blood.

Adenomas

These neoplasms are derived from either the ductal epithelium or myoepithelial cells, although most are a mixture of both.

Pleomorphic Adenoma

Pleomorphic adenoma (benign mixed tumor) is the most common salivary gland tumor and is composed of a mixture of myoepithelial cells with a few ductal-cystic structures and abundant myxoid cartilaginous stroma. Ductal or cystic structures are composed of ductal cells surrounded by many myoepithelial cells. These form sheets or cords that show complex ramification. Solid cords of myoepithelial cells are common and may be mistaken for epithelial cells. The stroma is a loose, blue, bubbly, ground substance containing spindle or stellate (metaplastic) myoepithelial cells. Often, fibrous zones that have scant cellularity or foci of cartilage formation may be present.

Cytologically, both stromal and ductal-cystic structures are seen. The stroma component almost always predominates. The background of the smear is filled with a mucoid or fibromyxoid ground substance that is bright pink or magenta on Romanovsky stain and bluish purple on Papanicolaou stain. Some stromal tissue may have more cellular areas composed of spindle-shaped myoepithelial cells. Cellular, branching cords of myoepithelial cells mimic epithelial fragments. Cartilage is infrequently encountered and usually appears as a deep purple, irregular fragment on Papanicolaou stain. The less frequent ductal-cystic structures are spherical and lie free or are encased in fragments of stroma. Myoepithelial cells can show nuclear atypia: primarily enlargement and nuclear membrane folding. Some of these neoplasms are almost monomorphic populations of myoepithelial cells without other elements. Scattered giant cells can be seen in a few cases.

Monomorphic Adenomas

These rare tumors are composed of cells of a single type, either epithelial or myoepithelial. They may represent an early phase in the development of a mixed tumor. They are most common in the minor salivary glands, followed by the parotid. Clinical features are similar to those of the mixed tumors.

Histologically, most monomorphic adenomas are composed of small, regular oval cells with scant cytoplasm and uniform chromatin similar to that of basaloid cells. These cells form trabecular cords, solid nests, or ductal structures. Areas of squamoid whorls may be present. The connective tissue is collagenous or loose with fine strands and may be acellular.

In aspirates, the basaloid cells shed as fragments and single cells in a monomorphic pattern in which cellular uniformity is striking. The stromal component associated with mixed tumors is absent.

Warthin Tumor

Warthin tumor (papillary cystadenoma lymphomatosum) comprises 6 to 10% of parotid gland tumors and is thought to arise from benign ductal inclusions within lymph nodes situated in or around the parotid, usually in the tail or lower edge of both lobes. These present as a painless, slow-growing, soft, cystic mass in or around the parotid in patients between 40 and 70 years old. They occur mainly in men and rarely in blacks or outside of the parotid gland. In some cases the cystic portion becomes infected, as does a branchial cleft cyst.

Warthin tumors are usually well-defined, encapsulated cystic masses (average size 3.5 cm) that routinely contain a mucoid brown fluid. At times they may be solid. Microscopically, they consist of lymphoid stroma with occasional germinal centers and spaces lined by an oxyphilic double-layered or pseudostratified columnar (oncocytic) epithelium. There is a lower layer of cuboidal to polyhedral cells and an upper layer of tall columnar to clavate cells with mitochondria-rich, bright, eosinophilic cytoplasm on H and E. The nuclei are oval or round and uniform in size. The cystic areas are filled with cellular debris. Infrequently, the epithelium may contain foci of mucus goblet cells or sebaceous cells.

Because the cystic areas contain fluid with debris from degenerating epithelial cells, the aspirate may consist of a fluid material that fills the syringe. This may even appear purulent, as if an abscess were being aspirated. In this instance, material should be retained for microbiologic studies. Sampling should be repeated in an attempt to secure more epithelium and the lymphoid material from the wall of the cystic area. On low power the smears appear very thick because of abundant necrotic debris from the cystic regions of the neoplasm. Suspended throughout the debris are orangeophilic or eosinophilic cells with columnar, cuboidal, or stellate shapes. These are exfoliated, degenerated oncocytic cells. They have uniform, round, degenerated, pyknotic nuclei. Occasionally, small sheets or fragments of columnar cells, seen en face, may be observed.

Neutrophilic leukocytes may also be seen in the necrotic debris. Depending on the amount of lymphoid stroma present, there may be variable numbers of lymphoid cells seen in the background of the smear. This population consists of the same cells seen in reactive lymph node aspirates.

Oncocytic Tumors

Oncocytic tumors (oncocytoma) are very uncommon, accounting for less than 1% of all salivary gland tumors. Although Warthin tumor contains true oncocytic epithelium, it is not classified among the oncocytic tumors because of the presence of a lymphoid component.

Malignant Neoplasms

Mucoepidermoid Carcinoma

Mucoepidermoid carcinoma shows a spectrum of cellular composition, gross appearance, and grades of malignancy. Next to the parotid gland, the most common site for this type of carcinoma is the hard palate.

These malignant tumors comprise a mixture of cell types. The most common is a mucus-secreting columnar cell, but goblet cells, squamous cells, and intermediate cells are also frequently seen. If the tumor is cystic, it contains more mucous cells and is defined as a low-grade neoplasm. Morphologically uniform mucus-secreting columnar and goblet cells predominate, and mitotic activity is low. In some areas of the tumor, squamous epithelium and intermediate cells may line portions of the cysts. Infiltrative growth may be seen. Intermediate-grade lesions are more solid in appearance with more squamous and intermediate cells and areas of unequivocal cellular pleomorphism.

High-grade tumors are characterized by considerable anaplasia, predominantly squamous differentiation, and a solid growth pattern. The mucus-secreting cells may be so uncommon in high-grade tumors that several tissue sections may result in an erroneous diagnosis of squamous cell carcinoma. In these cases a more complete sampling reveals the neoplasm's true character as a high-grade mucoepidermoid carcinoma.

Aspirates from these tumors reflect the histologic picture, but distinguishing low-grade from intermediate-grade and intermediate-grade from high-grade lesions can be difficult. In low- to intermediate-grades, abundant mucus is seen in the background of the aspirate. It appears blue to purple on Papanicolaou stain and pink on Romanovsky stain. It is often associated with foamy histiocytes, cellular debris, and degenerating cells. The mucus-secreting goblet cells and columnar cells are morphologically uniform in a low-grade tumor and predominate in the smear, often as small fragments and monolayered sheets. The mucus-secreting goblet cells may display a signet ring appearance with small, uniform, eccentrically placed nuclei and a foamy, almost perfectly round cytoplasm. Intermediate cells may appear as sheets of small cuboidal or pyramidal cells with regular nuclei and small nucleoli.

Squamous cells are less common in the low-grade tumors but are usually seen in sheets with parabasal cell differentiation and nuclei with single prominent nucleoli. Prominent intercellular bridges may be observed in some cases. Fragments of epithelium may contain tightly packed, intermediate, columnar, or squamous cells in which scattered goblet cells are present. The more clear, spherical goblet cell cytoplasm is distinctive and stands out in the background of smaller cells that have a higher N/C ratio. Nuclear atypia is lacking in the low-grade lesions but is expected in intermediate-grade tumors. High-grade neoplasms have predominantly squamous differentiation with marked pleomorphism, large nuclei, and prominent nucleoli. The cytoplasm is thin and abundant. In mucoepidermoid tumors, squamous epithelium with pearl formation or keratinization is less common than in an aspirate from nonkeratinizing squamous carcinoma. Occasional mucus-containing intracytoplasmic vacuoles within squamoid cells indicate coexistent glandular differentiation.

Adenoid Cystic Carcinoma

Adenoid cystic carcinoma, which probably arises from the intercalated ducts of the peripheral portion of the salivary glands, composes approximately 35% of all minor salivary gland carcinomas and 4% of major salivary gland carcinomas. The tendency for early nerve invasion results in pain and facial nerve paralysis in nearly one third of the patients. Patients may present with localized pain, a vaguely palpable mass, and negative computed tomography (CT) scans.

This neoplasm has two distinctive components: epithelial cells and characteristic stromal material. The epithelial portion consists primarily of uniform small cells with a high N/C ratio (basaloid cells). These cells have oval regular nuclei, appear hyperchromatic, and have a scant amount of cytoplasm. They may occur in solid nests or masses but most often form anastomosing cords, festoons, or gland-like spaces. Equally characteristic is the stroma, which is either hyaline and eosinophilic or myxoid and light blue to purple in appearance on H and E. The stroma is composed of reduplicated basement membrane produced by the cells. Portions of a benign mixed tumor may have small myoepithelial or ductal cells with a hyaline stroma, which may mimic the so-called cylindromatous pattern seen in adenoid cystic carcinoma.

Cytologically, the stroma of this neoplasm is the most striking feature. Large spheres and elongated cylinders of semitranslucent light blue, acellular stroma on Papanicolaou stain are present with scattered uniform cells lightly clinging to the outer surface of the stromal cores. A similar pattern is seen on Romanovsky stains, except the stroma stains a bright pink or magenta. The basaloid cells have uniform, oval, hyperchromatic nuclei with a scant amount of cytoplasm and present as single cells or cells arranged in loose syncytial fragments. Occasionally, they may occur in small rosette-like structures. In aspirates, the epithelial cells are dyshesive, and only a few adhere to the stromal cores.

Acinic Cell Carcinoma

Acinic cell carcinoma (acinous cell carcinoma) probably arises from the terminal portions of intercalated ducts where these cells are known to have the ability to differentiate into the secretory acinous type cell. These are uncommon neoplasms that comprise between 2 and 4% of parotid tumors and are equally rare in other salivary glands. Histologically, the acinar cells grow in solid, tubuloglandular, papillary, microcystic, or acinar-lobular formations. Various degrees of differentiation may be present, but usually the cells have relatively uniform, moderately enlarged nuclei and abundant granular cytoplasm, similar to the secretory cells of salivary gland acini. It is not uncommon to observe a lymphoid infiltrate in the stroma.

Aspiration of these tumors typically yields clusters, loosely formed tubules, acini, or solid groups of cells. There is a lack of fat or ducts in the sample. The cells have many similarities to normal acinar cells, except for nuclear enlargement and some anisonucleosis. The nuclei are usually eccentric in location. The cytoplasm is polygonal, cyanophilic, and granular in appearance on Papanicolaou stain and pale and granular on Romanovsky stain.

Adenocarcinoma

These glandular malignancies cannot be specifically classified with the other carcinomas and usually grow in papillary, tubular, or signet ring cell patterns. Adenocarcinomas exhibit mucin production in most cases. Histologically, they are similar to the adenocarcinomas of the gastrointestinal tract and are composed of columnar cells forming either ductal or papillary structures. Papillary structures may often project into a large cystic lumen.

In aspirate specimens, these tumors resemble quite closely the adenocarcinomas that involve the gastrointestinal tract, with ductal, tubular, and papillary structures formed by mucin-producing columnar cells. A signet ring cell pattern can be also be seen. Pleomorphism is related to the histologic grade.

Undifferentiated Carcinomas

Undifferentiated carcinomas are relatively uncommon in the salivary glands. They are highly malignant carcinomas that have a spectrum of appearances. They are usually seen in patients in the sixth and seventh decades of life, and there is no sex preference. About one third of the cases are superimposed upon a previously diagnosed benign mixed tumor, which may have been present for many years.

The cells are usually poorly differentiated, with high N/C ratios, and form solid or trabecular patterns. Spindle cell types are frequently seen. These tumors are very similar to small-cell undifferentiated carcinoma of the lung and frequently contain neurosecretory granules.

In aspirates, these neoplasms are similar to the histologic pattern. Poorly differentiated cells with scant cytoplasm, moderate to large nuclei, and variable nucleoli are typical. On Papanicolaou stain, the cells are occasionally seen in cohesive groups, and a tumor diathesis is present in the background. On Romanovsky stain, the absence of lymphoglandular bodies may be important to exclude lymphoma.

Uncommon Malignancies

Squamous Cell Carcinoma. Primary squamous cell carcinoma of the parotid gland and other major salivary glands is rare and represents less than 1% of all salivary gland neoplasms. Most believe that these arise from the large excretory ducts. Extensive sampling of every tumor thought to be purely squamous cell carcinoma must be done to exclude high-grade mucoepidermoid carcinoma. One feature besides the lack of mucus production useful in differentiating these tumors is that the squamous component is more likely to show keratinization and pearl formation than is a true mucoepidermoid carcinoma.

Lymphoma. Cervical lymph node involvement is much more common as a presentation of primary lymphoma in the head and neck than is salivary gland involvement. To qualify as a primary lymphoma of the salivary gland, no extrasalivary gland lymph nodes may be involved, and pseudolymphomatous hyperplasia must be ruled out. Large-cell and cleaved cell (small-cell cleaved and mixed) lymphomas comprise over 80% of primary salivary gland lymphomas. Lymphomas may also arise in benign lymphoepithelial lesions. Glands may be massively enlarged and floridly infiltrated with lymphoid cells for years prior to the lymphoma. Although statistics are difficult to assess, it is believed that less than 0.5% of all lymphomas of the head and neck are primary salivary gland lymphomas. The histologic and cytologic appearances are similar to lymphomas in other sites.

MISCELLANEOUS LESIONS OF THE HEAD AND NECK

Cystic Lesions of the Head and Neck

A variety of reasonably common lesions that arise in the head and neck region present as palpable masses and are suitable for aspiration cytology. Many of these lesions are cystic on aspiration and not associated with any specific organ, e.g., salivary gland, lymph node, or thyroid. Since they may require surgical intervention for resolution of the mass and its effects, it is prudent to briefly discuss their clinical and cytologic presentations.

Cystic lesions of the head and neck (excluding thyroid masses) have been evaluated by aspiration cytology for nearly three decades. Specifically, branchial cleft cysts (BCC), thyroglossal duct cysts (TGDC), and epidermal inclusion cysts (EIC) have been encountered and their cytologic presentation described. More recently, lymphoepithelial cyst (LEC) has been described in HIV infected patients. Branchial cleft and thyroglossal duct cysts are congenital cysts. BCCs have their origins in the embryologic branchial apparatus in the lateral neck, just anterior to and below the ear. Most BCCs are situated anterior to the sternocleidomastoid muscle. They usually arise from the second branchial cleft as the result of fistula tract formation during embryologic development. They present as painless, smooth masses usually less than 5 cm in diameter in patients between 10 and 40 years old. TGDCs similarly originate from the failure of the embryologic thyroglossal duct to involute during the sixth and seventh weeks of intrauterine life. They are usually located in the midline of the neck in the region of the hyoid bone but may occasionally extend to a more lateral position. They are typically smaller than BCCs and are seen in patients in the first to third decades of life as painless, slowly enlarging masses.

LECs are cysts that apparently arise from duct inclusions within lymph nodes in the parotid tail area or intraparotid lymph nodes. (This is similar to the origin of Warthin tumor.) LECs are seen in HIV-infected individuals and present as a unilateral or bilateral soft, prominent, painless swelling of the parotid gland. Aspirates consist of clear to slightly cloudy yellow fluid and aspiration results in partial collapse of the lesion. The swelling generally returns within a few days.

Histologically, BCCs are true cysts that are usually lined by squamous epithelium. Ciliated columnar epithelium may also be observed in these cysts and overlies abundant lymphoid tissue frequently with germinal center formation.

TGDCs are lined by either pseudostratified ciliated columnar or squamous epithelium. Thyroid follicles and/or mucous glands are frequently seen in the cyst wall. Occasionally, this epithelial lining may be replaced by histiocytes. A prominent lymphoid wall is also present in most TGDCs. LECs are large, fluid-filled spaces within a lymph node lined by a thin squamoid wall. The lymphoid tissue has a benign reactive pattern.

Cytologically, the fluid from a BCC is usually thick and composed of mature polygonal squamous cells, sometimes with evidence of keratinization. Lymphoid cells may also be observed in aspirates of these cysts but are an infrequent finding. Degenerative changes may occur in these cysts as may inflammatory processes, both of which may produce atypical features in the component cells. Nuclei in the affected cells usually do not have features of malignancy and are small and pyknotic.

This cytologic pattern is similar to that seen in TGDCs except that the epithelial lining cells tend to be scanty and are usually of the glandular type. Ciliated columnar cells are occasionally seen, as are lymphoid cells.

Epidermal inclusion cysts are occasionally aspirated since they present as an undefined mass in the head and neck. Called "sebaceous cysts" for years, these keratinous cysts are lined by cornified squamous epithelium and probably originate in the infundibular portion of hair follicles. Aspirates contain a mixture of degenerated squamous cells and amorphous material, occasionally with inflammatory cells if rupture has occurred. LECs have a "watery" fluid with mainly reactive lymphoid elements. Scattered lymphohistiocytic aggregates (see Chapter 14) are seen. The cyst wall is very attenuated and few or no cells from it may be seen on smears. If seen, these cells appear as spindle or squamoid cells with bland features.

Skin Neoplasms and Metastatic Lesions

Although uncommon, a few skin neoplasms and metastases can be seen in the head and neck region and require differentiation from salivary gland lesions. Four lesions are discussed very briefly (without histologic description) and illustrated.

Pilomatrixoma. This primary skin tumor is most common in the head and neck and is frequently located just over the parotid gland. Being a neoplasm of the germinative hair follicle epithelium, it contains small to intermediate-sized cells with high N/C ratios that can be cytologically interpreted as malignant. Four components are seen: (1) ghost cells from the atypical keratinization, (2) multinucleated giant cells as a granulomatous foreign body reaction to keratin debris, (3) clusters of tightly cohesive germinative epithelium, and (4) isolated cells with a high N/C ratio and bare nuclei from degenerate germinative cells. The latter cells can be mistaken for a poorly differentiated malignancy.

Lymphoepithelial Carcinoma. This malignancy is generally a primary nasopharyngeal squamous carcinoma of limited differentiation that metastasizes to cervical lymph nodes, often as a primary clinical presentation. These small germinative-like epithelial cells can blend into the lymphoid population in an aspirate specimen similar to histology. Cellular cohesion and the monotonous clusters help in differentiating the neoplasm from the reactive lymphoid background.

Basal Cell Carcinoma. This neoplasm is rarely sampled by aspiration. However, the technique can be employed to document a mass recurrence that arises after radiation therapy or under a skin graft. Basal cell carcinomas have a characteristic uniform small-cell population with high N/C ratios, cohesion, and nuclear molding. Many times the groups are so cohesive that only a few large clusters are present with very limited numbers of isolated cells.

Melanoma. Melanoma is very well described in the cytologic literature. Two cases are illustrated here to demonstrate both pleomorphic and uniform cellular patterns. Generally, little cohesion is seen. Binucleation, eccentric nuclei, prominent nucleoli, and intranuclear cytoplasm inclusions are often present. In metastases, melanin pigment is usually absent. If melanin is present, it is much more easily seen on Papanicolaou stain than on Romanovsky stain.

Bibliography

Finfer MD, Gallo L, Perchick A, et al.: Fine needle aspiration biopsy of cystic benign lymphoepithelial lesion of the parotid gland in patients at risk for the acquired immune deficiency syndrome. Acta Cytol 34:821–826, 1990.

Frable WJ: Thin Needle Aspiration Biopsy. Philadelphia: W. B. Saunders, 1983.

Kline TS: Handbook of Fine Needle Aspiration Biopsy Cytology. St. Louis: C.V. Mosby, 1981.

Koss LG, Woyke S, Wlodzimierz O: Aspiration Biopsy. Cytologic Interpretation and Histologic Bases. New York: Igaku-Shoin, 1984.

Linsk JA, Franzen S: Fine Needle Aspiration for the Clinician. Philadelphia: J.B. Lippincott, 1986.

Qizibash AH, Young JEM: Guides to Clinical Aspiration Biopsy, Head and Neck. New York: Igaku-Shoin, 1988.

Woyke S, Wlodzimierz O, Eichelkraut A: Pilomatrixoma: A pitfall in the aspiration cytology of skin tumors. Acta Cytol 26:189–194, 1982.

NORMAL GLAND

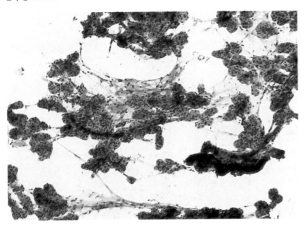

FIGURE 16–1A. Normal Salivary Gland (Parotid). This Papanicolaou stain shows a normal salivary gland, mostly acini, with a few ducts and fatty tissue (× 33).

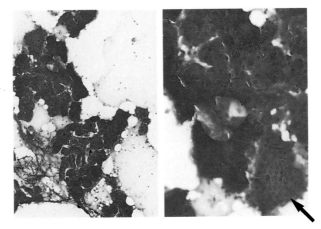

FIGURE 16–1C. Normal Salivary Gland. This Romanovsky stain depicts normal salivary gland tissue. Note on low power the fatty tissue and on high power the acinar units with a small sheet of ductal cells (arrow) (× 25/ × 50).

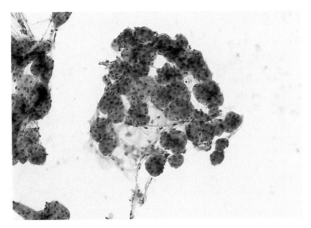

FIGURE 16–1B. Normal Salivary Gland. This intermediate power shows a Papanicolaou stain of acinar cells with some fatty tissue. Notice the loose arrangement of the acini and a few intact fat cells (× 50).

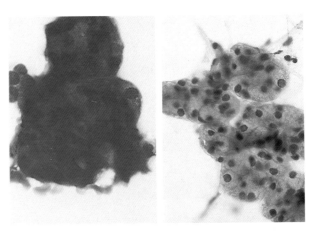

FIGURE 16–1D. Normal Salivary Gland Acini. This figure (Romanovsky and Papanicolaou stains) depicts acinar cells. Note the limited pink stroma around the acini on the Romanovsky stain. On the Papanicolaou stain notice the uniform spherical acini with peripherally placed nuclei and well-defined cytoplasmic borders (× 150/× 150).

CHRONIC OBSTRUCTIVE SIALADENITIS

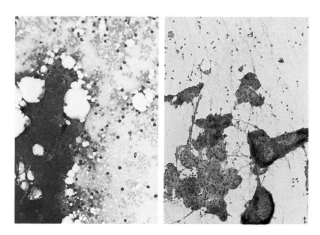

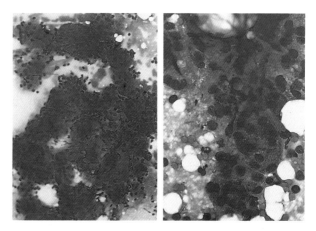

FIGURE 16–2A. Typical pattern of **Chronic Obstructive Sialadenitis**, low power. These Romanovsky and Papanicolaou stains show a background of bare acinar nuclei and clusters of benign-appearing salivary gland tissue. On the Papanicolaou stain, several large dilated ducts are seen, an uncommon finding in a normal salivary gland (Romanovsky stain × 33/Papanicolaou stain, × 50).

FIGURE 16–2C. Chronic Obstructive Sialadenitis with Periacinar Fibrosis. This Romanovsky stain shows the advantages of this stain in defining fibrosis in chronic obstructive sialadenitis. Bands of pink-staining dense connective tissue consistent with fibrosis are seen encircling the acini. In addition, there is a decreased amount of intact fatty tissue (× 50/× 150).

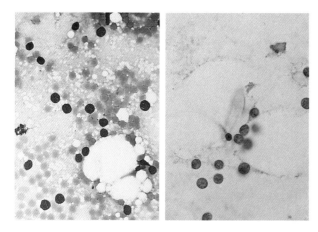

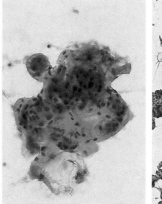

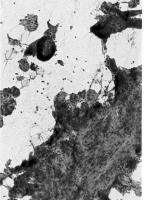

FIGURE 16–2B. Bare acinar nuclei from **Chronic Obstructive Sialadenitis**. These bare nuclei are common in the background of chronic obstructive sialadenitis and may be mistaken for lymphocytes. The Romanovsky stain shows the lack of lymphoglandular bodies seen in a lymphoid population. On the Papanicolaou stain, the chromatin pattern is not typical for a lymphocyte and is typical of acinar cell nuclei (Romanovsky stain, × 150/Papanicolaou stain, × 198).

FIGURE 16–2D. Chronic Obstructive Sialadenitis with Fibrosis. This Papanicolaou stain shows an end-stage chronic obstructive sialadenitis with dense fibrosis entrapping acini. In addition, numerous large sheets of ductal cells and a large fragment of fibrotic salivary gland tissue are seen (× 80/× 33).

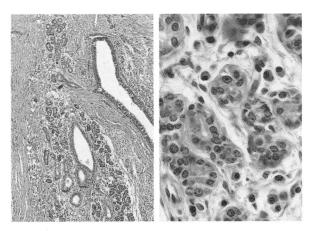

FIGURE 16–3A. Chronic Obstructive Sialadenitis with Fibrosis and Secondary Ductal Cyst. These tissue sections show a hematoxylin and eosin stain of chronic obstructive sialadenitis with dense fibrosis and ectatic, cystic ducts. Note the periacinar fibrosis and minimal chronic inflammation (plasma cells) on the high-power view (× 16/ × 150).

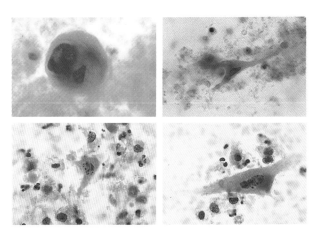

FIGURE 16–3C. Chronic Obstructive Sialadenitis with Secondary Cyst and Sialometaplasia. These photographs depict cells from several cystic lesions that followed an acute sialadenitis. These squamoid cells show "atypia" in a background of acute inflammatory cells, mucus, and crystalline debris (Papanicolaou stain, × 240/× 150/ × 150/×150).

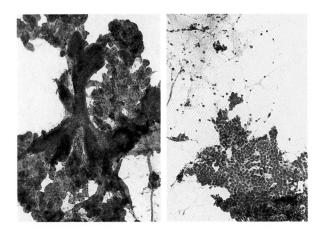

FIGURE 16–3B. Chronic Obstructive Sialadenitis with Duct Ectasia. This aspirate shows periacinar fibrosis with enlarged dilated ducts in one frame and a background of mucus with sheets of ductal cells and occasional mucus goblet cells in the other (× 25/× 40).

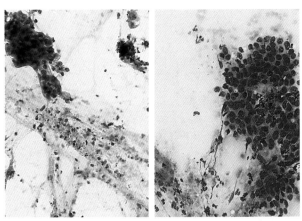

FIGURE 16–3D. Chronic Obstructive Sialadenitis with Mucous Cysts. This aspirate shows Papanicolaou- and Romanovsky-stained sheets of ductal cells in a background of mucus. These specimens were composed of two to four drops of mucoid material that fill the needle hub (× 66/ × 66).

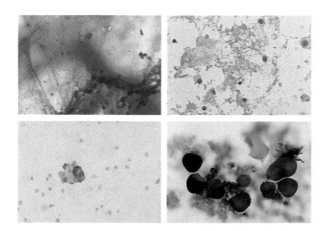

FIGURE 16–4A. Chronic Obstructive Sialadenitis with Mucus, Cysts, and Calcospheres. These figures show mucus on Romanovsky and Papanicolaou stains as well as some calcospheres seen in a cystic lesion. Note: the mucus is often associated with foam cells (Romanovsky stain, × 50/Papanicolaou stain, × 80/Romanovsky stain, × 50/Papanicolaou stain, × 66).

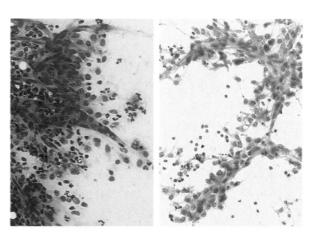

FIGURE 16–4C. Acute Sialadenitis with Microabscess and Granulation Tissue. These Romanovsky and Papanicolaou stains show complex blood vessels and acute inflammatory cells from the walls of a microabscess (× 66/× 66).

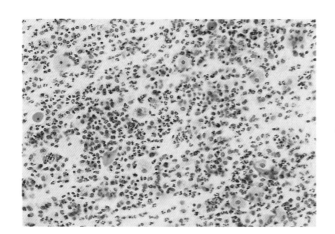

FIGURE 16–4B. Acute Sialadenitis. This aspirate depicts acute inflammation and squamous metaplasia (sialometaplasia) associated with microabscesses in acute sialadenitis (Papanicolaou stain, × 66).

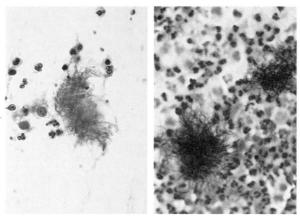

FIGURE 16–4D. Actinomyces and Acute Sialadenitis. This material is from the same case as Figure 16–4C. The Papanicolaou stain shows *Actinomyces* organisms, which were difficult to visualize in many areas. The Gram stain shows typical Gram-positive beaded rods of *Actinomyces* species (× 160/× 160).

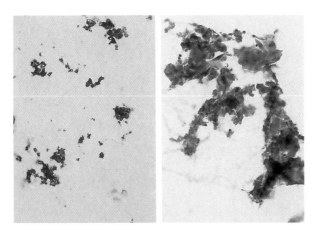

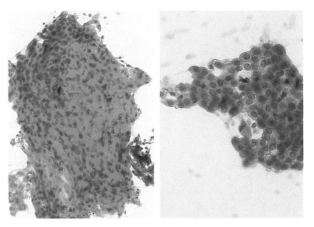

FIGURE 16–5A. Sialolithiasis with Reactive Changes. These Romanovsky and Papanicolaou stains depict calcified material from a stone in the parotid gland. The Romanovsky stain is primarily calcified debris and the Papanicolaou stain shows proteinaceous material with areas of refractile red material representing calcium (× 66/× 66).

FIGURE 16–5C. Sialolithiasis with Reaction. This Papanicolaou stain shows two fragments of tissue: 1) a dense area of squamous metaplasia, and 2) a sheet of glandular cells with numerous goblet cells. These two patterns of tissue are quite similar to that seen in a low-grade mucoepidermoid carcinoma. A reaction such as this necessitates gland excision to make the final diagnosis (× 50/× 100).

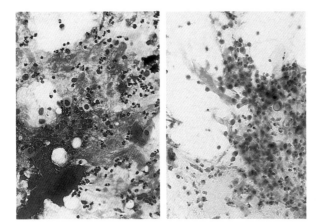

FIGURE 16–5B. Sialolithiasis with Reaction. These Romanovsky and Papanicolaou stains show a mucous background with metaplastic squamous cells, acute inflammation, and intracytoplasmic mucus (× 66/× 66).

BENIGN LYMPHOEPITHELIAL LESION AND LYMPHOEPITHELIAL CYSTS

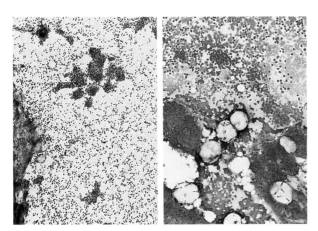

FIGURE 16–6A. Benign Lymphoepithelial Lesion. This photomicrograph depicts a lymphoid background with a few scattered fragments of recognizable salivary gland tissue (Papanicolaou stain, × 33/Romanovsky stain, × 25).

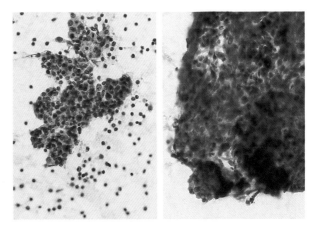

FIGURE 16–6C. Benign Lymphoepithelial Lesion. These Papanicolaou stains depict an aggregate of lymphoid cells and a myoepithelial island. The lymphoid cells are cohesive because of entrapment by stroma (Papanicolaou stain, × 80).

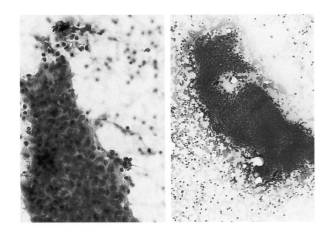

FIGURE 16–6B. These Papanicolaou and Romanowsky stains depict large **Myoepithelial Islands** (× 80/× 25).

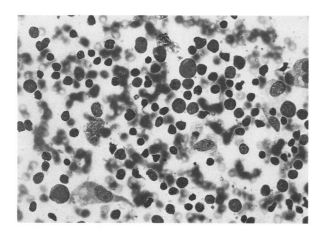

FIGURE 16–7A. Lymphoepithelial Cysts. This aspirate from a patient whose serum was positive for the human immunodeficiency virus shows a typical reactive lymphoid background with scattered histiocytic-appearing cells (Romanovsky stain, × 132).

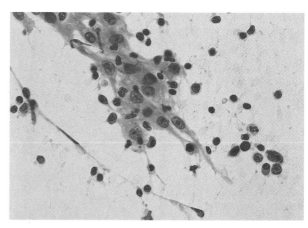

FIGURE 16–7B. Lymphoepithelial Cyst. This field depicts spindle cells, either from stroma or representing reticular cells (histiocytes) from a lymphohistiocytic aggregate (Papanicolaou stain, × 130).

HEMANGIOMA

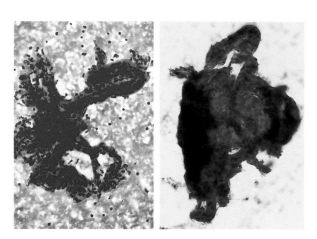

FIGURE 16–8A. Hemangioma. These Romanovsky and Papanicolaou stains show a cluster of coils of small blood vessels in a background of blood. This sample had minimal fragments similar to this, as is characteristic of a hemangioma (× 50/× 50).

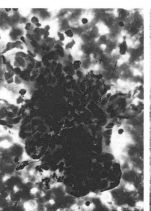
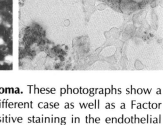

FIGURE 16–8B. Hemangioma. These photographs show a Romanovsky stain on a different case as well as a Factor VIII stain showing the positive staining in the endothelial cell fragments (Romanovsky stain, × 100/Factor VIII, × 250).

WARTHIN TUMORS (PAPILLARY CYSTADENOMA LYMPHOMATOSUM)

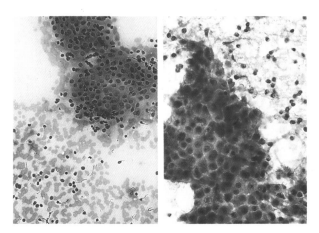

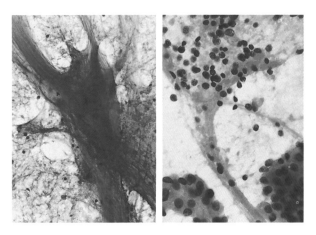

FIGURE 16–9A. Warthin Tumor. This low-power view shows Papanicolaou and Romanovsky stains of the oncocytic epithelium with a background of lymphocytes (Romanovsky stain, × 50/Papanicolaou stain, × 100).

FIGURE 16–9C. Warthin Tumor. This is an example of a Warthin tumor with mucinous material. The left panel is a low-power view of thick mucus strands, and the right panel shows lymphocytes and fragments of oncocytic epithelium (Papanicolaou stain, × 66/× 132).

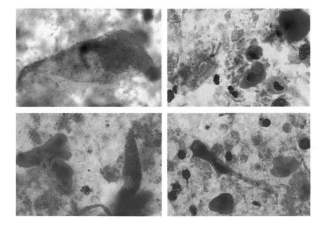

FIGURE 16–9B. Warthin Tumor. This panel shows several areas of the cystic debris from Warthin tumor, which stain variably with the EA portion of the Papanicolaou stain. When less than 8 to 10 minutes in stain is used, the degenerating oncocytes are a granular red in appearance. These cells mimic pleomorphic squamous cells. In these slides such eosinophilic cells are seen. In the left lower panel, a degenerating cell in a smear stained for over 10 minutes shows the slight red granular cytoplasm with a ghost of the nucleus, which appears almost like a hole in the center of the cell. To the left of that cell are other degenerate glandular forms, which stain deep blue with the EA (× 330/× 198/× 198/× 198).

PLEOMORPHIC ADENOMA (BENIGN MIXED TUMOR)

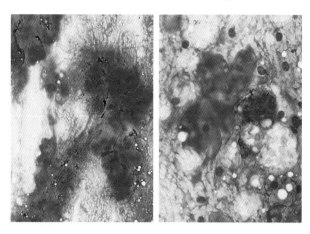

FIGURE 16–10A. Pleomorphic Adenoma. These Romanovsky stains depict the typical appearance of magenta-stained myxoid stroma. This material is so abundant and intensely stained that the cellular components appear very pale unless the staining time is extended (× 25/× 100).

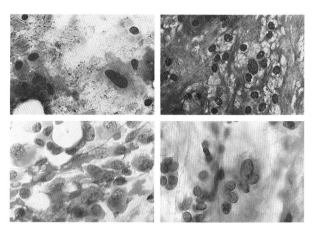

FIGURE 16–10C. Pleomorphic Adenoma with Nuclear Atypia. These Romanovsky and Papanicolaou stains show two cases with nuclear atypia, which is common in this tumor. Generally, the nuclei are enlarged but have a chromatin pattern similar to that seen in normal-sized nuclei (Romanovsky stain, × 100/× 100; Papanicolaou stain, × 150/× 150).

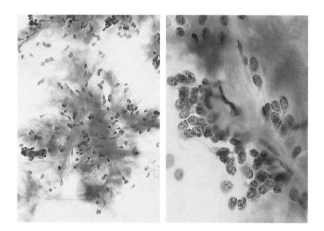

FIGURE 16–10B. Pleomorphic Adenoma. This Papanicolaou stain shows the typical background of violet-stained myxoid tissue with delicate, branching groups of myoepithelial cells (× 50/× 150).

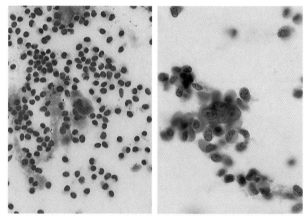

FIGURE 16–10D. Pleomorphic Adenoma with Isolated Cells and Giant Cells. This case depicts a cellular pleomorphic adenoma with numerous isolated myoepithelial cells, some of which are morphologically similar to plasma cells. Occasional giant cells are seen (Romanovsky stain, × 66/Papanicolaou stain, × 150).

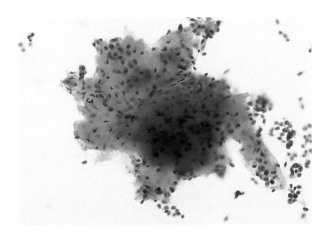

FIGURE 16–11A. Pleomorphic Adenoma with Cartilage. This fragment of cartilage is typical for pleomorphic adenomas but is infrequently observed in aspirate samples (× 66).

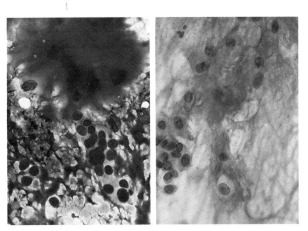

FIGURE 16–11C. Pleomorphic Adenoma with Mucinous Background. This case shows a typical pattern on Romanovsky stain but a more mucinous-appearing background on Papanicolaou stain. This pattern is occasionally seen in this neoplasm (× 132/× 132).

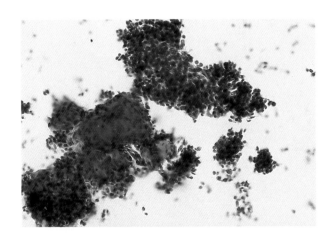

FIGURE 16–11B. Pleomorphic Adenoma with Cellular Areas. This Papanicolaou stain shows cellular groups of myoepithelial cells and some early cartilage formation (× 50).

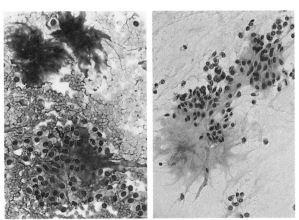

FIGURE 16–11D. Pleomorphic Adenoma with Spindle Cells. Occasionally, the myoepithelial cells of this tumor have a spindle configuration. This is usually more apparent on the Papanicolaou stain (× 66/× 66).

MUCOEPIDERMOID CARCINOMA

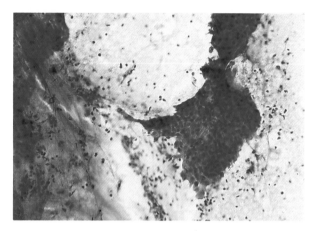

FIGURE 16–12A. Low-Grade Mucoepidermoid Carcinoma. This neoplasm generally presents as a predominantly mucoid specimen with small and large sheets of glandular cells. Histiocytes and isolated degenerating glandular cells and mucous goblet cells are seen in the background (Papanicolaou stain, × 50).

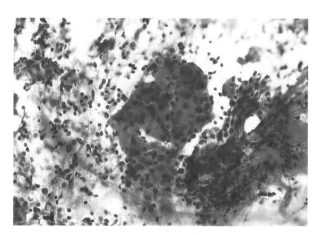

FIGURE 16–12C. Low-Grade Mucoepidermoid Carcinoma. This case depicts a central group of cells showing squamous metaplasia and goblet cells. Dense, intracytoplasmic mucus can sometimes be seen (× 80).

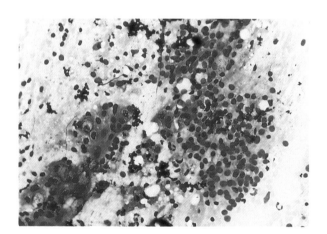

FIGURE 16–12B. Low-Grade Mucoepidermoid Carcinoma. This Romanovsky stain is from the same case as seen in Figure 16–12A. Notice the sheet of bland glandular cells. A group of cells adjacent to this sheet contains goblet cells (× 80).

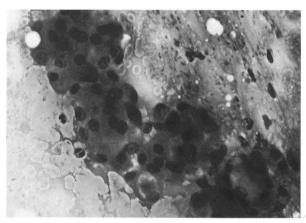

FIGURE 16–12D. Low-Grade Mucoepidermoid Carcinoma. This Romanovsky stain shows clusters of bland glandular cells, some of which are clearly goblet cells (× 132).

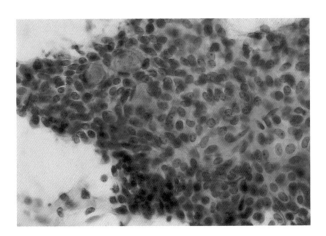

FIGURE 16–13A. Mucoepidermoid Carcinoma, Intermediate Grade. This sample contains tissue fragments from the solid variant of this tumor. Note the higher N/C ratios in some of the cells (intermediate cells) and occasional goblet cells in this fragment (Papanicolaou stain, × 132).

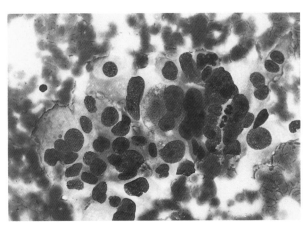

FIGURE 16–13C. High-Grade Mucoepidermoid Carcinoma. This Romanovsky stain shows a pleomorphic fragment of epithelium from a high-grade neoplasm of this type. Note that the cells are clearly malignant and one cell in the center has a magenta cytoplasmic vacuole from mucin production (× 132).

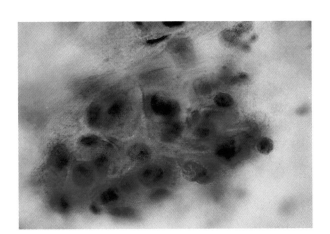

FIGURE 16–13B. Mucoepidermoid Carcinoma, Intermediate Grade. This is a fragment of squamous epithelium from one of these neoplasms. Note the intracellular bridges between these squamous cells and the relatively prominent nucleoli. This is a common finding in this neoplasm (× 330).

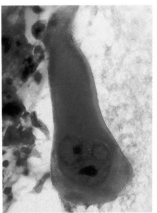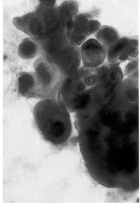

FIGURE 16–13D. High-Grade Mucoepidermoid Carcinoma with Pleomorphic Squamous Forms. These two panels show a Papanicolaou stain of pleomorphic squamous cells from the same neoplasm that was seen in Figure 16–13C (× 132/× 132).

ADENOID CYSTIC CARCINOMA

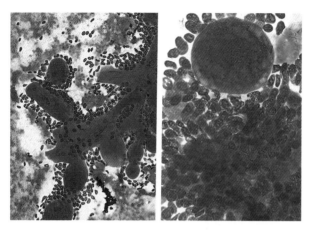

FIGURE 16–14A. Adenoid Cystic Carcinoma. These low- and high-power Romanovsky stains show the characteristic magenta-colored stroma with the small uniform cells that have limited cytoplasm. Note that there are no cells within the stroma, as would be expected with a benign mixed tumor (× 50/× 150).

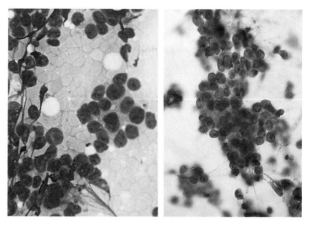

FIGURE 16–14C. Adenoid Cystic Carcinoma, Solid Type. This solid adenoid cyst carcinoma showed very limited stroma. The smears did show a couple areas of stroma but they are not included in these photographs. Note the small clusters of cells with small nucleoli and larger size than seen in the more typical adenoid cystic carcinoma (× 150/× 150).

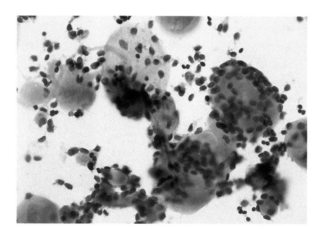

FIGURE 16–14B. Adenoid Cystic Carcinoma. This Papanicolaou stain shows the variable staining of the stroma of an adenoid cystic carcinoma. Note how the cells lack cohesion (× 132).

ACINAR CELL CARCINOMA

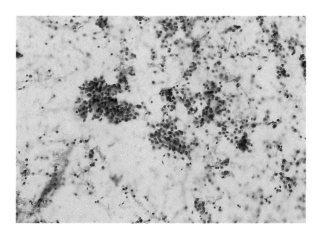

FIGURE 16–15A. Acinar Cell Carcinoma. This low-power Papanicolaou stain shows the ubiquitous cellular population of well-differentiated glandular cells without ducts, fat, or good acinar organization (× 50).

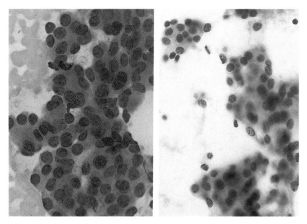

FIGURE 16–15B. Acinar Cell Carcinoma. These Romanovsky and Papanicolaou stains show the high-power pattern of these uniform cells, with eccentric nuclei and abundant cytoplasm. Again note the lack of typical acinar formation and ductal components (Romanovsky stain, × 132/Papanicolaou stain, × 150).

UNDIFFERENTIATED CARCINOMA

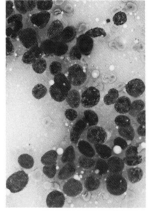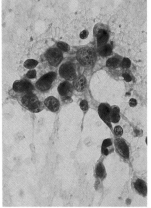

FIGURE 16–16. Undifferentiated Carcinoma. This high-power picture shows the atypical cells of an undifferentiated carcinoma. They are small to medium-sized cells, with the scant cytoplasm associated with some cellular necrosis. Aspirates are often abundantly cellular and necrotic, and only occasional cohesive areas are seen. This type of carcinoma must be differentiated from lymphoma. On Romanovsky stain, the lack of the lymphoglandular bodies is helpful (Romanovsky stain × 132/Papanicolaou stain, × 198).

ADENOCARCINOMA

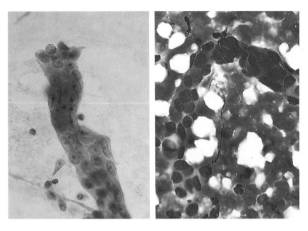

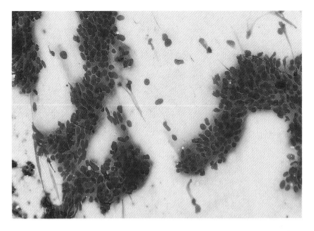

FIGURE 16–17A. Adenocarcinoma, Tubular/Ductal Type. This figure illustrates a case of the more solid-growing tubular or ductal type of carcinoma. These are small-celled carcinomas but have significant nuclear atypia and very abnormal cell growth compared with normal salivary gland ducts (Papanicolaou stain, × 150/Romanovsky stain, × 150).

FIGURE 16–17C. Adenocarcinoma, Papillary Type. This Romanovsky stain shows papillary fragments from an adenocarcinoma (Romanovsky stain, × 50).

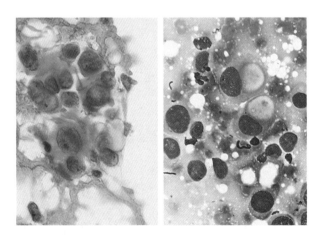

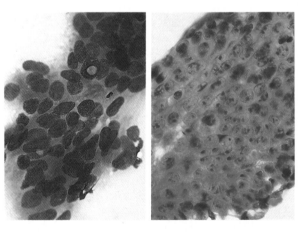

FIGURE 16–17B. Adenocarcinoma, Signet Ring Cell Type. This shows a typical example of a signet ring cell carcinoma, which mainly consists of isolated cells or cells in loose clusters. The cells have cytoplasmic vacuoles and eccentric nuclei. On the Romanovsky stain, purple to pink debris in the vacuoles is typical of mucin (Papanicolaou stain, × 198/Romanovsky stain, × 132).

FIGURE 16–17D. Adenocarcinoma, Papillary Type. Note the oval nuclei, disorganization, and nuclear atypia (Romanovsky stain, × 150/Papanicolaou stain, × 150).

CYSTIC LESIONS IN THE HEAD AND NECK AND SALIVARY GLAND AREA

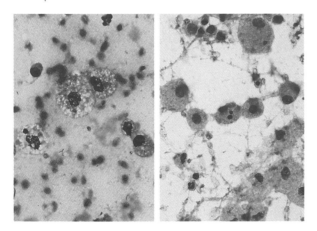

FIGURE 16–18A. Mucocele. These slides show the typical pattern of a mucocele. On both the Romanovsky and Papanicolaou stains, histiocytes are seen with a mucinous background. This mucin may be light staining and somewhat watery, with thicker, more tenacious areas. Grossly, the lesion may partially collapse and have a mucoid character (Romanovsky stain, × 132/Papanicolaou stain, × 132).

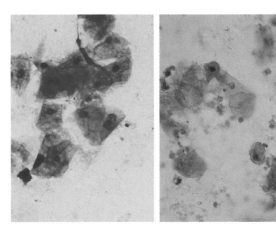

FIGURE 16–18C. Branchial Cleft Cyst. Generally, these are specimens that are milky to mucoid or purulent in appearance. These Romanovsky and Papanicolaou stains show the typical bland squamous cells present in one that is free of inflammation. Generally, these squamous cells are quite large and may be associated with scattered immature metaplastic cells. Most of the squamous cells have intact nuclei. If inflamed, these lesions can have significant squamous atypia, making it difficult to exclude a well-differentiated squamous cancer (Romanovsky stain, × 66/Papanicolaou stain, × 66).

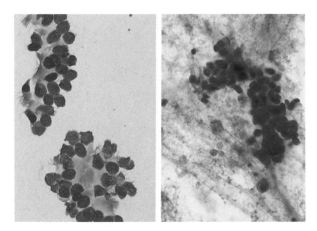

FIGURE 16–18B. Thyroglossal Duct Cyst. These Romanowsky and Papanicolaou stains show cell fragments that are scattered throughout a specimen from a thyroglossal duct cyst. Generally, these are mucoid specimens, either with a background of histiocytes as seen in a mucocele, with limited cellular material, or at times with acute inflammation. Ciliated columnar cells may be found scattered throughout the specimen. In some cases, a squamous cell lining may be encountered. Even with a squamous lining, there is generally a mucoid yellow to clear appearance to the fluid (Romanovsky stain, × 132/Papanicolaou stain, × 132).

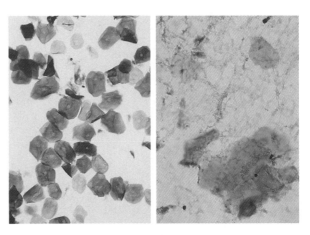

FIGURE 16–18D. Epidermal Inclusion Cyst. These cysts are generally attached to the skin but may be quite deep and overlie the parotid gland and mimic a parotid lesion. When aspirated, they generally have anucleated squames in abundance. Occasionally, a granulomatous reaction may be present as a result of cyst rupture (Romanovsky stain, × 33/Papanicolaou stain, × 66).

MISCELLANEOUS SKIN AND METASTATIC LESIONS IN THE HEAD AND NECK

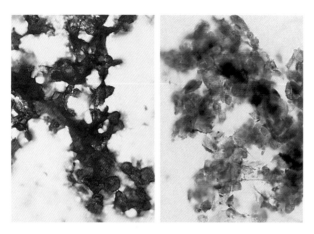

FIGURE 16–19A. Pilomatrixoma. We have seen this lesion overlie the parotid gland on numerous instances, most often in younger patients. Many of the samples contain degenerated ghost squamoid cells, as seen on these photographs. Note the lack of nuclei in these degenerate squamoid forms (Romanovsky stain, × 100/Papanicolaou stain, × 100).

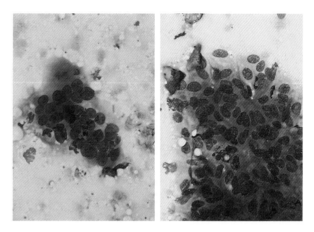

FIGURE 16–19C. Pilomatrixoma. On occasion, giant cells and cells with more generous cytoplasm (basaloid cells) are seen (Romanovsky stain, × 132/Papanicolaou stain, × 100).

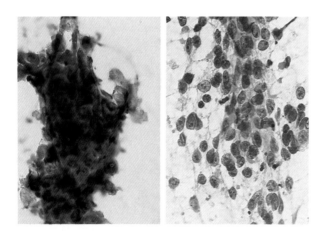

FIGURE 16–19B. Pilomatrixoma. In addition to the changes seen in Figure 16–19A, scattered clusters of epithelial cells, often with very high N/C ratios, may cause significant concern that this is a malignant neoplasm. These are in tight clusters, as seen in one panel, or in loose aggregates, often with degenerate features producing bare nuclei. Areas of necrosis (histiocytes and debris) are common in aspirates of these lesions (Papanicolaou stain, × 132/Romanovsky stain, × 132).

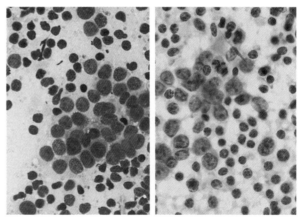

FIGURE 16–19D. "Lymphoepithelial Carcinoma" or Poorly Differentiated Squamous Carcinoma Metastatic to the Lymph Nodes. This shows a typical pattern of a poorly differentiated or so-called undifferentiated squamous carcinoma, metastatic to the head and neck nodes. This tumor was primarily in the nasopharynx. Notice the loose clusters of cells intermingled with the background of reactive lymphoid tissue (Romanovsky stain, × 132/Papanicolaou stain, × 198).

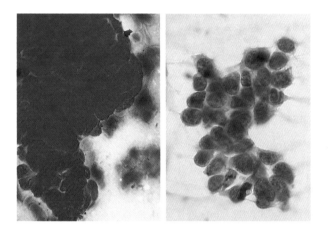

FIGURE 16–20A. Basal Cell Carcinoma. This sample shows a pattern seen in basal cell carcinoma as a recurrent nodule in the skin after radiation therapy for an extensive neoplasm. Note on the Romanovsky stain the very tight clusters of cells with limited cytoplasm. The Papanicolaou stain shows these germative cells with minimal nuclear enlargement and minute nucleoli (Romanovsky stain, × 198/Papanicolaou stain, × 250).

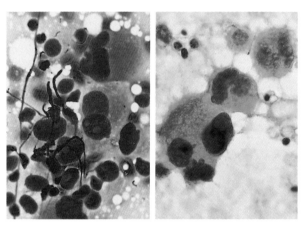

FIGURE 16–20C. Melanoma, Metastatic. Malignant melanoma has the same pattern in metastases as it does in primary neoplasms. The one exception is that metastases often lack pigment. This case shows a more pleomorphic melanoma, with binucleation, intranuclear vacuoles, and abundant cytoplasm with eccentric nuclei (Romanovsky stain, × 198/Papanicolaou stain, × 198).

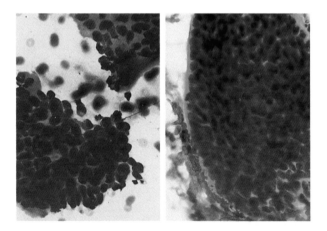

FIGURE 16–20B. Basal Cell Carcinoma. On some neoplasms, the neoplastic cells are in their typical nests on the aspirate, particularly when fibrosis is present (Romanovsky stain, × 132/Papanicolaou stain, × 132).

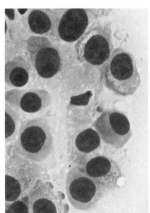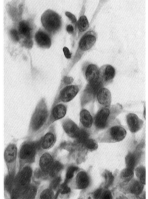

FIGURE 16–20D. Melanoma, Metastatic. These Romanovsky and Papanicolaou stains show a smaller-celled melanoma metastatic to an intraparotid node. Note the eccentric nuclei and large nucleoli on the Romanovsky stain. On the Papanicolaou stain, the cells have a more spindle shape and the nucleoli are not as impressive as on the corresponding Romanovsky stain (Romanovsky stain, × 198/Papanicolaou stain, × 198).

C·H·A·P·T·E·R

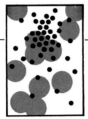

17

FINE NEEDLE ASPIRATION OF SOFT TISSUE AND BONE

L. Patrick James

Tumors and tumor-like lesions of soft tissue and bone represent a diverse group of clinical entities that vary considerably in morphology and biologic potential. Sarcomas, the primary malignancies in these sites, are treated aggressively; therefore, the correct diagnosis and classification of these tumors are essential for proper clinical management. The challenge to the cytologist engaged in the interpretation of aspiration biopsies from these sites is formidable. Establishing the correct diagnosis involves the separation of primary benign and reparative reactions from sarcomas and the distinction of primary lesions from metastatic tumors.

This chapter describes and illustrates the more common and clinically important tumors of soft tissue and bone as revealed in fine needle aspiration biopsy specimens. Guidelines for maximum accuracy and the explicit consideration of major differential diagnoses are emphasized. Following a section on general principles, soft tissue tumors, bone tumors, and metastatic tumors that may simulate a primary malignancy are discussed. The chapter concludes with recommendations on the practice of aspiration biopsy from these sites.

TECHNICAL CONSIDERATIONS

The techniques for obtaining and processing aspiration biopsy specimens from soft tissue are similar to those for specimens from most other body sites. The hard outer cortex of bone precludes use of a usual bore fine needle (22-gauge or smaller). In my experience, the use of trocars or other devices to break through an intact cortex has led to excessive discomfort for the patient and specimens that have been largely unsatisfactory for cytologic evaluation. Unless the cortex is at least partially eroded by the lesion, I do not advise aspiration biopsy. Since many sarcomas are not homogeneous and may be extensively necrotic, thorough sampling is critical in obtaining a representative sample. A minimum of two biopsies per site is recommended.

To a certain extent, preferences for processing and staining techniques reflect personal bias. My preference is to use the Diff-Quik variant of the Romanowsky stain and Gill's modified Papanicolaou stain for smears from all biopsies. I review a Diff-Quik preparation at the time of biopsy to ensure adequacy and to allow judicious allocation of the specimen. For routine preparations, I prefer cytospin preparations from the needle rinsings. If special stains or immunocytochemistry is anticipated, I have found greater stain reproducibility and reliability with the use of cell block preparations instead of smears or cytospins.

DIAGNOSTIC APPROACH

The diagnostic approach to aspiration biopsies from soft tissue and bone is similar for all patients and clinical settings: the correct biologic classification of a mass lesion. The task may be subdivided into the following questions:

1. Is the lesion a benign reactive or reparative process and not a true neoplasm?
2. If the lesion is a neoplasm, is it benign or malignant?
3. If malignant, is the tumor primary to this site or could it be a metastasis?
4. Does the cytologic diagnosis fit clinical and radiographic findings?

This sequential approach helps place diagnostic reasoning in the proper perspective, namely, that primary neoplasms of soft tissue and bone are uncommon. Primary malignant tumors are even less common. Adopt a skeptical approach in most instances; assume that a mass is benign or reactive until cytologic features prove otherwise. If malignant features are present, the possibility of a metastatic pleomorphic tumor should be excluded before entertaining the diagnosis of a primary sarcoma.

FINE NEEDLE ASPIRATION BIOPSY OF SOFT TISSUE

Strictly speaking, the soft tissues include all body sites except bone. By convention, though, soft tissues include supporting tissues such as fibrous connective tissue, fat, muscle, peripheral nerve, and blood vessels. Tumors and tumor-like conditions form a varied group in terms of clinical presentation, morphology, and clinical behavior. Most tumors present clinically as masses detected by either palpation or imaging. Symptoms may not reflect clinical behavior, but worrisome features include rapid growth, location in deep soft tissue compartments, and fixation to surrounding tissues.

The following points are important to keep in mind when dealing with a possible soft tissue sarcoma. Most soft tissue tumors are benign with a benign to malignant ratio of approximately 100 : 1. Metastatic carcinomas to soft tissue are more common than primary sarcomas. With certain exceptions (dermatofibrosarcoma protuberans and epithelioid sarcoma), lesions in the superficial soft tissues are unlikely to be soft tissue sarcomas. The cellularity of the specimen is an important clue to biology. Malignant tumors usually yield richly cellular biopsies. Avoid an unequivocal diagnosis of malignancy without appropriate clinical and radiographic correlation and technically excellent specimens. The cytologic features of most soft tissue sarcomas are rarely so distinctive that differential diagnostic considerations are not important, such as cellular reparative processes and pleomorphic carcinomas. Such tumors are referred to as pseudosarcomas. Common pseudosarcomatous lesions are listed in Table 17–1. Several soft tissue sarcomas display a peak incidence in various age groups. For instance, rhabdomyosarcoma is a tumor of childhood; clear cell sarcoma, epithelial sarcoma, and synovial sarcoma tend to occur in young and middle-aged adults; and malignant fibrous histiocytoma is a tumor of the elderly.

Space limitations preclude a detailed discussion of the tumors that may be encountered from soft tissue sites. My approach is to describe the more common entities grouped into differential diagnostic clusters of spindle cell, pleomorphic, and lipoblastic tumors. This is followed by a review of tumors of skeletal muscle and blood vessels. The degree of necessary diagnostic accuracy in practice largely depends on the clinical circumstances. Documentation of recurrent disease may require only comparison of the aspiration biopsy with prior material, but a newly diagnosed sarcoma may need extensive evaluation with immunocytochemical or electron microscopic studies.

Spindle Cell Lesions

Figure 17–1 shows fibroblasts with a spectrum of reactive features. In benign and reactive conditions, biopsies are sparsely cellular and may contain single fibroblasts with delicate features (Fig. 17–1A) or thick plugs of fibrous connective tissue (Fig. 17–1B). In biopsies from fibromatoses, fibroblasts are often arranged in web-like clusters and display greater nuclear atypia (Fig. 17–1C). Nodular fasciitis is perhaps the most easily recognized pseudosarcoma. The cytologic features of this superficial, rapidly growing reactive lesion are shown in Figure 17–2. Biopsies tend to contain few cells with a predominance of loosely cohesive spindle to epithelioid cells within an inflammatory and edematous background.

Aspiration biopsies from benign nerve sheath tumors display features that overlap with benign fibroblastic reactions. Findings from both schwannomas and neurofibromas are similar and include low cellularity and occasional clusters of bland spindle cells. Schwannomas tend to yield small fragments of spindle cells with indistinct cytoplasm. Figure 17–3A shows one clue to these tumors— twisted, croissant-like nuclei. Verocay bodies are formed by an apparent syncytium of palisaded nuclei and fused flame-shaped cytoplasm (Fig. 17–3B). When present, Verocay bodies represent excellent evidence for the diagnosis of schwannoma.

Neoplasms of fibroblasts exhibit a gradation of atypia and varying degrees of fibrohistiocytic differentiation. Dermatofibroma (Fig. 17–4A) is a common benign dermal tumor that contains both spindle and histiocytic cells. Note the occasional intranuclear cytoplasmic inclusion and abundant hemosiderin pigment. These features may be confused with melanoma.

Dermatofibrosarcoma protuberans (DFSP) is a fibrohistiocytic tumor of borderline malignant potential that usually occurs in the dermis or subcutaneous tissues. Aspiration biopsies are cellular and may contain characteristic pinwheel or storiform arrangements of the spindle cells (Fig. 17–4B). Nuclei are somewhat uniform and delicately hyperchromatic.

Fibrosarcoma is the prototype for spindle cell sarcomas. Aspiration biopsies are cellular, and in lower-grade tumors, many atypical spindle cells may be arranged in dense fascicles (Fig. 17–5A). The malignant cells have elongated, tapered nuclei that are hyperchromatic and irregular (Fig. 17–5B). Cytoplasm is indistinct and offers little diagnostic information.

Kaposi sarcoma (Fig. 17–6A) shares many features with low-grade fibrosarcoma. Helpful discriminating features are a hemorrhagic background and intracytoplasmic hemosiderin pigment in Kaposi sarcoma (Fig. 17–6B).

Leiomyosarcoma may be encountered as a primary tumor in the retroperitoneum, gastrointestinal tract, or pelvis. Similar to fibrosarcoma, aspiration biopsies from this tumor are highly cellular and show fascicular arrangements (Fig. 17–7A). Individual cells, however, display nuclei with rounded contours, and the cytoplasm may be fibrillar with focal metachromasia and perinuclear vacuoles (Fig. 17–7B). Immunocytochemical stains for desmin and smooth muscle actin are usually positive.

Malignant schwannoma and synovial sarcoma also may present as predominantly spindle cell sarcomas. Malignant schwannoma is associated with von Recklinghausen disease and is difficult to diagnose specifically in cytologic preparations. The malignant cells are fusiform and may exhibit a serpentine arrangement (Fig. 17–8). Nuclei are often curved or twisted. Markers for S-100 protein and Leu-7 are positive sometimes. Synovial sarcoma typically arises around the knee and ankle joints in young adults. It is one of the few spindle cell sarcomas that regularly has calcified areas. Both biphasic and monophasic patterns have been described. In aspiration biopsies, the glandular foci in the biphasic form often appear as poorly formed acinar structures (Fig. 17–9A). In my experience, the monophasic spindle pattern is more common and may simulate malignant schwannoma with the presence of curved and twisted nuclei (Fig. 17–9B). Stains for acid mucopolysaccharides, cytokeratins, and CEA may be helpful and allow distinction from other spindle cell sarcomas.

Malignant fibrous histiocytoma (MFH) is the most frequently diagnosed sarcoma and has incorporated tumors previously described as pleomorphic liposarcoma and pleomorphic rhabdomyosarcoma. Several subtypes exist and may be recognized in aspiration biopsies. Figure 17–10A displays the cytologic features of the storiform pleomorphic subtype, which is the most common and characteristic type. The storiform arrangements of spindle cells are similar to those seen with DFSP, but nuclear pleomorphism is more prominent. Figure 17–10B represents biopsy findings from the inflammatory subtype and shows the bizarre malignant histiocytoid cells that are the hallmarks of malignant fibrous histiocytoma. The myxoid subtype (Fig. 17–10C) contains a similar pleomorphic cellular population and also has a distinctive metachromatic myxoid matrix. No currently available immunocytochemical markers are absolutely specific for malignant fibrous histiocytoma, and other pleomorphic tumors, such as melanoma, must be excluded.

Tumors of Fat

Normal adult adipose tissue is a common finding in most aspiration biopsies that traverse body cavities or involve the breast or subcutaneous tissues. The primary cytologic feature of adult fat cells is abundant neutral fat in the cytoplasm. This fat appears as a single vacuole and disperses the delicate nucleus to the periphery of the cell (Fig. 17–11). The major reactive and reparative process in this site is fat necrosis. Like most benign reactions in soft tissue, the cellular yield from aspiration biopsy is low and has an admixture of reactive and regenerating fat cells and macrophages (Fig. 17–12A). In contrast to normal fat, the fat cells in fat necrosis may have large nuclei, prominent nuclei, and multiple cytoplasmic fat vacuoles (Fig. 17–12B). Diagnostic pitfalls include mistaking these regenerating cells for the lipoblasts of liposarcoma or for vesicular cells of other tumors, such as renal cell carcinoma. Lipomas occur in the superficial soft tissues and yield fragments of benign fat cells on aspiration biopsy (Fig. 17–13A). Such fragments cannot be distinguished from normal fat, and clinical correlation is required for the diagnosis. Rare atypical lipomas may contain spindle or multinucleated giant cells. They usually occur in the subcutaneous tissues of the neck and shoulder region of older men.

Liposarcoma is the second most common soft tissue sarcoma in adults. At the time of detection, these tumors are often large and bulky. They arise in the deep soft tissues, most commonly in the lower extremities and retroperitoneum. Current classifications divide liposarcoma into well-differentiated, myxoid, round cell, and pleomorphic subtypes. Well-differentiated liposarcomas are not well described in aspiration biopsy material and probably cannot be consistently recognized at this time. Pleomorphic liposarcoma is indistinguishable from malignant fibrous histiocytoma in routine preparations. The myxoid subtype is the most common and most readily recognized in aspiration specimens. Three features are paramount to the diagnosis: a delicate capillary network, a filmy extracellular matrix, and the presence of lipoblasts (Figs. 17–13B to 17–13D).

Lipoblasts are large cells with variably sized hyperchromatic nuclei and multiple fat vacuoles in their cytoplasm. Nuclei are frequently scalloped by adjacent fat vacuoles. In round cell liposarcoma, the neoplastic cells are smaller and display greater nuclear atypia (Fig. 17–13E). In the absence of lipoblasts, this tumor may not be recognizable as liposarcoma. When lipoblasts contain a single fat vacuole, they may simulate signet ring carcinomas. Differential diagnostic considerations include fat necrosis, chordoma, and mucinous carcinomas. It should be emphasized that special stains for fat are of little help in establishing the diagnosis of liposarcoma. Most tumors of fat show focal staining for S-100 protein.

Other Soft Tissue Sarcomas

Normal skeletal muscle is also not an infrequent finding in aspiration biopsies that penetrate muscle bundles. Figure 17–14A illustrates the characteristic syncytial groupings with prominent cytoplasmic striations and peripherally located bland nuclei. Regeneration and repair in skeletal muscle typically follow trauma and are usually only sampled by aspiration biopsy when they create a deep-seated mass. In Figure 17–14B, a cluster of atypical fusiform cells displays central cytoplasmic fusion and atypical nuclear features. This biopsy was from a mass in the psoas muscle that developed after a skiing accident. The keys to the diagnosis of skeletal muscle repair were the very sparse cellularity and cells in the smears that showed evidence of progressive maturation toward normal muscle (Fig. 17–14C). Subsequent radiographs documented complete resolution over a three-month period.

With the virtual elimination in recent years of the diagnosis of pleomorphic rhabdomyosarcoma, the diagnosis of rhabdomyosarcoma beyond the pediatric age group has become a rarity. Two subtypes have been described: embryonal and alveolar rhabdomyosarcoma. Although differences between the types exist both in their morphology and clinical behavior, this chapter focuses on their overlapping cytologic characteristics. Aspiration biopsies from these tumors are cellular. Although small cells may predominate, there is usually an admixture of larger cells with myoblastic differentiation and scattered multinucleated giant cells (Fig. 17–15A). The binucleate cell in Figure 17–15B shows nuclear polarity, nuclear atypia, and focal cytoplasmic metachromasia; these findings overlap with regeneration and repair. The diagnoses can be distinguished by the cellularity of the specimen and the association with the small tumor cells of rhabdomyosarcoma. A number of immunocytochemical markers such as desmin are available to demonstrate myogenic differentiation (Fig. 17–15C).

Tumors derived from blood vessels are among the most frustrating of the soft tissue group for the cytologist to identify. This frustration is due in large part to the lack of specific features of vascular differentiation in most biopsy specimens. Hemangiomas are the most common vascular tumors. They usually arise in superficial soft tissues and the liver. Aspiration biopsies usually yield the nonspecific findings of abundant blood and rare spindle and polygonal cells (Fig. 17–16A). Intact, dilated vessels are a helpful but inconsistent finding. Like lipoma, the diagnosis of hemangioma by aspiration biopsy requires clinical correlation.

Angiosarcoma is a highly malignant sarcoma that arises in the liver, breast, and subcutaneous tissues of the elderly. The histologic hallmark of angiosarcoma is the formation of irregular vascular channels lined by atypical endothelial cells. Immunocytochemical stains for Factor VIII antigen may be helpful. Aspiration biopsies are hemorrhagic and cellular. The malignant endothelial cells are arranged in loosely cohesive clusters that are usually admixed with erythrocytes (Fig. 17–16B). Large oval nuclei with prominent nucleoli are characteristic. Cytoplasm may be angular (Fig. 17–16C) and offers no specific features of differentiation at the light microscopic level. Hemangiopericytoma may simulate angiosarcoma in aspiration specimens. This sarcoma occurs in the deep soft tissues, most commonly in the lower extremities. Smears are hemorrhagic and contain loose clusters of cells similar to angiosarcoma. Individual cells tend to be smaller and have more of a fusiform contour (Fig. 17–16D). Both of these sarcomas are difficult to diagnose specifically by aspiration biopsy.

Epithelioid sarcoma is an insidious tumor that violates many of the generalizations about sarcomas. It is a tumor of the superficial soft tissues that usually forms multiple nodules rather than a large bulky mass. The histologic features are bland and may mimic necrotizing granulomatous inflammation. The clinical course tends to be protracted but relentless. In aspiration smears, atypical polygonal and epithelioid cells are often clustered around metachromatic necrotic material (Fig. 17–17A). Binucleate cells are common, and multinucleated giant cells are an occasional finding (Fig. 17–17B). The cytologic similarities to granulomatous inflammation are obvious. The tumor should be suspected in aspirations that appear granulomatous from the extremities of young adults. Stains for epithelial markers such as cytokeratins are usually positive in epithelioid sarcoma and may be crucial in establishing the diagnosis.

A final topic regarding aspiration biopsy of soft tissue tumors relates to the sarcomas created in the laboratory. Figure 17–18A shows an apparent fascicular arrangement of malignant spindle cells similar to many of the sarcomas already discussed. Figure 17–18B displays the true cytologic features of this small-cell carcinoma. Any carcinoma with delicate cytoplasm may be artifactually transformed into a pseudosarcoma by excessive pressure during preparation of smears.

FINE NEEDLE ASPIRATION BIOPSY OF BONE

Because of the many cell types in normal bone, lesions affecting it are many and varied. With the exception of lymphoma and myeloma, lesions of the hematopoietic system are not discussed. Only those metabolic diseases producing a mass are mentioned. Bone is a favored site for metastatic tumors. Indeed, approximately 80% of clinically apparent bone tumors are metastatic rather than primary. Most of these metastases are derived from carcinomas of the breast, prostate, lung, kidney, and thyroid. The number of primary bone tumors may seem overwhelming, and the difficulty is compounded by a confusing nomenclature. My approach organizes these tumors into categories associated with matrix production (bone or cartilage) and cell size (giant cell tumors of bone and small-cell tumors). As with soft tissue, the discussion begins with some general principles followed by a discussion of normal bone and reactive and reparative conditions.

Correlation with clinical and radiographic findings is even more critical with tumors of bone. A review of the relevant imaging studies should be considered a routine part of the preparation for a biopsy. This review is essential in selecting appropriate sites for biopsy to avoid necrotic areas and regions of periosteal reaction. Knowledge of the patient's age and the location and radiographic features of a tumor usually limit diagnostic considerations to three or four entities. The radiographic characteristics of the more common benign primary bone tumors such as nonossifying fibroma and osteochondroma are so typical that usually biopsy confirmation is unnecessary. Imaging studies also provide an important quality assurance check for the cytologic diagnosis.

Normal Bone

Bone is important for support, mineral homeostasis, and hematopoiesis. Osteoblasts are cells responsible for the production of the extracellular matrix called osteoid. When this matrix is mineralized, it becomes bone, and osteoblasts mature into osteocytes. Osteoblasts may be encountered in many reactive and reparative lesions of bone as well as in primary bone tumors. Figure 17–19A depicts a group of reactive osteoblasts from an aspiration biopsy of a fracture site. The biopsy needle strips these cells from their alignment along osteoid seams, and they tend to appear in loose aggregates or picket-fence arrangements in smears. Note their marked nuclear polarity and abundant cytoplasm with an eccentric zone of clearing, which corresponds to a well-developed Golgi complex. These cells may be confused with plasma cells. Osteoblasts are distinguished by their tendency to occur in groups and to have a larger size, columnar orientation, and zone of cytoplasmic clearing, which tends to be located further from the nucleus. Osteoid is sharply defined and brilliantly metachromatic in Romanowsky-stained smears (Fig. 17–19B). Its density and woven texture set it apart from chrondroid matrix.

Hematopoietically active bone marrow is diffuse in children but usually limited to the axial skeleton and proximal femur and humerus in adults. Cells of the erythroid, myeloid, and megakaryocytic cell lines proliferate and mature in these sites. When these areas are sampled by fine needle aspiration, a polymorphous population of immature cells may result (Fig. 17–20A). Recognition of a maturation sequence and characteristic cellular types like megakaryocytes (Fig. 17–20B) helps avoid a false-positive diagnosis of malignancy. Despite their large hyperchromatic nuclei, well-preserved megakaryocytes can readily be distinguished from metastatic large-cell tumors (Fig. 17–20C). Osteoclasts (Fig. 17–21) are other giant cells that must be distinguished from malignant and granulomatous lesions. These multinucleated giant cells are important in bone remodeling and mineral homeostasis. They are encountered in small numbers as a reaction to metastatic tumor and may be the dominant cell in hyperparathyroidism and giant cell tumors of bone.

Bone possesses tremendous powers of regeneration. Osteoblasts are usually the most numerous cells with variable contributions from osteoclasts and fibroblasts. A number of lesions may lead to repair in bone. Trauma, infection, and reaction to tumor are some of the more common ones. In aspiration specimens, these reparative reactions may be termed osteoblastic reactions with features similar to those seen in Figure 17–19A. Clues to the etiology rest with other cells present in the smears.

Both benign and malignant primary tumors of bone show a remarkable tendency to occur in certain age groups and in specific locations. Osteosarcoma, chondrosarcoma, Ewing sarcoma, and malignant giant cell tumors comprise the bulk of malignant bone tumors. Osteosarcoma tends to occur in the long bones during the most active periods of skeletal growth—childhood and adolescence. It arises in the metaphyseal region of long bones. Ewing sarcoma, possibly a primitive neuroectodermal tumor, arises in the diaphysis or shaft of long bones in young adults. Chondrosarcoma and giant cell tumors of bone occur during middle age. Chondrosarcoma commonly arises in the pelvis or metaphysis of long bones. The favored site of origin for giant cell tumors is the end or epiphysis of long bones in the extremities. Figure 17–22 summarizes the location of the more common tumors of bone. This tendency of tumors to occur in well-defined locations during specific periods of skeletal maturation has been termed the "field theory of bone tumors" and is an extremely powerful tool for defining differential diagnostic considerations.

Fibrous dysplasia is a benign lesion of bone that may be encountered in aspiration specimens. This lytic-appearing mass probably reflects abnormalities in remodeling of bone and may lead to fractures and confusion with metastatic carcinoma. Dense fibrous connective tissue and poorly formed woven bone are characteristic features. Aspiration biopsies (Fig. 17–23) are sparsely cellular and contain aggregates of reactive fibroblasts and collagen. Usually, fragments of bone are not present in aspiration smears. Cytologic findings are quite similar to the fibromatoses seen in soft tissue sites.

Osteosarcoma

Osteosarcoma is second only to multiple myeloma as the most common primary malignant tumor of bone. It is a highly malignant tumor whose pleomorphic morphology usually underscores its biology. Figure 17–24 illustrates the many facets of this tumor as seen in aspiration specimens. In addition to the presence of atypical cells with osteoblastic differentiation, osteoid is required to establish the primary diagnosis of osteosarcoma. Figures 17–24A and 17–24B display osteoid as seen in Romanowsky- and Papanicolaou-stained smears. Notice that textural features are more clearly detailed with the Romanowsky stains, and there is less obscuring of cellular detail by the osteoid. Polygonal and spindle cells predominate in most osteosarcomas (Figs. 17–24C and 17–24D). Parosteal osteosarcoma is a well-differentiated subtype that is associated with a better prognosis (Fig. 17–24E).

Chondrosarcoma

Chondrosarcoma is the next most common sarcoma of bone in most series. This tumor is distinct from osteosarcoma in several respects: it affects older patients, more commonly originates in the axial skeleton, and has a better prognosis. Because the tumor is soft and gelatinous, it presents less of a technical challenge in obtaining an adequate biopsy sample by aspiration. Chondrosarcomas tend to be large, bulky, lobulated masses at the time of diagnosis. Figure 17–25 presents a composite of the cytologic features of chondrosarcoma. Observe that the chondroid matrix has a less distinct, filmy appearance compared with osteoid, and the density of staining varies throughout the smear (Figs. 17–25A and 17–25B). In general, the cells of chondrosarcoma display less pleomorphism than do those of osteosarcoma, and their cytologic features overlap with benign cartilaginous tumors such as enchondroma. Less well-differentiated tumors (Figs. 17–25C and 17–25D) show obvious malignant features and must be differentiated from other myxoid tumors such as chordoma and metastatic renal cell carcinoma.

Several variants of chondrosarcoma exist. The myxoid subtype is one of the most distinctive in aspiration specimens (Fig. 17–25E). The initial diagnosis of chondrosarcoma should be made with great caution and only when the clinical, radiographic, and cytologic features are all consistent with that diagnosis. An additional hazard with chondrosarcoma is that a slimy matrix may lead to seeding of the needle track if a large needle or poor technique is used for the aspiration biopsy.

Chordoma is a primary tumor of bone that closely mimics chondrosarcoma in aspiration specimens. This low-grade sarcoma is derived from notochord remnants and arises most commonly in the skull and sacrum. The cytologic findings include a delicate myxoid matrix that contains lobules and syncytial arrangements of large vacuolated cells (Fig. 17–26). These bubbly physaliperous cells contain voluminous cytoplasm and eccentric nuclei that often lack significant pleomorphism. Depending on cytoplasmic features, these cells may resemble signet ring cells or the lipoblasts of liposarcoma. Like chondrosarcoma, chordoma usually stains for S-100 antigen but also stains for epithelial markers such as cytokeratin and epithelial membrane antigen in many cases.

Round Cell Tumors of Bone

Less common than osteosarcoma and chondrosarcoma, Ewing sarcoma is the prototype for highly malignant round cell tumors that may affect bone. This tumor may arise in any bone but has an affinity for the diaphysis of long bones. It is typically a tumor of adolescence and young adulthood. Unlike the previously discussed sarcomas of bone, the cells of Ewing sarcoma are not associated with an extracellular matrix and usually are arrayed in cohesive, epithelial-like clusters. Figure 17–27 shows typical cytologic features. The specimens from aspiration biopsies tend to be cellular, with cells arranged in rosettes, irregular clusters, and singly. Nuclear molding, hyperchromasia, and scanty indistinct cytoplasm are the cytologic hallmarks of Ewing sarcoma. Nuclear size and shape are often described as round and monotonous, but there may be considerable variation in individual cases (Fig. 17–27B). The presence of cytoplasmic glycogen (Fig. 17–27D) and the age of the patient help distinguish Ewing sarcoma from metastatic neuroblastoma.

Of the primary hematopoietic malignancies of bone, only lymphoma and myeloma are discussed in this chapter. Their inclusion is deserved because they form mass lesions and enter into the differential diagnosis of small round cell tumors of bone. Primary lymphoma of bone is uncommon and typically affects older adults. Primary lymphomas of bone are often B-cell lymphomas of the large cleaved and noncleaved types (Fig. 17–28). Single cells predominate in aspiration biopsies, and nuclear irregularities are more common than in Ewing sarcoma. A panel of immunocytochemical markers is useful to establish a definitive diagnosis. Myeloma is the most common primary solid tumor of bone. This is a tumor of older adults that shows a predilection for the axial skeleton and ribs. Aspiration biopsies yield cellular samples with a heterogeneous collection of polymorphous plasma cells (Fig. 17–29). A relatively pure population of plasma cells and the presence of atypia permit separation of myeloma from chronic osteomyelitis. Immunocytochemical stains for kappa and lambda light chains are helpful and can document the monoclonality of the tumor.

The nonlipid histiocytoses and Hodgkin disease are often included in the differential diagnosis of round cell tumors of bone. Both of these lesions contain a population of inflammatory cells in which eosinophils may be numerous and are characterized by a specific type of giant cell. Eosinophilic granuloma is the most common histiocytosis of bone. This lesion occurs in adolescents and young adults. Favored sites are the flat bones of the skull, spine, and ribs. True granulomas are not found; rather, Langerhans histiocytes and eosinophils comprise the cellular population. The Langerhans histiocyte contains abundant cytoplasm and an oval or reniform nucleus that has one or more clefts or indentations (Fig. 17–30A). These histiocytes stain for the S-100 antigen, and electron microscopy discloses the characteristic Birbeck granule. Hodgkin disease is the most important diagnostic consideration and can be separated from eosinophilic granuloma when classical Reed-Sternberg cells are present (Fig. 17–30B). These cells possess large atypical nuclei that may be bilobate and prominent nucleoli.

Giant Cell Tumor of Bone

Giant cell tumor of bone is one of the few tumors that originates in the epiphyseal region of long bones. Most of these tumors occur in middle adulthood. Of all bone tumors, the biology of giant cell tumors is the most difficult to predict. This tumor presents a particularly difficult diagnostic challenge because many benign and malignant lesions of bone may contain a large complement of giant cells. Figure 17–31A shows the numerous multinucleated, osteoclast-like giant cells that form the major diagnostic criterion for this tumor. These giant cells often have the appearance of budding from delicate fibrovascular cores. Smaller mononuclear cells form the second cellular population and complete the classic biphasic appearance of this tumor. Their nuclei are delicate and frequently cleaved (Fig. 17–31B). This tumor must be distinguished from the brown tumor of hyperparathyroidism, which can be accomplished by correlation with clinical laboratory studies and the location of the lesion within bone. Other tumors that may contain large numbers of giant cells include chondroblastomas, aneurysmal bone cysts, and giant cell sarcomas. In the absence of typical clinical and radiographic features, most giant cell lesions may be best characterized in aspiration specimens as giant cell reactions and tissue studies are pursued.

Metastatic Tumors to Bone

When considering the diagnosis of a primary malignancy in bone, it is imperative to exclude the much more likely possibility of metastatic carcinoma. Common tumors such as carcinomas of the lung, breast, or prostate commonly metastasize to bone. Frequently, the clinical setting and radiographic features point to the correct diagnosis. Figure 17–32 illustrates cells aspirated from an osteolytic lesion in the metaphysis of the humerus in an elderly male. The location of the tumor and the degree of pleomorphism suggest the possibility of osteosarcoma. The age of the patient, radiographic features, and the presence of cohesive arrangements of the cells point to the correct diagnosis of metastatic carcinoma. An occult primary tumor was detected in the lung.

Less common tumors may show a remarkable tendency to metastasize to bone. For some patients, this may be the first manifestation of malignancy. Tumors from the kidney, thyroid, or gastrointestinal tract and melanoma may display this behavior. Renal cell carcinoma (Fig. 17–33) mimics cartilaginous tumors and myxoid malignancies such as chordoma. In most instances, routine preparations and clinical correlation are sufficient. In some cases, immunocytochemical panels for epithelial markers are extremely helpful in defining the correct diagnosis.

CONCLUSION

This chapter has surveyed the major categories of lesions encountered in fine needle aspiration biopsy of soft tissue and bone. My review illustrated only the major diagnostic considerations and their principal differential diagnoses. Brief consideration about the proper role of aspiration biopsy in these sites is a fitting way to conclude the discussion.

In the cytologic literature, rates for diagnostic specificity and sensitivity are usually quoted in the 80% range or better for aspiration biopsy specimens from soft tissue and bone. Perhaps a better approach to gauge the effectiveness of this tool is to compare results with clearly identified objectives. If an objective is to use aspiration to document the presence of tumor recurrence or metastases from previously diagnosed sarcomas, the task is relatively straightforward and requires careful evaluation and comparison with previous tissue studies. A greater challenge involves determining the basic biology—benign or malignant—of a newly discovered lesion in soft tissue or bone. If this determination can be made, further definitive classification then awaits additional tissue studies. The most daunting task confronts the cytologist who attempts to make a definitive diagnosis upon which therapy may proceed. Despite the emergence of powerful aids to morphologic diagnosis, this role for aspiration biopsy in these sites is controversial and is not recommended outside the realm of metastatic tumor or the diagnosis of multiple myeloma.

Bibliography

Akerman M, Rydholm A, Persson BM: Aspiration cytology of soft-tissue tumors. Acta Orthop Scand 56:407–412, 1985.
Enzinger FM, Weiss SW: Soft Tissue Tumors, 2nd ed. St. Louis: Mosby, 1988.
James LP: Cytopathology of mesenchymal repair. Diagn Cytopathol 1:91–104, 1985.
Koss LG, Woyke S, Olszewski W: The bone. In Koss LG, Woyke S, Olszewski W (eds.): Aspiration Biopsy. Cytologic Interpretation and Histologic Bases. New York: Igaku-Shoin, 1984, pp 422–441.
Layfield LJ, Anders KH, Glasgow BJ, Mirra JM: Fine needle aspiration of primary soft tissue lesions. Arch Pathol Lab Med 110:420–424, 1986.
Mirra JM: Bone Tumors. Philadelphia: Lea and Febiger, 1989.

Table 17–1. PSEUDOSARCOMAS OF FIBROUS CONNECTIVE TISSUE

Tissue	Age	Site	Differential	Keys
Nodular fasciitis	20–50 years	Extremities	Fibrosarcoma Malignant fibrous histiocytoma	Cellularity
Proliferative fasciitis	>50 years	Extremities	Fibrosarcoma Malignant fibrous histiocytoma	Cellularity, giant cells
Fibrosis	Any age	Any site	Fibromatosis Fibrosarcoma	Cellularity, uniformity
Spindle cell carcinoma	Adults	Head and neck	Spindled sarcomas	Cohesion markers
Giant cell carcinoma	Adults	Any site	Pleomorphic sarcomas	Cohesion markers
Melanoma	Adults	Any site	Pleomorphic sarcomas	Melanin markers
Lymphoma	Any age	Any site	Small-cell sarcomas	Markers

BENIGN CONDITIONS

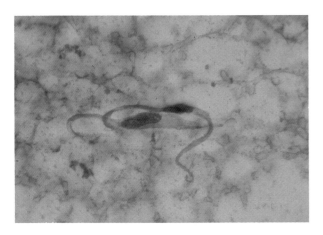

FIGURE 17–1A. Reactive Fibroblasts. Two spindled fibroblasts with mild variation in nuclear size and delicate chromatin pattern (Papanicolaou stain, × 225).

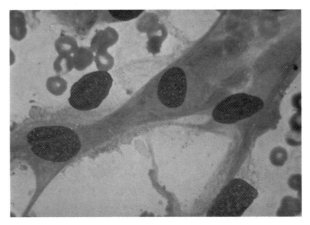

FIGURE 17–1C. Reactive Atypical Fibroblasts. Aspiration from fibromatosis. Low cellularity with reticular arrangement of fibroblasts that exhibit nuclear enlargement and a coarse chromatin pattern (Diff-Quik, × 400).

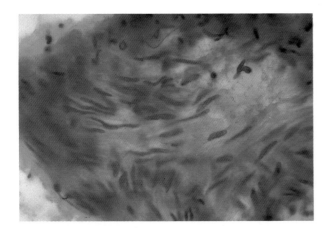

FIGURE 17–1B. Reactive Fibroblasts. Thick aggregate of reactive fibroblasts. Tapered wavy nuclei are set within indistinct cytoplasm and collagen (Papanicolaou stain, × 160).

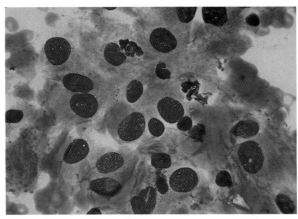

FIGURE 17–2. Nodular Fasciitis. Cluster of plump reactive fibroblasts and inflammatory debris (Diff-Quik, × 630).

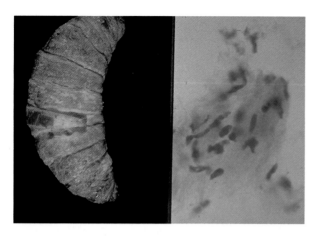

FIGURE 17–3A. Schwannoma. Low cellularity, tight clusters, and elongated, twisted, croissant-like nuclei characterize benign tumors of nerve sheath. As seen in the right hand figure, the nuclei resemble croissants (see left-hand figure). (Papanicolaou stain, × 400).

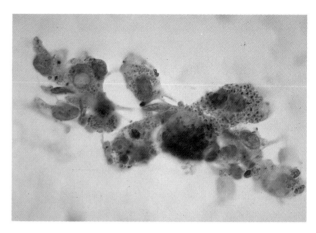

FIGURE 17–4A. Dermatofibroma. Admixture of bland fibroblastic and histiocytic cells with prominent intracytoplasmic hemosiderin pigment (Papanicolaou stain, × 225).

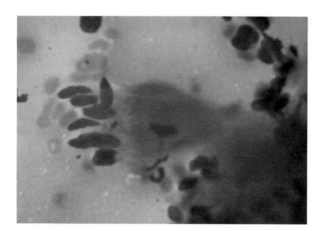

FIGURE 17–3B. Verocay body in **schwannoma**. Alignment of plump spindle nuclei and fusion of cytoplasm into a flame-shaped mass (Diff-Quik, × 630).

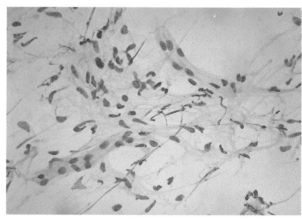

FIGURE 17–4B. Dermatofibrosarcoma Protuberans. Cellular aspirate with cohesive fascicular arrangement of atypical fibroblasts (Papanicolaou stain, × 160).

MALIGNANT TUMORS

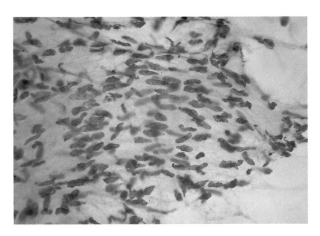

FIGURE 17–5A. Fibrosarcoma, grade 1 of 3. Cellular field with disorganized atypical spindle cells (Papanicolaou stain, × 225).

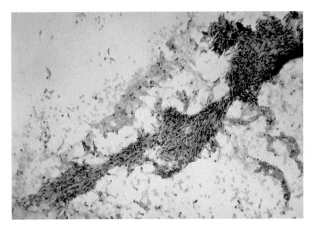

FIGURE 17–6A. Kaposi Sarcoma. Cellular fragments of spindle cells within a hemorrhagic background (Papanicolaou stain, × 100).

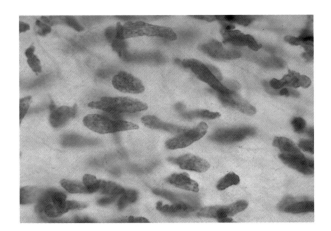

FIGURE 17–5B. Fibrosarcoma, grade 1 of 3. Field is dominated by coarsely hyperchromatic and irregular nuclei. Cyanophilic cytoplasm is indistinct (Papanicolaou stain, × 630).

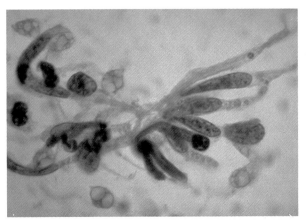

FIGURE 17–6B. Kaposi Sarcoma. Cartwheel-like formation of atypical spindle cells. Note hemorrhagic background and intracytoplasmic hemosiderin pigment (Papanicolaou stain, × 630).

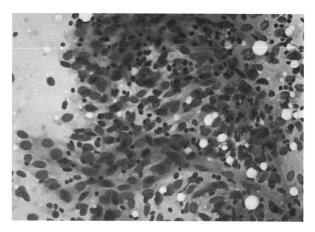

FIGURE 17–7A. Leiomyosarcoma, grade 2 of 3. Extremely cellular fragment of haphazardly arrayed spindle cells (Diff-Quik, × 225).

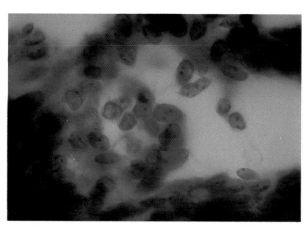

FIGURE 17–9A. Synovial Sarcoma, biphasic pattern. Organoid arrangement of moderately sized polygonal cells characterize the epithelial component of this tumor (Papanicolaou stain, × 630).

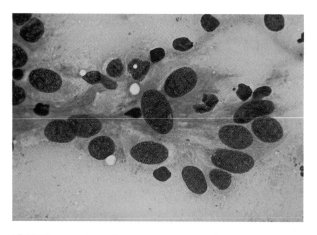

FIGURE 17–7B. Leiomyosarcoma, grade 2 of 3. Plump oval nuclei with coarse hyperchromasia. Note fibrillar and focally metachromatic cytoplasm (Diff-Quik, × 400).

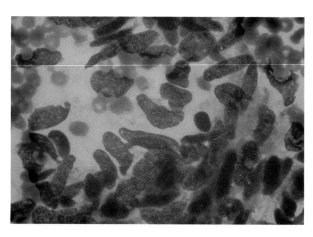

FIGURE 17–9B. Synovial Sarcoma, monophasic pattern. Spindle cells with irregular coarse nuclei and sparse cytoplasm (Diff-Quik, × 630).

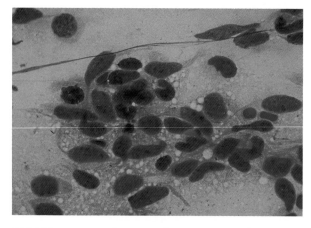

FIGURE 17–8. Malignant Schwannoma, grade 2 of 3. Atypical spindle cells with oval to curvilinear nuclei and delicate nucleoli (Diff-Quik, × 400).

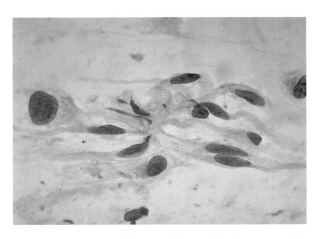

FIGURE 17–10A. Malignant Fibrous Histiocytoma. Admixture of malignant fibroblastic and histiocytoid cells (Papanicolaou stain, × 400).

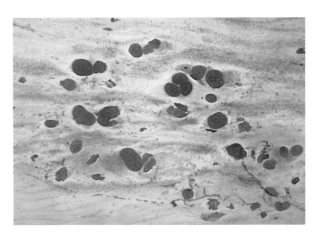

FIGURE 17–10C. Malignant Fibrous Histiocytoma, myxoid variant. Pleomorphic cells are separated by metachromatic myxoid matrix (Diff-Quik, × 400).

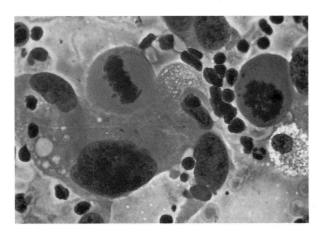

FIGURE 17–10B. Malignant Fibrous Histiocytoma, inflammatory variant. Marked pleomorphism is the cytologic hallmark of malignant fibrous histiocytoma. Note mitotic activity and evidence of phagocytosis. Lymphocytes may be prominent in the inflammatory variant (Diff-Quik, × 630).

NORMAL TISSUE

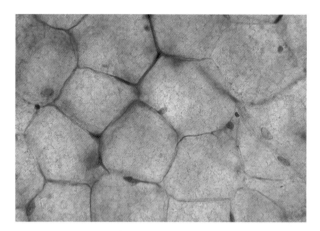

FIGURE 17–11. Normal Adipose Tissue. Note voluminous cytoplasm and small peripheral nuclei (Papanicolaou stain, × 225).

LESIONS OF ADIPOSE TISSUE

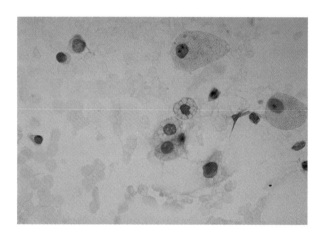

FIGURE 17–12A. Fat Necrosis. Clusters of reactive fat cells and histiocytes (Papanicolaou stain, × 225).

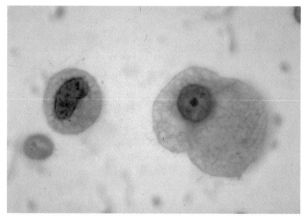

FIGURE 17–12B. Fat Necrosis. Reactive fat cells with small nucleoli and multivesicular cytoplasmic fat (Papanicolaou stain, × 400).

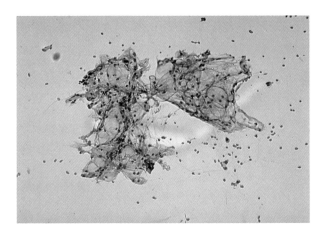

FIGURE 17–13A. Lipoma. Smears tend to show low cellularity with occasional clusters of uniform, bland fat cells. Naked nuclei may be common (Papanicolaou stain, × 100).

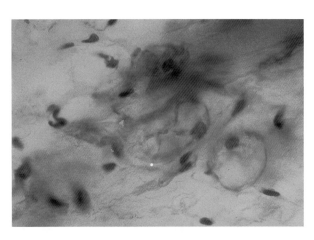

FIGURE 17–13C. Myxoid Liposarcoma. Lipoblasts are irregularly arrayed within a cyanophilic myxoid matrix (Papanicolaou stain, × 400).

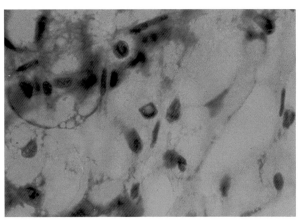

FIGURE 17–13D. Myxoid Liposarcoma. Dense cluster of lipoblasts. Note delicate nuclei and multiple fat vacuoles with cytoplasm (Papanicolaou stain, × 630).

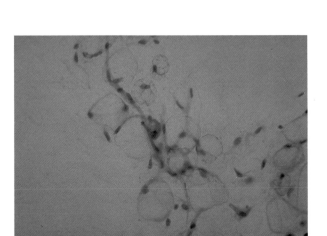

FIGURE 17–13B. Myxoid Liposarcoma. Large lipoblasts are closely aligned to a delicate capillary network (Papanicolaou stain, × 225).

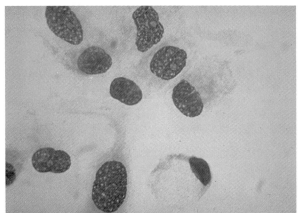

FIGURE 17–13E. Round Cell Liposarcoma. Loosely cohesive group of pleomorphic cells with prominent nucleoli. Only rare cells display lipoblastic differentiation (Diff-Quik, × 630).

NORMAL TISSUE AND LESIONS OF SKELETAL MUSCLE

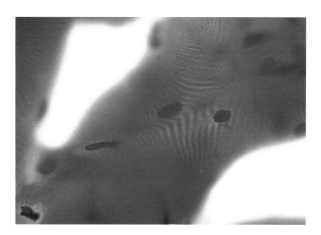

FIGURE 17–14A. Normal Skeletal Muscle. Small dark nuclei within a syncytium of coarsely striated cytoplasm (Diff-Quik, × 400).

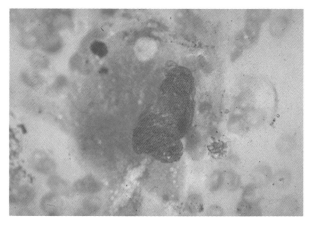

FIGURE 17–14C. Skeletal Muscle Regeneration. Large atypical cell showing an eccentric lobular nucleus and abundant cytoplasm (Diff-Quik, × 630).

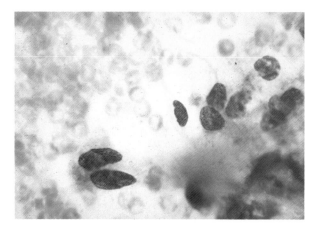

FIGURE 17–14B. Skeletal Muscle Regeneration. Aspirates contain few cells with a variable amount of cytoplasm and reactive nuclei (Diff-Quik, × 400).

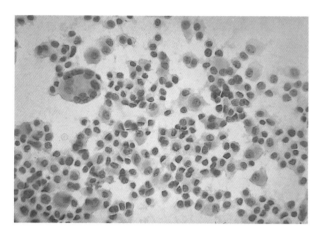

FIGURE 17–15A. Embryonal Rhabdomyosarcoma. Cellular biopsy showing a polymorphous mixture of small round cells and multinucleated giant cells (Papanicolaou stain, × 225).

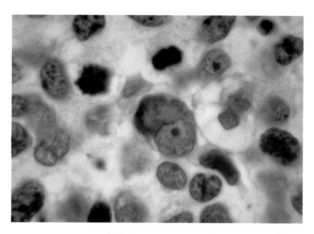

FIGURE 17–15C. Rhabdomyosarcoma. Immunocytochemical stains for desmin show strong cytoplasmic staining (Desmin, × 630).

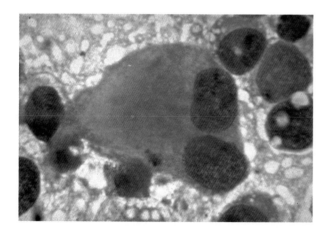

FIGURE 17–15B. Rhabdomyosarcoma. Large binucleate rhabdomyoblast with abundant cytoplasm that is focally metachromatic (Diff-Quik, × 630).

OTHER LESIONS

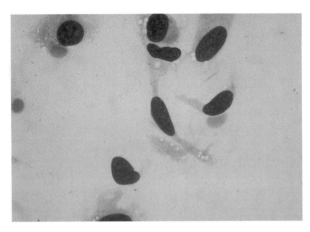

FIGURE 17–16A. Hemangioma. Aspirates contain few cells with nonspecific cytologic features. Spindle and polygonal cells predominate in this field (Diff-Quik, × 630).

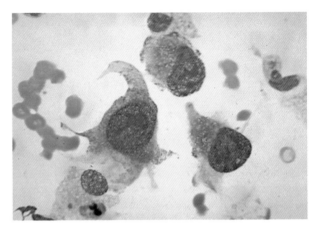

FIGURE 17–16C. Angiosarcoma. Moderately sized pleomorphic cells with eccentric nuclei, prominent nucleoli, and angular cytoplasm (Diff-Quik, × 630).

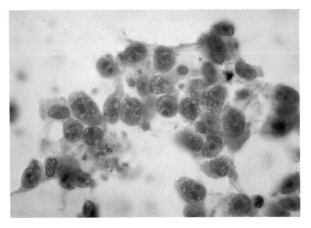

FIGURE 17–16B. Angiosarcoma. Cluster of undifferentiated polygonal cells within a hemorrhagic background (Papanicolaou stain, × 400).

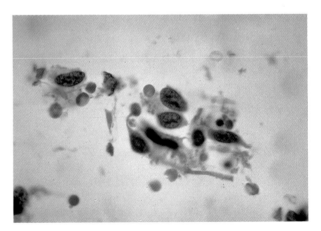

FIGURE 17–16D. Hemangiopericytoma. Small to intermediate-sized cells display spindle and polygonal forms. Smears are hemorrhagic (Papanicolaou stain, × 225).

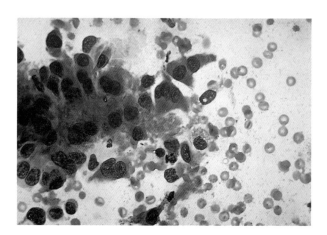

FIGURE 17–17A. Epithelioid Sarcoma. Cluster of metachromatic necrotic material surrounded by histiocytoid polygonal cells (Diff-Quik, × 225).

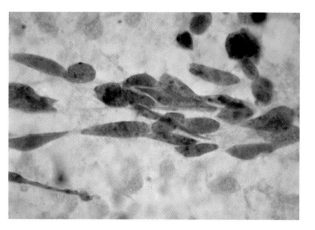

FIGURE 17–18A. Small-Cell Carcinoma of Lung Metastatic to Soft Tissue. Smear made with excessive pressure produced spindle cells with scant cytoplasm simulating a sarcoma.

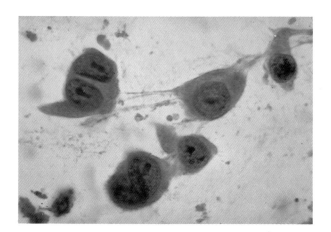

FIGURE 17–17B. Epithelioid Sarcoma. Polygonal cells with high N/C ratio and prominent nucleoli. Bi- and multinucleated cells may be seen (Papanicolaou stain, × 630).

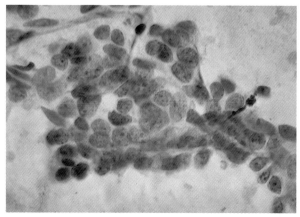

FIGURE 17–18B. Properly made smear displays characteristic features of **small-cell carcinoma** (Papanicolaou stain, × 630).

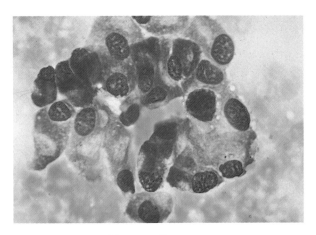

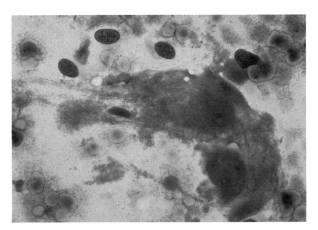

FIGURE 17–19A. Osteoblastic Reaction at fracture site. Cluster of reactive osteoblasts with columnar orientation and tendency toward alignment of nuclei. Abundant cytoplasm with characteristic peripheral cleared zone (Diff-Quik, × 400).

FIGURE 17–19B. Osteoid. Sharply demarcated, intensely metachromatic extracellular matrix with dense, woven texture (Diff-Quik, × 400).

BONE MARROW COMPONENTS

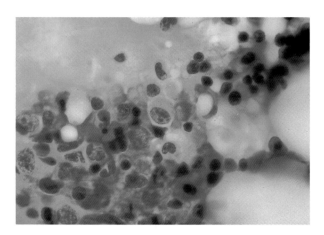

FIGURE 17–20A. Normal Hematopoietic Cells. Clusters of immature erythroid and myeloid precursors (Papanicolaou stain, × 400).

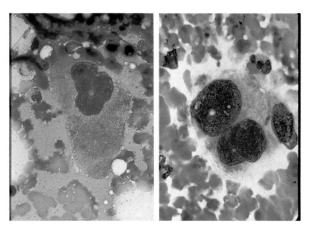

FIGURE 17–20C. Metastatic Large-Cell Carcinoma to bone contrasted with megakaryocyte. Note difference in N/C ratio and nuclear features (Diff-Quik, × 630).

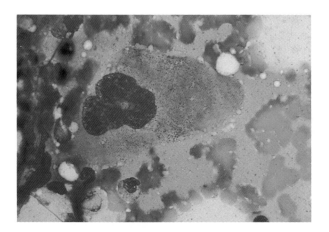

FIGURE 17–20B. Megakaryocyte. Large cell with eccentric, lobular nucleus and abundant granular cytoplasm (Diff-Quik, × 630).

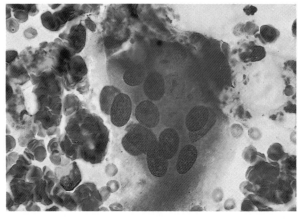

FIGURE 17–21. Osteoclast. Relative nuclear uniformity and delicate nucleoli characterize this large multinucleated cell (Diff-Quik, × 630).

BONE LESIONS

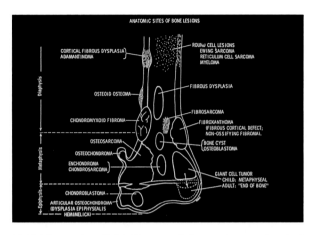

FIGURE 17–22. Field Theory of Bone Tumors. Typical location of primary bone tumors as exemplified in a long bone. Reticulum cell carcinoma is an older name for large cell lymphoma.

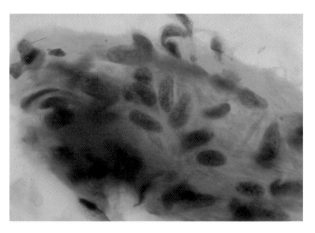

FIGURE 17–23. Fibrous Dysplasia. Thick aggregate of fibrous connective tissue. Fibroblastic nuclei are bland and uniform (Papanicolaou stain, × 400).

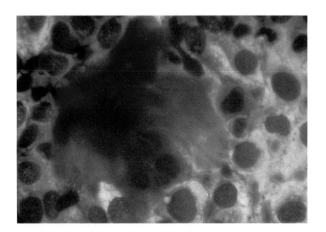

FIGURE 17–24. Osteosarcoma.
FIGURE 17–24A. Brilliantly metachromatic osteoid is encircled by polygonal osteoblasts (Diff-Quik, × 630).

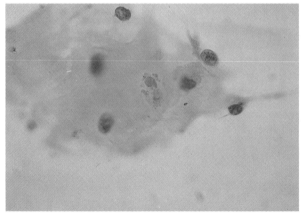

FIGURE 17–24B. Osteoid with embedded malignant osteoblasts. Note obscuring effect of osteoid in Papanicolaou-stained smears (× 400).

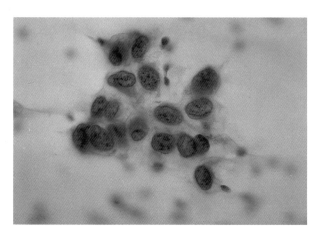

FIGURE 17–24C. Undifferentiated malignant osteoblasts (Papanicolaou stain, × 630).

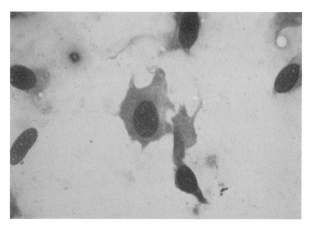

FIGURE 17–24E. Parosteal osteosarcoma. This low-grade tumor yields relatively bland neoplastic cells (Diff-Quik, × 630).

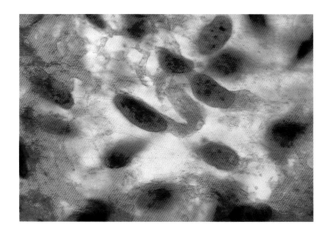

FIGURE 17–24D. Spindle cell variant of osteosarcoma (cell block, H&E, × high power).

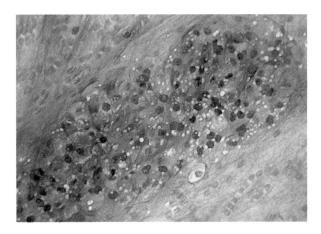

FIGURE 17–25. Chondrosarcoma.
FIGURE 17–25A. Malignant cells are dispersed within a hazy, metachromatic chondroid matrix (Diff-Quik, × 225).

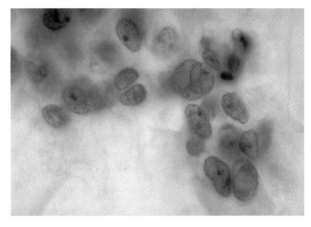

FIGURE 17–25C. Intermediate-grade chondrosarcoma. Malignant cells show large irregular nuclei and prominent nucleoli (Papanicolaou stain, × 630).

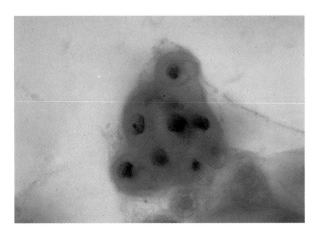

FIGURE 17–25B. Low-grade chondrosarcoma. Cluster of malignant chondrocytes with hyperchromatic nuclei and small nucleoli. Filmy chondroid matrix is less distinct with Papanicolaou stain (× 400).

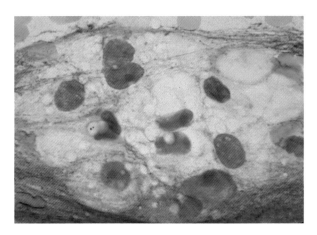

FIGURE 17–25D. High-grade chondrosarcoma. Large pleomorphic cells contain large nucleoli and copious vesicular cytoplasm (Diff-Quik, × 630).

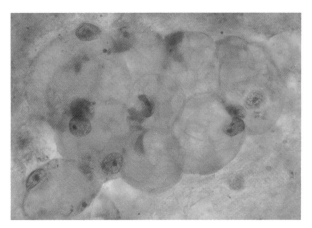

FIGURE 17–26. Chordoma. Group of large, bubbly (physalipherous) cells. Compare these bland nuclei and delicate nucleoli to Figure 17–25D (Papanicolaou stain, × 400).

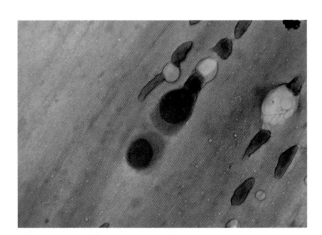

FIGURE 17–25E. Myxoid variant of chondrosarcoma. Metachromatic myxoid matrix predominates and contains scattered small oval cells with scant cytoplasm (Diff-Quik, × 630).

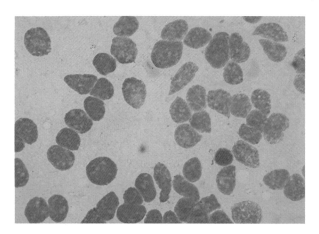

FIGURE 17–27. Ewing Sarcoma.
FIGURE 17–27A. Rosette-like array of small to intermediate cells. Anisonucleosis, nuclear molding, and indistinct cytoplasm are characteristic (Diff-Quik, × 400).

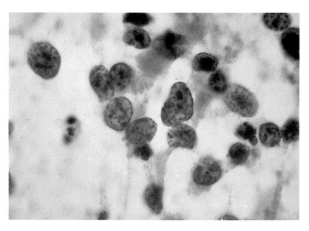

FIGURE 17–27C. Loosely dispersed cells and naked nuclei with coarse hyperchromasia (Papanicolaou stain, × 630).

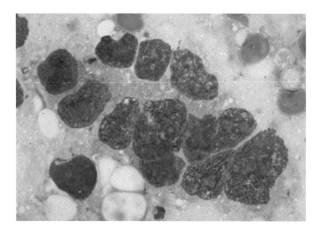

FIGURE 17–27B. Tightly cohesive grouping with irregular, coarsely hyperchromatic nuclei and large nucleoli (Diff-Quik, × 630).

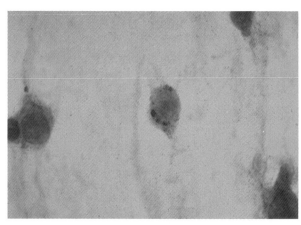

FIGURE 17–27D. Cytospin preparation stained by periodic acid–Schiff (PAS) method displays granular glycogen within cytoplasm (PAS stain, × 630).

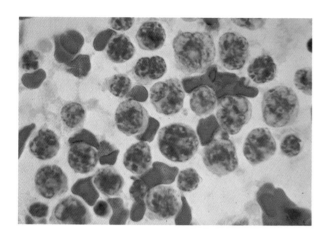

FIGURE 17–28. Primary Lymphoma of Bone. Large-cell lymphoma with both cleaved and noncleaved cells. Immunophenotyping demonstrated B-cell differentiation (Papanicolaou stain, × 630).

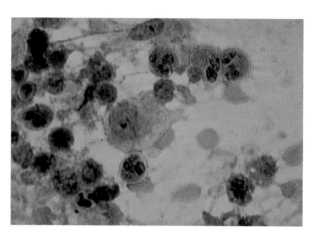

FIGURE 17–30A. Eosinophilic Granuloma. Characteristic Langerhans histiocyte is flanked by eosinophils. Note eccentric folded nucleus with delicate chromatin pattern (Papanicolaou stain, × 630).

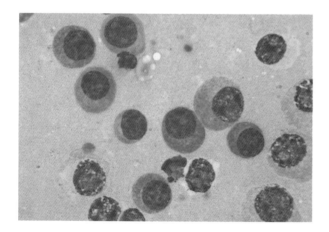

FIGURE 17–29. Myeloma. Polymorphous collection of neoplastic plasma cells. Note variation in size, degree of plasmacytic differentiation, and nucleolar prominence (Diff-Quik, × 630).

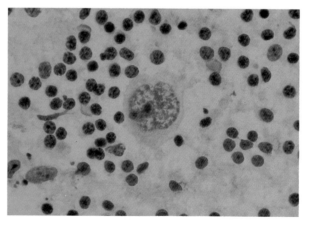

FIGURE 17–30B. Hodgkin Disease involving bone. Reed-Sternberg cell. Centrally located nuclei and large nucleoli dominate cell (Papanicolaou stain, × 630).

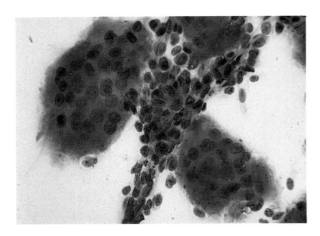

FIGURE 17–31A. Giant Cell Tumor. Osteoclast-like giant cells are juxtaposed to a sheet of mononuclear cells (Diff-Quik, × 225).

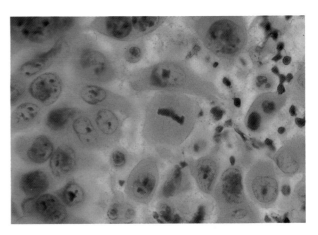

FIGURE 17–32. Metastatic Poorly Differentiated Carcinoma, occult primary. Clinical presentation was as an osteolytic lesion of bone. Note resemblance to osteosarcoma. Primary tumor was identified in lung (Papanicolaou stain, × 630).

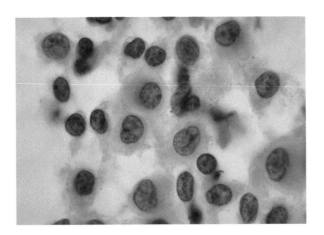

FIGURE 17–31B. Giant Cell Tumor. Mononuclear cells contain delicate cleaved nuclei and indistinct cytoplasm (Papanicolaou stain, × 630).

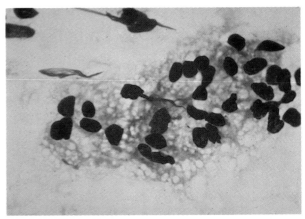

FIGURE 17–33. Renal Cell Carcinoma Metastatic to Bone. This tumor may initially present as a bone lesion and may cytologically mimic chondrosarcoma and chordoma. Note prominent nucleoli (Papanicolaou stain, × 400).

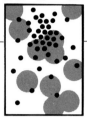

18

FINE NEEDLE
ASPIRATION OF THE
ORBIT

Scott Wang

NORMAL CELLS

Before describing the abnormal processes that occur in the orbit, one must be familiar with the normal cellular constituents in this site. The orbit is composed predominantly of adipose tissue within which are nerves, blood and lymphatic vessels, skeletal (ocular) muscle, and lacrimal glands. Normally, there is no significant lymphoid tissue within the orbit. Therefore, any lymphoid infiltrate aspirated is significant. A benign lacrimal gland may be aspirated and confused with a glandular tumor and should, therefore, be considered in any aspirate from the upper outer quadrant. A benign lacrimal gland should have a more orderly symmetry of the branching acini without crowding or overlap, in comparison with most adenocarcinomas. Benign lacrimal gland aspirates should not reveal abundant metachromatic stroma as seen in air-dried smears of pleomorphic adenoma (described later). The glandular acini from a benign lacrimal gland have regular spacing of cytoplasm between the nuclei, in comparison with the tight ball-like clusters of adenoid cystic carcinoma.

BENIGN CONDITIONS

A group of lesions that may lead to diagnostic confusion are those with a predominance of mixed inflammatory and histiocytic cells. Included in this group are abscess, nonspecific orbital inflammation, cholesteatoma, mucopyocele, degenerating cyst, and eosinophilic granuloma. Abscesses are fairly easy to diagnose by fine needle aspiration (FNA) as they are composed almost entirely of polymorphonuclear leukocytes with a dirty or necrotic background. Nonspecific orbital inflammation, in contrast, reveals fewer leukocytes, owing to the accompanying fibrosis, and the leukocytic population is more heterogeneous. Nonspecific orbital inflammation is frequently not diagnosed because of the paucity of cells and the lack of a recognizable cell population.

Cholesteatoma and benign degenerating cyst yield a mixture of histiocytes of varying size and nuclear number with leukocytes. A frequent finding in both of these benign cystic processes is the presence of hematoidin crystals resulting from the breakdown of red blood cell hemoglobin. These crystals are orange-yellow refractile rhomboids that are present both outside and within the accompanying foamy histiocytes. Cholesterol crystals can also be seen in degenerating cysts and cholesteatoma. The characteristic, polarizable, corner-notched, rectangular cholesterol crystals are usually only seen on immediate wet smears that have not undergone alcohol fixation.

Eosinophilic granuloma can be confidently diagnosed by FNA alone. The admixture of numerous eosinophils with mono- and multinucleated histiocytes with kidney-bean nuclei is pathognomonic. The cytoplasmic eosinophilic granules, which characterize eosinophils, are not usually apparent on Papanicolaou-stained smears. On these smears one must rely on the observation that the eosinophil has only two nuclear lobes, as opposed to the three or more lobes of a neutrophil. Another helpful clue to eosinophilic granuloma is the presence of refractile, elongated or needle-like, orange-red Charcot-Leyden crystals both outside and within histiocytes. These crystals are seen in both air-dried and alcohol-fixed smears.

LYMPHOID LESIONS

Lymphoid lesions, which should be subcategorized as reactive or lymphoma whenever possible, can at least be accurately identified as lymphoid when an adequate sample is present. Single mononuclear cells recognizable as lymphocytes comprise the majority of cells against a background of varying numbers of peripheral blood cells. The lymphoid nature of these mononuclear cells is best appreciated on air-dried Romanowsky-stained material. Although the exact subcategorization of these lymphoid lesions is always attempted, it is not a prerequisite for treatment, as a full oncologic work-up is undertaken in all cases to search for systemic lymphoma. Even with immunophenotyping, it may be difficult to distinguish a reactive process from a malignant one. Lymphomas are usually composed of atypical lymphoid cells of varying size and shape, which are either mixed or monotonous. Those cases of large-cell or poorly differentiated small-cell lymphoma characterized by a fairly monotonous atypical infiltrate of either enlarged or irregularly contoured nuclei are most easily diagnosed.

Cases revealing a mixture of lymphocytes of varying size and shape are more difficult to subcategorize as reactive versus lymphoma. Although plasma cells are frequently seen in reactive lymphoid lesions, plasmacytoid lymphocytes that exhibit atypical features suggest lymphoma or plasmacytoma. These atypical features include marked cell and/or nuclear enlargement or size variation, replacement of the typical clockface nuclear chromatin by a loose, immature chromatin distribution, or the presence of prominent and/or irregular nucleoli.

Immunoperoxidase or immunoalkaline phosphatase antibody procedures can be utilized to immunophenotype the lymphoid infiltrates obtained by FNA. Antibodies directed against T- and B-lymphocyte surface antigens, leukocyte common antigen plus kappa and lambda light chains are the most commonly used. Positivity with leukocyte common antigen is used to confirm the lymphoid lineage of malignant mononuclear infiltrates of uncertain etiology. The normal kappa to lambda light chain ratio of 2 : 1 is greatly altered or reversed in many cases of B-cell lymphoma, and it is not unusual to see a monoclonal proliferation. Reactive lymphoid infiltrates are usually characterized by a mixture of lymphocytes of varying size, such as mature lymphocytes and plasma cells, larger transformed lymphocytes, immunoblasts, and macrophages, including tingible-body forms that contain ingested cellular debris. The nuclei of both the larger and smaller lymphocytes are usually round, although occasional cells reveal irregular nuclear contours. Tingible-body macrophages are indicative of increased cellular proliferation and are seen in both benign reactive and high-grade malignant lymphoid lesions. Usually, it is not difficult to distinguish these latter two categories, as the background lymphocytes are nearly all atypical in a high-grade lymphoma, whereas the lymphoid population is mixed (as previously described) in reactive lymphoid lesions or pseudolymphomas. Unfortunately, it is not uncommon for a benign reactive lymphoid infiltrate to be present surrounding a malignant lymphoma.

MALIGNANT TUMORS OTHER THAN LYMPHOMA

Both primary and metastatic tumors may present in the orbit. The recognition of metastatic or primary carcinoma is aided by identifying coherent atypical epithelial cells. Further subcategorization is aided by observing either cytoplasmic or architectural differentiation. Cytoplasmic differentiation is best appreciated in squamous cell carcinoma. Clues to squamous differentiation are polygonal or tadpole-shaped cells and irregular, pyknotic, or inky nuclei, which are evident on both alcohol-fixed and air-dried slides. Adenocarcinoma displays glandular differentiation and has cuboidal to columnar cells that form tight balls or acini, which frequently form three-dimensional clusters. Metastatic prostate carcinoma frequently exhibits small acini, which may be arranged in a "back-to-back" or cribriform manner. There may be nuclear molding and often prominent nucleoli. Immunoperoxidase-labeled antibodies directed against prostate-specific antigen and prostatic acid phosphatase are available and are highly sensitive and specific for metastatic prostate carcinoma. Metastatic breast carcinomas may reveal patterns similar to those described for the prostate. Breast carcinomas may also reveal Indian-filing growth and nuclear molding. Metastatic colonic adenocarcinoma is frequently composed of columnar cells forming glands that sometimes demonstrate mucin positivity.

Among the primary orbital tumors, those of lacrimal gland origin are particularly challenging to diagnose. Pleomorphic adenomas and adenoid cystic carcinomas are the most frequently seen tumors in this group. Both demonstrate findings similar to the identical tumors that arise in the salivary glands.

Pleomorphic adenoma is characterized by a distinct myxocartilaginous stroma that stains a brilliant metachromatic pink-purple on air-dried smears but is frequently clear and easily overlooked on alcohol-fixed slides. Freely scattered ovoid myoepithelial cells may be seen in varying number within this stroma. The stroma surrounds coherent clusters of uniform duct cells.

Adenoid cystic carcinomas are composed of deceptively bland small round cells with scanty cytoplasm forming balls and circles. Metachromatic, pink-purple stromal material is again appreciated on air-dried slides within the balls or circles of duct cells. On alcohol-fixed slides the stromal material is less apparent, although the nuclear morphology can be better appreciated. The nuclei are small, regular, and round, and only occasionally have prominent nucleoli that might mistakenly suggest a benign proliferation. The key to the recognition of adenoid cystic carcinoma lies in the identification of the ball-like clusters.

A number of malignant tumors can present in the orbit and simulate lymphoma, being composed of a fairly monotonous population of single mononuclear cells with a paucity of differentiation features. Included in this differential are leukemia, neuroblastoma (including the olfactory variant), retinoblastoma, glioma, melanoma, rhabdomyosarcoma, nasopharyngeal carcinoma, and lymphoepithelioma, among others.

Rhabdomyosarcomas, which occur predominantly in the young, closely resemble a large-cell lymphoma. Most cells resemble large immature lymphocytes with scant cytoplasm and prominent nucleoli. One must search diligently for cells that reveal muscle differentiation. Although cytoplasmic cross-striations are the hallmark, even on histology they are rare and in cytologic material even rarer. Instead, one encounters scattered cells with eccentrically placed nuclei and elongated, somewhat tapered cytoplasm. Immunoperoxidase stains directed against muscle-derived proteins, such as myoglobin, can be used to confirm the diagnosis of rhabdomyosarcoma.

Gliomas likewise can be expected to reveal a varying number of cells with cytoplasmic tails or processes. Cell clustering with rosette formation suggests primitive neuronal differentiation as seen in neuroblastomas or retinoblastomas.

Melanoma cells usually possess more abundant cytoplasm than lymphomas and more frequently reveal bi- and multinucleation. If cytoplasmic pigment consistent with melanin is discovered, the diagnosis is easy.

In all of these cases the key to the proper diagnosis is a diligent search for evidence of cellular differentiation, which is usually stimulated by a clinical suspicion that one may be dealing with a nonlymphoid malignancy.

Nasopharyngeal carcinoma or lymphoepithelioma is another instance in which immunoperoxidase studies can aid in the diagnosis. Like lymphoma, the majority of the cells are single and have enlarged nuclei and prominent nucleoli. A cytologic clue to the diagnosis is the presence of some adherent cells or cellular clustering indicative of the epithelial origin. Immunoperoxidase studies using antibodies directed against keratin strongly stain the cytoplasm of these epithelial-derived cells. Antibodies directed against lymphoid markers stain the accompanying reactive lymphocytes but not the malignant cells.

Optic nerve tumors may be diagnosed by FNA, but a word of caution is necessary and applies to both FNA and biopsy. Optic gliomas are frequently associated with marked meningothelial hyperplasia of the optic nerve sheath that can simulate meningioma. Therefore, careful clinicopathologic correlation with other studies should be undertaken before diagnosing meningioma, even when numerous characteristic meningothelial whorls are present.

BENIGN TISSUE AND REACTIVE LESIONS

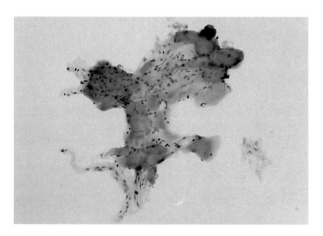

FIGURE 18–1. Skeletal Muscle. Even at low power these tissue fragments can be recognized as skeletal muscle by identifying the peripherally placed sarcolemmal nuclei that surround the dense round to polygonal muscle fibers. This is a normal finding in an orbital aspirate and does not indicate a pathologic lesion (Papanicolaou stain, × 240).

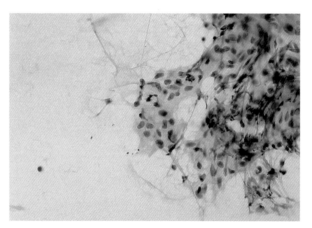

FIGURE 18–2. Benign Lacrimal Gland. Coherent epithelial cells with fairly abundant cytoplasm and evenly separated round to oval nuclei adjacent to cells distorted by "crush artifact" are present. Acinar formation is suggested where cells are present surrounding a central space. Although difficult to recognize in this smear, benign lacrimal gland should be considered in the differential diagnosis when epithelial cell clusters devoid of malignant features are seen in aspirates from the upper outer quadrant of the orbit (Papanicolaou stain, × 360).

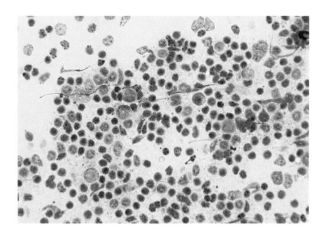

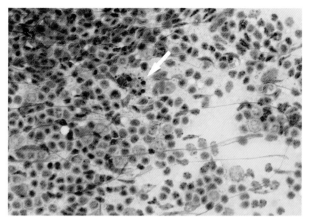

FIGURE 18–3. Reactive Lymphoid Lesion. Admixture of small mature lymphocytes, larger transformed lymphocytes, and intermediate-sized lymphocytes. Most cells have round nuclei with occasional cells revealing plasmacytoid features. This population corresponds to the lymphocytes seen in a reactive germinal center. Although lymphomas may also contain an admixture of lymphocytes of varying size, there is usually either a predominant population of atypical lymphocytes or a mixed population of lymphocytes with irregular nuclear features. In lymphomas, it is unusual to obtain a mixture of cells that would correspond to a normal germinal center. This lesion was confined to the orbit and resolved with radiation therapy (Diff-Quik, × 200).

FIGURE 18–4. Reactive Lymphoid Lesion. Mixture of lymphocytes (as in Fig. 18–3) with tingible body macrophages (arrow) revealing dark intracytoplasmic granules of varying size, which correspond to ingested cellular debris. These macrophages are seen in lymphoid lesions with a high rate of cell turnover, which include both reactive lesions and high-grade or aggressive lymphomas. Therefore, one must rely on the evaluation of the remaining lymphoid cells to determine if the infiltrate is benign or malignant (Diff-Quik, × 200).

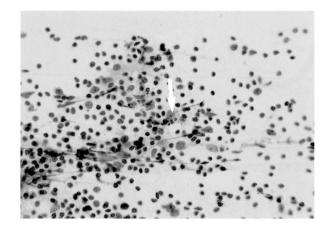

FIGURE 18–5. Reactive Lymphoid Lesion. Scattered intermediate-sized lymphocytes with irregular nuclear contours may be seen in reactive lymphoid lesions because they are part of the lymphoid population of the normal germinal center. The presence of tingible body macrophages with ingested debris (arrow) suggests that this is a reactive lymphoid lesion. If this had been a lymphoma of the small cleaved cell type, it would be composed of a predominant population of irregular intermediate-sized lymphocytes without tingible body macrophages, since these lymphomas are not associated with a high rate of cellular turnover (Papanicolaou stain, × 200).

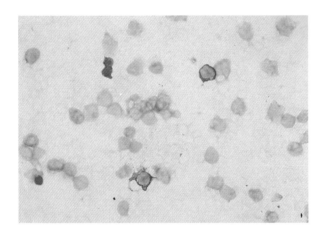

FIGURE 18–6. Reactive Lymphoid Lesion. Positive cytoplasmic staining for kappa light chain (red) seen in a few small and large lymphocytes. Normally, there is an admixture of both kappa- and lambda-positive lymphocytes in a reactive lymphoid lesion in approximately a 2 : 1 ratio. Although this ratio may be altered in a small sample, one would not expect to see a marked predominance of lymphocytes positive for only one light chain in a polyclonal or reactive proliferation (immunoalkaline phosphatase–labeled technique directed against kappa immunoglobulin light chain with hematoxylin counterstain, × 128).

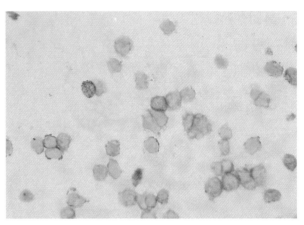

FIGURE 18–7. Reactive Lymphoid Lesion. Positive cytoplasmic staining for lambda light chain (red) is seen in more than half of the lymphocytes in this field (sample from the same patient as in Fig. 18–6). Although lambda-positive lymphocytes predominate in this field, they do not constitute a sufficient overall majority of the entire sample to suggest monoclonality. Greater emphasis should be given to apparent monoclonality when the lymphocytes, which stain as one light chain type, also reveal cytologic atypia. Benign reactive lymphocytes should be recognized and not included in the determination of possible monoclonality. One should be cautious placing too much emphasis on the results of light chain staining in the determination of both monoclonality and, in turn, malignancy. Although monoclonality is strongly suggestive, it is not diagnostic of lymphoid malignancy (immunoalkaline phosphatase–labeled technique directed against lambda immunoglobulin light chain with hematoxylin counterstain, × 128).

LYMPHOMA

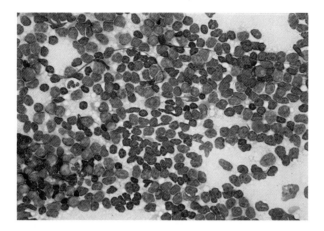

FIGURE 18–8. Orbital Lymphoma, Small Cleaved Cell Type. A monotonous infiltrate of intermediate-sized lymphocytes is seen here. Note the small mature lymphocytes and neutrophils in the background for size reference. There are irregular nuclear contours or protrusions on these malignant lymphocytes as opposed to the smooth and regular nuclei of mature lymphocytes seen in chronic inflammation. This lymphoma was diagnosed in the orbit and subsequently became systemic (Diff-Quik, × 128).

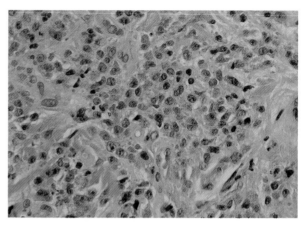

FIGURE 18–10. Biopsy of Plasmacytoma from Right Arm (sample from same patient with orbital FNA shown in Fig. 18–9). Mono- and occasional binucleated lymphocytes with malignant plasmacytoid features are seen infiltrating between the collagen bundles of the dermis (H&E stain, × 400).

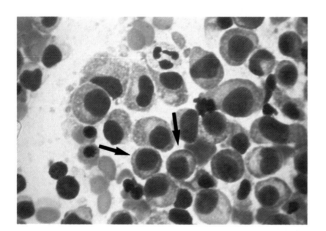

FIGURE 18–9. Orbital Plasmacytoma in a Patient with Multiple Myeloma. Two mature plasma cells (arrow) can be compared to the remaining enlarged lymphoid cells. These larger cells also reveal plasmacytoid differentiation with eccentrically placed nuclei and perinuclear clearing. In contrast to the mature plasma cells, these larger cells exhibit atypical or malignant nuclear features with irregular, rather than round, nuclear contours, marked nuclear enlargement, and size variation plus prominent nucleoli (Diff-Quik, × 400).

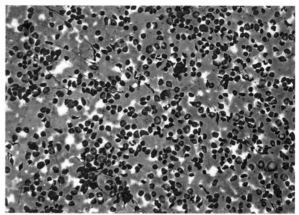

FIGURE 18–11. Orbital Lymphoma. Air-dried smear reveals a monotonous infiltrate of malignant mononuclear cells with artifactual nuclear distortion secondary to excessive force used in smearing, which impairs evaluation. Although lymphoma was favored, poorly differentiated metastatic carcinoma from the prostate (which this patient was know to have) could not be excluded. An additional aspirate was therefore performed so that immunoperoxidase studies could be done to document the suspected lymphoid origin of these cells (Diff-Quik, × 80).

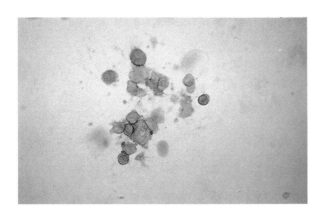

FIGURE 18–12. Orbital Lymphoma (sample from the same patient as in Fig. 18–11). Positive cytoplasmic staining for leukocyte common antigen confirms the lymphoid origin of these cells. Positive staining with this antibody does not discriminate between a benign and a malignant lymphoid lesion (immunoperoxidase-labeled antibody to common leukocyte antigen, × 240).

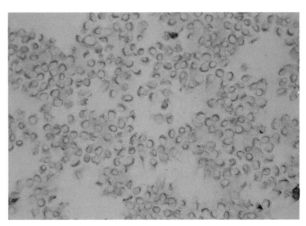

FIGURE 18–14. Orbital Lymphoma. Only a rare mature reactive lymphocyte reveals positive cytoplasmic staining for kappa light chain (red). Nearly all the lymphocytes were monoclonal lambda phenotype as seen in Figure 18–13 (immunoalkaline phosphatase–labeled antibody technique directed against kappa immunoglobulin light chain with hematoxylin counterstain, × 128).

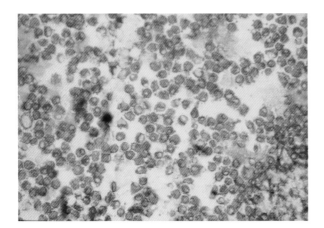

FIGURE 18–13. Orbital Lymphoma. Positive cytoplasmic staining for lambda light chain (red) in nearly all lymphocytes is consistent with a monoclonal proliferation, which usually indicates a lymphoma (immunoalkaline phosphatase–labeled antibody technique directed against lambda immunoglobulin light chain with hematoxylin counterstain, × 128).

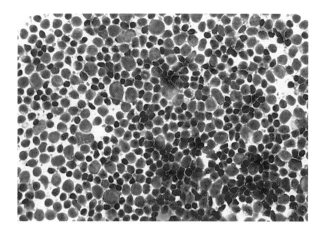 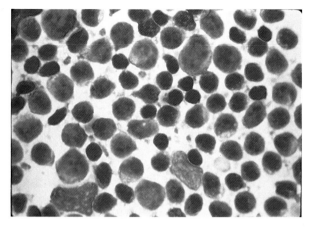

FIGURE 18–15. Abnormal Lymphoid Infiltrate in the Orbit. FIGURE 18–15A. Admixture of small, mature lymphocytes with larger, round lymphocytes. There is a notable absence of plasma cells and tingible body macrophages, which are frequently seen in reactive lymphoid lesions. Note the presence of the small, round extracellular blue "lymphoglandular bodies," frequently seen in lymphoid lesions. Although this lesion is suspicious for mixed cell lymphoma, this admixture might be present in a pseudolymphoma (Diff-Quik, × 128). **FIGURE 18–15B.** Higher magnification of Figure 18–15A. This infiltrate was confined to the orbit and resolved following radiation therapy (Diff-Quik, × 320).

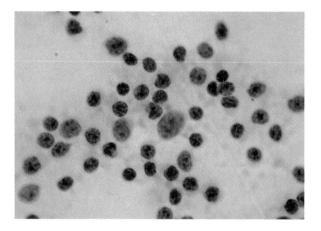

FIGURE 18–16. Abnormal Lymphoid Infiltrate in the Orbit (sample from the same patient as in Fig. 18–15). Admixture of small lymphocytes, some revealing a plasmacytoid or clockface chromatin distribution whereas others have irregular nuclear contours, and larger lymphocytes containing prominent nucleoli. If these larger lymphocytes were the predominant population, one would consider the possibility of lymphoma, but not in this setting when a mixed lymphocytic population is present (Papanicolaou stain, × 320).

OTHER CONDITIONS

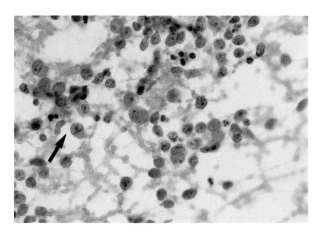

FIGURE 18–17. Orbital Rhabdomyosarcoma. Fine needle aspiration revealing single mononuclear cells of varying size and shape with occasional prominent nucleoli, which closely resemble lymphoma cells. A few cells such as the one at the arrow have eccentric nuclei and elongated, tapering cytoplasm suggesting myogenic differentiation (Papanicolaou stain, × 320). (Courtesy of Andrew Dekker, M.D., University of Pittsburgh.)

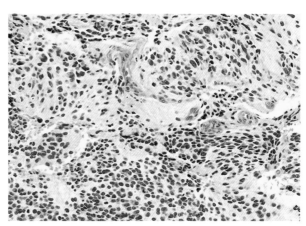

FIGURE 18–19. Orbital Rhabdomyosarcoma (sample from same patient as in Fig. 18–17). Biopsy revealing the classic alveolar pattern of rhabdomyosarcoma consisting of nests of round to spindle cells. Scattered cells are again noted with cytoplasmic extensions (H&E stain, × 320). (Courtesy of Andrew Dekker, M.D., University of Pittsburgh.)

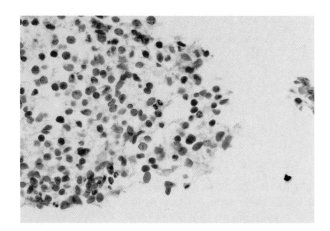

FIGURE 18–18. Orbital Rhabdomyosarcoma (sample from same patient as in Fig. 18–17). Fine needle aspiration revealing positive (brown) cytoplasmic staining in a few cells for myoglobin, which supports the muscle derivation of this tumor (immunoperoxidase labeled–antibody directed against myoglobin with hematoxylin counterstain, × 128). (Courtesy of Andrew Dekker, M.D., University of Pittsburgh.)

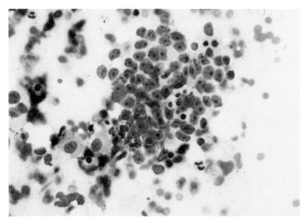

FIGURE 18–20. Orbital Extension of Nasopharyngeal Lymphoepithelioma. Fine needle aspiration revealing a cluster of mononuclear cells with prominent nucleoli and scant cytoplasm. Note the mature lymphocytes for size reference. The differential diagnosis includes both poorly differentiated carcinoma and lymphoma. The tight clustering, which is focally present, suggests a carcinoma (Diff-Quik, × 320).

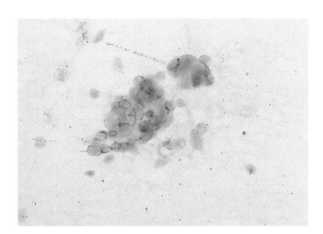

FIGURE 18–21. Orbital Extension of Nasopharyngeal Lymphoepithelioma. Fine needle aspiration revealing positive cytoplasmic (brown) staining for keratin, confirming the epithelial origin of these clustered cells (immunoperoxidase-labeled technique directed against low-molecular-weight keratin, × 128).

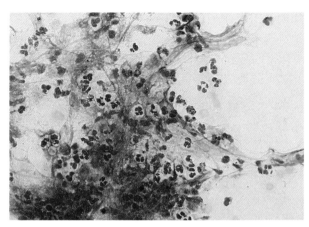

FIGURE 18–23. Orbital Abscess. Fine needle aspiration with numerous neutrophils, stringy blue fibrinous material, and necrotic debris in the background. These findings could be seen in any lesion with necrosis and acute inflammation, including a malignancy. Therefore, a thorough search of the background for neoplastic cells is necessary (Diff-Quik, × 320).

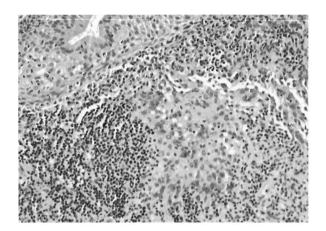

FIGURE 18–22. Orbital Extension of Nasopharyngeal Lymphoepithelioma. Biopsy of nasopharyngeal mass showing admixture of coherent groups of mature lymphocytes and carcinoma cells (H&E stain, × 320).

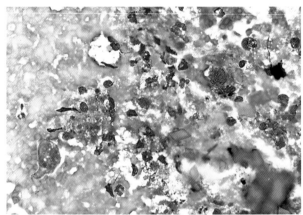

FIGURE 18–24. Orbital Cholesteatoma. Fine needle aspiration reveals foamy histiocytes with intra- and extracellular hematoidin crystals derived from the breakdown of red cell hemoglobin. These crystals are refractile, stain orange, and have a rhomboidal shape. These findings are not specific for cholesteatoma and can be seen in any degenerating cystic process (Diff-Quik, × 320).

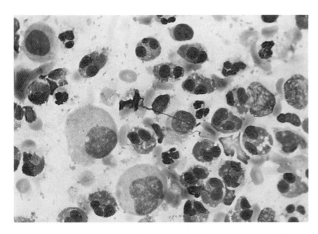

FIGURE 18–25. Eosinophilic Granuloma. Fine needle aspiration with a mixture of eosinophils and histiocytes. Cytoplasmic eosinophilic granules are only apparent on air-dried (not alcohol-fixed) slides. The recognition of eosinophils is most helpful in determining the etiology of the histiocytic cells (Diff-Quik, × 320).

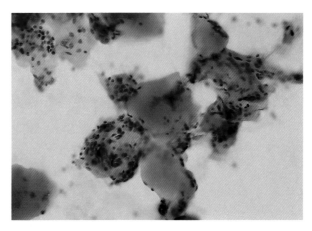

FIGURE 18–27. Orbital Plasmacytoma with Abundant Amyloid. Another FNA where numerous multinucleated histiocytes are noted. In this case, the histiocytes are present surrounding thick amorphous amyloid, which was confirmed on Congo red staining (H&E stain, × 240).

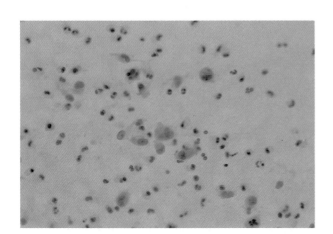

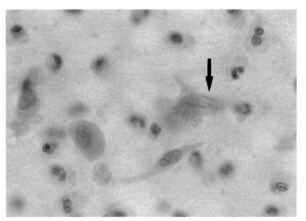

FIGURE 18–26. Eosinophilic Granuloma. FIGURE 18–26A. Binucleated eosinophils, as seen here, fail to show granules on alcohol-fixed smears, which may mask their identity. Polymorphonuclear leukocytes, nevertheless, can usually be distinguished from eosinophils on these smears because they typically have three or more nuclear lobes. The histiocytes are larger and round to oval, with one or more kidney-bean–shaped nuclei. Note mitotic figure in histiocyte at edge of field (Papanicolaou stain, × 320). **FIGURE 18–26B.** Intracytoplasmic orange crystal fragments in histiocytes (arrow) are fragments of Charcot-Leyden crystals from degenerating eosinophils, another clue to eosinophilic granuloma. Histiocytes are seen in many different lesions besides eosinophilic granuloma, including infectious granulomas and foreign body reponses. Attention to the remaining cells and structures is crucial to more accurately identify these lesions (Papanicolaou stain, × 1000).

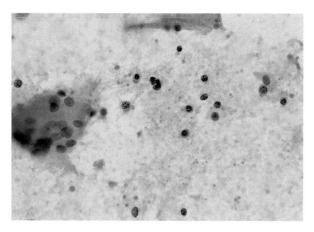

FIGURE 18–28. Orbital Plasmacytoma with Abundant Amyloid. Fine needle aspiration showing a multinucleated histiocyte together with only a few scattered plasma cells and mature lymphocytes. There were an insufficient number of plasma cells in this lesion to identify it as a plasmacytoma. Nevertheless, a lymphoid lesion might be suspected if the amyloid was recognized because amyloid deposition is frequently associated with lymphoplasmacytic processes (H&E stain, × 320).

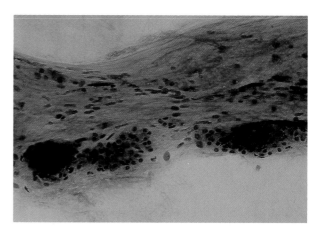

FIGURE 18–30. Pleomorphic Adenoma of Lacrimal Gland Origin. Fine needle aspiration revealing metachromatic pink stroma surrounding clusters of uniform duct cells. Ordinarily, one does not see this stroma in aspirates of a benign lacrimal gland, although it may occasionally be seen in cases of adenoid cystic carcinoma (Diff-Quik, × 240).

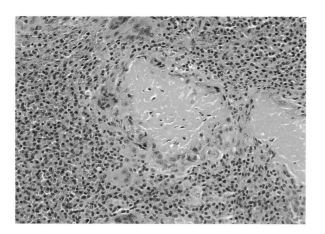

FIGURE 18–29. Orbital Plasmacytoma with Abundant Amyloid. Biopsy revealing amyloid with surrounding multinucleated giant cells and sheets of plasma cells, which were not evident in large number on the preceding FNA (H&E stain, × 320).

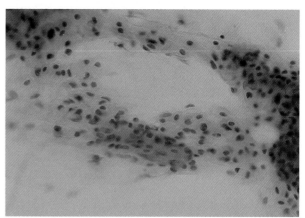

FIGURE 18–31. Pleomorphic Adenoma of Lacrimal Gland Origin. Fine needle aspiration showing light green stroma with scattered, ovoid myoepithelial cells surrounding the uniform duct cells. The stroma is usually clear to pale green on alcohol-fixed smears, as opposed to the more obvious metachromatic pink stroma seen on air-dried smears (Papanicolaou stain, × 360).

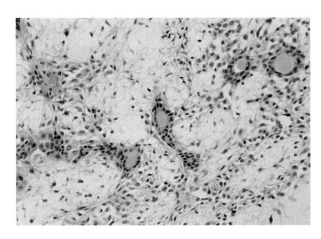

FIGURE 18–32. Pleomorphic Adenoma of Lacrimal Gland Origin. Abundant myxochondroid stroma with scattered ovoid myoepithelial cells surrounding clusters of uniform duct cells present on biopsy (H&E stain, × 240).

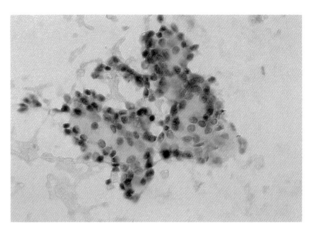

FIGURE 18–34. Adenoid Cystic Carcinoma of the Orbit. Fine needle aspiration with clear to light green concretions surrounded by uniform duct cells with occasional small nucleoli that appear deceptively benign. As in pleomorphic adenoma, alcohol-fixed smears do not bring out the extracellular stromal material, in contrast to air-dried smears, which mask their presence (Papanicolaou stain, × 240).

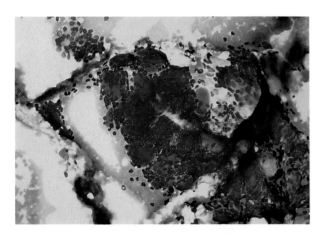

FIGURE 18–33. Adenoid Cystic Carcinoma of the Orbit. Fine needle aspiration revealing round concretions of metachromatic pink material surrounded by fairly uniform, basaloid cells. The metachromatic material is usually within small cellular clusters or present freely as small balls, as opposed to the abundant extracellular material present in pleomorphic adenoma (Diff-Quik, × 240).

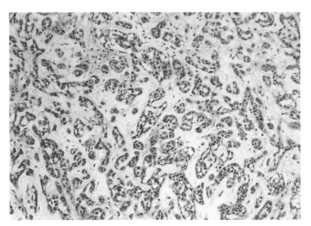

FIGURE 18–35. Adenoid Cystic Carcinoma of the Orbit. Biopsy of orbital tumor with cribriform nests of small and uniform duct cells within and surrounding the dense extracellular material (H&E stain, × 120).

CARCINOMA

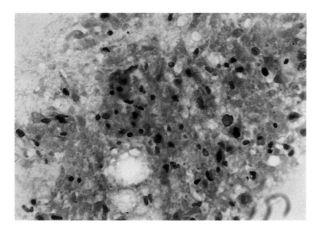

FIGURE 18–36. Locally Invasive Squamous Cell Carcinoma from the Maxillary Sinus. Fine needle aspiration reveals orange staining of the cytoplasm of several cells consistent with keratinization. Orange staining of the cytoplasm may also be seen as an artifact secondary to air-drying on alcohol-fixed smears. Therefore, one should rely on other features of squamous differentiation, such as polygonal or tadpole-shaped cells or densely staining irregular nuclei, to accurately identify the cells (Papanicolaou stain, × 180).

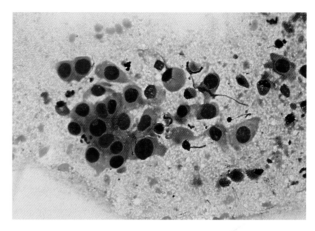

FIGURE 18–38. Metastatic Squamous Cell Carcinoma. Cells on air-dried FNA smears are recognizable as squamous by their polygonal shape. Although nuclear preservation is inferior to alcohol-fixed smears, sufficient nuclear size variation and atypia are present to suspect malignancy. Keratinization is not obvious on air-dried smears as opposed to alcohol-fixed fixed slides. A deep blue cytoplasm, as seen in the small cell in the center, usually corresponds to keratinization (Diff-Quik, × 240).

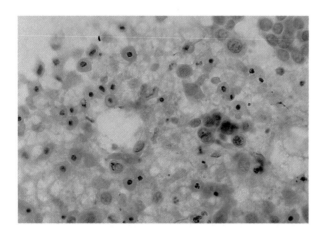

FIGURE 18–37. Metastatic Squamous Cell Carcinoma. Fine needle aspiration with single and cohesive polygonal cells with dense cytoplasm consistent with squamous differentiation. Nuclei are either pyknotic or variably enlarged with prominent nucleoli (Papanicolaou stain, × 240).

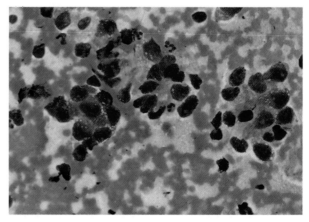

FIGURE 18–39. Metastatic Prostatic Adenocarcinoma. Air-dried smear of orbital FNA revealing acinar formations with nuclear molding. Almost any origin of an adenocarcinoma could yield this appearance. The small nuclear size and prominent molding are frequently seen in breast and prostatic adenocarcinomas as well as in neuroendocrine and neuroepithelial malignancies (Diff-Quik, × 360).

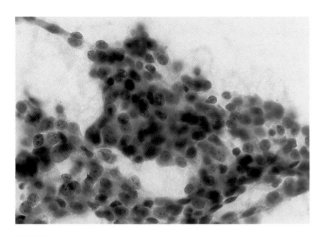

FIGURE 18–40. Metastatic Prostatic Adenocarcinoma. Alcohol-fixed orbital FNA showing back-to-back acini of irregular, small cells, with distinct nucleoli in many cells. The prominent nucleoli, which are not as apparent on the air-dried smears, suggest the prostate as a possible site of the primary tumor; this can be confirmed with immunoperoxidase stains (Papanicolaou stain, × 360).

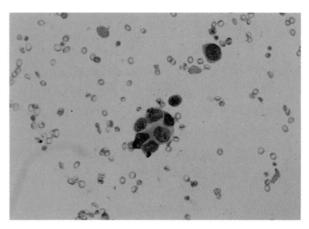

FIGURE 18–42. Metastatic Breast Carcinoma. Fine needle aspiration showing cells present both singly and in a duct formation. The marked variation in nuclear size and shape supports a diagnosis of carcinoma, although it would be difficult to determine if this represented a primary or metastatic lesion. In this case, the presence of single cells with retained cytoplasm suggested the possibility of a breast carcinoma. Therefore, the breasts were examined and an ulcerate tumor was discovered and aspirated (see Fig. 18–43) (Diff-Quik, × 360).

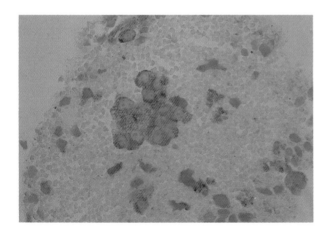

FIGURE 18–41. Metastatic Prostatic Adenocarcinoma. Cell block from orbital FNA revealing positive cytoplasmic staining (red) for prostate-specific antigen. This antibody is quite sensitive and specific for prostate origin, especially when combined with antibody to prostatic acid phosphatase, as in this case (immunoperoxidase-labeled antibody technique directed against prostate-specific antigen, × 240).

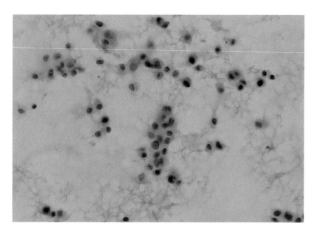

FIGURE 18–43. Fine Needle Aspiration of Ulcerated Breast Tumor (sample from same patient as in Fig. 18–42). Cohesive and single duct cells with retained cytoplasm exhibiting marked variation in nuclear size and shape confirming a diagnosis of breast carcinoma (Papanicolaou stain, × 360).

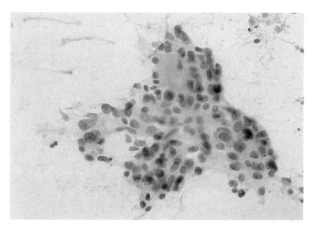

FIGURE 18–44. Metastatic Colonic Adenocarcinoma. Fine needle aspiration reveals glandular clusters of ovoid to columnar cells with marked nuclear size and shape variation, prominent nucleoli, and cellular overlap confirming a diagnosis of adenocarcinoma. Although not specific, the presence of columnar cells in the clusters should suggest the possibility of a metastatic intestinal adenocarcinoma (Papanicolaou stain, × 360).

MENINGIOMA

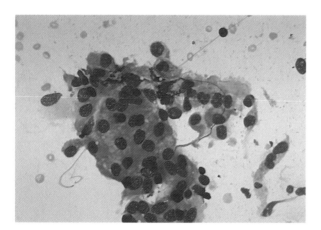

FIGURE 18–45. Optic Nerve Meningioma. Fine needle aspiration with cohesive clusters of round to oval cells with uniformly rounded nuclei. Occasional cells (not shown) revealed intranuclear cytoplasmic inclusions suggestive of meningothelial origin. Similar clusters may be seen in reactive meningothelial proliferations overlying the optic nerve when involved with other neoplasms. Close correlation with radiologic studies and the clinical impression is vital to avoid this pitfall (Diff-Quik, × 128). (Courtesy of John Keltner, M.D., University of California at Davis.)

C·H·A·P·T·E·R

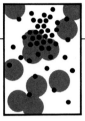

19

OCULAR CYTOLOGY

Hormoz Ehya

Various neoplastic and non-neoplastic diseases of the eye can be diagnosed by cytologic techniques. Whereas some methods, such as conjunctival scraping, can be employed in any clinical setting without the need for sophisticated equipment, others require technical expertise as well as a sound knowledge of ophthalmic pathology and cytopathology, thus restricting their application to highly specialized centers. In this chapter, cytologic techniques used in the evaluation of ophthalmic diseases are reviewed, and the cytomorphologic features of the more common entities are described.

CYTOLOGIC METHODS

The types of specimens used for cytologic evaluation of the eye include conjunctival smears, vitrectomy specimens, aqueous humor, and fine needle aspiration of intraocular lesions.

Conjunctival and Corneal Scraping

Conjunctival and corneal scraping is used for evaluation of some inflammatory and ulcerative conditions of the conjunctiva and cornea. Normally, conjunctival smears contain sheets of small squamous or cuboidal cells and scattered goblet cells. In inflammatory conditions, the epithelial cells exhibit reactive and reparative changes. A more specific diagnosis can be made when organisms (e.g., bacteria, fungi, or parasites) or inclusions (e.g., chlamydial or viral infection) are found. Additionally, some conjunctival neoplasms, particularly squamous cell carcinoma and malignant melanoma, can be diagnosed by this sampling technique.

Vitreous Specimens

The vitreous is a gelatinous substance that occupies most of the intraocular space behind the lens. This transparent, viscous substance is practically acellular and consists of water, collagen, and hyaluronic acid. The vitreous is affected by various inflammatory, degenerative, and neoplastic conditions of the eye. The cytologic examination of the vitreous may provide specific diagnoses in several ophthalmologic disorders. A cytologic sample is obtained either by aspiration of a small amount of the vitreous or by a vitrectomy procedure. In the author's laboratory, small aspirated samples are processed by the membrane filtration technique, whereas on vitrectomy specimens cell blocks are prepared in addition to filters and smears. Conditions that can be diagnosed by this method include malignant lymphoma, leukemia, metastatic carcinoma, juvenile xanthogranuloma, infectious endophthalmitis, granulomatous inflammations, phacoanaphylaxis, bilateral acute retinal necrosis, amyloidosis, asteroid hyalosis, and epithelial downgrowth.

Aqueous Humor

Aqueous humor is a clear, acellular fluid that fills the anterior chamber (the space between the cornea and iris) and the posterior chamber of the eye (the space between the iris and lens). Specimens for cytologic examination are obtained by anterior chamber paracentesis under topical anesthesia using a 27-gauge needle. Such samples, which usually do not exceed one or two drops of the fluid, are processed by a membrane filtration or cytocentrifuge method.

Cytologic examination of the aqueous humor is useful in the diagnosis of a variety of eye diseases, particularly glaucoma, acute and chronic inflammation, and neoplasms. Some types of glaucoma, including blood-induced, tumor-induced, and phacolytic glaucomas, may be identified by cytologic study of the aqueous humor. Malignant lymphoma, leukemia, melanoma, and neoplasms metastatic to the iris may shed tumor cells into the aqueous humor and be detected by cytologic examination. Cytology is particularly helpful in distinguishing uveitis from metastatic disease in patients with a known malignancy. In one such case, we identified neoplastic plasma cells in the anterior chamber fluid of a patient with multiple myeloma who presented with a clinical impression of uveitis.

Fine Needle Aspiration of Intraocular Lesions

This method is used for obtaining cytologic samples from intraocular tumors or tumor-like lesions. The target is usually a mass in the choroid, ciliary body, or iris. Subretinal fluid collections also can be sampled by this technique. Aspirations are performed with a 25-gauge needle using an indirect ophthalmoscope or operating microscope. The aspirated material is usually confined to the lumen of the needle. It is flushed into 1 to 2 milliliters of a balanced salt solution. An aliquot of the material is prepared by membrane filtration technique and stained by a modified Papanicolaou method. After cytologic evaluation of filter preparations, additional smears are made as needed for histochemical or immunocytochemical studies.

In a collaborative effort, the ophthalmologists at Wills Eye Hospital of Philadelphia and cytopathologists in our laboratory have aspirated and interpreted over 500 intraocular lesions during the past decade. Our results indicate that, in experienced hands, fine needle aspiration (FNA) is an accurate and relatively safe procedure for the diagnosis of intraocular neoplasms. However, since the diagnostic accuracy of noninvasive techniques in the identification of ocular tumors is quite high, and because the potential complications of FNA include vitreous hemorrhage, traumatic cataract, and tumor seeding, this technique should not be used routinely on all ocular neoplasms. The indications for intraocular FNA include the following: (1) clinical suspicion of a metastatic neoplasm in the absence of a known primary cancer, (2) request by the patient for confirmation of a malignant clinical diagnosis prior to treatment, and (3) diagnostic uncertainty about the neoplastic nature of an ocular lesion.

CYTOMORPHOLOGIC FEATURES OF EYE LESIONS

Non-Neoplastic Conditions

Cytologic examination of the vitreous or aqueous humor is helpful in the diagnosis of several non-neoplastic diseases of the eye. Acute ophthalmitis is characterized by an inflammatory infiltrate of predominantly polymorphonuclear leukocytes, whereas lymphocytes, plasma cells, and histiocytes predominate in chronic inflammation. In granulomatous inflammation, epithelioid histiocytes, multinucleated giant cells, and lymphocytes are present. Eosinophils may be seen in parasitic infestations. The specific cause of infection may be identified in cytologic preparations. These include fungi (e.g., *Cryptococcus, Candida, Aspergillus*), parasites (e.g., *Toxocara canis*), and viral inclusions (e.g., cytomegalovirus, herpes simplex virus). Whenever infection is clinically suspected, a portion of the aspirated material should be sent for microbiologic evaluation.

Some causes of glaucoma are identified by cytologic examination of the aqueous humor or vitreous. Examples include glaucomas caused by hemorrhage or by disintegration of the lens. The latter condition, called "phacolytic glaucoma," is the result of the liquefaction of the lens secondary to a hypermature cataract. The lens protein leaks out of the intact lens capsule into the aqueous humor and elicits a phagocytic response. The blockage of the trabecular meshwork by macrophages results in glaucoma. Phacolytic glaucoma is diagnosed by the discovery of lens substance and large foamy histiocytes in the anterior chamber fluid. In blood-induced glaucoma, lysed erythrocytes (ghost cells), globules of extracellular hemoglobin, and macrophages are found in the aqueous.

Following penetrating trauma or ocular surgery, conjunctival or corneal epithelium may grow into the eye from the wound site. In this condition, called epithelial downgrowth, clusters of squamoid epithelial cells are found in the aqueous humor or vitreous.

Phacoanaphylactic endophthalmitis is a granulomatous inflammation that results from the rupture of the lens capsule. This inflammatory reaction is believed to be secondary to antibody-antigen reaction to the lens material. Cytologically, mixed inflammatory cells, histiocytes, multinucleated giant cells, and fragments of inflamed lens material are seen in the vitrectomy specimen.

Asteroid hyalosis and amyloidosis are two conditions that cause vitreous opacity. Asteroid hyalosis is a usually unilateral disorder of the eye, more common in the seventh and eighth decades of life, which may be associated with diabetes mellitus or hypercholesterolemia. It is characterized by the presence of spherical white deposits in the vitreous that contain mucopolysaccharide, lipid, and crystals. In cytologic preparations, small spherules are found in the vitreous that are birefringent with polarized light and react positively with periodic acid–Schiff (PAS).

The vitreous can be affected by the primary systemic amyloidosis, leading to a slowly progressive loss of visual acuity. This condition can be diagnosed by the presence of acellular globules in the vitrectomy specimen. Amyloid is more readily recognized in cell block preparations as an amorphous eosinophilic substance that reacts positively with Congo red and crystal violet stains and produces the characteristic green birefringence with polarized light when stained with Congo red.

Coats disease, a unilateral telangiectasia of the retina associated with massive retinal and subretinal lipid deposition, may be confused clinically with retinoblastoma. Fine needle aspiration enables establishment of a correct diagnosis of this childhood disease, and it prevents unnecessary enucleation of the eye. The aspirated material contains lymphocytes and large foamy macrophages with coarse granules of melanin.

Retinoblastoma

Retinoblastoma is the most common malignant intraocular neoplasm of childhood. The tumor usually occurs during the first three years of life and is rare after the age of 7 years. Most cases are diagnosed on the basis of the characteristic clinical presentation and noninvasive tests. In some cases, however, the neoplasm may mimic non-neoplastic conditions. For example, hemorrhage or permeation of tumor cells into the anterior chamber fluid may cause a secondary glaucoma or may produce the clinical appearance of the hypopyon and thus be mistaken for endophthalmitis. On the other hand, some benign conditions may mimic retinoblastoma. Examples include persistent hyperplastic primary vitreous (the failure of the primary vitreous to regress, thus forming a vascular mesenchymal tissue behind the lens), retrolental fibroplasia, uveitis, and Coats disease. Fine needle aspiration is extremely helpful in establishing a correct diagnosis in these circumstances.

The FNA material from retinoblastomas is highly cellular and usually contains necrotic debris. Tumor cells are small with scant cytoplasm and are arranged singly or in cohesive clusters, occasionally forming rosettes. The nuclei are round or irregular, have evenly dispersed chromatin, and tend to mold in cell clusters. Nucleoli are generally absent. Cytologically, retinoblastoma may be difficult to distinguish from the malignant variant of another childhood neoplasm, medulloepithelioma. However, these two neoplasms can be easily distinguished on the basis of their clinical presentations since medulloepithelioma characteristically arises from the ciliary body.

Melanocytic Tumors of the Uvea

Benign nevi of the uvea are common in adults. They present as single or multiple flat pigmented lesions, usually under 3 mm in size. Nevi are usually diagnosed correctly on a clinical basis and are rarely subjected to FNA. A variant of nevus called "melanocytoma," which presents as a heavily pigmented nodule in the uvea or optic disc, may be mistaken for malignant melanoma. On FNA, clusters of relatively large cells with abundant cytoplasm and finely granular melanin are seen. Nuclei are small, uniform, and regular with small nucleoli. The small nuclear to cytoplasmic ratio is the most helpful feature in distinguishing this tumor from malignant melanoma.

Malignant melanoma is the most common malignant tumor of the eye. The majority of ocular melanomas arise from the choroid. Melanomas of the eye are composed of one or more of the following three cell types:

1. *Spindle A cells* appear in FNA material as cohesive clusters of cells with ill-defined borders and, occasionally, as single elongated cells. The nuclei are spindle-shaped and uniform and frequently display longitudinal grooves. Nucleoli are not visible, and mitoses are rare.
2. *Spindle B cells* are plumper than spindle A cells and appear in FNA specimens both singly and in cohesive clusters. The nuclei are oval, and single nucleoli are usually evident. Chromatin clumping and occasional intranuclear inclusions (cytoplasmic invaginations) are seen.
3. *Epithelioid cells* are round or polygonal and exhibit a higher degree of pleomorphism than spindle cell neoplasms. In needle aspirates, the cells occur singly or in poorly cohesive sheets and evince chromatin clumping, irregularity of the nuclear membrane, prominent nucleoli, and occasional intranuclear invaginations. Multinucleated cells and mitoses are frequently seen.

The amount of melanin pigment is variable. When present, the pigment is dispersed as fine granules, unlike melanophages, wherein the pigment granules are coarse and of variable size. Sometimes the tumor cells are so heavily pigmented that nuclear characteristics are not visible prior to bleaching.

The prognosis of ocular melanoma is greatly dependent upon the cytologic type of the tumor. Epithelioid melanomas have a poor prognosis, whereas pure spindle A melanomas have an excellent prognosis with a generally benign clinical course. Thus, a preoperative cytologic diagnosis of these tumors is highly valuable in selecting an appropriate treatment. However, pure spindle A and pure epithelioid tumors are uncommon; the majority of ocular melanomas are either spindle B cell or mixed cell type (epithelioid and spindle cells).

Intraocular Lymphoma and Leukemia

Most intraocular lymphomas affect the retina and vitreous. Involvement of the uvea by malignant lymphoma is exceedingly rare. The clinical diagnosis of this disease is difficult, and it is usually mistaken for uveitis with exudative retinal detachment. The delay in diagnosis usually results in central nervous system involvement and death. Successful treatment has been reported with early diagnosis and aggressive therapy. Cytologic examination of the vitrectomy specimen is the method of choice for diagnosis. The tumor cells are round and single with scant cytoplasm and a high nuclear to cytoplasmic ratio. The nuclei have irregular outlines, clumped chromatin, and prominent nucleoli. Necrotic tumor cells and mitoses are commonly present.

Acute leukemia commonly involves the uvea. Leukemic cells may be found in the vitreous or aqueous humor and exhibit characteristics similar to those seen in the blood or body cavity fluids.

Metastatic Neoplasms

Most neoplasms metastatic to the eye occur in the posterior uvea, the most common sources being the breast and lung. Metastatic tumors are sometimes confused clinically with amelanotic melanoma. Since the prognoses for metastatic tumors to the eye are much worse than those of primary ocular melanomas, and because the methods of treatment are completely different, establishing a correct diagnosis by FNA is essential. Cytomorphologic features of metastatic carcinomas are similar to those of their primary tumors, which are detailed in other chapters.

Bibliography

Augsburger JJ, Shields JA: Fine needle aspiration biopsy of solid intraocular tumors: Indications, instrumentation and techniques. Ophthalmic Surg 15:34–40, 1984.

Augsburger JJ, Shields JA, Folberg R, et al.: Fine needle aspiration biopsy in the diagnosis of intraocular cancer: Cytologic-histologic correlations. Ophthalmology 92:39–49, 1985.

Char DH, Miller TR, Ljung B-M, et al.: Fine needle aspiration biopsy in uveal melanoma. Acta Cytol 33:599–604, 1988.

Czerniak B, Woyke S, Domagala W, Krzysztolik Z: Fine needle aspiration cytology of intraocular malignant melanoma. Acta Cytol 27:157–165, 1983.

Engel HM, Green WR, Michels RG, et al.: Diagnostic vitrectomy. Retina 1:121–149, 1981.

Ljung B-M, Char D, Miller TR, Deschenes J: Intraocular lymphoma: Cytologic diagnosis and the role of immunologic markers. Acta Cytol 32:840–847, 1988.

NORMAL CELLS

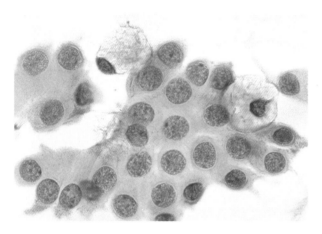

FIGURE 19–1. Normal Conjunctiva. Monolayer sheets of medium-sized polygonal cells in a conjunctival smear. The cells have uniform round nuclei. Scattered goblet cells (having pink cytoplasms) are evident (Papanicolaou stain, × 1000).

INFECTIOUS CONDITIONS

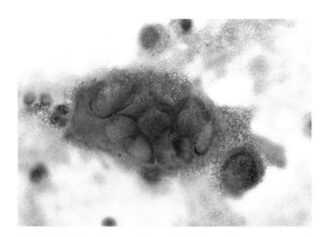

FIGURE 19–2. Herpes Virus Infection. This conjunctival smear exhibits a large multinucleated epithelial cell with ground-glass appearance, margination of the chromatin, and nuclear molding (Papanicolaou stain, × 1000).

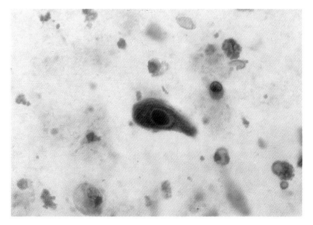

FIGURE 19–3. Cytomegalovirus Infection. This intraocular fine needle aspiration (FNA) of an immunosuppressed patient exhibits a cell with a large intranuclear inclusion forming the characteristic target-shaped appearance. Scattered inflammatory cells and degenerated cells are present in the background (Papanicolaou stain, × 1000).

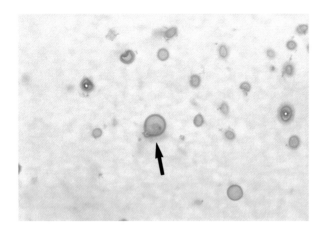

FIGURE 19–4A. *Cryptococcus neoformans.* The FNA of an intraocular lesion in a patient who was treated with corticosteroids for polyarteritis nodosa. Variable-sized pale yeast forms are evident, one of which contains an early bud (arrow) (Papanicolaou stain, × 1000).

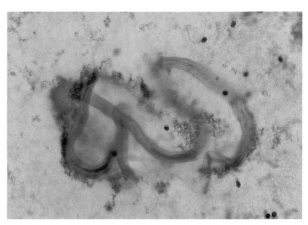

FIGURE 19–5. *Toxocara canis.* An intact larva approximately 400 μ long and 15 to 20 μ in diameter. The alimentary tract is visible. Involvement of the eye by the larvae of *Toxocara canis* (a common ascarid of the dog) or *Toxocara cati* (a common ascarid of the cat) may produce a clinical picture mimicking retinoblastoma. When the infective eggs of these nematodes (present in dog or cat excrement) are ingested, the larvae hatch in the small intestine, enter into the circulatory system, and migrate to various organs, including the eye. The larvae then die and elicit an inflammatory reaction (vitrectomy specimen, Papanicolaou stain, × 400).

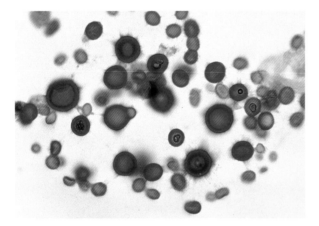

FIGURE 19–4B. *Cryptococcus neoformans.* The same case illustrating numerous budding organisms. The thick mucicarminophilic capsule is characteristic of *Cryptococcus* (mucicarmine stain, × 1000).

OTHER NON-NEOPLASTIC CONDITIONS

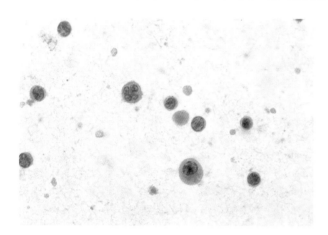

FIGURE 19–6. Chronic Endophthalmitis. Lymphocytes and occasional neutrophils and plasma cells are present. Malignant lymphoma can be ruled out because of the absence of atypical lymphocytes (vitrectomy specimen, Papanicolaou stain, × 1000).

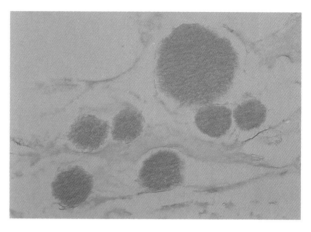

FIGURE 19–8A. Asteroid Hyalosis. Amorphous spherules of varying sizes seen in the vitrectomy specimen of a 72-year-old man with vitreous opacity. These structures contain mucopolysaccharide, lipid, and crystals (vitrectomy specimen cell block, H&E stain, × 400).

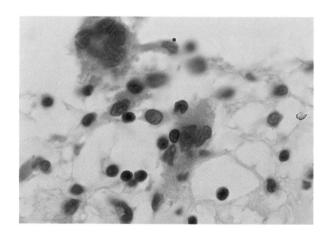

FIGURE 19–7. Granulomatous Endophthalmitis. Note lymphocytes, histiocytes, and multinucleated giant cells. The cause of granulomatous inflammation cannot be determined on the basis of cytologic examination alone, unless the infectious organisms (e.g., tuberculous bacilli or fungi) or lens fragments (seen in phacoanaphylactic endophthalmitis) are identified (vitrectomy specimen cell block, H&E stain, × 1000).

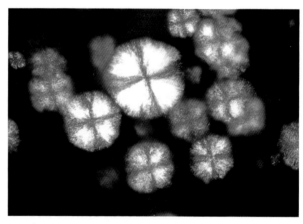

FIGURE 19–8B. Asteroid Hyalosis. The same case exhibiting characteristic Maltese cross birefringence with polarized light (vitrectomy specimen, Millipore filter, H&E stain, × 400).

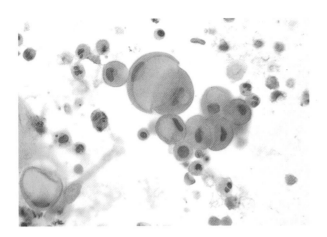

FIGURE 19–9. Epithelial Downgrowth. Groups of round epithelial cells with abundant cytoplasm and small, frequently eccentric nuclei. These squamoid cells are derived from downgrowth of conjunctival or corneal epithelium following penetrating wounds (vitrectomy specimen, H&E stain, × 400).

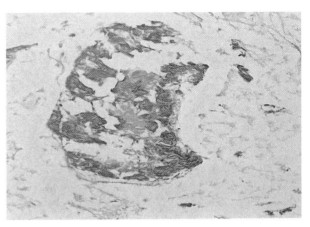

FIGURE 19–10B. Amyloidosis. The positive reaction with Congo red stain (vitrectomy specimen cell block, Congo red stain, × 200).

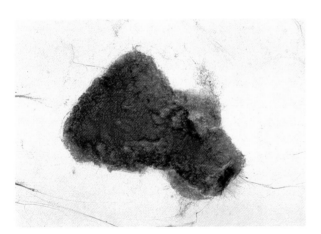

FIGURE 19–10A. Amyloidosis. An acellular globule of amorphous material against a clean background. This patient with a history of primary systemic amyloidosis presented with decreased visual acuity. It is difficult to recognize amyloid in the Papanicolaou-stained material without the help of histochemical stains (vitrectomy specimen, Millipore filter, Papanicolaou stain, × 40).

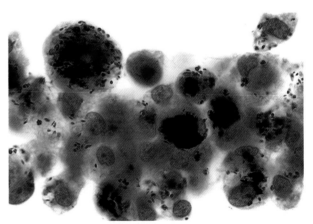

FIGURE 19–11. Coats Disease. A group of large macrophages containing melanin pigment. Scattered lymphocytes were also present in this specimen but are not seen in this field. This childhood disease, which clinically may mimic retinoblastoma, can be easily diagnosed by FNA cytology (Papanicolaou stain, × 1000).

NEOPLASTIC CONDITIONS WITH NORMAL CELL COMPARISONS

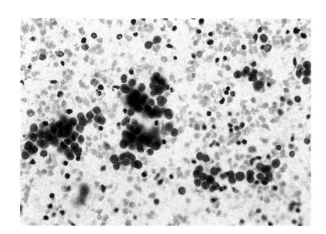

FIGURE 19–12A. Retinoblastoma. Fine needle aspiration of a white retrolental mass in a 2-year-old boy. The smear is highly cellular and contains numerous single cells and clusters of small cells in a background of necrotic debris (Papanicolaou stain, × 400).

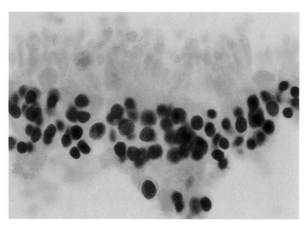

FIGURE 19–13. Normal Retinal Cells. This photograph depicts a group of retinal photoreceptor cells (rods and cones) found in the FNA of a choroidal lesion. The crowded nuclei of these cells may be mistaken for a small-cell tumor by the novice. The uniformity of the nuclei, lack of nuclear molding, the orderly arrangement and polarity of the cells, and the presence of cytoplasmic processes are helpful in distinguishing these cells from malignant neoplasms (Papanicolaou stain, × 1000).

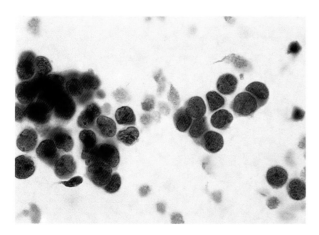

FIGURE 19–12B. Retinoblastoma. Higher magnification depicting clusters of small cells with scant cytoplasm. Nuclei are hyperchromatic, vary from round to irregular, lack nucleoli, and mold against each other. Cytologically, retinoblastoma cells are indistinguishable from metastatic small-cell carcinoma. However, the two neoplasms can be easily distinguished on the basis of the patient's age and clinical history (Papanicolaou stain, × 1000).

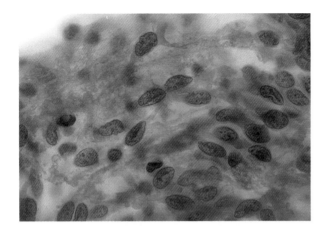

FIGURE 19–14A. Spindle A Melanoma. The FNA of a choroidal mass depicting a cluster of cohesive cells with ill-defined borders and spindle-shaped nuclei. Nuclei are uniform and lack nucleoli, and some have longitudinal grooves (Papanicolaou stain, × 1000).

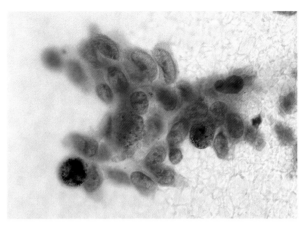

FIGURE 19–15A. Spindle B Melanoma. This FNA of a choroidal mass exhibits a cluster of cohesive cells with oval nuclei and visible nucleoli. Several cells contain cytoplasmic melanin. The presence of nucleoli is the most helpful feature to distinguish spindle B melanoma from spindle A type (Papanicolaou stain, × 1000).

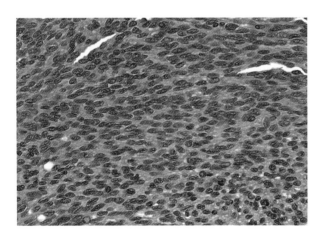

FIGURE 19–14B. Spindle A Melanoma. The histologic section of the same tumor as in Figure 19–14A. Note the ill-defined cell borders and the lack of nucleoli (H&E stain, × 400).

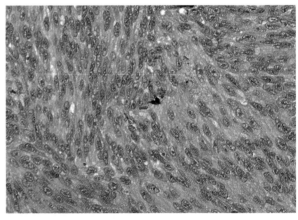

FIGURE 19–15B. Spindle B Melanoma. Note spindle cells with ill-defined borders, plump nuclei, and visible nucleoli in this histologic section (H&E stain, × 400).

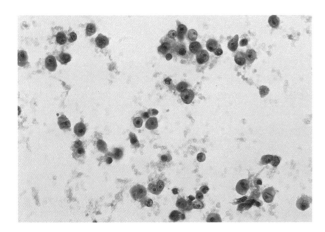

FIGURE 19–16A. Epithelioid Melanoma. This intraocular FNA contains tumor cells arranged singly or in poorly cohesive groups. Because of the poor cohesiveness of tumor cells, FNA of the epithelioid melanoma usually yields abundant cells that appear singly or in loose groups, whereas spindle melanomas have a tendency to form large clusters of cohesive cells (Papanicolaou stain, × 400).

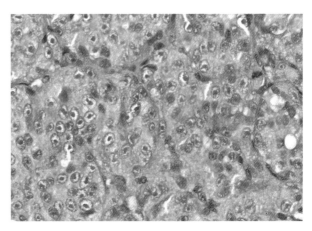

FIGURE 19–16C. Epithelioid Melanoma. Histologic section depicting epithelial-like cells with high nuclear to cytoplasmic ratios and prominent nucleoli (H&E stain, × 400).

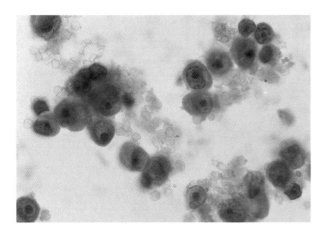

FIGURE 19–16B. Epithelioid Melanoma. Higher magnification depicting round medium-sized cells with large eccentric nuclei and prominent nucleoli. The cells of ocular melanomas are relatively uniform and rarely exhibit a significant degree of pleomorphism. Amelanotic melanomas may be difficult to distinguish from metastatic carcinomas without immunocytochemical stains (Papanicolaou stain, × 1000).

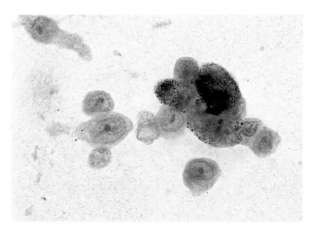

FIGURE 19–17. Malignant Melanoma, Mixed Cell Type. Ocular melanomas commonly have both spindle and epithelioid cell components. In melanoma cells the pigment is in the form of fine granules. Pigmented melanoma cells should be distinguished from retinal pigment epithelial cells and from melanophages (Papanicolaou stain, × 1000).

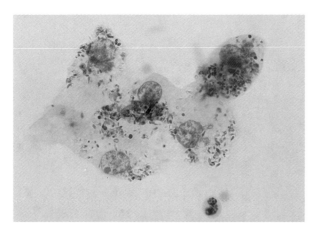

FIGURE 19–18. Retinal Pigment Epithelial Cells. Retinal pigment epithelium (RPE) is the outermost layer of the retina. The cells depicted in this photograph were present in the FNA smear of a metastatic carcinoma to the choroid. The melanin in RPE cells consists of spherical and fusiform granules that are larger than those in melanoma cells. Furthermore, in contrast to malignant melanoma cells, RPE cells have small nuclear to cytoplasmic ratios (Papanicolaou stain, × 1000).

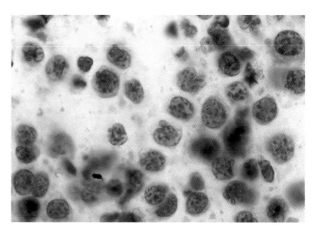

FIGURE 19–20. Primary Ocular Lymphoma. A monotonous population of single round cells with irregular nuclear outlines, occasional protrusions, and coarse chromatin pattern characteristic of large-cell lymphoma. A complete lack of cohesiveness is a helpful criterion for distinguishing lymphoma from metastatic carcinoma. However, immunocytochemical stains may be necessary to confirm the diagnosis (vitrectomy specimen, Papanicolaou stain, × 1000).

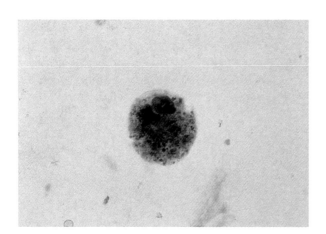

FIGURE 19–19. Melanophage. A large macrophage with small eccentric nucleus and abundant melanin. Melanophages that may be found in a variety of benign conditions can be distinguished from malignant melanoma cells by their small nuclear to cytoplasmic ratio and variable-sized pigment granules (Papanicolaou stain, × 1000).

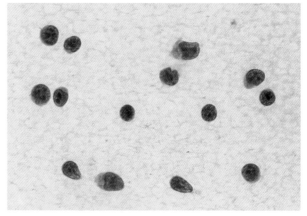

FIGURE 19–21. Leukemic Infiltrate. Single round cells with a very high nuclear to cytoplasmic ratio and prominent nucleoli are consistent with the patient's known history of acute lymphoblastic leukemia. These findings are in contrast to the polymorphous cell population seen in chronic inflammation (anterior chamber fluid, Papanicolaou stain, × 1000).

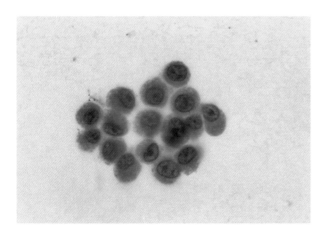

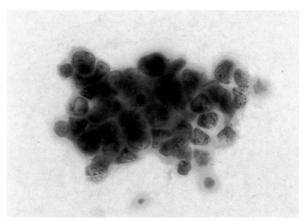

FIGURE 19–22. Plasma Cell Myeloma. A group of single round cells with eccentric nuclei and prominent nucleoli. The patient had a history of multiple myeloma and presented with an iridic infiltrate simulating uveitis. Immunocytochemical studies demonstrated the presence of a monoclonal population of cells containing immunoglobulin G, kappa chains thus confirming the diagnosis of plasma cell myeloma. On the basis of cytomorphologic features alone, this tumor is difficult to distinguish from epithelioid melanoma or malignant lymphoma (anterior chamber fluid, Papanicolaou stain, × 1000).

FIGURE 19–24. Metastatic Small-Cell Carcinoma. The FNA of a nonpigmented choroidal mass in a 64-year-old man who also had a right lower lobe lung mass extending to the mediastinum. This photograph depicts a cluster of cells with scant cytoplasm and irregular hyperchromatic nuclei that mold against each other and lack nucleoli. Morphologically, the tumor cells resemble retinoblastoma, but the two neoplasms are easily distinguished on the basis of clinical presentation and age (Papanicolaou stain, × 1000).

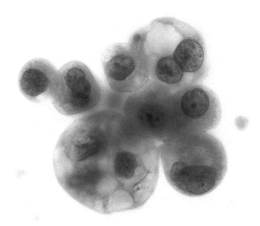

FIGURE 19–23. Metastatic Adenocarcinoma. The FNA of a metastatic pulmonary adenocarcinoma exhibiting large cells with irregular nuclei, abnormal chromatin pattern, and prominent nucleoli. The presence of cytoplasmic vacuoles and marked pleomorphism of the cells are against the diagnosis of primary ocular melanoma (Papanicolaou stain, × 1000).

CASE STUDIES

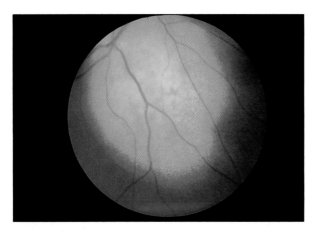

FIGURE 19–25. Case A: Metastatic Adenocarcinoma. A 58-year-old man without a previous history of malignancy presented with a nonpigmented choroidal nodule. Fine needle aspiration of the mass was performed.

FIGURE 19–25A. Photograph of the fundus depicting a nonpigmented choroidal tumor.

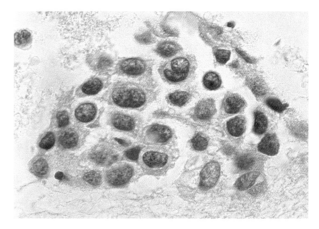

FIGURE 19–25C. This photograph depicts negative immunocytochemical staining for S-100 protein. The stain for melanoma-specific antigen was also negative.

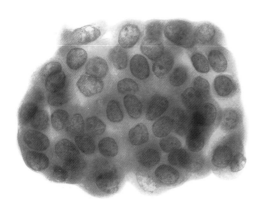

FIGURE 19–25B. A large cluster of cells with hyperchromatic nuclei and occasional nucleoli suggestive of metastatic adenocarcinoma (Papanicolaou stain, × 1000).

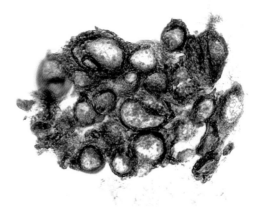

FIGURE 19–25D. Immunocytochemical stains were positive for cytokeratin (shown in this photograph) and epithelial membrane antigen, supporting the diagnosis of metastatic carcinoma. On follow-up, the patient was found to have pulmonary adenocarcinoma.

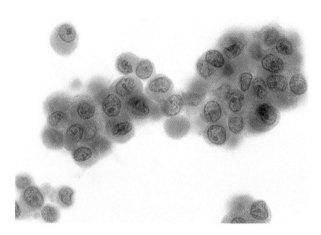

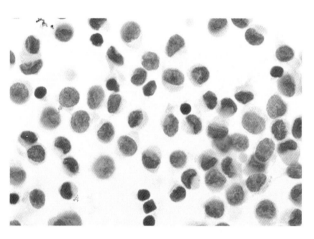

FIGURE 19–26. Case B: Choroidal Malignant Melanoma. A 60-year-old woman with a history of breast carcinoma presented with a nonpigmented choroidal mass. Fine needle aspiration was performed.

FIGURE 19–26A. This photograph depicts poorly cohesive medium-sized tumor cells with a high nuclear to cytoplasmic ratio and small nucleoli. No melanin is present. The differential diagnosis is amelanotic melanoma versus metastatic mammary carcinoma (Papanicolaou stain, × 1000).

FIGURE 19–26C. The stains were negative for epithelial membrane antigen (shown in this photograph) and cytokeratin.

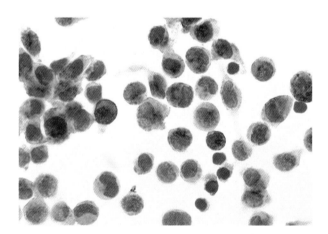

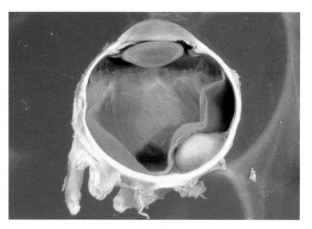

FIGURE 19–26B. Positive immunocytochemical staining for melanoma-specific antigen (shown in this photograph) and S-100 protein supported the diagnosis of malignant melanoma.

FIGURE 19–26D. A cross section of the enucleated eye, exhibiting an amelanotic malignant melanoma of the choroid.

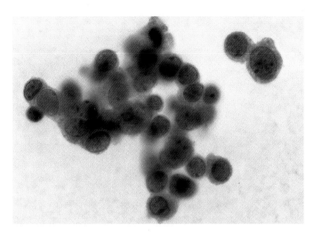

FIGURE 19–27. Case C: Metastatic Carcinoid Tumor. This 70-year-old woman presented with bilateral amelanotic choroidal masses. There was no previous history of a malignant neoplasm. Fine needle aspiration was performed.

FIGURE 19–27A. This photograph depicts medium-sized round tumor cells with a high nuclear to cytoplasmic ratio. In addition to the three-dimensional clusters shown here, the cells were arranged singly and in loosely cohesive groups. There is no pigment or cytoplasmic vacuoles. The chromatin is evenly dispersed. Some nuclei contain chromocenters, but nucleoli are not evident. The cytologic features are suggestive of a metastatic neoplasm, particularly carcinoid tumor (Papanicolaou stain, × 1000).

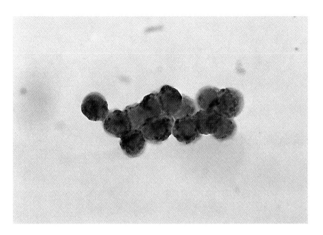

FIGURE 19–27C. Positive immunostaining for chromogranin (shown here) supported the cytologic impression of metastatic carcinoid tumor. Stains were also positive for cytokeratin and epithelial membrane antigen.

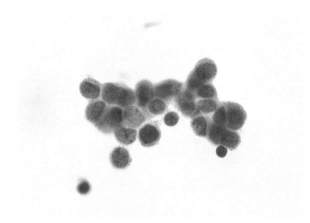

FIGURE 19–27B. The immunocytochemical stains were negative for S-100 protein (shown in this photograph) and melanoma-specific antigen.

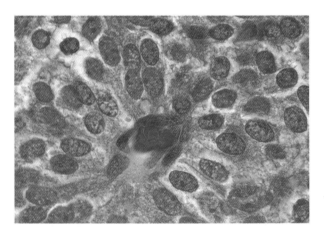

FIGURE 19–27D. A subsequent computed tomography of the thorax revealed a mediastinal mass that proved to be a metastatic carcinoid tumor in lymph nodes, as shown in this photograph (H&E stain, × 1000).

INDEX

Note: Numbers in *italics* refer to illustrations;
numbers followed by (t) indicate tables.